High-Risk
Parenting

High-Risk Parenting:

Nursing Assessment
and
Strategies
for the
Family at Risk

Suzanne Hall Johnson, R.N., M.N.

Director, Health Update
Lakewood, Colorado

J. B. Lippincott Company
Philadelphia
New York   Toronto

ISBN 0-397-54312-3

Library of Congress Catalog Card Number 79-14522

Printed in the United States of America

2 4 6 8 9 7 5 3 1

Library of Congress Cataloging in Publication Data

Main entry under title:

High-risk parenting.

   Includes bibliography and index.
   1. Nursing.   2. Family—Health and hygiene.
3. Pediatrics nursing.   I. Johnson, Suzanne Hall.
RT42.H53   610.73′6   79-14522
ISBN 0-397-54312-3

To My Family

Contents

Contributors

The following contributors were chosen for their clinical nursing expertise for each chapter. I would like to thank them for their contributions.

CLAUDIA J. ANDERSON, R.N., M.N.
Doctoral Candidate, University of Texas, Austin, Texas. Previously Nurse Clinician and Clinical Instructor, University of Kansas, Kansas City, Kansas.

SALLY FELGENHAUER BAIRD, R.N., M.S.N.
Clinical Nurse Specialist, Young Family Resource Center, University of Texas School of Nursing, San Antonio, Texas.

CATHERINE CROPLEY, R.N., M.N.
Neonatal Nurse Educator, Charles R. Drew Post Graduate Medical School, Los Angeles, California. Previously Neonatal Clinical Nurse Specialist, Children's Hospital, Los Angeles, California.

KATHLEEN KNUDSEN DeSANTIS, R.N., M.N.
Instructor, Humboldt State University, Arcata, California. Previously Clinical Nurse Specialist, Daniel Freeman Hospital, Inglewood, California.

CHARLOTTE C. ELSBERRY, R.N., M.S.N., C.N.M.
Lecturer, Yale University School of Nursing, Nurse Midwife for Young Mothers Program and Staff Nurse Midwife, Yale New Haven Hospital, New Haven, Connecticut.

CHERYL HALL HARRIS, B.S.N.
Staff Nurse, The Children's Mercy Hospital, Kansas City, Missouri. Previously Supervisor, Neonatal ICU, Children's Mercy Hospital, Kansas City, Missouri. Lecturer in Medicine, University of Missouri, Kansas City, Missouri.

LYNDA LAW HARRISON, R.N., M.S.N.
Instructor, University of Tennessee, Knoxville. Previously Public Health Nurse, Minneapolis, Minnesota.

MARY BREWER JONES, R.N., B.A.
Physiology student. Previously Perinatal Instructor, Bexar County Hospital District, San Antonio, Texas.

CAROLE K. KAUFFMAN, R.N., M.P.H.
Public Health Nurse Coordinator, Children's Hospital National Medical Center, Washington, D.C.

CAROLYN HILL KRONE, R.N., M.S.
Mental Health Nurse, Women's Hospital. Previously Hospital-Community Nurse, Adult Psychiatry, Neuropsychiatric Institute. University of Michigan Medical Center, Ann Arbor, Michigan.

PRISCILLA ADRIENNE LESTER, R.N., M.N.
Assistant Professor and Practitioner/Teacher, Special Care Nursery, Rush-Presbyterian St. Luke's Medical Center, Chicago, Illinois. Chairman, Illinois NAACOG.

ANNE MALLEY-CORRINET, R.N., N.S., C.N.M.
Assistant Professor, Yale School of Nursing, New Haven, Connecticut, and Coordinator, Young Mothers' Program, Yale University, New Haven, Connecticut.

MARGARET SHANDOR MILES, R.N., Ph.D.
Associate Professor and Pediatric Cardiology Nurse Specialist, University of Kansas, Kansas City, Kansas.

MARIE J. MILLINGTON, R.N., M.P.H.
Assistant Professor, University of Wisconsin, Oshkosh, Wisconsin. Previously Community Health Specialist on Maternal and Infant High Risk Projects, U. of Wisconsin Extension, Wisconsin.

CAROL EDGERTON MITCHELL, R.N., M.S.
Deceased, previously Assistant Professor, Mental Health and Community Nursing, University of California, San Francisco, California.

CAROL M. MURPHY, R.N., M.S.
Assistant Professor, California State University, Long Beach, California. Previously Inservice Director, Children's Hospital at Stanford, Palo Alto, California.

MARY KATHLEEN NEILL, R.N., M.A.
Psychiatric Nurse Clinician, Children's Hospital National Medical Center, Washington, D.C.

VIRGIL PARSONS, R.N., M.S.
Assistant Professor, San Jose State University, San Jose, California and D. N. S. student, University of California, San Francisco.

SELCUK T. SAHIN, R.N., Ed.D.
Assistant Professor, University of Massachusetts, Amherst, Massachusetts.

EDITH A. TANKSON, R.N., M.P.H.
Public Health Nurse Clinician, Ramsey County Public Health Nursing Service. Previously Maternity Nurse Clinician, St. Paul-Ramsey Hospital, St. Paul, Minnesota.

MARIE A. WACHT, R.N., B.S.N.
Public Health Nurse, Developmental Disability Prevention Services Golden Gate Regional Center, San Francisco, California.

JANE C. WILLIAMS, R.N., M.S.W.
Chairperson, Health Occupations, Moraine Park Technical Institute, Fon du Lac, Wisconsin.

DONNA L. WONG, R.N., M.N., P.N.P.
Nurse Counselor in Private Practice, Tototowa, New Jersey. Formerly Assistant Professor, Seton Hall, College of Nursing, South Orange, New Jersey.

LENI WRIGHT ZIEBELL, B.A.
Perinatal Social Worker, Theda Clark Regional Medical Center, Neenah, Wisconsin.

Consultants

I would like to thank the following people for their consultation during the development of High-Risk Parenting.

George Barrett
  Clinical Psychologist
  Alameda County Health Care Agency
  Oakland, California

Rosemarian Berni, R.N., M.N.
  Associate Professor
  Department of Rehabilitation
  University of Washington
  Seattle, Washington

M. Sandra Bourbon, R.N., M.S.
  Director, Rural Nurse Practitioner Program
  University of Nevada
  Reno, Nevada

Ann Bender Browning, R.N., B.S.
  Public Health Nurse
  Children's Hospital National Medical Center
  Washington, D.C.

Joan L. Brundage, R.N., M.S.
  Senior Instructor
  University of Colorado
  Denver, Colorado

Rose Broeckel Cannon, R.N., M.N.
  Instructor
  Emory University
  Atlanta, Georgia

William Carey, M.D.
  Private practice in Penna.
  Associate in Pediatrics
  U. of Pennsylvania Medical School
  Philadelphia, Pennsylvania

Monica Wolcott Choi, R.N., M.S.N.
  Assistant Professor
  University of Pennsylvania
  Philadelphia, Pennsylvania

Mecca S. Cranley, R.N., M.S.
  Lecturer
  University of Wisconsin
  Madison, Wisconsin

Sharon L. Cross, R.N., M.S., P.N.A.
  Instructor

University of Minnesota
  Minneapolis, Minnesota

Marcene Powell Erickson, R.N., M.N.
  Associate Professor
  University of Washington
  Seattle, Washington

Renée Euchner, R.N., M.A.
  Staff Nurse
  Stanford University Hospital
  Stanford, California

Betty Rae Eyles, M.A.
  Psychologist, Child Development Clinic
  Children's Mercy Hospital
  Kansas City, Missouri

Judy Pierson Grubbs, R.N., M.S.
  Senior Planning Associate
  Bobrow/Thomas Associates
  Los Angeles, California

Cheryl Hall Harris, R.N., B.S.
  Staff Nurse
  Children's Mercy Hospital
  Kansas City, Kansas

David J. Harris, M.D.
  Chief Genetic Counseling Center
  Children's Mercy Hospital
  Kansas City, Kansas

Sandra Hanson, R.N., M.Ed.

  Instructor
  University of Kansas
  Kansas City, Kansas

LaVohn Josten, R.N., M.N.
  Consultant
  Minneapolis Health Department
  Minneapolis, Minnesota

Sandra F. Kubarych, R.N.
  Clinical Coordinator
  University of Louisville
  Louisville, Kentucky

Susan Woolf Leonard, R.N., M.S.
  Assistant Professor

Texas Woman's University
Dallas, Texas

Mary Kolassa Lepley, R.N., M.S.N., P.N.P.
Assistant Professor
University of Colorado
Denver, Colorado

Roberta Marquart, R.N., M.P.H.
Instructor, School of Public Health
University of Minnesota
Minneapolis, Minnesota

Katharyn Antle May, R.N., M.S.N., N.P.
Doctoral Student
University of California
San Francisco, California

Lee J. Parsons, R.N., M.N.
Consultant Pediatric Nursing
Fort Collins, Colorado

Mary Ellen Morse Pendergrast, R.N., M.N.
Consultant Public Health Nursing
Atlanta, Georgia

Janice Marie Petrella, R.N., M.S.N.
Instructor of Nursing

Wagner College
Staten Island, New York

Nancy Ann Pickrell, R.N., B.S., P.N.P.
P.N.P. Associate
Alameda County Health Agency
Oakland, California

Karen Roach, R.N., B.S.
Supervising Public Health Nurse
Alameda County Health Agency
Oakland, California

Elizabeth D. Taft, R.N., M.S.
Director Patient Placement
Stanford University Medical Center
Stanford, California

Candace G. Woelk, R.N., M.N.
Nursing Consultant and Instructor
Kansas University Medical Center
Kansas City, Kansas

Rothlyn P. Zahourek, R.N., M.S.
Clinical Specialist and Consultant
Creative Health Services
Denver, Colorado

Preface

With today's attention to high-risk individuals such as the high-risk infant, abusive parent, or the terminally ill family member, two important questions arise: What are the parenting and other family difficulties when a family member is at risk? What are the nursing strategies for the high-risk family?

The purpose of this book is to identify family difficulties resulting from situations placing a child or parent at risk and to suggest nursing strategies for preventing and reducing these family problems.

The Introduction describes the framework for the book; the first part on assessment suggests ways to identify family members' potential problems behavior; the second and third parts discuss family difficulties related to child or parent risk situations; the fourth part applies many nursing strategies to the risk family; and the Conclusion discusses the commonalities for the family at risk for any reason and suggests further nursing directions.

There are three aspects to the holistic focus of *High-Risk Parenting*. First, the whole family is seen as the target client for the nurse when any family member is at risk. Second, some common potential problems are recognized among many families in different specific risk situations, thus suggesting the broader concept of the family at risk.

Third, *High-Risk Parenting* is intended for nurses working with families at risk in any setting. The book is not exclusively for any one nursing specialty, but instead draws upon and is intended for many specialties including pediatric, obstetric, medical, surgical, mental health, and community health nursing. The family at risk exists in each specialty and requires a holistic view encompassing all specialties to identify family difficulties and nursing strategies.

This book's style is designed for clarity and conciseness in communicating the main ideas. The pronoun "she" is used rather than the more awkward "he/she" style, with the understanding that the nurse may be either a man or woman. Clinical examples clearly show the point while unrelated family characteristics and names have been changed to protect the family. In addition to the references, each chapter lists pertinent organizations and addresses for the reader who would like additional information. A self-study guide for continuing education credit is included in the appendix.

Introduction: High-Risk Parenting

Suzanne Hall Johnson, R.N., M.N.

Specific views about high-risk situations, their effects on the family system, and holistic nursing care are the basis for the ideas presented in *High-Risk Parenting*. What is high-risk parenting? What are the common characteristics of high-risk situations? What nursing actions are needed?

The nursing profession has long been aware of the concept of the *high-risk infant* or child whose life or developmental abilities are threatened, and the *high-risk pregnancy* in which there is a threat to normal fetal development and the possible death of the mother or child. However, as we have undertaken a holistic approach to patient care we have become increasingly aware that a high-risk situation which threatens any one member of the family will affect all its members. In the *high-risk family* the ability of the family members to function appropriately within the family unit and the ability of the family unit as a whole to maintain its normal function are threatened. Parenting involves many stresses and the learning of new roles; *high-risk parenting* involves even greater stress and more complex role changes. These stresses can result in the poor development of the family members and the dissolution of the family unit.

Nursing trends toward holistic care, consumer demands for respectful coordinated care, and present community pressures on the family all focus on the need for a family viewpoint and new strategies to care for the high-risk family. This book presents the concept of high-risk parenting, reviews practices of expert nursing clinicians for risk families, and suggests new directions for nursing care.

High-risk parenting occurs when either the child or a parent is the symptomatic person as a result of a risk situation. For example, a child at risk because of a congenital anomaly influences the family and places it at risk; the high-risk parent such as the alcoholic parent influences the family members and the family unit. Either a child or a parent at risk places the family at risk of abnormal development or disunity.

This book covers the most common high-risk conditions that nurses are confronted with. Although these conditions are considered to be potentially the highest risks for the family, it is not an exclusive list and other conditions may cause family disunity. It is also possible for these situations to occur with very minor or no disruptive effects on the family. Indeed, the nurse's goal is to help prevent the situation from causing disruptive effects on the family.

Most high-risk situations have a high incidence. It is difficult to determine the exact number of families in high-risk situations because the various situations are usually studied separately. A rough estimate of the incidence of families at high-risk involves adding the rates of incidences for the separate types of risk situations. A composite of the estimated incidence for each risk situation is in Table 1.

There are significant numbers of families at risk due to perinatal, childhood, or parental risk situations. Although it is difficult to collect reliable data in the same statistical format in order to project the exact incidence of high-risk parenting, a relatively high incidence of each situation contributing to high-risk parenting clearly demonstrates that most families will experience at least one high-risk situation and many families will experience several.

High-risk families are seen in many nursing settings. Obstetric and neonatal nurses see the families at risk due to pregnancy and infant problems, pediatric nurses work with families with high-risk situations caused by child difficulties, medical and surgical nurses see high-risk families with parent difficulties, while community and mental health nurses see high-risk families with child or parental difficulties.

Since the symptomatic family member is usually the reason for the first visit to the medical

Table 1.   Incidence of Risk Situations

Risk Situation	Approximate Incidence
At-risk pregnancy	
infant mortality	1.8% of live births[13]
neonatal mortality	1.3% of live births[13]
post-neonatal mortality	.5% of live births[13]
Premature infant	
low birh weight infants	8% of births[2]
Physically or mentally handicapped child	15% of the newborn population[3]
Failure to thrive child	1% of pediatric admissions at Boston Floating Hospital[5]
Hyperactive child	4% of children below 12 years of age[7]
Terminally ill child	
cancer	4,000 deaths per year[1]
accidents	14,000 deaths per year[9]
sudden infant death	9,000 per year[8]
Abusing/battering parent	1 million[6]
Alcoholic parent	9 million problem drinkers[12]
Addicted parent	300,000 addicts[11]
Adolescent parent	6% of births[15]
Single parent	10% of births[2]
Emotionally disturbed parent	2.5% of the population[16]
Terminally ill parent	
cardiovascular and renal diseases	450 per 100,00 deaths[14]
cancer	175 per 100,000 deaths[14]
accidents	45 per 100,000 deaths[14]

team, the past focus has been on the specific risk member rather than on the high-risk family as a whole. Today, the nurse's role is to identify the family unit at risk, prevent family difficulties, and reduce family problems. The information on assessment of the family members, potential family difficulties, and nursing strategies described in this book will help the nurse meet this goal.

There are many advantages to categorizing high-risk families as a group and looking at the family in any risk situation. Seeing these families as a unit provides a conceptual framework for nurses' clinical, teaching, and research practice for the high-risk family. Considering the commonalities of families at risk suggests common areas for assessment for any family. When problems from many high-risk families are identified, possible problems can be predicted and the difficulties prevented or reduced for other families. If one risk situation creates a certain family problem, the nurse is encouraged to look for these previously ignored problems in families with other risk situations. Also, by applying interventions developed to reduce a family problem for one risk situation to families with similar problems in another risk situation, new and specific interventions are created and tested.

Ultimately the advantages of a conceptual framework for clinical, teaching, and research practice and advantages in assessment, problem identification, and intervention for the high-risk family are reflected in nursing care that prevents and reduces high-risk family problems and results in increased satisfaction and bonding between family members.

CHARACTERISTICS OF HIGH-RISK SITUATIONS

The high-risk situations discussed in this book were chosen because they have the following characteristics. These characteristics are similar regardless of the exact cause of the risk situation. The common characteristics of high-risk situations may cause the main difficulties for the family and explain the many common difficulties for families in different types of risk situations.

Complex Causation

Many high-risk situations result from a very complex and often unknown cause. For example, although many causes of premature birth are identified, such as a multiple pregnancy or placenta previa, there are many unknown factors leading to prematurity. This unknown complex causation makes it very difficult to anticipate all high-risk situations and to prevent their occurrence. Some causes of congenital anomalies are known, but many are still undetermined. The causes of alcoholism and drug abuse are extremely complex; some of the causes of child abuse are only beginning to be identified. The unknown complex causation of the high-risk situation makes prevention difficult and emphasizes the need for strategies to reduce and treat family difficulties resulting from the high-risk problem when they appear.

In addition, family reactions to the risk situation are also influenced by complex and unknown factors. Since families react differently to risk situations, it is often difficult to anticipate the types and extent of problems for the family. As nurses focus on the family, identify family difficulties, and suggest possible causes for the family problems, more preventive nursing measures will be developed.

Multiple Crisis Situations

Unfortunately, a family with one risk situation is more likely to experience additional risk situations. Certain risk problems may actually cause other risk situations. For example, premature birth has been shown to be associated to later child abuse.[10] Families in which one of the parents is alcoholic are more likely to end in divorce than nondrinking families and therefore more likely to have a single parenthood problem.[4] A high-risk fetal situation frequently leads to a premature birth or an infant with a congenital anomaly. Adolescent pregnancy and single parenthood frequently occur together. The nurse identifies signs of the initial risk situation so that she can help reduce the initial problem, prevent family difficulties and therefore prevent any resulting risk situations.

The more high-risk situations occurring in a

family, the more stress there will be on the family. For example, an adolescent mother may have enough difficulties learning to care for her child, but she will have additional stresses if she is a single parent rather than married, and even more stresses if the child is premature or has a congenital defect. Although any one situation places the family at risk of abnormal development and disunity, the combination of high-risk situations causes more or greater problems.

Critical Nature

Another characteristic of any high-risk situation is its critical nature. Resolution of the high-risk situation is critical to the future of the family. The parents' response to the high-risk situation can lead either to growth and increased closeness or to poor adaptation and disintegration of the family unit. One family in a high-risk situation may be able to communicate its difficulties, jointly solve its problems and become closer because of the stressful situation. Another family in the same situation may display anger and blame toward each other and demonstrate no sharing of difficulties or mutual identification of family problems, resulting in the potential disruption of the family unit. It is the nurse's goal to help the family to adapt to the high-risk situation so that the family members will experience growth and closeness rather than the maladaptation and disintegration of the family.

Whether or not an event is critical enough to place a family at risk depends on four factors. 1) The uniqueness of the situation itself affects the family. A premature birth may affect a family very differently from an alcoholic parent. 2) The family's past experiences in coping with stresses influence the outcome of the high-risk situation. Parents who have already adapted to other stressful conditions such as the loss of a job or moving are more likely to have developed communication lines and problem identification skills that will help them to cope with the present high-risk situation. 3) The parents' relationship before the risk situation also influences the outcome. Parents who already have an established relationship of mutual support

and communication of problems will be able to use this close relationship to help solve the high-risk problems. 4) The assistance of professionals may also influence the outcome of the risk situation. A nurse's discussion of the premature infant's abilities and behavior as well as his difficulties helps the parents to become less fearful of all the child's behavior and to enjoy interacting with their child.

Long-Term Duration

Another characteristic of most high-risk situations is that they are long-term problems. Congenital anomalies and mental disability are both life-time risk situations. The potentially terminal illness of a child or a parent may be long term with intermittent periods of remission followed by recurrence and crisis. Alcoholism, abuse, and mental disability of the parent are all long-term conditions with intermittent difficulties.

Multiple crises may occur during the high-risk situation when the parents are temporarily unable to cope and reduce the stress. For example, in a premature birth situation the parents' fear for the child's life is the initial crisis. Later crisis periods may occur, such as the first visiting of the baby with fear of his appearance, first caring for the baby with fear of hurting the child, the mother returning home without the child to a lonely house, the returning of the child home to the mother who is fearful she may not be able to give him adequate care, and the development of parental overprotectiveness which may create problems for both the parents and the child for years to come. This is a typical characteristic; there may be multiple crises over a prolonged period of time during the risk situation.

NURSING MANAGEMENT OF THE HIGH-RISK FAMILY

The nurse is in an optimum position to provide preventive and supportive care for the high-risk family. Some families already see the nurse as concerned about their health and their families. The nurse is frequently in contact with the family during the initial stages of the crisis and can easily continue to follow the family after the medical crisis has been resolved but while the family is still dealing with their high-risk difficulties. The family focus is consistent with the nurse's role and many schools of nursing are recognizing the family as the main client of nursing care. In addition, nurses are in the many different locations where the high-risk families are identified. Nurses in many settings such as hospital and community health settings can plan together for the families' care. Therefore, nurses not only can take care of the family during its medical crises, but can follow the family after the crisis to help in working through the high-risk family difficulties.

The nurse's abilities make her an essential health professional for caring for the high-risk family. She has learned sensitive assessment skills for physical ailments, behavioral difficulties and family problems, which help her to identify the high-risk family. The nurse's empathy and concern for the family results in her sensitivity and ability to identify difficulties which might otherwise be overlooked during the medical treatment of the symptomatic family member. In addition, her ability to actively include the family members in their own decisions about health care makes her valuable in helping them to identify ways to reduce their own problems.

The nurse has two main goals in working with the high-risk family. First the family members will jointly plan and carry out ways to prevent, reduce, or adapt to their high-risk situation. A second goal is for the family to achieve a feeling of satisfaction and closeness from working together on the problem rather than anger, resentment, and the disruption of the family unit. The nursing strategies are aimed at helping the family to identify the stresses of a high-risk situation and to work together to adapt to them.

The Family Is the Client

Since a health problem of any one of the family members will influence all of the family members, it is essential for the nurse to identify the

primary health problem, recognize the changes in each of the family members, and identify the family's abilities to continue to meet the needs of the family.

Although in many high-risk situations one family member has obvious symptomatic problems, a closer look will show that all family members are having difficulties. For example, a child with a congenital anomaly originally appears to be the symptomatic family member. Upon closer observation, the nurse will see that the parents may have symptoms of extreme guilt, fear of the child's death and difficulty seeing their child's abilities, and that a sibling is fearful that he has lost his parents' love because of the time they are spending with the disabled child. In another example, the terminally ill parent has the obvious symptoms of weakness and pain. At a closer look, however, the other family members frequently can be seen to experience guilt at the way they previously treated the ill parent and physical ailments related to stress.

In any high-risk situation, the nurse must identify the family as the client, the center of attention. The individual problems of the mother, the father, the children, and their related family problems must be identified, prevented, or reduced.

A health problem of one family member changes that member's behavior and role in the family and in turn influences all the other family members' behavior and their roles. Some of the effects of health problems on the families can be seen in subtle changes while others can be seen in more drastic changes. For example, the hyperactive child who is displaying very active bodily motions in the living room may influence the other family members by preventing them from concentrating on working on their own projects. Drastic family changes leading to actual disintegration of the family occur in some high-risk situations, such as the increased incidence of divorce and family disunity in the family with an alcoholic parent.

Not only does a health problem influence family members, but family members influence health problems. It is commonly recognized that family members participate in the treatment and support for a family member during illness, such as the mother providing fluids and comfort for her child during an illness. Family members' actions are also very important in the prevention and diagnosis of health problems. For example, family members who recognize the importance of adequate nutrition for the pregnant mother will support her by helping to prepare and joining her in eating nutritious meals. A family member's observation frequently draws attention to a symptom and a possible diagnosis for a problem. This family recognition of the first signs of a problem can encourage the family member to seek professional care. Family members who do not observe changes of other members or who believe symptoms are not serious or the result of a magical power will delay the diagnosis for a medical illness. In addition, presently health professionals are helping family members adopt an important role in the terminal care of a family member. This family care and influence during the terminal period of a family member's life can greatly influence the quality of the health care given to him and his satisfaction during this period.

PARTICIPATING IN THE HEALTH CARE TEAM

The nurse works as part of the health care team in providing the optimum health care for the high-risk family. She works with social workers, physicians, psychologists, nutritionists, and other health care professionals. In addition, she works with other nurses in the team such as the nurses on each shift caring for the patient and family, the primary nurse following the family, the clinic or outpatient nurse who may see the family for follow-up visits, and the community health nurse who may be following the family at home.

The nurse can take many different roles within the health care team. The role she takes should be developed from a coordination of 1) her own abilities; 2) the abilities of the other health team members; and 3) the needs of the family. The goal in any team is for the person who is best quali-fied to perform the needed action. The team should be flexible so that the best qualified person will perform the action needed; however, they should also be coordinated to prevent gaps in coverage of the care. The team must be coordinated not only to ensure provision of the necessary services at a particular time, but also to avoid gaps in treatment during the critical or follow-up stages.

The underlying concern shown by all members of the team is for the welfare of the family. All health team members must respect the abilities of the other members, use specific observations and data rather than assumptions to communicate problems, follow up and evaluate their strategies, base their interventions on a plan that complements the interventions of the other health team members, communicate the plan, and provide mutual support.

Although the physician is frequently the coordinator of the medical plan for the symptomatic high-risk family member such as the at-risk fetus or terminally ill child or parent, the nurse may be the best qualified person to coordinate the health care for the entire family. Because of the nurse's family focus, ability to talk to the family and presence in many settings, she is one of the most important figures for coordination of care.

The center of the team must always be the family. The family members frequently can best identify the problem, determine alternatives, and actually carry through programs to help reduce the difficulties for the family. The health care team recognizes that the family members are not only part of but the heart of a team.

Assessment

Previously, the nurse identified the high-risk family through the symptomatic family member. The presence of the premature infant or alcoholic parent indicated the potential family problems. Although this is the most certain method of identifying risk families, the risk situation is always past before the family is identified.

Presently nurses are developing more sensitive family assessments which will identify the family before the risk condition occurs. For example, an assessment of maternal attachment showing a mother with difficulty coordinating her mothering behaviors with the infant's needs and rising frustration may warn the nurse of a possible child abuse family. With additional information of a history of the mother's parents frequently hitting her when she was small, the nurse has more reason to suspect a potential abuse family. This early assessment of risk factors allows the nurse to institute preventive measures.

The assessment chapters in this book will help the nurse to assess family members and identify maladaptive behaviors. Although the assessment of factors leading to risk situations is still being developed, the present assessment guidelines help identify the family at risk before the risk situation occurs.

Identifying Family Difficulties. Unfortunately, the nurse may not be able to prevent the risk situation. The nurse must then identify the presence of a family difficulty through a thorough assessment of the changes in all family members due to the high-risk situation.

All too often professionals link the occurrence of a high-risk situation with a standard family difficulty and assume that the family is having that difficulty. For example, the family with a mentally retarded child has potential difficulty in allowing the child freedom to solve the problems of which he is capable. Although this is a potential problem for families in that situation, it may not be a problem for all such families. Assumption of a family difficulty that is not present not only prevents the nurse from intervening in the actual difficulties, but frequently alienates the family from her. Since the difficulties listed in the chapters to follow are all potential difficulties for families in the risk situations under discussion, the nurse must determine whether or not they exist for the individual family.

Ideally, the early signs of a difficulty can be identified by the nurse before the situation becomes complex. The signs of family difficulties and potential problems are described in later chapters. Since a difficulty with one family member can cause difficulties in the other family members, early recognition and intervention for a problem can prevent further difficulties. In the example of the premature infant whose mother is experiencing guilt, if the guilt reaction continues, the husband may also start blaming her for the premature birth. The initial symptom would therefore have disrupted the family system and resulted in more complex family problems.

The nurse openly discusses the family difficulty so the family members will be able to identify their own changes and problems and begin to concentrate on ways that they may be able to solve the family problem. One of the main nursing actions is to help the family to identify their own behavior so that they can mobilize their resources to help resolve the problem. For many families the nurse's help in identifying the family difficulty has been all they needed to generate solutions and solve the problem. For example, in a single parent family, Barry was unaware that some of his anger and tenseness was due to a lack of private time for himself. When a nurse helped him recognize that the lack of time alone was a cause of his irritability, he planned some quiet times for himself and found that his understanding and patience with other family members increased.

With early identification of the observed problems and sharing of these with the family, frequently more complex situations can be prevented and movement toward resolution begun.

Nursing Interventions

There are many types of specific intervention strategies used for high-risk families, such as counseling, crisis intervention, teaching, and other strategies discussed in later chapters. All nursing interventions for the high-risk family are aimed at preventing the original high-risk situation, preventing family difficulties, and reducing the effects of the high-risk situations.

Preventing the Original High-Risk Situation. The nurse's first area of intervention for the high-risk family is in the prevention of the high-risk situation. Unfortunately, this is frequently impossible. Prevention is centered on reducing the causes of the specific risk situation. For example, the premature birth risk situation is prevented by optimum nutrition and health of the mother. However, there are many other possible causes, such as a multiple pregnancy, which cannot be avoided. Since many of the high-risk situations have unknown or complex causes, preventing them is very difficult or even impossible at this time.

Although it may not be possible to prevent all of the risk situations, certainly some of the known causes can be reduced and some additional high-risk situations can be prevented. For example, although all the causes for parental abusing of a child are not known, one of the known contributing factors is a critical incident where the parent is angry at the child and batters him. Some prevention approaches which are now being used are crisis lines which enable parents to talk about their anger and ask for help in dealing with a crisis situation and day care centers where a child can be left if the parents feel that they cannot take the strain of caring for the child at that time.

Prevention is certainly the best and most valuable approach for dealing with high-risk situations and family difficulties. However, until all high-risk situations can be prevented, the nurse must have additional techniques for helping the family already in the high-risk situation.

Preventing Family Difficulties. If a nurse cannot prevent the situation from occurring, she may be able to prevent the resulting family difficulties. This is a relatively new area of intervention for the nurse working with high-risk families. In order to prevent the difficulties, the nurse must know the potential difficulties, the individual family reactions, and strategies to reduce the anticipated difficulties.

All the potential difficulties for the family in a high-risk situation have unfortunately not been identified at this time. Some difficulties are known, however many new ones may be identified by nurses carefully interviewing families in high-risk situations. In the chapters on high-risk situations, the contributors' clinical experiences with families in the specific risk situations result in clear descriptions of potential family difficulties.

The nurse identifies which potential difficulties would be most likely for the individual family. Assessment of the family members' behaviors and past coping experiences helps the nurse to anticipate how the family may react to the high-risk situation. Some families may be more inclined to have guilt reactions while others might be more inclined to have anger reactions.

After identifying the potential family difficulties for the individual families the nurse acts to prevent the family difficulties. Many preventive actions are described in later chapters. For example, in the premature situation, if the mother has been very conscientious and is always very careful with her other children, the nurse may anticipate that she will wonder what she did wrong and feel guilty about the premature labor. The guilt may be prevented if the nurse discusses the known cause of the premature birth before the mother has spent energy blaming herself for actions causing the birth.

Reducing the Effects of High-Risk Situations. If the family difficulties cannot be or have not been prevented, the nurse helps the family to reduce their problems related to the high-risk situation. Unfortunately, many families have already experienced the risk situation and its resulting difficulties before they have contact with the nurse. For example, the alcoholic parent frequently first has medical care for chronic physical symptoms related to years of alcohol abuse. In many cases the nurse starts with interventions to reduce already present problems for the family.

When the nurse commonly sees families after a high-risk situation, she must identify ways to develop and provide prevention strategies for future families. With the situation of adolescent pregnancy, a nurse that works with pregnant adolescents and helps them to reduce their difficulties related to the pregnancy can also recognize that ways for preventing the pregnancy from occurring in adolescence help reduce the incidence of high-risk families. Thus she can arrange for birth control information and supplies for adolescents.

At the present, strategies used to reduce family difficulties seem to be limited to specific situations. Such strategies as behavior modification, used in some high-risk situations, might be valuable in other risk situations but are seldom used. There are some nursing interventions used in specialty areas such as pediatrics for including families in the child's care that are seldom used in such other areas as the medical surgical units to include the child in the parent's care.

The nurse needs a repertoire of many possible strategies for application to the individual high-risk family. Her strategies can combine the knowledge and experiences from pediatric, obstetric, medical-surgical, community health, and mental health nursing practice. A cross-fertilization among specialty categories in nursing will tend to broaden the repertoire of intervention choices in any one situation. Although specialization is very important in identifying the very specific interventions for certain problem areas, nurses must also have an overview of all the available strategies in order to select the ones most useful for the individual family. The strategies presented in the strategy chapters of this book will help the nurse to develop such a repertoire. These strategies are applied to many high-risk situations and emphasize clinical application of the concepts.

Evaluation of Nursing Management

Since families react in individual ways and nursing interventions that are successful for one family may not be successful for another, evaluation of nursing actions is essential. A specific and continuous evaluation is needed to determine the extent of success of the nursing intervention for the high-risk family.

The evaluation is based on the specific assessment of the difficulties for the risk family, so the changes in the family after the intervention will be apparent. For example, a problem behavior and its frequency of occurrence for a hyperactive child is identified before an intervention is used to make the evaluation of the change in behavior clear.

Since the family difficulties related to risk situations frequently occur over a long period of time, the evaluation must be a continuous process. Parents with a premature infant may be afraid for the life of their child at many times during the child's normal development. The nurse must continue to evaluate the interventions aimed at reassuring the parents even after the initial crisis stage is over.

Assessing and intervening in the family difficulties of the high-risk family are new actions for the nurse and are continually being developed. Since the family difficulties are very complex and the nursing strategies have only recently been developed, the nurse will find that even some well-planned strategies may not work for a family. Rather than be discouraged, the nurse can use this feedback to refine the strategies further until they do reduce the family problems. This process of assessment, planned interventions, evaluation, and refinement of interventions leads not only to actions that help the family but also to further development of the nursing care for the high-risk family.

SUMMARY

The nurse's role with the high-risk family is to identify and prevent potential family difficulties and to assess and reduce actual family problems. The chapters in the Assessment, High-Risk Situation, and Strategy parts of this book will guide the nurse in assessment, identification, intervention, and evaluation for the family at risk.

REFERENCES

1. Atkinson, L. "Is Family Centered Nursing a Myth?" *MCN*, 1 #4, July 1976, 256–259.
2. Babson, S. G. and R. C. Benson. *Management of High-Risk Pregnancy and Intensive Care of the Neonate.* St. Louis: C. V. Mosby Co., 1971, 1–8.

3. Barnard, K. and M. Erickson. *Teaching Children with Developmental Problems: A Family Care Approach.* St. Louis: C. V. Mosby Co., 1976.

4. Crawford, C. O. *Health and the Family.* New York: Macmillan Co., 1971, 11, 121, 122, 236.

5. Hannaway, P. "Failure to Thrive." *Clinical Pediatrics,* 9, 1970, 96–99.

6. Helfer, R. and C. H. Kempe. *Child Abuse and Neglect: The Family and the Community.* Cambridge: Ballinger Publishing Co., 1976, XVII–XVIII.

7. Millichap, J. G. *The Hyperactive Child with Minimal Brain Dysfunction.* Chicago, Ill.: Year Book Medical Publishers, 1975, 4.

8. Ray, G. et al. "Analysis of the Problem." *Pediatric Annals* 3:11, November 1974, 9.

9. Rudolph, A. *Pediatrics.* New York: Appleton-Century-Crofts, 1977, 764.

10. Stern, L. "Prematurity as a Factor in Child Abuse." *Hospital Practice,* 8, #5, May 1973, 117–123.

11. —. *Dealing with Drug Abuse.* New York: Praeger Publishers, 1972, 288.

12. —. *Facts about Alcohol and Alcoholism.* Rockville, Md.: National Institute on Alcohol and Alcoholism, 1974, 5.

13. —. *Infant, Maternal, and Childhood Mortality.* Rockville, Md.: DHEW Publication, 1975.

14. —. National Center for Health Statistics, Department of Health, Education and Welfare.

15. —. *Population Bulletin: Adolescent Pregnancy and Childbearing.* Population Reference Bureau, Inc., Vol. 31 #2, September 1976.

16. —. *Provisional Data on Patient Care Episodes in Mental Health Facilities.* U.S. National Institute of Mental Health, 1973, 127.

ADDITIONAL READINGS

1. Eyres, P. J. "The Role of the Nurse in Family Centered Nursing Care." *Nursing Clinics of North America,* 7, March 1972, 27–39.

2. Fawcett, J. "The Family as a Living Open System: An Emerging Conceptual Framework for Nursing." *International Nursing Review,* 22, July/August 1975, 113–116.

3. Kaplan, D. M. et al. "Predicting the Impact of Severe Illness in Families." *Health and Social Work* 1 #3, August 1976, 72–82.

4. Sedgwick, R. "The Family as a System: A Network of Relationships." *Journal of Psychiatric Nursing,* 12, March/April 1974, 17–20.

Assessment of the Family at Risk

PART ONE

Early and continuous assessment of risk families is crucial to preventing or reducing their difficulties. The assessment can identify three stages of difficulties for the risk family. First, the nurse can identify behaviors which indicate a pending risk situation, such as bonding difficulties warning of later failure of the child to thrive. Second, the nurse can identify the presence of a risk situation previously unrecognized, such as early signs of battering or alcoholism. Third, the nurse can identify family problems resulting from difficulty coping with a risk family member, such as sibling aggression following a high-risk birth of a new infant. Thus these assessments can lead respectively to prevention of the risk situation, early treatment, and reduction of family difficulties. Specific guidelines for assessing mothering, fathering, and children's behavior with a focus on identifying problem behaviors are described in the following three chapters.

Assessment of Mothering Behaviors

Catherine Cropley, R.N., M.N.

CHAPTER ONE

A newborn infant emerges totally dependent on someone else to meet his needs. As this dependency continues for a period of months, the nature of the relationship developed between the infant and mother can have a profound effect on the child's physical, psychological, and intellectual development.

The development of maternal attachment is a complex and continuous process, beginning with knowledge of conception and proceeding throughout the relationship of mother and child. Although problems with maternal attachment may occur at any time in the relationship, the neonatal period is a particularly critical time when high-risk situations and other factors can temporarily alter or permanently damage the relationship. By identifying as early as possible those mothers who are having difficulty attaching to their infants, corrective measures can be taken by nurses or other professionals to prevent the consequences of maladaptive parenting. Early intervention can increase the mother's satisfaction with her infant, her new role, and her mothering capabilities.

The birth of a high-risk infant or of a child to parents with physical or emotional difficulties can threaten the development of maternal attachment, increasing the potential for problems and leading to future risk situations such as child abuse or failure to thrive. Therefore, early assessment of maternal behaviors in the high-risk family is essential for preventing later developmental problems.

Present approaches for the high-risk family include anticipating and preventing physical problems in the fetus and newborn. Genetic studies, amniocentesis, ultrasound, and fetal monitoring are diagnostic tools that help identify and/or prevent problems such as fetal distress, congenital abnormalities, respiratory distress syndrome, and prematurity. There is, however, a lack of approaches for identifying potential behavioral problems within the family. Presently no diagnostic tool is routinely used for assessing the mother-infant relationship in order to identify the child and mother who may be at risk for the consequences of mothering disorders. Too often disorders of the mother-infant relationship are recognized only after problems have become obvious.

Although nurses are often able to identify mothers who react passively or negatively toward their infants, their observations may be based on intuition rather than on a systematic assessment of behaviors. This prevents problems from being specifically defined and communicated to other health team members, thus decreasing the chances of establishing a plan of action. Nurses need to recognize the bonding process and assess maternal behaviors to identify and reduce potential maternal-infant relationship problems for the risk families. Nurses in obstetric, pediatric, and community health settings can identify problems using these assessment tools.

BASIC MATERNAL ATTACHMENT CONCEPTS

For the purposes of our discussion, the term "mother" will be used to designate the individual primarily responsible for the infant's care. Although the principal caretaker is usually the mother, it is recognized that the father, grandmother, foster or adoptive mother may be the primary caretaker. Since the nonmother caretaker must meet the individual needs of the child in a manner similar to that of the mother, the caretaker's behaviors must similarily be based on attachment with the child and coordination with the child's needs.

Development of Maternal Attachment

Maternal attachment begins during pregnancy as a result of the mother's fantasies about her expected infant and the sensations created by fetal movement. With the emergence of the infant at birth, fantasies give way to reality and the mother begins the process of getting to know her infant and deciding how she feels about him. The infant's responses to the mother play an important role in the bonding process. The process of maternal attachment develops throughout the prenatal, birth, and postpartum periods.

Antepartum Period. Early in the pregnancy the mother begins to imagine what the infant will be like, based on her sensations, her attitudes about the pregnancy, and her own fantasies. Once quickening occurs, the infant's reactions add to her fantasies as she begins to attach positive or negative meanings tc his movements. By the end of the pregnancy, the mother may have fantasies about many of her infant's characteristics, such as facial features, temperament, strength, sex, and size. If the fetus is quite active, the mother may picture a strong healthy boy. With a fetus who is less active, the mother may fantasize a girl or a passive infant with an easygoing disposition. Mothers often fantasize about specific features, such as large eyes, dimples, or a full head of hair. One mother related, "It never occurred to me to buy a baby brush because I always imagined the baby would be bald." Fantasies regarding appearance can result from family baby pictures, features of previous offspring, or features the mother values.

Past experiences, guilt or low self-esteem can contribute to a mother's fantasizing about an infant who is less than the ideal. A mother of four boys may view the fifth baby as a boy in order to prepare herself for the disappointment of not having a girl. If a previous infant was born with an abnormality, a mother may have difficulty picturing a normal infant.

The mother's attitudes about the pregnancy itself may influence her feelings about her infant. Most women initially experience some degree of ambivalence, because the infant will impose some changes in her lifestyle and in her relationship with the father and other family members. Ambivalence may be intensified by an unplanned pregnancy, especially one which occurs in a very young girl or in a woman near the end of her childbearing years. It may also be intensified by a pregnancy which is likely to impose an emotional, physical, or economic strain on the mother or family. The presence or lack of support from others can also affect a mother's attitude toward her unborn child.

If a mother is able to resolve the ambivalence and view the pregnancy favorably, her feelings and fantasies about the infant are more likely to be positive, fostering her attachment to the expected infant. On the other hand, if the ambivalence continues or her feelings about the pregnancy are predominantly negative, she may view the infant in negative terms and be less attached to the baby at birth. For example, a mother who is concerned that an infant might alter her relationship with her husband may display few attachment behaviors at birth, and may remain ambivalent toward the baby well into the neonatal period. This was the case with one mother who discussed her baby infrequently during the pregnancy and kept the infant in a bedroom most of the time during the first several weeks at home. Once reality proved that her relationship with her husband had not changed significantly, the infant eventually was integrated into the family. If a discussion of the anticipated impact of the infant on the family had occurred during the prenatal period, the mother would have had an opportunity to ventilate her anxieties, receive reassurance, and more realistically anticipate her husband's response.

Intrapartum and Postpartum Period. The actual presence of the infant at birth is a powerful initiator of maternal feelings. There is a unique period shortly after delivery in which mothers seem to be particularly receptive to involving themselves emotionally with their infants. Immediately after birth, infants are particularly alert and responsive to their environment. The time period encompassing the first several hours following delivery has been labeled the "maternal sensitive period" because of the lasting effects that events which occur during this time can have on the mother-infant relationship. Klaus emphasizes the importance of maximizing the maternal sensitive period to foster maternal bonding. He has recommended that the mother and her nude infant be placed together under a radiant heater for 30 to 45 minutes after the delivery, to allow the mother to explore her infant and the two to interact. He also suggests delaying the application of silver nitrate to the infant's eyes so that the mother can look into her child's eyes without the interference of the baby's swollen eyelids caused by the medication.[13]

Although high-risk infants may require special care following delivery, interventions for physical contact and eye-to-eye encounters can still be provided. If a mother is unable to visit the nursery the first few hours or days, perhaps because of cesarean section or hypertension, premature or sick infants can frequently be taken to the mother's bedside in an incubator for short visits, and the mother can be encouraged to reach in and touch her baby. If an infant is unable to leave the nursery because of the need for oxygen or special equipment, the mother should be encouraged to visit the baby in the nursery, even if she is restricted to a wheelchair or stretcher. It is especially important for a mother to see and touch her baby if the infant is to be transferred to another hospital for care.

At birth the mother begins to compare her infant with the fantasized child. If the two are similar, attachment is likely to progress with little interruption. If there is considerable discrepancy, the mother may grieve over the loss of the fantasized child, which will delay or inhibit her attachment to the infant. Major discrepancies may occur if the infant is premature or born with an obvious defect.

In order to become familiar with them, mothers visually and physically "explore" their babies. An orderly progression of behaviors used by mothers when becoming acquainted with their new infants has been identified. The mother initially uses her fingertips on the infant's face and extremities progressing to massaging and stroking the infant with her fingers. This is followed by palm contact of the trunk and eventually drawing the infant toward her, holding the infant's body against hers.[16]

As mothers attempt to get to know their infants by touching and looking, they also express interest in interacting with them through eye-to-eye contact.[15] Mothers can frequently be seen changing their position or the infants' in order to assume the "en face" position. In this position the mother's and infant's eyes meet in the same vertical plane. Eye-to-eye contact gives a real identity to the baby, as well as providing the mother with a rewarding experience as shown in Figure 1-1.

At the same time the mother is getting acquainted with her infant, she is concerned with the infant's acceptance of her. Positive responses from the infant can foster maternal bonding. Positive feelings toward the baby are stimulated when the infant looks at her, holds on to her finger, or turns his head toward her. If, on the other hand, the infant cries, will not open his eyes, or withdraws his hand

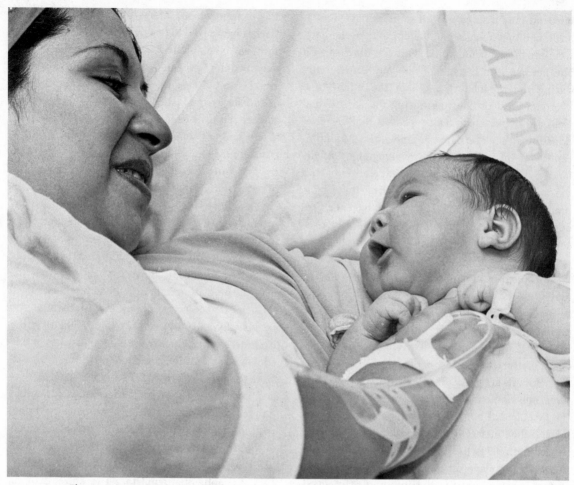

Figure 1-1. Nonverbal communication between mother and infant in en face position.

when touched, she receives negative reinforcement and may interpret the behavior to mean she has hurt the child. It is more likely that the infant cried because he was cold, withdrew his hand because her finger was cold or he became startled, or failed to open his eyes because they were sensitive to the bright lights or irritated from the silver nitrate solution. The mother uses the infant's reactions to evaluate her success at mothering.

If reasons for the infant's behavior are explained to the mother, she will not feel that she has done something to make the baby unhappy or that the baby is displeased with her. At the same time, the nurse might help the mother receive a more positive response from the baby by suggesting that

she shield the baby's eyes from the bright lights, or that she talk to the baby before touching him, so that he will not be startled.

The rapid development of maternal attachment is currently believed to be related to the behavioral exchanges between mother and infant and the infant's personality is thought to play an active role in the bonding process. For attachment to progress to a healthy maternal-infant relationship, the mother must be able to elicit responses from the infant which are rewarding to her, and the infant must be able to elicit from the mother behaviors which are satisfying to him. If a fussy infant quiets, looks at his mother, and smiles when she bends over and talks to him, the mother is reinforced, her self-concept is enhanced, and she is more likely to repeat the behavior. Similarly, the infant is rewarded by the pleasing sound of her voice and by observing her facial expression which has been brought within his visual field. When both mother and infant receive pleasure from their interactions, they have established a communication system unique to themselves. This keeps them physically close during a time when the infant is dependent on the mother for all of his needs.

Disorders of Maternal Attachment

Awareness of a high incidence of abandonment or death of infants who had been separated from their mothers for prolonged periods following birth led to the recognition of the importance of maternal attachment. It was discovered that mothers often lost interest in their premature babies when they had no opportunity to participate in their care. Fanaroff found that there was a significantly increased incidence of mothering disorders in high-risk infants when there were fewer than three maternal visits in a two-week period.[9] Some recent studies have also suggested that there is an increase in maladaptive mothering behaviors when birth defects, adoption, or multiple births occur.[2,13] A lack of maternal attachment and the inability to develop a mothering role based on the child's abilities and needs has been shown to lead to serious consequences. Some authors have suggested that high-risk situations such as failure to thrive, child abuse and neglect, and the vulnerable child syndrome are often related directly to disorders of maternal-infant attachment.[1,10,12] It is probable that there are many other problems as yet unidentified which result from disorders of maternal attachment.

In addition, disorders of mothering lead to serious family consequences. The inability to develop a mother-child relationship based on mutual satisfaction of needs results in an unsatisfied mother.[11] Since the family members' roles are related, the unmet needs of the child and mother affect the entire family. Behaviors of the infant, other children, and the father must be assessed along with those of the mother.

Factors which Inhibit the Attachment Process

The complexity of maternal-infant attachment has been recognized only in recent years. It was once thought that maternal feelings were present and fully developed at birth. Although maternal bonding can still be viewed as a natural and unconscious process between a mother and her infant, it is now apparent that attachment is continually developing and sensitive to many factors which can contribute or interfere with its formation. As the nurse is often aware of factors in a particular family which may inhibit or delay attachment, she is frequently in a position to intervene to prevent or minimize their effect on the mother-infant relationship.

Many of the factors that inhibit or delay attachment are present for high-risk families. Some of these factors are related to the mother while others are related to the infant, father, or hospital practices.

Maternal Factors. Physical and emotional energy may be diminished in a new mother at a time which is critical for becoming involved with her infant. Many of the medical, physical, sociological, and psychological factors which can disrupt attachment are listed below.

1. Narcotics, sedatives, and some forms of anesthesia interfere with a mother's initial alertness and responses to her infant. These drugs also make the infant depressed and unresponsive and may further interfere with bonding by creating the need for resuscitative measures at birth.

2. Physical problems resulting from the pregnancy, a prolonged labor, difficult delivery, or chronic illness may limit the physical and emotional energy a mother has to devote to her infant, as well as the care she is physically able to provide. Maternal illnesses such as preeclampsia not only create high-risk situations for the health of both mother and child, but increase the risk to maternal attachment as well. Discomfort and preoccupation with thoughts of a traumatic and painful delivery or of postpartal complications seriously interfere with a mother's relating to her infant.

3.   Lack of previous experience with infants increases a mother's anxiety in caring for her infant. Uncertainty about how to perform the mothering procedures and what to expect from the infant can increase the mother's fears about hurting her baby or not meeting her infant's needs. A primipara who has had no exposure to infants and is overwhelmed with all that she has to learn, may lack time and energy to enjoy her baby.

4.   Learned maternal behaviors may have both positive and negative influences on maternal bonding. Mothers frequently imitate the behaviors of their own mothers. A mother may concentrate only on the physical aspects of care, keeping the infant meticulously clean and on a rigid feeding schedule with minimal cuddling or verbal interaction, if that was how she was cared for or how she observed her mother caring for other children in the family. Histories of mothers who batter their children often reveal that they themselves suffered physical abuse as children.

5.   A negative self-concept can affect a mother's confidence in herself and in how she feels others (including her new infant) view her. If she sees herself as being unlovable or incapable of performing the mothering role, the mother-infant relationship can be seriously affected. Teenage mothers commonly have difficulty developing a mutually satisfying mothering role because of their normal identity and self-esteem crises.

6.   Lack of a positive support system deprives the mother of physical and emotional support at a time when she needs it most. Moral support from others is important, for it makes the mother feel that she and her baby are important and can instill confidence in her mothering abilities. Support may come from the father, friends, or parents. The fewest attachment behaviors occur in mothers who state they have no one they can count on or relate to easily.[8] Single mothers who are not married or who are recently widowed, separated, or divorced may need help in seeking positive personal support.

7.   Grieving over a significant loss, such as the loss of a spouse, parent, previous offspring, or close friend, may interfere with the normal bonding process. Attaching to a new infant and detaching from a lost loved one do not occur easily. Sometimes the new infant is seen as a "replacement" for a previous infant who has died. This seriously interferes with the mourning process and places unrealistic expectations on the new baby.

8.   Anticipatory grieving over the imagined loss of the infant prevents emotional investment in the baby. Anticipatory grieving may occur prenatally due to a pregnancy problem or postnatally due to a delivery or neonatal complication. One mother who grieved the loss of the baby during her complicated pregnancy later revealed she had been so prepared for the infant to die that she found it upsetting to visit and see him alive. She was relieved when he died four weeks later.

9.   Psychological unpreparedness for attachment may occur with premature delivery. The unexpected delivery of a premature infant can place the mother in a state of shock and disbelief which may delay the development of maternal attachment.

Infant Factors. Maternal attachment is fostered when the infant closely resembles the fantasized child. It is further reinforced by the interactions of the mother and infant. Both of these situations are violated if the infant is born prematurely, is born with a defect, or suffers neonatal complications. Intensive care or hospitalization following the mother's discharge separates the mother and infant at a critical time. Incubators, monitors, respirators, and oxygen hoods frequently restrict a mother to fingertip touch and may prevent an infant from responding to the mother's voice. The complete separation created by hospitalization and the partial separation created by the presence of equipment inhibit the mother-child attachment. Just as it is important to provide special medical care for the high-risk infant, it is also important to provide special interventions to foster maternal-infant bonding.

Some infant characteristics that can delay maternal attachment are presented here. The family difficulties associated with these particular risk situations are described in later chapters.

1.   Neonatal complications in full-term in-

fants can have a profound effect on the bonding process regardless of the severity of the condition. For example, the necessity for phototherapy for several days for an otherwise healthy infant can produce considerable anxiety and fear in the mother.

2. Infants with abnormalities may be unable to interact normally with the mother, depending on the nature of the defect. For example, a child with meningomyelocele may be able to lie on his abdomen on his mother's lap, but cuddling and eye-to-eye contact are difficult. Besides the acute grief experienced during the newborn period by mothers of infants with abnormalities, a state of chronic sorrow may continue throughout the child's life.[18]

3. Because of their immaturely developed reflexes, premature infants exhibit different behavioral responses from those seen in full-term infants. Johnson and Grubbs describe the dissatisfaction and confusion experienced by mothers of premature infants as a result of these differences.[11]

4. Multiple births can have several effects on the bonding process. The infants are frequently premature, requiring separation and special care. The mother may be mourning the death of one while trying to invest in the other(s).

Paternal Factors. Marital difficulties or the inability of the father to adjust to his new role can interfere in many ways with the maternal-infant relationship. The mother may not only be deprived of physical and emotional support from her husband, but may incur additional stresses as well. Fathers who have difficulty adjusting to the responsibility of a new dependent may compete with the infant for the mother's attention, may fail to relate to the newborn, or may use escape mechanisms, such as drinking or spending excessive time away from home. All of these responses make maternal attachment more difficult. Fathering behaviors, including specific adjustments that must be made by the new father, are described in the next chapter.

Hospital Factors. Hospital care practices and behaviors of health team members can have a significant influence on maternal bonding. These factors are more easily changed than the characteristics of the mother, infant, or father. Although many of the following occur with normal newborns as well as high-risk infants, the other stresses of the risk situation interfere with maternal attachment and make these factors even more significant.

1. Separation from the infant immediately after birth, at night, and for long periods during the day minimizes mother-infant interaction and negates the maternal sensitive period.

2. Policies which prohibit unwrapping and exploring the infant decrease a mother's knowledge about her baby and restrict interaction. When the infant is presented to the mother nude rather than wrapped, the mother progresses more rapidly from using her fingertips on the infant to enfolding the baby in her arms and holding him against her body.[5]

3. Limited caretaking by the mother interferes with attachment. When infants require special care, the maternal caretaking role is of necessity altered, but mothers are frequently restricted more than is necessary from providing care to their infants. Most units encourage touching, holding, and feeding infants, but mothers also enjoy and can be taught to participate in bathing, weighing, changing diapers, dressing and wrapping their babies, giving vitamins, and assisting with gavage feedings.

4. Restrictive visiting policies limit a mother's support from those who are most important to her.

5. Nonreinforcing staff behaviors can create feelings of inadequacy in the mother. When mothers are asked to perform caretaking tasks without proper instruction, for example, the chances of maternal lack of confidence and failure are increased.

6. The intensive care environment can be frightening and overwhelming even to the most confident mother. The strange sounds, sights, activity, and lack of privacy can stifle maternal feelings and behaviors.

Compounded Factors. Although any one of the factors mentioned has the potential of inhibiting maternal-infant bonding, certainly a combination of several factors increases the difficulty of achieving maternal attachment. In the high-risk family there is often a combination of many maternal, paternal, infant, and hospital factors which interfere with attachment. For example, the mother who is an adolescent may suffer from a lack of self-esteem, no husband to share the parenting, and premature delivery. The prevalence of many of these factors for the family at risk frequently makes attachment difficult. Since there are so many factors which may be compounded in risk situations, it is important for nurses to develop and use assessment tools to identify potential maladaptive mothering behavior.

NURSING APPROACHES

Although most risk situations cause stresses that interfere with bonding, the mother's ability to adapt to these stresses influences her ability to bond to her infant. Through sensitive observation and planned assessment, the nurse can identify the mothers with maladaptive mothering behavior and plan interventions to foster maternal-infant bonding.

Determining Adaptive and Maladaptive Mothering Behaviors

Maternal behaviors have been categorized in Table 1-1 as adaptive or maladaptive. *Adaptive behaviors* are those which are indicators of maternal-infant attachment and meet both the infant's and the mother's needs. *Maladaptive behaviors* are those which indicate a lack of maternal-infant attachment and result in unmet infant and/or mother's needs.

Only recently has attention been given to identifying maternal behaviors which are most conducive to the optimal development of the child. It is still not known which behaviors are the most valid indicators of maternal attachment.

Cultural differences in maternal behaviors must also be considered. Behaviors are not of equal importance in all cultures. While visual, auditory, and affective modes of interaction are important in Western industralized nations, continuous body-to-body contact with decreased emphasis on eye-to-eye contact predominates between mother and infant in other cultural groups. The behaviors presented in Table 1-1 are seen in contemporary Western society.

Another problem in defining adaptive behaviors is that a behavior may be adaptive in one situation and not in another. A mother may decline an offer to hold her premature infant who has just undergone a series of diagnostic procedures and is asleep in the incubator. She may be concerned about further disturbing and cooling the infant. This is adaptive behavior in this instance, as the mother is attempting to meet the infant's needs. But not holding a baby may be maladaptive if the mother emphatically declines to hold her infant even though he is in stable condition and awake. Another example is the mother who expresses a desire for eye-to-eye contact, but initiates it only when the infant is sleepy or agitated, rather than when the infant is in a quiet, alert state. Attempting to elicit behaviors when the infant is unable to respond produces a negative interaction for the mother.

Assessing attachment based on one observational period can be misleading. Single deviations in maternal behaviors are not as important as consistent patterns of behavior. On a particular occasion, a mother may not feel well or may be extremely tired and allow her infant to cry himself to sleep, rather than use soothing measures as she normally would. A mother who is busy preparing breakfast and lunches for school children and is confronted with a hungry baby who awakens early may on an occasion prop the infant's bottle.

For these reasons, the following list (Table 1-1) should be used only as a *guide* to assist the nurse in observing and evaluating mothering behaviors. The list does not contain all potential adaptive or maladaptive behaviors, but those which are most frequently observed in clinical practice and are felt to be indicators of attachment or nonattachment, if consistently performed. The nurse also must be alert for other behaviors, evaluating them in light of their effect on the infant and mother.

Table 1-1. Potential Adaptive and Maladaptive Mothering Behaviors

Time/Situation	Adaptive	Maladaptive
Delivery	Attempts to position head to see infant as soon as delivered and while infant is on warming table.	Does not position head to see baby. Stares at ceiling.
	When shown infant: Smiles. Keeps eyes on infant, looking at all parts exposed. Attempts en face position. Uses fingertip touch on face and extremities. Asks to hold baby. Partially opens blanket to see more of infant. Talks to baby. Asks questions about baby.	When shown infant: Frowns. Stares at baby without expression. Does not assume en face position. Turns head away. Does not touch baby. Does not ask to hold baby. Declines offer to hold. If infant placed in her arm, lies still, and does not touch or stroke face or extremities. May not look at infant. Does not talk to baby. Asks few or no questions.
	Makes positive statements about baby: "She is so cute." "He is so soft!"	Makes no comments or makes only negative statements: "She looks awful." "He's ugly."
	May cry out of joy or relief that infant is normal or of desired sex.	May cry, appearing unhappy or depressed.
	May smile and cry at the same time. To differentiate from crying out of disappointment, must note facial expressions and verbal statements.	When asked why she is crying, states being disappointed in baby.
	Expresses satisfaction with or acceptance of sex of infant. "We really wanted a girl, but it is more important that he is healthy." "I can't believe, a boy at last!"	Expresses dissatisfaction with sex of baby. "Not another girl. I should have known better than to have tried again for a boy." "I don't even want to see him." May use profanity when told sex.
	Predominant affect—appears pleased and happy.	Predominant affect—appears sad, angry, or expressionless.
	Suddenly decides she wants to breast feed.	Suddenly decides against breast feeding.
First Week	Initially uses fingertips on head and extremities. Progresses to using fingers and palm on infant's trunk. Eventually draws infant toward her, holding infant against her body.	Uses fingertip touch, without progressing to using palm on trunk or drawing infant toward her body.
	Snuggles infant to neck and face.	Does not hold infant to neck or face.
	Makes spontaneous movements, kissing, stroking, rocking.	Makes few or no spontaneous movements with infant.
	Attempts to establish eye contact by moving infant, assuming en face position, or shielding infant's eyes from light.	Does not use en face position or attempt to establish eye-to-eye contact.
	Handles and holds baby at times other than when giving direct care.	Handles only as necessary to feed or change diapers.
	Talks to infant.	Does not talk to infant.
	Smiles at baby frequently—changes affect appropriately, such as when infant cries.	Rarely smiles at baby. *or* Smiles all the time without change in affect.
	Makes many specific observations of infant: "Her eyes look like they might turn brown." "One foot turns in just a bit."	Makes no observations. Makes few observations which are either general or negative.

Time/ Situation	Adaptive	Maladaptive
First Week (cont)	Discusses infant's characteristics attempting to relate them to others in the family: "He has my ears, but his daddy's chin." "She really doesn't look like either of our baby pictures, she just looks like herself."	Does not discuss infant's characteristics in relation to characteristics of family members.
	With a positive affect and affectionate manner, uses animal characteristics to describe baby: "She is just like a cuddly little kitten." "His hair feels like down."	In a negative or hostile manner, uses animal characteristics to describe baby: "She looks awful, just like a drowned rat." "He looks just like an ape to me."
	Asks questions about caring for infant after discharge.	Asks no questions about care.
	By the time infant is discharged, has obtained basic supplies for caring for infant.	Has made no plans for obtaining basic supplies.
First Few Weeks	*If infant remains hospitalized after mother is discharged*	
	Calls every 1–2 days.	Calls less frequently than every other day, or not at all.
	Visits minimum of twice a week.	Visits less frequently than twice a week, or not at all.
	Visits minimum of 30 minutes.	Visits fewer than 30 minutes.
	Asks specific questions about infant's condition.	Asks specific questions. Asks very few questions. Asks inappropriate questions.
	Spends most of visit looking at and handling infant.	Spends most of visit observing unit activities and other infants (this may be normal behavior first 1 or 2 visits). Has little or no interaction with infant during visits.
	Becomes involved with care when encouraged and supported by staff.	When encouraged by staff to participate in care, refuses, terminates visit, or does only minimal care.
	Although visits are frequent and last longer than 30 minutes, makes statements about missing infant, e.g., expresses that she misses baby at home or that she wishes she could visit more often and stay longer.	Makes no statements about missing infant. *or* States she misses baby at home and wishes she could visit more often, but comments are not validated by frequent or lengthy visits.
	Expresses reluctance to terminate visit.	Leaves nursery with little hesitation.
	Waits until infant is asleep before leaving. Touches or talks to baby just before leaving. May stand outside window and look at baby before leaving unit.	Frequently asks nurse to complete feeding, or to change and settle infant.
First Months	Holds infant close to her body.	Does not hold infant securely against body.
	Supports infant's trunk and head in position of comfort.	Head and body of infant are not well supported.
	Muscles in arms and hands are relaxed and conform to curvature of infant's body.	Shoulder, arm, and hand muscles appear tense. Hands and fingers to not conform to infant's body.
	During feedings, holds infant in well-supported position against her body.	Holds infant away from body during feedings, or props infant or bottle.
	Positions during feedings so eye-to-eye contact can occur.	Position during feeding prevents eye-to-eye contact.

Table 1-1. Potential Adaptive and Maladaptive Mothering Behaviors (continued)

Time/ Situation	Adaptive	Maladaptive
First Months (cont)	Minimizes talking to infant while he is sucking.	Continues talking to infant during feeding, even though infant is distracted and stops sucking.
	Refers to infant using given or affectionate name.	Refers to infant in impersonal way, e.g., "the baby," "she," or "it."
	Plays with infant at times unrelated to direct care.	Handles infant mainly during caretaking activities.
	When infant is in infaseat, playpen, etc. frequently interacts with him.	Leaves infant for long periods in infaseat, playpen, or crib interacting only after baby becomes fussy.
	Places infant, when awake, in an area where he can observe and interact with others.	Leaves infant, when awake, alone for long periods of time in bedroom or isolated area.
	Occasionally leaves infant with someone else.	Frequently leaves baby with someone else. *or* Refuses to leave baby with someone else.
	Uses discretion in selecting babysitter and provides her with instructions on baby's routines, likes, and dislikes.	Does not use good judgment in selecting babysitter. Provides inadequate or no instructions for care.
	Provides infant with routine well-baby care.	Fails to provide infant with well-baby care, seeking medical assistance only after problems arise. *or* Keeps all appointments, and makes additional phone calls or additional visits to physician or emergency room for imagined or insignificant problems.
	Carries out medical plan for management of specific problems or conditions, e.g., thrush, anemia, or an ear infection.	Fails to or is inconsistent in carrying out medical plan for specific problems.
	Remains close to infant during physical exams, and attempts to soothe baby if he becomes distressed.	Remains seated at a distance from the exam table. Does not soothe infant during exam. Frequently arranges for someone else to take infant for medical appointments.
	Makes positive statements about mothering role.	Makes negative statements about mothering role.

Maternal Assessment Tools

The following four assessment tools guide the nurse in assessing maternal behaviors to help her identify specific bonding difficulties. Use of these tools does not replace good nursing practice to encourage mother-infant bonding, but guides the nurse in designing individualized approaches for the families most at risk of developing maladaptive mothering patterns.

The assessment tools should be used along with sensitive observation and interactive skills.

Assessment of mothering should take place over many observations and in different settings, since an observation made at one time is not necessarily indicative of mothering behavior all of the time.

The Dual-Purpose Tool for Assessing Maternal Needs and Nursing Care. The Dual-Purpose Tool is a comprehensive six-part form used to record antepartum, intrapartum, and postpartum information.[4] The tool provides areas under each part for writing an assessment, a plan of action, and the results of interventions, as shown in Figure 1-2. As the tool

ASSESSMENT OF MATERNAL NEEDS AND NURSING CARE

I. Maternal History: Antenatal, Labor, and Delivery

A. Antenatal

  1. first prenatal visit (data) _____

  2. preparation classes _____

  3. follow-up visits (regular) _____

  4. lowest hematocrit _____

  5. blood type _____

  6. serology _____

  7. prescribed medications _____

  8. other medications, drugs _____

  9. significant family history _____

    _____

    _____

  10. significant personal history _____

    _____

    _____

  11. past OB history _____

    _____

    _____

  12. problems with this pregnancy _____

    _____

    _____

B. Labor

  1. date and time of onset _____

  2. EDC _____ Week gest. _____

  3. rupture of membranes (art. or spon.) _____

    time _____

  4. stimulation of labor (type) _____

  5. medications (drug, dose, route, and time) _____

    _____

  6. fetal heart rate (pattern, lowest and highest) _____

    _____

  7. signs of fetal distress _____

  8. length of first stage _____

  9. significant patient behaviors _____

    _____

    _____

C. Delivery

  1. type _____

  2. presentation _____

  3. difficulties _____

  4. length of second stage _____

  5. anesthesia and analgesia _____

    _____

  6. Apgar _____

D. Placenta

  1. length of third stage _____

  2. problems _____

ASSESSMENT (actual and potential problems) _____

_____

_____

NURSING INTERVENTION (S) _____

_____

_____

RESULTS OF INTERVENTION (S) _____

_____

_____

II. Maternal Characteristics and Behaviors

A. Age _____ B. Marital status _____

C. Parity _____ D. Ethnic group _____

E. Religion _____ F. Socioeconomic _____

G. Pregnancy planned _____

H. Affect (smiles freq., etc.) _____

  _____

I. Activity level (lethargic, nervous) _____

  _____

J. Expectations regarding infant _____

  _____

K. Physical complaints _____

L. Acceptance of femininity (Consider complaints such as those regarding absence from work; feelings about breast-feeding; complaints of coital pain or dysmenorrhea.

  Note appearance.) _____

ASSESSMENT _____

_____

_____

NURSING INTERVENTION (S) _____

_____

_____

RESULTS OF INTERVENTION (S) _____

_____

_____

Figure 1-2. Cahill's Assessment of Maternal Needs and Nursing Care. Permission from *JOGN Nursing,* 4, 1975, 28–32. Copyright © 1975, Harper & Row, Publishers, Inc., Hagerstown, Md.

III. Infant Characteristics and Behaviors

A. Frank anomalies _____

B. Prematurity, LGA, SGA _____

C. Activity level

    1. sleep patterns _____

    2. random activity: minimal_____moderate _____

       extreme _____

D. Crying

    1. number of hours _____

    2. character: coarse, guttural _____

       weak, whining _____

E. Feeding

    1. uncoordinated sucking _____

    2. regurgitates _____amount _____

    3. tonicity when nursing _____

ASSESSMENT _____

_____

_____

NURSING INTERVENTION (S) _____

_____

RESULTS OF INTERVENTION (S) _____

_____

_____

IV. Parental-Infant Interaction

A. Simulation of infant by mother or father

    1. passive with little physical contact _____

    2. attempts to elicit response _____

    3. physically overstimulates infant (slaps, bites, hits, pokes) _____

B. Communication

    1. calls baby by name _____

    2. calls baby "it" _____

    3. talks to infant _____

    4. looks at infant _____

C. Attitude toward, and concern for, infant

    1. immediately meets infant's needs _____

    2. talks to others about infant _____

3. is happy about infant's sex _____

4. focuses more on self than infant _____

_____

D. Infant's behaviors (already listed in Part III, C, D, E) in response to mothering behaviors _____

_____

_____

_____

ASSESSMENT _____

_____

NURSING INTERVENTION (S) _____

_____

RESULTS OF INTERVENTION (S) _____

_____

_____

V. Maternal Physical Condition

A. Vital signs _____

B. Fundus _____

C. Lochia (color, odor, # pads) _____

D. Breasts _____

    1. type of feeding _____

    2. engorgement _____

    3. nipples

       a. extended or inverted _____

       b. condition _____

E. Episiotomy

    1. type _____

    2. lacerations _____

    3. condition _____

F. Hemorrhoids _____

ASSESSMENT _____

_____

NURSING INTERVENTION (S) _____

_____

RESULTS OF INTERVENTION (S) _____

_____

VI. Knowledge and Education Needs

A. Prenatal preparation _____
   1. classes _____
   2. reading _____
   3. physical (exercises, breast care) _____
   _____

B. Breast care (breast feeding)
   1. nipple care _____
   2. breaking suction _____
   3. alternating breasts _____
   4. supplemental feedings _____
   5. law of supply and demand _____
   6. diet _____
   7. let down reflex _____
   8. supportive bra _____
   9. technique of expressing milk _____
   10. drugs and breastfeeding _____
   11. weaning _____

C. Bottle feeding
   1. type of formula _____
   2. preparation _____
   3. vitamins and iron _____

D. Feeding variables
   1. rooting reflex _____
   2. demand scheduling _____
   3. length of feeding _____
   4. amount of fomula per feeding _____
   5. positioning _____
   6. burping _____
   7. introduction other foods _____

E. Infant care
   1. bath _____
   2. cord care _____
   3. circumcision care _____
   4. diapering _____
   5. temperature _____
   6. diaper rash _____
   7. pediatric followup _____

F. Birth control
   1. type _____
   2. understanding _____

G. Diet (nutritionist referral?) _____

H. Exercise
   1. received instruction postpartum _____
   2. received written information _____

I. Supports
   1. layette _____
   2. father of child at home? _____
   _____
   3. assistance from friends, relatives _____
   _____
   4. professional assistance _____
   _____
   5. financial status _____

ASSESSMENT _____

_____

NURSING INTERVENTION (S) _____

RESULTS OF INTERVENTION (S) _____

Remarks _____

_____

_____

_____

_____

_____

_____

_____

_____

_____

_____

includes observations of mother and infant interactions, it is particularly applicable to units that have rooming-in or primary nursing where the same nurse is responsible for both mother and baby. Data and observations requested are self-explanatory, requiring a minimum amount of instruction for use of the data-collection portion of the form.

The disadvantages of the form are its length, the need to collect data from the prenatal period through the postpartum period, and the knowledge required to properly assess the data and plan interventions. These can be overcome by initiating the form during the antepartum period so that it is completed over time by several nurses, or providing for the data to be recorded by one level of staff and assessed by another. Some of the information could be recorded by a unit clerk or practical nurse and assessed by a registered nurse.

The Family-Staff Interaction Guide. This interaction guide is a one-page form designed for use in a nursery which cares for high-risk infants.[7] It provides a continuous record of parent-infant and parent-staff interactions, as shown in Figure 1-3. It is an objective tool, based on recording the occurrence of prestated behaviors and parent teaching. Its brevity and simplicity minimize the need for instruction and foster increased compliance by staff. Unlabeled areas permit individualizing the form for patients with varying medical problems and complex parent-teaching needs. It facilitates communication among disciplines, as it provides for recording by all persons who interact with the family. It also provides current readily available data for interdisciplinary conferences and discharge planning.

The main disadvantage is that the tool provides only for the collection of data. A written assessment or plan of action, as well as additional information about the family, can be recorded in the patient's progress notes. The tool is particularly applicable as a means of providing data where a problem-oriented method of charting is used.

Neonatal Perception Inventory. This inventory is a questionnaire consisting of six questions related to what a mother believes is true of the "average" baby and six related to what she perceives in her own baby.[2,6] A scale rating system is used for each question with values from one for none to five for a great deal. The total score for how the mother perceives her infant is subtracted from the score for how she sees the average baby, with a negative score indicating the mother has more difficulty with her baby than she expects of the average baby. This indicates a potential risk situation. The inventory (shown in Figure 1-4), can be used through the first several months, and has a number of positive features: it can be used to screen for potential maladaptive mother-infant relationships, providing an opportunity for intervening before deviant mothering occurs; it does not require professional skill or knowledge to administer or interpret; and it can be given more than once to determine changes in a mother's perception of her infant.

The Observation Guide for Maternal Behaviors. The observation guide in Figure 1-5 lists specific basic maternal behaviors which are felt to be indicators of maternal bonding. It has been designed by the author for use with mothers of normal full-term infants during the first week and mothers of high-risk infants throughout the infant's hospitalization.

The tool can be used to record behaviors during a specific short observational period, such as during the mother's first interaction with her infant, or when she is feeding or bathing him. If used on more than one occasion with a particular mother, the number of behaviors observed can identify a progression or regression in maternal attachment behaviors. The tool can also be used by a primary care nurse to record behaviors which occur over a period of time, such as during an entire shift or during a mother's postpartum stay.

Specific advantages include: 1) its use as a screening mechanism to identify mothers who show few attachment behaviors and who will require additional assessment or immediate interventions and 2) its use in determining the effect of specific interventions.

The behaviors are organized in blocks according to a conceptual framework stressing important components of attachment, such as observing ap-

FAMILY–STAFF INTERACTION GUIDE
SPECIAL CARE NURSERY

MARTIN LUTHER KING, JR. GENERAL HOSPITAL
County of Los Angeles • Department of Health Services

DATE	CALLED	VIEWED	TOUCHED	HELD	BOTTLE FED	BREAST FED	DIAPERED	WRAPPED	BATHED		INIT.

RECORD ALL PARENT VISITS. USE CODES & INITIALS

M – MOTHER   **F** – FATHER   **P** – PARENT

O – OTHER (GIVE NAME) –

ADMISSION DATE	BIRTH WEIGHT

INFORMATION DISCUSSED	NURSE	M.D.	LIAISON NURSE	CHW MSW
VISITING & PHONING				
ENCOURAGED TO VISIT AFTER DISCHARGE				
SCRUBBING TECHNIQUE				
FACTORS PREDISPOSING TO PREMATURITY				

MEDICAL PROBLEMS

EXPLANATION OF & NEED FOR

- INCUBATOR
- MONITOR
- IV EQUIPMENT
- OXYGEN EQUIPMENT
- RESPIRATOR
- BILI LITES

DISCHARGE TEACHING

- BATH DEMONSTRATION
- CORD CARE
- CIRC CARE
- FORMULA PREPARATION
- SIBLING RIVALRY
- INFANT CARE, ROUTINE WHEN TO BATHE, FEED, ETC.
- ACTIVITIES OF THE MOTHER
- ENCOURAGED TO TREAT AS NORMAL INFANT
- DISCHARGED MEDICATION

FOLLOW-UP APPOINTMENTS

OTHER TEACHING

PATIENT IDENTIFICATION
NAME
MLK NO.

MLK-793 (9-73)

Figure 1-3. *Family-Staff Interaction Guide.* Reproduced with permission from *Pediatrics,* vol 55, #2, February 1975. Copyright 1975, American Academy of Pediatrics.

Figure 1-4. Neonatal Perception Inventory II

Average Baby

Although this is your first baby, you probably have some ideas of what most little babies are like. Please check the blank you think best describes the AVERAGE baby.

How much crying do you think the average baby does?

| a great deal | a good bit | moderate amount | very little | none |

How much trouble do you think the average baby has in feeding?

| a great deal | a good bit | moderate amount | very little | none |

How much spitting up or vomiting do you think the average baby does?

| a great deal | a good bit | moderate amount | very little | none |

How much difficulty do you think the average baby has in sleeping?

| a great deal | a good bit | moderate amount | very little | none |

How much difficulty does the average baby have with bowel movements?

| a great deal | a good bit | moderate amount | very little | none |

How much trouble do you think the average baby has in settling down to a predictable pattern of eating and sleeping?

| a great deal | a good bit | moderate amount | very little | none |

Your Baby

You have had a chance to live with your baby for a month now. Please check the blank you think best describes your baby.

How much crying has your baby done?

| a great deal | a good bit | moderate amount | very little | none |

How much trouble has your baby had feeding?

| a great deal | a good bit | moderate amount | very little | none |

How much spitting up or vomiting has your baby done?

| a great deal | a good bit | moderate amount | very little | none |

How much difficulty has your baby had in sleeping?

| a great deal | a good bit | moderate amount | very little | none |

How much difficulty has your baby had with bowel movements?

| a great deal | a good bit | moderate amount | very little | none |

How much trouble has your baby had in settling down to a predictable pattern of eating and sleeping?

| a great deal | a good bit | moderate amount | very little | none |

Reproduced with the permission of Brunner/Mazel, New York, 1971.

Figure 1-5. Observation Guide for Maternal Behaviors

Critical Attachment Tasks	Criteria of Attachment Indicators	Observed Behaviors (√)
	Spends time looking at baby, other than when providing care.	☐
Observes Infant's Appearance	Inspects or reviews head, trunk, and extremities.	☐
	Partially unwraps or undresses baby to observe body features.	☐
	Comments on baby's features, e.g., size, sex, hair, etc.	☑
Observes Infant's Behaviors	Talks to baby or smiles in response to infant's movements.	☑
	Comments on baby's behavior, e.g., opening eyes, grasping with hand.	☐
	Comments on infant's bodily functions, e.g., wetting, sucking, burping, etc.	☐
Identifies Infant's Physical Condition	Makes realistic statements about condition. "Her eyes are not so puffy today." Or, "He looks so pale."	☐
	Asks questions about condition, e.g., "What is the mark on her head?" Or, "Is he getting better?"	☐
Sees Infant as Another Human Being	Has selected a name for the baby.	☐
	Uses given or affectionate name when talking to or about baby.	☐
	Associates infant's characteristics with human characteristics, e.g., "He looks like a football player." Or, "She looks like a real baby now."	☑
Includes Infant in the Family	Attempts to associate infant's characteristics with those of other family members, e.g., "She has her daddy's eyes." Or, "He doesn't look like anyone else in the family."	☐
Talks to Infant	Talks or sings to infant.	☑
Establishes Eye Contact	Uses en face position.	☑
	Changes own position or that of infant to establish eye contact.	☑
	Stimulates infant to open eyes by shielding them from the light or by using other maneuvers.	☐
Demonstrates Physical Closeness	When handed infant, reaches out to receive baby.	☑
	Uses fingertips on head and extremities.	☑
	Uses palms on infant's trunk.	☐
	Enfolds infant in arms and holds against her body.	☐
	If infant hospitalized after mother discharged, visits a minimum of twice a week, for not less than thirty minutes per visit.	☐

Figure 1-5. Observation Guide for Maternal Behaviors (continued)

Critical Attachment Tasks	Criteria of Attachment Indicators	Observed Behaviors (√)
Changes Behaviors in Response to Infant's Behavior	When infant is fussy, attempts to soothe by patting, cuddling, rocking or talking to baby.	☐
	Does not continue behaviors which upset infant, or behaviors to which infant does not respond.	☐
	When infant is quiet and alert, makes eye contact and talks to baby.	☑
	Meets infant's needs prior to her own, e.g., "I'll feed him now and have breakfast later."	☐
Recognizes Infant's Needs and Provides Appropriate Care	Readily participates in care when asked.	☐
	Recognizes baby's needs and attempts to meet them or communicate them to someone who can, e.g., changes shirt after baby spits up, or changes wet diaper.	☐
	Handles baby in a manner which is comfortable for infant, e.g., infant's head and body are well supported and infant is handled gently with smooth rather than jerky movements.	☐
Plans for Ways to Care for infant at Home	Has obtained basic supplies for infant's care; prior to infant's discharge.	☐
	Asks questions about care, e.g., feeding schedule, formula preparation, cord care, etc.	☐
	Has made plans for or asks assistance with plans for well baby care.	☐
Perception of Infant	Comments about baby are predominantly positive.	☑
	Smiles frequently when looking at infant or when talking to or about baby.	☑
Perception of Self	Comments about self are predominantly positive.	☐
	Expresses satisfaction with mothering role.	☐

Total Number of Behaviors Observed   `11`

Date _____ 8-9-77 _____   Time _____ 4 P.M. _____

Situation __First interaction with infant following delivery__

pearance, behaviors, and others. When blocks of behaviors are not observed, this can be helpful in defining problems and selecting appropriate interventions. For example, if no behaviors are demonstrated in the area of "Identifying Baby's Condition," this may represent the mother's fear of something being wrong with her baby or it may result from a perceived unwillingness on the part of staff to answer the mother's questions. Another instance in which the conceptual framework can be helpful is in identifying a mother who does not talk to her baby. The mother may have had no experience with newborns and may need to be taught the importance of talking to an infant and also shown how her infant responds to a voice. Role modeling would be an important intervention with this mother.

The main disadvantage of the tool is that some behaviors may not be equally applicable in all situations, so several observations may be needed. For example, behaviors requiring interaction with a staff member, such as making comments or asking questions, may not be observed if there is a language barrier or if the mother is shy, young, or intimidated by the hospital environment.

The tool is presented here, with clinical observations of a mother's first interaction with her infant, shortly after delivery. This mother demonstrated attachment behaviors which are marked on the assessment tool. The lack of attachment behaviors related to recognizing physical condition and providing physical care alerts the nurse to reevaluate these at a later time and to provide interventions to foster attachment in these areas.

Fostering Maternal Attachment

Frequent assessment of maternal behavior during the first few days, weeks, and months of an infant's life is essential to identifying maternal-infant relationships which are at risk. Because patterns of behaviors are most important, data accumulated at one time should be recorded in the patient record for comparison with future assessments. This has become particularly important because of the increasing number of agencies and health team members interacting with families. The tools which have been presented can be used individually or together to guide the nurse in assessing mothering behaviors and in initiating and evaluating interventions.

Maternal attachment can be fostered by interventions which either reduce the factors inhibiting it, or increase those promoting it. Obstetrical and neonatal nurses can have a significant influence on the development of maternal attachment because

they are present when the mother begins to relate to her infant. Through initiating changes in routine procedures and practices, they can create an environment which is therapeutic to the development of maternal-infant bonding and one which accommodates to the needs of individual mothers and babies.

Maximum opportunity should be given during the postpartum period for a mother to get to know her infant and to begin developing confidence in meeting her child's needs. Such opportunities are afforded in hospitals which provide rooming-in. There should be no restrictions to a mother's unwrapping or undressing her infant, as long as the baby is protected from unnecessary cooling.

Just as a mother needs to become familiar with her infant's physical characteristics, she needs to become familiar with how her infant expresses his needs. If she is unable to perceive her infant's needs correctly, she may become frustrated and angered by his responses. When the mother is able to recognize her infant's needs and meet them adequately, the result is satisfaction and responsiveness in the infant. This, in turn, increases the mother's confidence and promotes pleasure in her mothering.

The rarity of extended family support and the established routine of many physicians of waiting until the infant is two to four weeks old before seeing him contribute to a serious lack of support and education for new mothers at a particularly critical time. Many mothers fail with breast feeding or become frustrated with an infant's excessive crying the first few weeks because they have not had guidance in handling problems which arise during the early newborn period. The impact of changes in lifestyle also are felt at this time, and may adversely affect all family members. When couples who had participated in childbirth education classes were asked several weeks after delivery about their need for classes during the early neonatal period, 82 percent felt small group classes would have been helpful. The majority of these couples stated that further information given prenatally about picking up cues from the baby or managing particular problems of the newborn would not have met their needs.[17] Health team members and nonprofessional individuals knowledgeable in the area of infant care can help parents become more successful in interpreting and meeting their infant's needs and in adjusting to their new roles.

Understanding an infant's basic personality or behavioral style is important in learning to identify an infant's needs and to appreciate his uniqueness. A number of temperaments have been noted in newborns shortly after birth.[3] A mother who expected a passive, cuddly, and easily satisfied infant will become frustrated if her baby is extremely active, naps for short periods at irregular intervals, and is not easily pacified. If these behaviors can be interpreted to the mother as part of the infant's unique personality, she can better understand her baby and more appropriately respond to his needs. Most important, she will not feel his behavior results from inadequate mothering.

Special interventions are frequently needed for mothers who experience a traumatic delivery or postpartum complications. During the postpartum period these mothers have been noted to direct conversation and thoughts toward themselves with decreased discussion of the baby.[6,14] They may also have no contact or decreased contact with their infant as a result of physical discomfort or the mother being isolated with an infection. Initial interventions should include encouraging these mothers to talk about their delivery or postpartum experience. Interactions with the infant should be encouraged, and during infant visits the mother should be rested and made as comfortable as possible so she is free to attend to the baby. Supportive assistance during the early mother-infant interactions is often needed to help overcome the handicaps encountered by these mothers in becoming acquainted with their infants.

Numerous interventions have been described for mothers of premature and other high-risk infants, most of which are aimed at increasing contact between mother and infant. It is essential that the mother be made to feel important during her infant's hospitalization even after the mother has returned to her home. This can be done by encouraging her to phone, visit, and handle her baby as often as she desires. To promote bonding and prevent feelings of helplessness and inadequacy, mothers should be encouraged to share in caretaking as early as possible. A mother of a two-pound infant can be taught to change his diaper, brush his hair after a bath, or to burp him following a gavage feeding.

One mother reduced the frequency and length of her visits at a time when her three-pound baby was no longer sick, but was not ready for bottle feeding. She became bored and frustrated during visits as she sat stroking and observing her sleeping infant. As an intervention, the baby's bath time was changed to coincide with her visits. The mother thoroughly enjoyed seeing changes in her son's movements and facial expressions as he sat in a small tub of water inside the incubator. After the first night, she expressed a desire to give all baths until discharge. Accordingly, this was incorporated into the baby's care plan. As a result, the length and frequency of her visits increased, and she appeared happier during visits.

An important skill for nurses working in special care nurseries is to be able to assess maternal readiness for participating in care and to provide the type of instruction and support the mother needs to feel successful in her task. If a premature infant is put to breast too early, or without sufficient help, he may refuse to suck. A mother who is asked to bottle feed an infant who poorly coordinates sucking and swallowing may become frightened and lose confidence in her ability to care for her infant if the baby should choke or develop cyanosis.

The mother of a premature infant or an infant with one or more abnormalities may have difficulty relating to her child because of his appearance. Very immature infants are often skinny, jaundiced, bruised, and they may have had part of their hair shaved for intravenous infusions. In an infant with a congenital defect, the abnormality may prevent the mother from noting features in the child which are normal. For instances when the infant's appearance is thought to inhibit maternal bonding, one large neonatal unit maintains a wardrobe of clothes which can be used to dress infants during parent visits. The clothes are made by staff and range from flannel pajamas and overalls to colorful dresses and sunsuits. Mothers frequently ask permission to keep their infant's first outfit and volunteer to replace it with another to maintain the unit's supply. The clothes are individually packaged and gas autoclaved by the hospital's central supply.

The importance of a community health nurse in supporting parents of high-risk infants during the infant's hospitalization as well as following discharge cannot be overstated. A referral to the community health nurse should be initiated soon after the infant's admission to a special care unit. Additional information received from the community health nurse about the family and home environment can be helpful to the hospital staff. The mother will feel more secure at the time of discharge if she has developed a relationship with someone she can call and count on to visit her during the first few days the baby is home.

If a high-risk infant dies, the community health nurse can support the family throughout the grieving process, reduce guilt by interpreting factors contributing to the death, and assist the family with realistic plans if another child is desired.

Interventions for reducing family difficulties related to specific high-risk situations are discussed in Parts Two and Three, while nursing strategies for increasing maternal-infant bonding, such as crisis intervention and counseling, are described in Part Four of this book.

SUMMARY

Over the past several years, considerable insight has been gained into the mother-infant dyad. Although no standardized tools exist for assessing this relationship, there are significant guidelines to help the nurse identify mothers who are having difficulty developing a positive relationship with their infants. These guidelines are especially useful in assessing the family at risk for abnormal development and disruption.

Further research is needed to develop methods of assessing and fostering maternal bonding in order to avert the consequences of mothering disorders and maximize the pleasure shared by mother and child.

REFERENCES

1. Blodgett, R. "Growth Retardation Related to Maternal Deprivation." In *Modern Perspectives in Child Development*, ed. A. J. Solnit and S. A. Provence. New York: International Universities Press, 1963.
2. Broussard, E. R. and M. Hartner. "Further Considerations Regarding Maternal Perception of the First Born." In *Exceptional Infant*, ed. Jerome Hellmuth. New York: Brunner/Mazel, Vol 2, 1971, 444–445.
3. Brown, J. B. "Infant Temperament: A Clue to Childbearing for Parents and Nurses." *American Journal of Maternal Child Nursing*, July/August 1977, 228–232.
4. Cahill, A. S. "Dual-Purpose Tool for Assessing Maternal Needs and Nursing Care." *JOGN Nursing*, January/February 1975, 28–32.
5. Cannon, R. B. "The Development of Maternal Touch During Early Mother-Infant Interaction." *JOGN Nursing*, March/April 1977, 28–32.
6. Clark, A. L. "Recognizing Discord Between Mother and Child and Changing it to Harmony." *American Journal of Maternal Child Nursing*, March/April 1976, 100–106.
7. Cropley, C. and R. Bloom. "An Interaction Guide for a Neonatal Special-Care Unit." *Pediatrics*, 55, February 1975, 287–290.
8. Cropley C. et al. "Assessment Tool for Measuring Maternal Attachment Behaviors." *Current Practice in Obstetric and Gynecologic Nursing*, 1, 1976, 16–28.
9. Fanaroff, A. et al. "Follow-up of Low Birth Weight Infants—The Predictive Values of Maternal Visiting Patterns." *Pediatrics*, 49, February 1972, 287–290.
10. Green, M. and A. Solnit. "Reactions to the Threatened Loss of a Child: A Vulnerable Child Syndrome." *Pediatrics*, 34, July 1964, 58–66.
11. Johnson, S. H. and J. P. Grubbs. "The Premature Infant's Reflex Behaviors: Effect on the Maternal-Child Relationship." *JOGN Nursing*, May/June 1975, 15–21.
12. Kempe, C. H. "Pediatric Implications of the Battered Baby Syndrome." *Archives of Disease in Childhood*, 46, February 1971, 28–37.

13. Klaus, M. H. and J. H. Kennel. *Maternal-Infant Bonding.* St. Louis: C. V. Mosby Co., 1976.
14. Mercer, R. T. "Postpartum: Illness and Acquaintance—Attachment Process." *American Journal of Nursing,* July 1977, 1174–1178.
15. Robson, K. S. "The Role of Eye-to-Eye Contact in Maternal-Infant Attachment." *Journal of Child Psychology,* 8, 1967, 13–25.
16. Rubin, R. "Maternal Touch." *Nursing Outlook,* II, November 1963, 828–829.
17. Williams, J. K. "Learning Needs of New Parents." *American Journal of Nursing,* July 1977, 1173.
18. Young, R. K. "Chronic Sorrow: Parent's Response to the Birth of a Child with a Defect." *American Journal of Maternal Child Nursing,* January/February 1977, 38–42.

ADDITIONAL READINGS

1. Bishop, B. "A Guide to Assessing Parenting Capabilities." *American Journal of Nursing,* November 1976, 1784–1787.
2. Harrison, L. L. "Nursing Intervention with the Failure-to-Thrive Family." *American Journal of Maternal Child Nursing,* March/April 1976, 111–116.
3. Klaus, M. H. et al. "Human Maternal Behavior at First Contact with Her Young." *Pediatrics,* 46, 1970, 187–192.
4. Morris, M. G. "Maternal Claiming-Identification Processes: Their Meaning for Mother-Infant Mental Health." In *Parent-Child Relationships.* Continuing Education Program by A. Clark et al. New Brunswick, N.J.: Rutgers, The State University of New Jersey, 1968, 34–35.

PERTINENT ORGANIZATIONS

NATIONAL
- *American Society for Psycho-Prophylaxis in Obstetrics, Inc.* (ASPO)
  1523 'L' Street, N.W., Suite 410
  Washington, D.C. 20005
  Provides classes on prepared childbirth which include care of the newborn.
- *La Leche League International*
  9616 Minneapolis Avenue
  Franklin Park, Illinois 60131
  Offers practical advice and encouragement to mothers who want to breast feed.
- *National Mothers of Twins Club Inc.*
  5402 Amberwood Lane
  Rockville, Maryland 20853
  A social and educational group for mothers of twins and other multiple births.

LOCAL
- *YWCA, Red Cross, Park and Recreation Departments and various Churches.* Frequently sponsor classes in prenatal education, mother-child interaction, and parenting.
- *Special Parent Groups.* There are an increasing number of parent groups being developed in some of the larger cities to meet the needs of parents of children with special problems.

Assessment of Fathering Behaviors

Carol M. Murphy, R.N., M.S.

CHAPTER TWO

American society is a dynamic force, and with movement comes growth. The recent women's movement has begun to liberate women personally and professionally. The integrated nature of American society dictates that changes in the role of women must be accompanied by complementary role changes for men.

Traditionally, the father's role in the family has been primarily that of "breadwinner." He often worked away from home, traveled long distances, and worked long hours; thus contact with his children was limited. The role of disciplinarian may have been thrust upon him by a wife who had been parenting all day and needed support in her efforts to set limits for the children.

In contrast, as more mothers enter the work force each year, the father's role in family life expands. Many young working couples report that they have developed well-balanced daily routines for sharing household and child-rearing responsibilities. Many men can perform "women's work" and enjoy it, without fear of stigma. As the working relationship between mother and father improves and their common experiences and concerns increase, communication is enhanced.

The blending of female and male roles is significantly altering personal and group values. Progressive educators are attempting to facilitate nonsexist attitudes and experiences in the classroom. Boys who are raised in a nonsexist environment may be better prepared to assume an expanded fathering role. The rapid evolution of sexual role equality is producing a host of novel male as well as female roles and responsibilities. Therefore, reevaluation of man's role as father is imperative.

In this chapter the development of fathering behavior and "fatherliness" will be traced and compared to mothering behavior. A brief exploration of personal, social, and environmental high-risk factors which facilitate or deter the development of mutually satisfying father-child relationships will be highlighted. Adaptive and maladaptive fathering behaviors will be identified and incorporated into an assessment tool for use by the nurse in clinical practice. The presentation will conclude with a discussion of the clinical nurse's role in prompting adaptive fathering behaviors through intervention and teaching.

FATHERING CONCEPTS

Nursing research in the area of maternal-child relationships is abundant and scholarly, but there is a dearth of literature concerning fathering behaviors. As described in most classical maternal-infant literature, the father's role was to support the mother as she nurtured the child. The fathering role was accorded neither a primary function nor autonomy.

However, recent literature demonstrates the recognition of the mother-father-child triad as a dynamic relationship and the essential participatory role of fathers in child-rearing. There is evidence that many fathers consistently make themselves available to their children, are responsive to their cues, and interact positively with them. The father acts as a sexual role model for his sons and daughters, affecting their sex role adoption.[1] Many fathers are very concerned with school performance, cultural value adoption, and morality, thus influencing the values of their children.[2] It is well documented that father-absent homes are more likely to produce children with delinquency and school failure problems.[5]

Much of the current research recognizes the significance of the father's role in the delivery room and in immediate postpartum interaction with the infant. Prenatal and delivery room experiences shared by both parents have helped to foster positive paternal attitudes and have increased fathers' willingness to participate in child care activities. Many new fathers experience "engrossment," defined as the father's bond to his newborn, during the first few days of his infant's life.[2] Some new fathers report feeling emotionally high—that they see their baby as attractive and individual. When the infant grasps the father's finger, the infant is communicating with him. It is possible that paternal-infant bonding is occurring during the engrossment period. One study suggests that the "engrossed" father has an increased sense of self-esteem, adequacy, and worth.[2]

It is interesting to note that a common deterrent to paternal participation in child care is maternal reluctance to relinquish caretaking responsibilities. Fathers may desire to assume an active child care role, yet they have been found to meet the expectations of their wives regarding the amount of responsibility they actually assume.[8] The father who is not invited to participate in the care of a newborn often feels unimportant and jealous.

Further research is needed to broaden the base of fathering theory. Potential areas of focus include identification of critical attachment periods, father-child interaction, communication patterns throughout childhood, and the effects of stress on the father-child relationship.

Development of Fathering Behaviors

A father's ability to actively participate in his child's life is influenced by several personal factors. The quality of a man's relationship with his own father and the fathering behaviors to which he was exposed during childhood affect a man's fathering potential. Fathers tend to discipline their children in a manner reflecting the discipline imposed on them by their own fathers. A man's ordinal position may influence his parenting capabilities. Men who have had exposure to children, including siblings, express more positive attitudes toward child care and having several children.[7]

Cultural and Socioeconomic Factors. The cultural milieu of a man's upbringing strongly affects his personal values, role expectations, and practices. A man's personality type, educational level, and career choice can affect fathering behaviors.

For example, Karl, a four-year-old boy was hospitalized for treatment of pneumonia and was constantly attended by his parents. The father had taken time off from his job as an efficiency consultant for a large firm. The father was the eldest son of a large German family and had been in this country for ten years. He was obviously the leader of this family unit, and it was observed that the mother and child rarely interacted. The father initiated caretaking behavior more often than the mother, and the behaviors he demonstrated most often were feeding, washing, and generally tidying the boy. His values and beliefs were reflected in his expression of fear that the child would lose weight if he were not fed. The father described himself as meticulous and efficient, which helped explain his job choice as well as the care-taking behavior in his fathering role. Through conversations with the father, the nurse recognized his dominance in the family and care-taking behavior were strongly linked to his cultural background.

The lower and middle socioeconomic groups tend to have different attitudes toward child-rearing. Attitudinal studies have shown that middle-class men are more involved in child care and have a greater influence over family life than do lower-class men. Middle-class wives expect their husbands to support the children, while lower-class husbands are expected to restrain and discipline them.[5]

Critical Periods. It is possible to speculate that there are critical periods for development of the father-child relationship similar to those in mother-child attachment. A critical period is defined as a distinct time period during which an individual is most receptive to specific learning experiences. If an individual is not exposed to the necessary learning experiences during the receptive time period, adequate behaviors may be more difficult to learn.

A potential critical period for father-child bonding is the "engrossment" period, from birth to three days of infant life. Fathers need exposure to infants during their most active, alert periods so that the infants' behavior and responses will trigger and reinforce bonding.[2] Father-infant bonding suffers when an infant is immediately and continuously separated from the parents after birth, as frequently occurs with high-risk infants.

There is also evidence that the critical period for father acceptance of the child and child acceptance of the father is quite early in the preschool years. Fathers and children who are separated for long periods during the first few years of life often have extreme difficulty in adjusting to one another when reunited. Separated fathers and children may both show signs of frustration and emotional distress. The children, especially boys, may have problems with sex role identity, while the fathers express distaste that the boys seem effeminate.[7]

Touching Behaviors. The comparative wealth of literature concerning mothering behavior can be utilized as a basis for observation of fathering behavior. A classic paper presented by Reva Rubin 15 years ago describes the orderly sequence of touch behaviors from fingertips to palm to body contact which can be observed as a mother becomes acquainted with her newborn. The touch acquaintance process is an observable aspect of the bonding process. Factors which influence the rate of progression of touch behaviors include the mother's self-confidence in her new role, the infant's response, environmental stress factors, the presence of birth defects in the infant, or illness in the mother.[9]

This well-described progression of touching behaviors is observable in many situations which involve acquaintance. Fathers, grandparents, and siblings also seem to display this touch pattern when introduced to a new infant. The pattern recurs when parents are reunited with their children after a long separation or when parents visit a hospitalized child whose appearance has been altered, either by accident or through the use of medical equipment such as endotracheal tubes or bandages.[9]

The nurse who is aware of these touch patterns can observe father-child interaction in an organized fashion. Maladaptive behaviors, such as holding the child a distance from the father's body or no touching, as in separation of a risk child from the parents, signify the need for further data collection and interventions.

Play Activities. Fathering behaviors may differ significantly from mothering behaviors in some cases; this seems to be true in father-child play activities. Play activities are an important aspect in a child's daily life. It has been demonstrated that fathers have a unique and special role in playing with their children. Fathers usually tend to play rough, tumbling, and unpredictable games with children, in contrast to mothers who play more conventional and less active games.[5] Mothers tend to hold children more frequently for the purpose of caretaking activities, whereas fathers hold children more for the purpose of lap play. Children of both sexes respond positively to the type of physical contact they have with their fathers during play activities. Observing fathers and children at play is potentially productive, in that the type of play and the child's response may provide the nurse with insight into the father-child relationship.

For example, a mother, father, and ten-month-old female infant who had been hospitalized for Wilms' tumor, a malignant abdominal tumor, were observed. The child was awake and lying in bed. The mother encouraged the child to take a rattle, moved the child's mobile, and encouraged her to speak. The father tickled the baby and used his hands to roll her from side to side in the crib. The child responded with smiles and active movement of extremities to both forms of play. She responded more vigorously with squeals and laughter to the father's interactions. Observing play activities can provide an understanding of the family members' reactions to each other and may provide insights into existing adaptive or maladaptive behaviors.

Adaptive and Maladaptive Fathering Behaviors

Adaptive fathering behaviors are defined as constructive father-child interactions which demonstrate a father's integrated awareness of his own needs paralleled with his child's needs. Maladaptive fathering behaviors are nonconstructive, neglectful, or harmful actions which demonstrate a father's lack of awareness of the child's needs or a predominance of his own needs.

Fathering behaviors are easily observable by the nurse who has contact with the father and child; the nurse may then analyze this data in assessing adequacy of paternal behavior. The consistency with which any behavior is displayed is significant. Adaptive behaviors should be seen most of the time.

Parenting high-risk factors interfere with the father's ability to develop adaptive fathering behaviors and increase the risk of the development of maladaptive behaviors. For example, the birth crisis and grief related to the birth of a premature, genetically defective, or physically handicapped infant may prevent normal interactive behaviors from occurring during the critical period of father-infant bonding. The family crisis and instability related to parental risk situations such as divorce, alcoholism, or abuse may foster the father's protective coping behaviors and prevent a close reciprocal relationship with the child.

For example, Bobby J. was born prematurely, at 32 weeks gestation, and had an extensive cleft lip and palate. His parents had limited financial resources and had expressed a strong desire to have this child, but also had some misgivings about incorporating a child into their lifestyle. The baby had a mild case of Respiratory Distress Syndrome, required oxygen therapy, intravenous feedings, and an incubator, but his condition improved rapidly. The parents were told that the cleft lip and palate would be repaired when he was older. The parents visited the nursery together each evening. They were very hesitant to touch the child and would reach into the incubator only after being strongly encouraged by the nursing staff. The father would touch the baby's feet and the top of his head, stating that "he looks so fragile." Neither parent verbalized their concerns about the child's cleft lip and palate, but it was noted that the father rarely touched or looked at the child's face. The nursing staff, aware that the parents were exhibiting few attachment behaviors, initiated a care plan aimed at increasing both parents' participation in the child's care. A clinical nurse specialist who works with parents who have experienced a loss began counseling the parents and provided them with an outlet for their anger and grief about the baby's disfiguring defect.

Though initially, the parents exhibited few adaptive behaviors, with time and counseling, they began to touch and talk to the baby frequently. The father would hold the child if it was suggested by the nursing staff. The parents were taught to feed the child using a special nipple. By the time of discharge, both parents were involved in the child's care, responding to his cries, holding him securely, and relating with him in a positive manner. Had the child been discharged before the parents were able to work through their grief and move toward attachment, it is conceivable that the family may have been vulnerable to future risk situations such as child abuse or neglect, marital discord, depression, and emotional problems.

Table 2-1. Potential Adaptive and Maladaptive Fathering Behaviors

Time/Situation	Adaptive	Maladaptive
Touches Child	freely, uses whole hand, gentle	infrequent, uses fingertips, rough
Holds Child	holds close to body, relaxed posture	holds distal from body, unrelaxed
Talks to Child	positive manner, tone; uses appropriate language, speed, content	uses curt, loud, inappropriate language or content
Facial Expression	makes eye contact, expresses spectrum of emotions	makes limited eye contact, little change in expression
Listens to Child	active listener, gives feedback	is inattentive or ignores child
Demonstrates Concern for Child's Needs	active, involves others, seeks information	indifferent, asks few questions
Aware of Own Needs	expresses feelings about self in relation to child	gives no expression about self
Responds to Child's Cues	responds promptly to verbal, nonverbal cues	has limited awareness and response
Relaxed with Child	posture, muscle tone relaxed	posture rigid, tense, fidgets
Disciplines Child	initiates reasonable, appropriate discipline	does not initiate or uses measures too severe or too lax
Spends Time with, Visits Child	routinely, utilizes time so that child is involved	has no routine, no emphasis on child during time spent
Plays with Child	uses appropriate level of play, active, both enjoy	uses inappropriate play, no obvious enjoyment
Gratification after Interaction with Child	father states, appears gratified	gives no statement or display of gratification
Initiates Activity with Child	frequently	infrequently
Seeks Information and Asks Questions about Child	concerned, asks frequent, appropriate questions	asks few questions, needs prompting
Responds to Teaching	positive, reinforces instructor, seeks more information	has low interest
Knowledge of Child's Habits	is knowledgeable	has little knowledge
Participates in Physical Care	feeds, bathes, dresses	allows others to perform tasks
Protects Child	aware of environmental hazards, actively protects	protective behaviors not exhibited
Reinforces Child	gives verbal/nonverbal responses to child's positive behaviors	does not notice or acknowledge child's behaviors
Teaches Child	initiates teaching	no teaching
Verbally Communicates with Mother about Child	uses positive, frequent verbal encounter	gives negative, infrequent communication
Verbally and Nonverbally Supports Mother	demonstrates support—reassures, touches, guides	support not obvious
Mother Supports Father, Father Responds	gives positive response	responds negatively, no response
Speaks of Other Children	responds when asked, initiates, shows interest	shows no interest, no initiation

A list of adaptive and maladaptive fathering behaviors such as the one in Table 2-1 directs the nurse in observing the father-child relationship and in identifying possible maladaptive behaviors. However, this must be used only as a guide for observations and not an absolute list. Maladaptive behavior for fathers in many circumstances may be adaptive behavior for fathers with other cultural backgrounds and in different situations. The nurse must determine the result of the fathering behavior in order to determine its actual adaptive or maladaptive nature.

NURSING APPROACHES

Current practices in maternal-child nursing reflect the societal trends which emphasize liberation of the individual and involvement of the individual in humanistic causes. Dramatic philosophical and practical changes in patient care have taken place during the last decade. Fathers are assisting mothers in the delivery room; fathers are staying overnight with and participating in the care of their hospitalized children; and family members are able to visit postpartum and pediatric patients at almost any time. In progressive institutions both parents and children are being included as essential members of the treatment team, since it is apparent that their involvement in the plan directly influences the outcome. Staff in newborn and pediatric intensive care units, where space is usually limited by equipment, now attempt to find room for the fathers as well as the mothers and encourage their participation in child care.

These changes are positive and progressive. By making such changes, health professionals have demonstrated that they are cognizant of fathers' needs and father-child dynamics, can utilize pertinent research findings, and can promote preventive as well as restorative family health care. The progress to date is gratifying and should give nurses incentive for continuing assessment and subsequent modification of practices.

Clinical Nursing Interventions

The clinical nurse's goals in working with fathers include the following:

1. To recognize the father's role as an essential, contributing family member.
2. To accurately assess adaptive and maladaptive behavior patterns.
3. To assess the effect of fathering behaviors on child response.
4. To assess the effect of child behaviors on fathering response.
5. To assist the father in the development of adaptive behavior patterns.
6. To reinforce and support adaptive fathering behaviors.
7. To provide feedback and alternatives to fathers who exhibit maladaptive behaviors.
8. To foster the growth of mutually satisfying father-child relationships and family interactions.

In order to meet these goals, the nurse must be able to assess the father-child relationship to identify difficulties and to institute preventive measures that reduce fathering difficulties in high-risk situations.

Assessment Tool

The fathering assessment tool in Figure 2-1 was designed for use by clinical nurses in hospital settings and public health nurses in home settings to guide the observation of fathers' adaptive and maladaptive behaviors. It could also be adapted for use by family nurse practitioners, psychiatric nurse therapists, or any nurse working with families. The tool is easy to complete and allows for a significant amount of data collection in a relatively short time period. It is suggested the nurse complete the tool during several interactions with the father, gathering more information with each meeting. When behaviors are observed over time, the data collected is likely to be more reliable than data collected in a limited period. Good observation and interview skills are essential to the completion of the tool.

The nurse begins by collecting some baseline

family data from the father. Notations of high-risk factors are indicated. Some examples of risk factors which increase stress on fathers and may precipitate crisis states are children in the custody of the newly divorced man; a sick neonate who is transferred to a hospital away from his home; child abuse, drug abuse, or psychiatric problems in a family. The specific family difficulties related to these problems are discussed in subsequent chapters.

The adaptive and maladaptive fathering behaviors are categorized in the assessment tool and the nurse is asked to be alert for these behaviors as she works with the father and child. The tool enables the nurse to systematically assess fathering behaviors and identify strengths and weaknesses in individual and related groups of behaviors.

There are four potential uses for this tool in nursing practice:

1. As a personal awareness tool, by the nurse who wishes to increase her awareness of fathering behavior patterns.
2. As a primary tool, by the nurse who needs to collect data about clients with actual or potential problems in the father-child relationship, so that interventions can be planned.
3. As a high-risk identification tool, by the nurse who needs to identify potentially hazardous father-child situations, so that preventive or restorative interventions may be instituted promptly.
4. As an adjunctive tool, by the nurse in a therapeutic relationship with a family unit, who needs supportive data relating to the fathering behaviors.

The tool was developed because the author felt a need for a guide to promote systematic observation of fathering behaviors. Once collected, the data needed to be in a format that could be easily shared with other members of the health team. The available fathering theories plus the author's own observations of fathers in high-risk nurseries, pediatric hospitals, and community settings contributed to the formulation of the tool. The tool was tested in

these same settings and was found to be a useful guide to the collection of specific, pertinent data regarding fathering behaviors. The tool was not developed as a research device, though with modification this is possible, but as a trigger for clinical nursing assessment and intervention. It was designed to allow easy reassessment of fathering behaviors, using the same tool at different times for comparison of behavior changes. The father can then be given concrete feedback regarding his development.

It is important to remember that, although active participation in child care seems to be a current societal trend, some men still prefer the traditional role of being less involved in actual caretaking behaviors than the mother. Fathers who choose the traditional role should be supported in their decision, as long as it is rewarding and productive for them and their families. Fathers who are not active in child care are not necessarily exhibiting maladaptive behaviors. Their individual fathering behaviors need to be assessed nonjudgmentally in order to identify the strengths and weaknesses of their fathering patterns.

In the example in Figure 2-1, the tool helped the nurse identify high-risk factors and assess the frequency of adaptive fathering behaviors. The tool was completed during this child's two-week hospital stay and was kept on file for use during subsequent admissions. The assessment tool enabled the nurse to identify the following family risk factors: divorced parents with mother as primary caretaker, child with long-term and potentially terminal illness, child with mental disability, financial difficulties secondary to health care costs. Using the tool for observation of the father's behavior as he interacted with the family during the ill child's hospitalization assisted the nurse in identifying specific adaptive and maladaptive fathering patterns. The father stated that he is fearful of caring for an ill child, yet comfortable and gratified by caretaking of the child when she is well. The assessment tool findings may reflect this fear. The observer noted strongly adaptive behaviors in the talking, play, eye-contact, teaching, and reinforce-

Figure 2-1. Fathering Assessment Tool

Case Example

FAMILY DATA SECTION

Names of Father: _____ Don _____ **Mother** _____ Alice _____ **Child** _____ Tina _____

Reason for Nursing Care: _____ newly diagnosed acute lymphoblastic leukemia _____

Father's Age: 20   (30)   40   50

Marital Status: Single   Married   Widowed   (Divorced)

Ethnic Backgrounds: Father: _____ Italian/American _____ Mother: _____ Italian/American _____

Occupations: Father: _____ housepainter _____ Mother: _____ homemaker _____

Financial Status: good   fair   (needs assistance)

Number of Children in Family: 1   2   (3)   4   5

Age and Developmental Level of Child: _____ 4 years old, lags in cognitive, verbal and fine motor skills _____

Special Problems of Child: _____ has Down's Syndrome _____

Identified Risk Factors: _____ divorced, terminally ill child with developmental handicap, financial difficulties secondary to hospital bills. _____

Father's Description of His Child Care Role: _____ states he takes an active part, enjoys having Tina stay with him, communicates with her easily, is fearful of caring for her when ill _____

Mother's Description of Her Child Care Role: _____ states she is primary caretaker, has few activities outside household unless children stay at father's house. _____

If Hospitalized:

Expected Visiting Hours for Father: _____ evenings, will spend the night _____

Mother: _____ most of the day _____ Siblings: _____ after school 3–5 p.m. _____

Figure 2-1

FATHERING BEHAVIORS

The nurse observes the father/child interactions to note the frequency of adaptive behaviors.

Fathering Behavior	adaptive behavior	Frequency			maladaptive behavior
		always adaptive	usually adaptive	rarely adaptive	
father-child interaction					
touches child	freely, gentle	○	●	○	rare, rough
holds child	close, relaxed	○	○	●	distal, unrelaxed
talks to child	appropriate	●	○	○	inappropriate
listens to child	attentive	○	●	○	inattentive
plays with child	active	●	○	○	passive
posture	relaxed	○	●	○	rigid
facial expression	expressive	●	○	○	inexpressive
eye contact	frequent	●	○	○	infrequent
response to cues	prompt	○	●	○	delayed
knowledge of child's habits	knowledgeable	○	●	○	not knowledgeable
participation in physical care	active	○	○	●	passive
protects child	aware, active	○	●	○	unaware, inactive
disciplines child	initiates, reasonable	○	●	○	passive or inappropriate
teaches child	initiates	●	○	○	no initiation
reinforces child	active	●	○	○	passive
role gratification					
initiates activity	active	○	●	○	passive
verbally expresses pleasure	frequent	●	○	○	infrequent
appears gratified	frequent	●	○	○	infrequent
growth potential					
seeks information	active	●	○	○	passive
response to teaching	positive	●	○	○	negative
family support					
aware of own needs	aware, expressive	○	●	○	unaware, inexpressive
verbally supports mother	active	○	○	●	passive
verbally supported by mother	active	○	○	●	passive
speaks of other children	frequent	●	○	○	infrequent

ment interactions between father and child. Touch, listening, posture, and cue response were less adaptive, while holding and participation in child care were rarely adaptive. The assessment tool demonstrates that his father's role gratification and growth potential behaviors are strongly adaptive while family support behaviors are frequently maladaptive.

Utilizing the nurse's observation and interview skills, the assessment tool, and the nursing process, an appropriate care plan can be developed for this father-child dyad. See Table 2-2 for an example of a portion of the care plan developed for use with this father.

It is suggested that the nurses caring for a family reassess the fathering behaviors utilizing the tool with every admission, as the behaviors should become more adaptive in response to the nursing interventions. The care plan, too, needs frequent revision to make it move with the father. The nurse should be aware that the father may exhibit an increasing number of maladaptive behaviors during crisis times, for example when the child suffers medical complications, and will need additional support and reinforcement during these times.

Preventive Interventions

The nurse's ability to foster adaptive fathering behaviors and prevent maladaptive patterns is contingent upon cooperation with other disciplines. Prevention of maladaptive behaviors for fathers in high-risk situations may require the services of a multidisciplinary health care team. It is likely that the nurse will identify high-risk potential in a family situation through her contact with parents in prenatal clinics, well-baby clinics, during home visits, or on hospital wards. The information may need to be shared appropriately with physicians, social workers, or child protection agencies. The nurse who is aware of maladaptive fathering behaviors and high-risk factors will be able to initiate intervention early, possibly preventing family crisis.

"Pregnant Fathers." The nurse working with prenatal classes, in labor and delivery, or in post-partum units has the opportunity to reach out to the "pregnant father" who tends to be neglected while energy and support are directed to his wife.[4] A fairly common occurrence among "pregnant fathers" is the "couvade" syndrome in which the man exhibits physical symptoms similar to those experienced by the pregnant woman, including nausea, vomiting, abdominal pain, and weight gain.[4] In one case, the husband gained 20 pounds during the course of the pregnancy. This man frequently complained about his weight gain in a joking manner, yet it was not until the eighth month of the pregnancy that a nurse heard his quiet cry for help and directed some energy and support toward him. The "pregnant father" has needs similar to his wife's, including preparing for the baby's arrival, considering the baby's individual place in the family unit, and having touch experiences with the newborn to facilitate bonding.

An important ongoing nursing role in maternity units is support of current practices of father participation and stimulation of further liberalization of hospital policies. The father needs to have ongoing contact with his new child during the immediate postnatal period for bonding to begin. Nursing practices must encourage the mother-father-child triad to begin to relate as a family unit. The father needs caretaking opportunities similar to those offered to the mother during hospital stay.

A nurse must address the father as well as the mother to teach him feeding and bathing techniques, to answer questions, and to give him feedback about his child care performance. Figure 2-2 shows one father caring for his high-risk infant. The nurse has the opportunity to assess engrossment, bonding, and parenting behaviors during the teaching sessions. Public health nurse referral can be made if additional teaching or assessment of parenting behaviors is needed.

The Father and the Child at Home. The nurse has a supportive and teaching role when working with fathers who participate actively in child care at home.

Fathers who assume the role of primary child caretaker need a great deal of support, as do hus-

Table 2-2. Initial Nursing Care Plan

Goal: To increase the number of adaptive fathering behaviors; to support adaptive father-child interaction.

Assessment	Nursing Diagnosis	Interventions	Evaluation
Father has high motivation to participate in child care. Displays adaptive talk, play, eye contact, reinforcement behaviors. Reluctant to touch, hold, physically care for ill child.	Adaptive behaviors are strong and consistent. Maladaptive behaviors reflect lack of confidence in caring for ill child, fear of ill child.	1. Verbally reinforce the father's adaptive behaviors: consistent visiting pattern, warm, playful manner, ability to teach child and talk with her appropriately.	Father smiles when specific adaptive behaviors are praised. Responds less to general statements about his fathering skills.
Actively seeks and is receptive to teaching.	Father has high potential to learn additional adaptive behaviors.	2. Point out the child's responsive behaviors—laughs and squirms during active games, reaches out for father's hand.	Father acknowledges that he, too, noted the child's response. He repeats those behaviors that elicit positive response from child.
		3. Initiate open-ended conversations about father's reaction to hospital setting. Reinforce that this reaction is normal.	Father initially seemed closed, embarrassed about his reaction. Will continue to give him the opportunity to verbalize, without pushing him.
		4. Introduce father to a "peer"—another father who visits at similar times.	Good results. Two fathers spend time talking each evening.
Fearful of tubes & equipment.		5. Explain equipment to father.	Father asked many questions about how equipment works, safety precautions.
		6. Demonstrate that touching the child is permissible despite tubes and equipment the child is attached to.	Works best when nurse demonstrates that child can be touched then leaves father to try it. Father able to hold child in lap if nurse assists with positioning equipment.
Long-term illness requiring frequent hospitalizations with high costs.	Financial burden secondary to hospital costs.	7. Ask social worker to interview family. Refer to appropriate agencies: Crippled Children's Services, American Cancer Society.	Father states that he is much less worried after hearing that Crippled Children's will assist.
Parents do not support each other. Large, Italian/American family is potentially supportive. Both will need support to face the long-term illness the child suffers (crisis state).	Severely maladaptive support behaviors between parents. Entire family needs to build a support system.	8. Early referral for family, couple or individual psychotherapy to assist family to cope with present crisis.	Father reluctant to participate in psychotherapy.
		9. Refer to "Parents' Group" that meets monthly at hospital.	Members of Parent's Group encouraged him to attend group meetings.
		10. Provide ongoing nursing support through verbal-nonverbal feedback.	Father relates well with nursing staff he knows. Uses them as supports. Ventilates to them.
Children demonstrate awareness of conflicts.		11. Reinforce extended family members' positive involvement in child's illness.	Grandparents are taking a more active role.

their children. The nurse might foster the development of adaptive behaviors by encouraging the fathers to perform the caretaking role in a variety of situations, for long and short periods, during pleasant and unpleasant times, and tune in to his, the mother's, and the child's reaction to each situation.

New fathers also need a good overview of normal child growth and development. The majority of men have had little opportunity to study normal development, thus they will be unprepared for the expected progression of behaviors in their child. Developmental guidelines are available in pamphlet form through health agencies and are often published in parents' magazines. The nurse might review the commonly used child-rearing guides and suggest a good title to the new father. This new knowledge will increase the father's abilities to care for the child, thus increasing his self-esteem.

Couples who share child-rearing responsibilities should be encouraged to share their ideas, techniques, and frustrations. When support is unavailable within the family framework, fathers may require alternate sources of support. Telephone "hot lines" have proven to be an effective outlet for mothers who are having difficulty dealing with a child-rearing situation. The "hot line" volunteers who allow mothers to ventilate their feelings and work toward solutions should also welcome calls from frustrated fathers. As husbands deal with children more, they may find themselves exhibiting more maladaptive behaviors and in need of help.

The Father and the Hospitalized Child. Hospitalization is a stressful experience for both parents and the child, thus it is essential that the nurse take steps to promote comfort by providing the family with a thorough orientation to the ward. A family-centered orientation program, in which the triad is addressed as a unit and not separately is desirable, for it fosters the child's trust and decreases his anxiety, allows the parents to hear the information that is given to the child so that they can reinforce it, and demonstrates that the nurse respects the integrity of the family unit.

Mothers and children are the focus of atten-

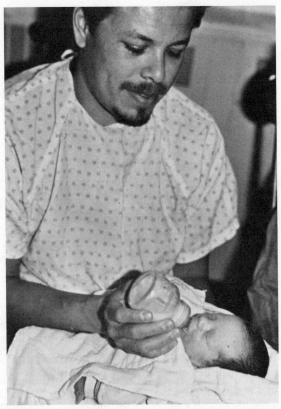

Figure 2-2. Fathers are encouraged to care for their risk infants.

bands that share child-rearing roles in high-risk situations. Clarification of the nurse's own values may be necessary, for it would be difficult for a nurse to be honestly supportive of a "househusband" if she holds traditional beliefs. Couples may work out a child care system which meets their needs but conflicts with the values of their peers.

For example, a physician husband and pharmacist wife decided to share equal child care responsibilities for their mentally disabled son. The physician was recently called from rounds because his son was ill and had been sent home from school. As he left the hospital to determine the extent of the child's needs, he noticed the obvious disapproval of the majority of his colleagues.

The nurse's teaching role is of particular importance when working with new fathers. Most fathers work and have limited time to spend with

tion in many hospitals and clinics. When a child is being admitted to the hospital, the mother generally responds to the admission interview questions. The father's participation even at this initial encounter is often overlooked and if his role in the family is that of an active participant, nursing staff run the risk of alienating him from the start by not including him. He may become angry and withdraw, denying himself and his child the rewards of their established relationship. The nurse may deny herself significant input by not actively including the father in the interview process.

The nurse has a role in explaining the institution's policies on parent rooming-in and care-by-parent. Most pediatric hospitals are liberalizing the traditional rules in order to promote the well-being of family members. Mothers and fathers generally want to stay with the hospitalized child and many formulate a schedule of shared responsibility. Common arrangements are the father spending the night with the child so he can work during the day, with the mother spending the day with the child and the night at home, or the father spending the weekend with the child while the mother takes the week days.

When the father is with the child, he should be allowed to assume those responsibilities which are familiar to him and take on new ones he shows interest in. The father and child should be encouraged to maintain their usual daily patterns as much as possible. The father who feels helpless in assisting his ill child is often pleased to learn a new caretaking behavior if the mother or nurse shows him what is needed. A common and often incorrect assumption made by nurses is that fathers, even those who room-in, do not want to assume responsibility for patient care. A father may be reluctant to initiate caretaking activities because he sees that the efficient nurse is handling everything.

With the high percentage of women personnel on pediatric wards, a father may feel alone or intimidated. One father who stayed with his ill son for several months communicated and socialized only with the janitor, one of the few male employees. Having a male nurse employed on this pediat-

ric ward would have provided this father with a role model he could more easily relate to and communicate with.

Parents often express a desire to meet other parents of children in the ward to form a peer group. Nurses can take the initiative in making parent-to-parent introductions. One father of a child with a long-term illness and frequent hospitalizations thought of selecting a "Parent of the Day" on the pediatric ward to help meet the needs of his peer group. The "Parent of the Day" is responsible for greeting and orienting any new parents and children admitted to the ward.

Through interactions with their peers, parents can share adaptive behaviors and support one another in times of stress to prevent maladaptive behaviors. The parents of children with leukemia in one hospital discussed the problems they faced in dealing with their reactions to the painful procedures, such as shots and lumbar punctures that their children frequently experienced. Parents reported that they often felt angry at the child as well as the person who performed the procedure; they sometimes withdrew from the child and were unable to adequately comfort him. The disclosure of these behaviors in an accepting atmosphere helped the parents to feel that they are normal and allowed them to work toward more adaptive behaviors.

When fathers of hospitalized children were asked to express their needs, their responses were concrete. They asked nurses to provide honest answers, simple explanations of the machines, a place to be alone, a chance to be with the child, someone to talk with, coffee, and a phone.

SUMMARY

Important changes in American society and in individuals are contributing to increased flexibility in the father's child-rearing role. His contributions to the family are significant, irreplaceable, and affect all members of the family.

Assessment of adaptive and maladaptive fathering behaviors with identification of high-risk factors is a key nursing role. Since high-risk situations interfere with the development of adaptive fathering behaviors and precipitate the development of maladaptive behaviors, early identification of high-risk families is essential. Timely and individualized interventions promote the well-being and adaptation of father, mother, and child.

REFERENCES

1. Biller, H. B. *Father, Child and Sex Role: Determinants to Personality Development.* Lexington, Mass.: Heath, 1971.
2. Greenberg, M. and N. Morris. "Engrossment: The Newborn's Impact Upon the Father." *American Journal of Orthopsychiatry,* 44 #4, July 1974, 520–531.
3. Hines, J. "Father—The Forgotten Man." *Nursing Forum,* 10 #2, 1971, 177–200.
4. King, E. "The Pregnant Father." *Bulletin of the American College of Nurse Midwifery,* 13 #1, February 1968, 19–25.
5. Lamb, M. E. (Editor). *The Role of the Father in Child Development.* New York: John Wiley & Sons, 1976.
6. Leonard, S. W. "How First-Time Fathers Feel Toward Their Newborn." *American Journal of Maternal Child Nursing,* November–December 1976, 361–365.
7. Nash, J. "The Father in Contemporary Culture and Current Psychological Literature." *Child Development,* 36, 1965, 261–297.
8. Reiber, V. D. "Is the Nurturing Role Natural to Fathers?" *American Journal of Maternal Child Nursing,* November–December 1976, 366–371.
9. Rubin, R. "Maternal Touch." *Nursing Outlook,* November 1963, 828–831.

ADDITIONAL READINGS

1. Anthony, E. J. and T. Benedek (Editors). *Parenthood: Its Psychology and Psychopathology.* Boston: Little, Brown and Company, 1970.
2. Arnstein, H. "The Crisis of Becoming a Father." *Sex Behavior,* April, 1972, pp. 42–47.
3. Gilbert, S. D. *What's a Father For?* New York: Warner Books, 1975.
4. Gollober, M. "A Comment on the Need for Father-Infant Postpartal Interaction." *Journal of Obstetrical, Gynecological, and Neonatal Nursing,* September–October, 1976, pp. 17–20.
5. Marquart, R. K. "Expectant Fathers: What Are Their Needs?" *American Journal of Maternal Child Nursing,* January–February 1976, pp. 32–36.
6. Parke, R. D. "Father-Infant Interaction." *Maternal Attachment and Mothering Disorders,* M. H. Klaus et al, Editors Johnson and Johnson, 1974, pp. 61–63.

Assessment of Children's Behavior

Cheryl Hall Harris, R.N., B.S.N.

CHAPTER THREE

Nurses who work with high-risk families are frequently requested to give their impression of a child's performance or to counsel parents on the best way to deal with their "problem" child. Rather than basing an assessment on intuition alone, the nurse can use several available tools which are carefully designed to delineate infant or child behavior and which provide specific information for effective problem solving.

The child's behavior is important in parent-child interactions, since it may affect parenting responses. If a child demonstrates specific mental or physical problems, his parents may respond to these problems rather than to the child's total emotional responses. The nurse may be able to help parents focus on their relationship with their child as a total individual by interpreting results obtained through her assessments.

Since the nurse may be one of the first health professionals to interact with the high-risk family, her initial assessments may prove to be invaluable. The nurse may use her assessment opportunities in a variety of ways. One important use is screening for children with potential problems, such as prematurity, birth defects, or emotional disturbances. For example, a delivery room nurse can perform physical examinations on an infant she suspects is a premature, providing, of course, the infant does not require resuscitative efforts and the nurse provides warmth and other necessary physical requirements before beginning her assessment. The nurse can observe the presence or absence of heel creases, the amount of cartilage formation in the ears, and so on, and report her findings to the physician. The nurse who is performing initial assessments of an infant's status may be the first to detect a birth defect. For example, in attempting nasal suctioning, the nurse may discover an infant with choanal atresia, or she might discover an infant with an imperforate anus. In a clinic setting, the nurse may be the first person in whom the parents confide their fears of their child's emotional instabilities. She may assess their reports and determine whether further testing is required.

The nurse may use assessment skills to assess individual characteristics of high-risk situations. The high-risk child, such as a child with birth defects, may have such overwhelming physical problems that his emotional difficulties are overlooked. For example, a child born with a meningomyelocele will probably require numerous hospitalizations, and the focus will be on providing for his physical disabilities. However, he may also have difficulties coping emotionally with his handicaps. The nurse may be in a position to assess his individual abilities and problems.

Another use of assessment skills is to help prevent problems from developing. If a nurse knows or suspects that parents abuse their children, she could begin early assessments of a new child's behavior patterns as well as any physical signs of abuse. Naturally, these parents should be receiving counseling for their former problems, but additional assessments may prove beneficial.

Assessment tools often prove to be invaluable teaching aids for the nurse in her attempts to help parents interact with their child. By utilizing the findings of the Brazelton Neonatal Scale, for example, the nurse can demonstrate to parents their infant's capabilities at an early age, and thereby increase their interest in stimulating their newborn. Parents who are having difficulty relating to their infant may discover through the use of the Carey Temperament Questionnaire that their infant's individual temperament characteristics influence their reactions and difficulties.

The nurse who works in a high-risk setting will utilize her assessment skills to determine potential difficulties which will require follow-up and referral. For example, a nurse who administers the Vineland Social Maturity Scale may discover a child with significant developmental delays. If a nurse makes such a determination, she should refer the child and his parents to a child-development clinic or other multidiscipline center which can provide further testing and evaluation. The child may require treatment or remedial training of some type, and these goals may be reached most effectively in a specialty setting.

The purposes of this chapter are to describe the child's influence on the parent-child relationship, to describe the necessity for nurses to assess children's behaviors at various developmental levels, to provide some general assessment guidelines, and to review some specific tools which the nurse may find useful in her work with high-risk families. While there are numerous tools available for assessing physical and intellectual parameters, this chapter will focus on several behavioral assessment tools and refer the reader to resources for other specific tools.

CHILD ATTACHMENT CONCEPTS

Parental-infant attachment is a reciprocal process. The mother brings to the relationship her prior experiences of care by her own mother, her educational level, and her socioeconomic status. The father brings to the situation his prior experiences, his expectations of his role, and his perceptions of how society expects him to act. And the infant has certain characteristics which elicit an attachment from his parents and other adults. While earlier chapters presented the mothering and fathering characteristics, this chapter focuses on the infant's role in the child-parent attachment process.

Infant Care-Eliciting Behavior[19]

There are several factors which cause parents to want to care for their infant. Some of the factors are parent initiated, such as seeing their infant as a duplication of themselves. Some of the factors are infant produced and are called care-eliciting behaviors. For example, one infant characteristic which causes adults to become attached to him is his physical appearance. His small stature, short extremities, and clumsy movements cause adults to want to protect and care for him. His parents realize their infant's total dependence upon them for his well-being, and this helplessness strengthens most parents' desire to care for him.

In addition to the physical characteristic, the infant may exhibit care-eliciting behaviors. Crying is one of the strongest of such behaviors an infant exhibits. His mother initiates several caretaking steps in response to his crying, such as changing his diapers, feeding him, or rocking him. In the initial interactions between parents and their infant, most of the parents' efforts are intended to stop his crying.

The infant responds to the care given him initially by cessation of crying, sucking, and later by smiling and babbling. These responses reinforce his parents desire to care for him. The parents and the infant suffer if the reinforcement from the infant does not occur. An infant who does not smile and babble, may be picked up less, or be held less frequently by his parents. Therefore, the infant receives less stimulation, and this may in fact affect his later social relationships.

An infant's responsive behavior toward his parents' ministrations is also important in helping them to feel competent in their caretaking abilities. When a mother believes she is capable, and her infant responds to her caretaking, she feels secure and competent. If the infant does not respond, his mother feels insecure, incompetent, and therefore unhappy in her caretaking role. The reciprocal nature of child-parent behaviors begins prenatally and continues throughout the lifelong interactions of the participants.

The nurse's assessment of the child's behaviors helps her to identify the infant's unique responses. This information helps the nurse to demonstrate the child's positive responses for his mother who is having difficulty attaching to her child. For example, a mother may not realize that her infant's smiling and cooing is actually a response to her actions. If the nurse points this out, it may improve the mother's image of her caretaking abilities and help strengthen her ties to her infant.

Infant Temperament

All children have temperamental characteristics at birth, although until recently there was little scientific documentation of this fact. An inventory of a child's temperament profile has been approached by Thomas and his associates, who organized a system of nine categories of temperament qualities.[21] These are:

1. Activity level—an assessment of the amount, frequency and tempo of the infant's motor activities.
2. Rhythmicity—the predictability of biologic cycles such as the sleep-wake cycle, eating patterns, bowel function, etc.
3. Approach or withdrawal—the infant's initial response to any new situation, such as a new toy, food, or people in his environment.
4. Adaptability—not the initial reaction, but subsequent response to a new situation; for example initially the infant did not like meat, but later developed a liking for it.
5. Intensity of reaction—assessment of mild or intense positive or negative reaction to external stimuli.
6. Threshold of responsiveness—the level of stimulus required to evoke a response.
7. Quality of mood—the amount of time an infant spends exhibiting happy, friendly behavior as opposed to the amount of time he demonstrates crying or unfriendly behavior.
8. Distractibility—whether or not an infant can easily be distracted from one activity by presenting him with another.
9. Attention span and persistence—the length of time an infant will continue to pursue an activity. Persistence is the quality of a child who continues to pursue an activity even though he has difficulty with it.

The value of organizing observations about a child's temperamental qualities into these categories is that it makes possible assessments of a child's strengths and weaknesses and facilitates discovering temperamental qualities which may lead to behavior problems. Carey and McDevitt have utilized these categories to develop an assessment tool for infants, which will be described later in this chapter.

The nurse must not view temperament as the primary cause of behavior problems, since there is a reciprocal effect of the parents' response to the child's temperamental qualities. Once a child's temperamental characteristics have been assessed, if a pathogenic interaction pattern by the parents is detected, the nurse can give them guidance in their approach. For example, if a child cries incessantly, and the parents become frustrated, they may begin abusing their child. If the nurse assesses that the infant's temperament difficulties are the cause of the problem, she may counsel the parents accordingly.

One value of assessing a child's temperament is that it helps those caring for him to recognize his uniqueness. The effect of environment on a child depends on his ability to incorporate the environment, given his temperamental characteristics. For example, a child with hyperative tendencies who is easily distracted may have difficulty concentrating on a specific task. If his mother becomes frustrated by his inability to concentrate, she may develop negative maternal patterns of behavior. If the nurse detects the child's peculiarity, through assessment of his temperament, she can point this out to the mother, as well as describe the manner in which the mother is setting unfair expectations for her child.

The newborn is neither unorganized nor passively receptive to his environment as was previously assumed. His temperament truly affects his parents and their perceptions of their caretaking abilities. If an infant is not "cuddly," and his mother has the need to cuddle him to feel adequate in her interactive skills, there may be a problem. Therefore, the assessment of this temperamental quality may be very important in helping the mother adjust her attitudes toward her infant, and thereby treat him as an individual, with needs of his own.

For example, a mother described her first child as having been such an "easy" baby. From her discussions with the mother, the nurse ascertained that the first child had demonstrated highly reliable rhythmic patterns of sleeping, eating, and so forth, and was a cuddly, responsive baby who seemed to adapt well to any situation. By contrast, the mother described her second child as crying almost constantly, and responding poorly to her attempts to soothe her. The nurse assessed the temperamental differences between the two children, and related this information to the mother. With further counseling, the mother realized that the difficulties were not a result of her being a poor mother incapable of caring for her second child, but rather were caused by the temperamental characteristics of that infant.

Child's Influence on Initial Maternal Attachment

The nurse should begin to assess the maternal-infant bonding pattern in the delivery room immediately following birth. Maternal attachment reactions are discussed in Chapter 1. The initial reactions of the infant are important in helping the mother form an attachment. If the infant is alert and active, his mother can begin to explore him and look into his eyes. If he is lethargic and unresponsive, the mother will not be able to interact with him, and she may begin to feel a sense of failure.

One rationale for restriction of the use of analgesics during labor is the effect such use has on the initial maternal-infant attachment. The use of analgesics during labor has been shown to produce a poor suck in infants for several days postdelivery.[15] Most mothers place great importance on their abilities to feed their infants, and they may feel guilty and inadequate if their infant demonstrates a poor suck and thereby a decreased ability to eat.

For example, a primiparous mother who had not received training in childbirth before labor was given large amounts of analgesics during labor. Following delivery, the infant was drowsy and unresponsive for several days. The mother complained that her baby did not like to eat. The nurses tried to help the mother wake her baby and encourage him to suck. The mother became very discouraged. At the first clinic visit, the infant had not gained weight appropriately and the mother expressed feelings that her infant did not like her and therefore would not eat. The clinic staff spent a great deal of time and effort helping the mother to overcome her rejecting behaviors and to point out the infant's positive behaviors to increase her interest in him. The nurse performed a Brazelton Assessment on the infant, and demonstrated to the mother how responsive the baby was, and the mother began to notice her infant's positive reactions, which increased her interest.

Child's Influence on Initial Paternal Bonding Patterns

Increased paternal involvement in prenatal and postnatal classes and the labor and delivery process has led to greater potential for paternal bonding in the initial stages. Naturally, the nurse should facilitate the father's bonding interactions with his newborn by encouraging him to hold the infant, cuddle him, and begin to use the en face position. The nurse may also point out the infant's responsive behaviors to his father. The infant's care-eliciting behaviors affect both parents. If the infant does not respond to the father's caregiving tasks, or if the father is unaware of the infant's positive responses, the father will begin to experience feelings of inadequacy and failure.

For example, an enthusiastic father who had attended prenatal classes helped his wife through labor and delivery. Initial disruptions in parental bonding occurred when the infant required resuscitation following delivery, and was later diagnosed as having severe aspiration pneumonia and placed in the Neonatal Intensive Care Unit (NICU). The parents visited their infant in the NICU, but expressed concerns over his condition and responded to the physical barriers required by his treatment, which prevented them from holding him. When the infant was discharged from the NICU, the father was still demonstrating difficulties in relating to his child. A visiting nurse was assigned to help the father establish his relationship with his child. The visiting nurse used information from a Carey-McDevitt Questionnaire to help the father notice his infant's temperament, and the Brazelton to demonstrate the infant's abilities. Recognizing the infant's positive behaviors, the father began to respond positively to his infant by holding and talking to him more.

Disruptions in Child-Parent Attachment

High-risk parents and their children are particularly susceptible to problems in their reciprocal behaviors. There are several categories of high-risk infants whose physical problems produce behavioral aberrations, in either the parents or child soon after birth or through the childhood period. The nurse must assess the high-risk infant or child's behaviors to determine their influence on the parent-child relationship.

Congenital Anomalies. There is a vast array of types and severities of congenital anomalies. Many of the physical problems associated with various anomalies produce emotional difficulties for the child and his parents. The parents' reactions to their child may be influenced by such variables as the type of defect, its severity, whether or not it is correctable, and whether or not it is visible. In response to these variables, the parents may exhibit symptoms of grief and mourning, extreme guilt, and depression over having produced such a child, as is discussed in later chapters. Obviously, when the parents approach their child with these feelings, they will affect his development.

Mental Disabilities. Children with various mental disabilities frequently demonstrate emotional problems which affect the parent-child relationship. The manner in which parents approach their child may be very important. For example, if they do not give him opportunities to learn a new skill because they assume he is incapable, they may frustrate him, as well as further retard his development. The child may respond by acting out his frustration with hostility, and the reciprocal relationship may develop problems. The nurse may be the first to assess these disruptions in parent-child interactions, and then she can take appropriate actions, such as referral to a psychologist.

Low Birth-Weight Infants. Premature or small-for-date infants may have weak or underdeveloped behavior patterns which affect the parent-child relationship. This lack of organized behavior and responsiveness may be one cause of the increased incidence of the Battered Child Syndrome among those who are of low birth weight.[12] The nurse who is involved in follow-up care for low birth-weight infants should pay careful attention in her assessments of his status to make certain he is not a victim of battering. For example, the nurse should pay special attention to bruises or other physical signs, as well as behavioral symptoms such as the infant drawing away from his mother, which might indicate poor attachment or signal possible child abuse.

Sick Newborns. The sick newborn's behavior may influence the parental attachment process. The physical separation from his parents and the fact that they cannot hold him or establish eye contact may cause initial disruptions. It is very important that parents be allowed free access to visiting their infant in the NICU to help minimize the negative aspects of physical separation. The nurse should point out what the infant does and discuss with his parents that he will probably demonstrate increased responsiveness as he overcomes his physical illness. As the infant does develop more interactive responses, the parents should be encouraged to stimulate him further and to develop bonding patterns.

NURSING APPROACHES

High-risk children demonstrate many abilities as well as specific problems which may be discovered through the use of various assessment tools. Some tools are designed to assess physical parameters and some are focused to delineate behavioral problems at various developmental levels. This section describes the nurse's role in performing assessments for high-risk children during their developmental stages.

Assessment at Various Developmental Levels

Newborn. Immediately following birth, numerous assessments must be made. There are obvious physical care requirements, such as providing the infant with a patent airway and a neutral thermal environment. Initial assessments of his condition would include the assignment of an Apgar score and performance of a physical examination to ascertain the presence of congenital anomalies or other physical problems. In a high-risk delivery, such as a cesarean section, multiple birth, or birth of a premature, even more careful attention to these assessments are necessary, since the infant may have been physically compromised.

In the immediate newborn period, the nurse will also begin to assess the infant's response to his new environment. She should assess his alertness, his response to noise and light, and his ability to suck if the mother wishes to nurse him in the delivery room. Some of the items from the Brazelton Neonatal Scale might be adapted for use in these assessments of newborn behavior. Naturally, during this period of initial assessment and acquaintance between parents and infants, the nurse should tend to the infant's physical requirement of warmth and determine that he is not otherwise physically endangered.

Neonatal to Toddler. The necessity for physical examinations including assessment of neurologic functions continues at this developmental level, because physical problems may lead to abnormalities in infant or toddler behavior. For example, if an infant demonstrates disabilities caused by neurologic damage, the parents may believe his inadequacies are due to an error in their parenting skills. If an infant does not sit or walk at the appropriate ages, the parents may believe they did not stimulate him enough, when his developmental lags are actually due to neurologic deficits. With specific assessment information, the nurse can help to reassure parents that they are not the cause of these developmental delays, as well as help them deal with the psychological impact these problems will have on them.

Besides the physical assessments for this age, the nurse can begin to test for an infant's temperamental characteristics at approximately four months of age. Normal infants and toddlers demonstrate variations in temperament. It is useful for parents to understand their child's temperamental individuality as soon as possible. Sometimes an infant's peculiarities of temperament may lead to a breakdown in parenting abilities.

There are some instances in which the nurse may be the first to detect a problem for a high-risk infant, such as failure to thrive, as she performs routine physical assessments during the course of a medical visit. There are some comprehensive tools such as the Denver Developmental Screening Test, some tools designed to primarily test intellectual skills, and some designed to detect behavioral problems. The nurse in a high-risk setting may use any or all of these tools in her practice.

Preschool. Comprehensive testing at this developmental stage provides a baseline for further assessment as the child gets older. Not only do physical evaluations continue, but also more definitive tests for intellectual-cognitive and motor skills can be administered. Since the normal child begins to develop social skills, such as an ability to relate to others, behavioral screening gains new significance.

Maladaptive behavior usually becomes apparent at this point, and this behavior often causes parents to seek professional help. Identification of parenting difficulties or child developmental lags at this time allows time for early interventions. Specific diagnostic tests are performed on the suspect child to further evaluate his problem and clearly define his problem. In the course of her performance of assessment tests, the nurse may discover a possible problem such as mental developmental lags. She should carefully reassess her findings, and then refer the child to a child-development clinic or other specialized center for more complete testing and evaluation.

School-age Child. Physical, behavioral, or intellectual problems may first become apparent when the child attends school and is observed along with other children. He may prove to have scholastic problems caused by underlying emotional distress.

For example, a nurse performing assessments for the school-age child might discover a child who is hyperactive. The parents might describe behavior which leads the nurse to suspect the child is hyperactive. At this point, the nurse could perform some preliminary assessments of the child's distractibility, his concentration time, and so forth, and if she determines he may be hyperactive, she should refer him for further evaluation and intervention.

Prevention and Teaching

Nursing assessment is the first step in prevention and teaching. Historically, high-risk patients who are followed in medical centers have benefited from numerous assessments. For example, a premature might be followed in a neonatal follow-up clinic associated with the NICU in which he was hospitalized. In addition to the assessments of his physical development, he would probably receive testing for behavioral and mental development as well. If the infant developed another problem, there are many other resources open to him, such as cardiac clinic, eye clinic, or hearing clinic, where he would receive further evaluation and care.

Currently, many middle-class parents are seeking screening before their essentially normal child enters preschool or school. For example, par-

ents of a normal child may wish to have additional physical examinations performed, such as tests for visual acuity and hearing abilities, which are not routinely done by their private physician. In addition, if the parents are concerned about some behavioral manifestation of their child, they may wish to have assessments of his behavior performed as well. The increased demand for screening seems to be related to the fact that parents are reading more books on child-rearing and therefore becoming more aware of potential problems. These parents seem to seek this type of behavioral testing from psychologists in private practice.

Testing

Nursing assessment requires careful administration of planned testing tools. The selection of a site for performing the assessments, the timing of the test, and the decisions regarding referral for further assessments are among the factors a nurse must consider in performing this role.

Home Testing. The nurse may choose to perform certain testing procedures in the home, which provides a more relaxed atmosphere, and allows her to observe the family in their own environment. The nurse has a valuable role in home testing since the visiting nurse is already accepted in the home. Use of the home site also helps the parent to concentrate on well-child care rather than sick-child care and may help the parent to perceive his child as not being at such high risk. In a high-risk clinic, all of the other children who are there for evaluation are also at high risk, and it is difficult for parents to separate their own child from the others. Also, within their own home, the parents can focus on their child and the abilities he has to perform normally in that environment, and, therefore, the nurse can point out his positive aspects more readily. In a clinical setting, which is unnatural, the child may react to the different setting resulting in unusual performances for him. Baseline assessments for behavior modification plans must be done in the usual environment to be accurate.

Medical Center Testing. Most assessments of high-risk children are performed within the medical center environment. This is certainly the most efficient place in terms of personnel time and energy. Specially trained professionals are available for more complex testing procedures. Within this setting, a pattern of testing at certain intervals is usually established.

The nurse may initially administer a test to a child in the newborn period and then use that information as a baseline to reassess his development from time to time. This technique not only gives a more accurate picture of the child's development, but also helps the nurse to assess whether or not a child is improving in an area of previous difficulty. In any case, a test should be administered more than once to ascertain the child's best performance.

Another use of assessments in the medical center setting is to provide an evaluation of a child's problem prior to any intervention, and then to periodically assess improvements after the implementation of specific health intervention. High-risk infants and children usually are recipients of one type of treatment or another, and it is helpful to assess the benefits of treatment.

Flexibility in Testing. The value of an assessment tool is only as great as the skill of the examiner who administers it. If the examiner is either unfamiliar with the test or unable to relate well to children, the validity of the test may be compromised. Therefore, a nurse who plans to administer assessment tools must be thoroughly trained in both the test items and the methods of administering it.

The examiner must give all instructions to the child in a clear and concise style which the child can readily understand. The examiner should be familiar enough with the test that he can change the pace or order of testing, depending on the child's reactions. The examiner needs to be alert to nuances of the child's response to various questions in the test, including his nonverbal communication.

Rapport with the child is very important. Many children are very sensitive to the way they are approached, and therefore it is important for the nurse to have skills as an adult relating to children. The nurse who wishes to administer a test to a child should spend some time talking with him about his interests and trying to acquaint herself with him as well as giving him the opportunity to feel comfortable with her before she begins the test. The primary nurse who has established trust by caring for the child over several days may be the best person to administer a general behavioral assessment.

Timing of Testing. The child's temperament and physical condition on the day of the test may affect his performance. The nurse should attempt to administer the test when the child is not tired, perhaps before the physical examination if the behavioral test is being performed during a routine clinic visit. If the nurse determines that the child is not physically well, or is overly tired or seems uncooperative, she should postpone the behavioral testing until another opportunity. The child deserves the chance to perform as well as possible, and therefore should not be forced to be tested under adverse conditions. If the child is not performing well, it may be because he cannot or will not do that which is required. The nurse may wish to utilize the parent to elicit a response, as frequently happens with the Denver Developmental Screening Test. Furthermore, there may be aspects of a child's temperament which cause him to react negatively to a testing situation. For example, if a child is easily distractible, the nurse may wish to administer portions of the test at different times in different settings.

Referral for Further Assessment. If a nurse detects a problem through the use of a screening device, she may wish first to retest the child and then, if her findings remain the same, she should refer the child to a setting where further testing can be done. Such a setting might be a child development clinic or the office of a child psychologist in private practice, where further tests can more carefully delineate the problem and treatment can be offered if necessary. For example, if the nurse discovers a child has unusual responsive behaviors indicative of severe emotional problem, which she realizes are beyond her intervention capabilities, she should refer that child to a psychologist or psychiatrist for further help. Another example would be referring a child found to be below his age level in verbal communication for hearing testing, while assessing the amount and type of verbal stimulation the parents provide. For legal reasons, a nurse must not make specific medical diagnoses which could be considered within the realm of medical practice rather than of nursing practice. She does make behavioral-nursing diagnoses as a basis for her nursing care.

Involving the Parents

Some tests utilize parents to complete questionnaires. Although there are advantages to this technique, such as that the parents observe their child more than a nurse could in the clinical setting, there are possible problems with this format. Aberrant behavior may be missed because it is not reported by the parents. Studies have shown that some parents tend to report their child as performing better than he actually does.[16] On the other hand, other parents may tend to be overly critical of their child. For these reasons, the child's behavioral profile should include direct professional observations as well as the completion of parental questionnaires.

Assessment can be very reassuring or distressing to parents, depending on the manner in which the nurse interprets the results. The nurse should report any negative findings, but should also point out the positive aspects of the child's development and stimulate the parent to help the child capitalize on his strengths. When doing her evaluation of results, the nurse should try not to alarm parents if there is a developmental lag in some area.

For example, a nurse was administering a Denver Developmental Screening Test to a 12 month old. The child did not play "peek-a-boo" and demonstrated some other questionable developmental delays. The nurse did not wish to alarm the mother, and asked her if her infant had ever played the game at another time. The mother replied that although he had been exposed to the game, he seldom played. The nurse asked the mother to observe and record his behavior at home before the next testing session. The nurse also sought to reassure the mother by stating that all

children develop at different rates. At the follow-up examination, the mother replied that the infant did not respond to her efforts to play peek-a-boo, and the nurse detected several other areas in which the child did not perform well, she therefore referred him to a child development clinic for further testing and evaluation.

Developing Research Tools

When an assessment tool is originally designed and tested, there is usually a population which serves as the test group to standardize the tool. For example, the Denver Developmental Screening Test initially used a group of children in the Denver, Colorado, area as the control.

Some tools are most useful in a clinical setting, while others are more appropriate for research. Tools used in a research setting are more carefully controlled. When a tool is used for research, the examiner must be meticulously trained and retested at periodic intervals to ascertain that his test results are still reliable. The Brazelton Scale, for example, has centers for training and reliability testing. Before a person can publish research using the Brazelton, he must pass reliability testing requirements and be certified. These same tools are used for clinical applications with less stringent application of reliability standards. However, the nurse must be properly trained to perform the tests if she is to trust her own findings and have other members of the health team rely on her conclusions.

CHILDREN'S BEHAVIORAL ASSESSMENT TOOLS

There are literally hundreds of tests which measure a variety of parameters in children. Figure 3-1 compares some general, social, behavioral, intelligence, and other types of tests which would be most useful for assessing high-risk children, indicates the populations they would test, and lists other requirements for use of the tools. The four most useful scales for nurses in dealing with high-risk families are reviewed in this section. They

Table 3-1. Some Children's Assessment Tools

Scale	Type	Child's Age	Focus	Materials Needed	Remarks
Denver Developmental Screening Test[9,10]	Comprehensive	Birth to 6 years	Personal-social, fine motor, adaptive, language and gross motor	Booklet, kit includes rattle, ball, etc.	Reviewed in this chapter
Developmental Screening Inventory (DSI)[13]	Comprehensive	4 weeks to 18 months	Gross and fine motor, language, personal-social	Test objects such as 4" hoop, child's picture book, etc. May substitute available materials	Based on work of Gesell; requires little training for nurses; based on history from parents + observation
Brazelton Neonatal Assessment Scale[3]	Comprehensive	Newborn	Physical and emotional	Booklet, rattle, safety pins, etc.	Reviewed in this chapter
Carey-McDevitt Infant Temperament Questionnaire	Behavioral	4 to 8 months	Temperament	Questionnaire, scoring and profile sheets	Reviewed in this chapter
Draw-A-Person[14]	Behavioral	Preschool and above	Emotional and developmental (mental abilities)	Drawing materials	Requires much training; nurse needs to be careful not to read in more than is there
Nurses Scale for Rating Neonates (Haar)[11]	Behavioral	Neonates	Behavior and personality characteristics of prematures	Scale consisting of 16 items	Designed for long-term observations
Bayley Scale of Infant Development[2]	Intelligence Motor Behavior record	Birth to 30 months	Intelligence, motor, some behavior	Manual and scale of 160+ items	Very complex
Gessell Developmental Scale (Revised)[10]	Intelligence	Birth to 5 years	Motor, mental, some behavior	Manual and kit items	
Infant Intelligence Scale (Cattell)[6]	Intelligence	2 months to 4 years	Motor, development	Formboard, pellets, ring, etc. and manual	Complex, generally superceded by Bayley
Apgar Scoring[1]	Physical	Birth	Cardiopulmonary function	Scale	In common usage
Gestational Age[1]	Physical	Birth to 3 days	Assessment of gestational level	Chart	In common usage
Vineland Social Maturity Scale[8]	Social/Emotional	Birth to adolescent	Assessment of social development	Manual and scale	Reviewed in this chapter
Rating-Ranking Scale for Child Behavior[7]	Social/Emotional	Preschool to adolescent	Emotionally disturbed	Scale	Developed for use by nurses, ward personnel and teachers
Maxfield Bucholz Scale Social Maturity[10]	Specific problem	Birth to 6 years	For use with blind children	Scale	Adaptation of Vineland
Picture Vocabulary for Deaf Children[18]	Specific problem	3 to 7 years	Language development of deaf children	Scale, 8 mm motion picture, cards, in kit	Part of battery developed by Galldaudet Col.

focus on the behavior of children, and although they all require some training time and effort, their worth justifies the effort required. All of these tests are useful in dealing with high-risk populations to screen for possible problems, more carefully define problems which are suspected, and determine the child's abilities.

Selecting the Assessment Tool

When considering which test to use, many factors must be taken into account, such as whether behavior or intelligence testing is required, the age of the child, and cultural limitations. Some tests require a great amount of training to develop proficiency, and probably should be performed by psychologists. With training, nurses can administer tests, but should be retested themselves at intervals to determine their proficiency in administering the test and interpreting the results to maintain reliability.

Other factors to consider in choosing which test to use are the cost of the tool and the amount of time it takes the nurse to administer the test. The cost of the test in terms of time spent by the tester to administer it may be prohibitive. Also, if a test takes more than approximately 40 minutes to administer, the child may become fatigued or bored, and may not respond as well near the end of the test.

Denver Developmental Screening Test

The Denver Developmental Screening Test (DDST) is a general scale which measures the personal and social aspects of a child's development, his language, and his gross and fine motor abilities.[9] This test is not designed to function as a diagnostic tool, but to identify potential problems which should receive further diagnostic evaluation. The DDST is designed to detect developmental delays during infancy and preschool years.

Nursing Application. The DDST was originally designed and standardized with a population of 1,000 children in the Denver, Colorado, area. Since its development, there have been numerous studies performed to assess the reliability and validity of the scale.

Most of those studies have recognized the usefulness of the DDST, although problems have been encountered when the test was used with children of lower socioeconomic status. Although a child from a minority ethnic group of a lower socioeconomic status may fail certain aspects of the DDST, and therefore be considered abnormal, he may actually be performing as well as can be expected of a child in his circumstances. For example, a child who cannot label a horse by looking at the picture may not be slow in all language development but rather may never have had the opportunity to see a horse. Therefore, when a nurse administers and interprets the results of the DDST, she must consider the social history of the child including the possibility of a broken home, adverse economic circumstances, and the child's prior educational experiences.[20] Efforts are being made to make the DDST more applicable to lower-income children and a Spanish tool is now available.

There are several positive aspects of the DDST regarding its use by nurses. It is a simple test for the nurse to administer, and requires approximately ten to 25 minutes. The nurse herself can be trained to administer the test in between a few hours and a few days, depending on her abilities and the availability of children in the proper age ranges to serve as practice subjects. There are self-instructional manuals, workbooks, and films available, which also contain a practice test and an evaluation of proficiency. In addition, the nurse should be periodically rechecked herself, to make certain she maintains proficiency and accuracy in evaluating her results.

The DDST is not designed to assign an IQ score or to label a child as being retarded or having cerebral palsy, but rather to provide a profile of developmental lags, as well as the areas in which a child performs above the norms. As any nurse who deals with high-risk populations knows, there are several problems associated with labeling children with specific disorders. Some problems arise when parents develop expectations for their child to behave in a certain way because he has been labeled as having a specific disorder. Therefore, one of the true benefits of the DDST is its avoidance of labeling.

Administration of the DDST. The manual which accompanies the DDST gives clear instructions for the administration of this test. The child is given a number of trials for each item on which he is to be tested. Figure 3-1a contains a copy of the DDST scoring sheet, which should help the nurse to organize her observations, and Figure 3-1b displays some basic directions. The manual also gives directions on scoring the items included in the DDST.

Training films, test kits, and other materials necessary for administration of the DDST can be obtained by writing: LADOCA, Project and Publishing Foundation, Inc, E. 51st Street and Lincoln Street, Denver, Colorado, 80216.

Usefulness with High-Risk Children. The DDST is very useful with high-risk populations. One of the values of the DDST is that it assesses several developmental parameters. The nurse should never give her general impression of a child without substantiating evidence. The DDST is designed to give her this evidence. The DDST also helps the nurse to interact with the parents about their child and to provide teaching opportunities to improve parenting skills.

For example, an 18-year-old father and 17-year-old mother of a nine-month-old male infant came to the well-baby clinic for the child's routine visit. They had failed to keep several clinic appointments, and a visiting nurse had been involved in the case to help them bring the baby to clinic. The clinic nurse was the first to see the infant in the clinic. The infant appeared thin, with poor weight gain, and behaviorally he seemed lethargic and disinterested in his surroundings. The nurse performed a DDST on the child and discovered that he did not play peek-a-boo, did not smile responsively, did not show any interest in toys, and generally gave the impression of being withdrawn. The nurse questioned the parents about whether the infant was usually more active than on this visit. The parents replied that he did not usually respond to many things—that he preferred to lie in his bed by himself. The nurse communicated her findings to the physician who was performing the physical examination. Both discussed the child and decided that the infant appeared to be socially deprived. They admitted the infant for further evaluation and tests.

Neonatal Behavioral Assessment Scale

Although it was previously assumed that infants are unable to react to their environment until they are several months of age, Dr. T. Berry Brazelton, M.D., developed a testing system to observe the interactive behavior of infants with their environment and parents.[3] Use of the Brazelton Scale demonstrates how the infant truly interacts with his environment and does not merely respond passively. The infant can not only see and hear as a newborn, but he can also shut out noxious stimuli. This scale helps the nurse observe subtle responses of the infant and the manner in which he causes his caretakers to respond to him. For example, if the infant can quiet himself by placing his hand in his mouth, the mother may notice that she does not always have to pick him up in order to quiet him.

One of the values of the scale is as a teaching tool for parents. For example, a mother may believe that her infant cries because he does not like her. By using the Brazelton Scale as a teaching device, the mother can be shown that her infant's crying behavior is part of his unique personality. Learning that her infant is difficult for others to console and has few self-quieting abilities may help the mother to develop a better concept of her mothering skills.

Nursing Application. The Brazelton Behavioral Assessment Scale is most beneficial as a scoring system for interactive behavior. Although it is not a formal neurologic examination, it does include some basic neurologic components. However, the major focus of this scale is behavioral, not neurologic. The Brazelton is more sensitive in predicting future development than the traditional neurologic evaluation tools. There seem to be fewer infants labeled as suspect who subsequently develop into normal infants with the use of the Brazelton than with some other tests.

There are, however, some difficulties with the

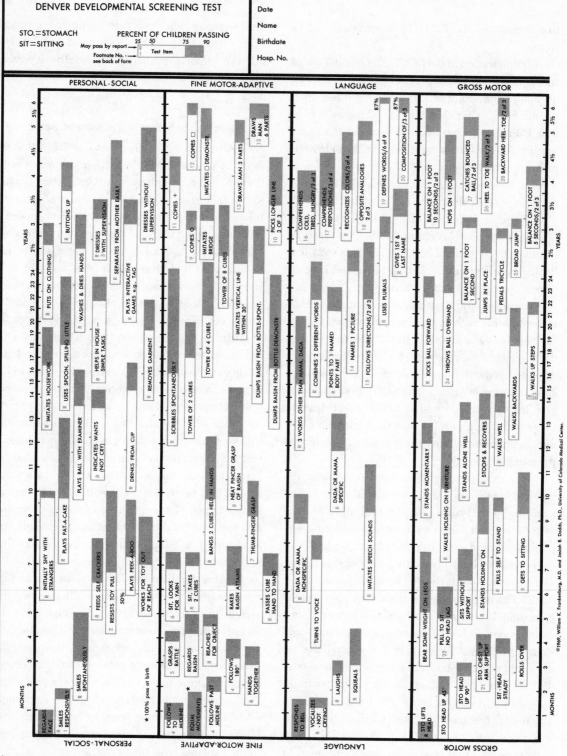

Figure 3-1a. Denver Developmental Screening Test Chart. Reproduced with permission of W. K. Frankenburg, M.D., University of Colorado Medical Center.

1. Try to get child to smile by smiling, talking or waving to him. Do not touch him.
2. When child is playing with toy, pull it away from him. Pass if he resists.
3. Child does not have to be able to tie shoes or button in the back.
4. Move yarn slowly in an arc from one side to the other, about 6" above child's face.
    Pass if eyes follow 90° to midline. (Past midline; 180°)
5. Pass if child grasps rattle when it is touched to the backs or tips of fingers.
6. Pass if child continues to look where yarn disappeared or tries to see where it went. Yarn
    should be dropped quickly from sight from tester's hand without arm movement.
7. Pass if child picks up raisin with any part of thumb and a finger.
8. Pass if child picks up raisin with the ends of thumb and index finger using an over hand
    approach.

 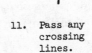 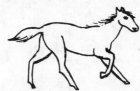 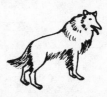 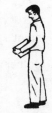

9. Pass any en-   10. Which line is longer?   11. Pass any   12. Have child copy
    closed form.   (Not bigger.) Turn   crossing   first. If failed,
    Fail continuous   paper upside down and   lines.   demonstrate
    round motions.   repeat. (3/3 or 5/6)

When giving items 9, 11 and 12, do not name the forms. Do not demonstrate 9 and 11.

13. When scoring, each pair (2 arms, 2 legs, etc.) counts as one part.
14. Point to picture and have child name it. (No credit is given for sounds only.)

15. Tell child to: Give block to Mommie; put block on table; put block on floor. Pass 2 of 3.
     (Do not help child by pointing, moving head or eyes.)
16. Ask child: What do you do when you are cold? ..hungry? ..tired? Pass 2 of 3.
17. Tell child to: Put block on table; under table; in front of chair, behind chair.
     Pass 3 of 4. (Do not help child by pointing, moving head or eyes.)
18. Ask child: If fire is hot, ice is ?; Mother is a woman, Dad is a ?; a horse is big, a
     mouse is ?. Pass 2 of 3.
19. Ask child: What is a ball? ..lake? ..desk? ..house? ..banana? ..curtain? ..ceiling?
     ..hedge? ..pavement? Pass if defined in terms of use, shape, what it is made of or general
     category (such as banana is fruit, not just yellow). Pass 6 of 9.
20. Ask child: What is a spoon made of? ..a shoe made of? ..a door made of? (No other objects
     may be substituted.) Pass 3 of 3.
21. When placed on stomach, child lifts chest off table with support of forearms and/or hands.
22. When child is on back, grasp his hands and pull him to sitting. Pass if head does not hang back.
23. Child may use wall or rail only, not person. May not crawl.
24. Child must throw ball overhand 3 feet to within arm's reach of tester.
25. Child must perform standing broad jump over width of test sheet. (8-1/2 inches)
26. Tell child to walk forward, heel within 1 inch of toe.
     Tester may demonstrate. Child must walk 4 consecutive steps, 2 out of 3 trials.
27. Bounce ball to child who should stand 3 feet away from tester. Child must catch ball with
     hands, not arms, 2 out of 3 trials.
28. Tell child to walk backward, 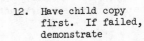 toe within 1 inch of heel.
     Tester may demonstrate. Child must walk 4 consecutive steps, 2 out of 3 trials.

DATE AND BEHAVIORAL OBSERVATIONS (how child feels at time of test, relation to tester, attention
span, verbal behavior, self-confidence, etc,):

Figure 3-1b. Denver Developmental Instruction Sheet. Reproduced with permission of W. K. Frankenburg, M.D.,
University of Colorado Medical Center.

scale. The examination takes about 30 minutes to complete and may be physically taxing to the examiner, and the infant may become tired and irritable before completion of the test. Repeated administrations of the test are necessary to provide the examiner with opportunities to observe the infant's optimal performance. For example, the nurse should probably administer the test once a day for two or three days, depending on how the infant responds. The scale is difficult for a potential examiner to learn, and the initial learning process may take some time. However, despite these negative aspects, the benefit which this tool can provide

to infant care and to improving parenting skills makes the effort spent worthwhile.

One of the criticisms of this scale is that the norms on which it is based do not comprise a broad spectrum of infants—that is, the sample population is too homogeneous. However, there have been numerous revisions to attempt to broaden the base and make the tool useful in virtually all situations and populations. There is an increased usage of this tool in testing preterm and other high-risk infants.

Administration of the Scale. One of the most important considerations in the administration of the Brazelton is the state of conciousness exhibited

Figure 3-2a. Brazelton Neonatal Behavioral Assessment Scale

Behavioral and Neurological Assessment Scale

Infant's Name _____ Sex _____ Age _____ Born _____
                                                                              Date   Hour

Mother's Age _____ Father's Age _____ Father's S.E.S. _____

                                                         Apparent Race _____

Examiner(s) _____ Place of Examination _____

Conditions of Examination: Date of Examination _____

  Birth weight _____ Current weight _____ Length _____ Head circ. _____

  Time examined _____ Time last fed _____ Type of feeding _____

  Type of delivery _____ Apgar _____

  Length of labor _____ Birth order _____

  Type, amount and timing of medication given mother _____

  _____

  Anesthesia? _____

  Abnormalities of labour _____

_____

Initial State (observe 2 minutes)

         1   2   3   4   5   6
       deep   light   drowsy   alert   active crying

Predominant States (mark two)

         1   2   3   4   5   6

Elicited Responses

	O*	L	M	H	A†
Plantar grasp		1	2	3	
Hand grasp		1	2	3	
Ankle clonus		1	2	3	
Babinski		1	2	3	
Standing		1	2	3	
Automatic walking		1	2	3	
Placing		1	2	3	
Incurvation		1	2	3	
Crawling		1	2	3	
Glabella		1	2	3	
Tonic deviation of head and eyes		1	2	3	
Nystagmus		1	2	3	
Tonic neck reflex		1	2	3	
Moro		1	2	3	
Rooting (intensity)		1	2	3	
Sucking (intensity)		1	2	3	
Passive movement					
Arms R		1	2	3	
L		1	2	3	
Legs R		1	2	3	
L		1	2	3	

* O = response not elicited (omitted)
† A = asymmetry

Descriptive Paragraph
(optional)

Attractive	0	1	2	3
Interfering variables	0	1	2	3
Need for stimulation	0	1	2	3

What activity does he use to quiet self?
    hand to mouth
    sucking with nothing in mouth
    locking onto visual or auditory stimuli
    postural changes
    state change for no observable reason
Comments:

---

by the infant at the time the test is given. There are six basic states: 1) deep sleep, 2) light sleep, 3) drowsy or semi-dozing, 4) alert, 5) general high activity level, and 6) intense crying. The nurse administers the test, when the infant is asleep, dressed and covered, and approximately halfway between feedings in a semi-darkened quiet room in which she will not be disturbed. Films and special training for administering the test are available and recommended for reliability.

The Brazelton assesses 27 different behavioral responses which are grouped into the following six categories:[3]

1. Habituation—These items are designed to detect how soon an infant diminishes his response to stimulation caused by light, pinprick to his heel, and sounds.
2. Orientation—The infant is given opportunities to respond to auditory and visual stimuli, and the examiner checks to see if he turns toward stimuli or gives other signs of responding to animate or inanimate stimuli.
3. Motor maturity—These items assess the infant's motor coordination and motor control.
4. Variation—Some of the scale items check the rate and quantity of an infant's changes in reaction during various periods of alertness. His color, activity, and peaks of excitement are noted, as well as his skin responses.
5. Self-quieting ability—These items determine an infant's ability to calm and quiet himself when he gets upset.
6. Social behavior—The infant's ability to smile and cuddle.

The manual for the Brazelton gives careful descriptions of the order of performance of the test maneuvers and the manner in which they may be varied if the infant is not in the proper state of consciousness for the particular test item. There is a score sheet which aids in organizing the test findings for interpretation. See Figures 3-2a and 3-2b for the scoring sheet from the Brazelton.

Figure 3-2b. Brazelton Neonatal Behavior Scoring Sheet

Behavior Scoring Sheet

Initial State . . . .

Predominant State . . . .

Scale (Note State)	1	2	3	4	5	6	7	8	9

1. Response decrement to light (2, 3)

2. Response decrement to rattle (2, 3)

3. Response decrement to bell (2, 3)

4. Response decrement to pinprick (1, 2, 3)

5. Orientation inanimate visual (4 only)

6. Orientation inanimate auditory (4, 5)

7. Orientation animate visual (4 only)

8. Orientation animate auditory (4, 5)

9. Orientation animate visual & auditory (4 only)

10. Alertness (4 only)

11. General tonus (4, 5)

12. Motor maturity (4, 5)

13. Pull-to-sit (3, 5)

14. Cuddliness (4, 5)

15. Defensive movements (4)

16. Consolability (6 to 5, 4, 3, 2)

17. Peak of excitement (6)

18. Rapidity of buildup (from 1, 2 to 6)

19. Irritability (3, 4, 5)

20. Activity (alert states)

21. Tremulousness (all states)

22. Startle (3, 4, 5, 6)

23. Lability of skin color (from 1 to 6)

24. Lability of states (all states)

25. Self-quieting activity (6, 5 to 4, 3, 2, 1)

26. Hand-mouth facility (all states)

27. Smiles (all states)

Figure 3-2a and 3-2b reproduced with permission from Brazelton, T. B., *Neonatal Behavioural Assessment Scale.* London: S.I.M.P./Heinemann Medical Books; Philadelphia: J. B. Lippincott Co., 1973, pp. 63–64.

The Brazelton *Neonatal Behavioral Assessment Scale* can be obtained from London: S.I.M.P./ Heinemann Medical Books; Philadelphia: J. B. Lippincott Co.

Usefulness with High-Risk Children. One of the benefits of the Brazelton is its use as an educational tool to alert parents to their infant's capabilities. The parents can be trained to observe some of the behavior that they might previously have missed. This increases the parents' awareness of their infant, a beneficial side effect of this tool. The parents also gain positive reinforcement for their efforts to stimulate their infant and are encouraged to continue this behavior. Obviously, high-risk parents need these types of experiences to improve their parenting skills, and their infants benefit from the increased stimulation as well.

There are several at-risk factors which have been discovered through research utilizing the Brazelton Scale to test the infants. Small-for-dates babies frequently exhibit developmental deficits when measured with the Brazelton Scale. Studies have also concluded that infants of mothers who had received meperidine during delivery scored lower on both elicited and emitted responses than did infants whose mothers had not received meperidine.[17] In deliveries where the mother had received anesthesia, infants showed more irritability and less motor maturity than infants whose mothers had not received anesthesia. The Brazelton Scale has also been used to follow infants whose mothers were drug addicts, infants of diabetic mothers, and many other high-risk maternal patients. The Brazelton has provided much needed and worthwhile information when used for high-risk infants.

For example, a nurse performed a Brazelton on a two-day-old male infant whose mother had received large dosages of analgesics and anesthetics during labor and delivery. In the delivery room, the infant was initially depressed, with Apgar scores of 5 and 9. The Apgar score had improved as a result of resuscitative efforts, including suctioning and administration of additional oxygen. The infant subsequently improved and demonstrated no problems in the nursery. The Brazelton showed the infant had poorly organized sleep patterns, a poor suck, and was less alert than he should have been. On day four, before the infant was dismissed, the nurse repeated portions of the Brazelton in the presence of his 23-year-old gravida three para three mother and his 25-year-old father. The parents had expressed concern about the initial resuscitation the infant had required. The nurse demonstrated how the infant oriented to sounds and light, his cuddliness, and his improving alertness. She cited his improvement in the past two days and encouraged the parents to continue to stimulate their infant.

Carey-McDevitt Infant Temperament Questionnaire

Parents often generalize their descriptions of their infant into an all-encompassing statement such as, "He cries all the time." With the use of the Carey-McDevitt Scale the parents can be helped to see that, although he may be fussy at times, he may have other more agreeable characteristics that should be appreciated and encouraged. High-risk parents can be helped to understand the "easy" aspects of their infant's temperament which may offset some of their more difficult characteristics. The Carey-McDevitt Questionnaire is based on the work of Thomas and associates.[21] The original version was published by Carey in 1970, and a revised version developed with McDevitt in 1977.

Nursing Application. The original research technique described in the book by Thomas and associates would take a nurse approximately one to two hours to interview the parents, and up to an hour to dictate and score their responses. The Carey-McDevitt tool can be completed by the mother in 25 minutes and scored by the nurse in ten to 15 minutes. The scale is designed to assess an infant's emotional reactivity or behavioral characteristics during the early months of his life.

One value of the test is that many mothers noted their perceptions about their infants were sharpened just from having completed the questionnaire. These mothers reported that they had not paid much attention to some aspects of their infants' behavior patterns before answering the questionnaire.

One of the criticisms of this scale is that the test population used in the standardization sample was largely middle class, although all levels of society were represented. Therefore the validity of the test for different types of populations needs to be shown. Perhaps this criticism will be answered when current studies using the questionnaire are published.

Administration of the Scale. The Carey-McDevitt Questionnaire is given to mothers whose infants are between four and eight months of age. Before four months some infant patterns have not appeared or stabilized and many items are unanswerable, therefore the tool does not have good predictive value if administered before this time.[4,5]

The scale is comprised of a questionnaire which the mother completes. The questionnaire contains 95 statements, each followed by six frequency options which describe to what extent the statement applies to the infant. The mother chooses the option which most accurately describes her child, and if none are applicable she crosses it out. For example, in response to an item about whether the infant wants his daytime naps at differant times, the mother is given the options of: 1) Almost never, 2) Rarely, 3) Variable, usually does not, 4) Variable, usually does, 5) Frequently, or 6) Almost always. The 95 items are checked off on the scoring sheet into the 9 categories of temperament: activity, rhythmicity, approach, adaptability, intensity, mood, persistence, distractibility, and threshold. There are several general areas of questioning, including sleep, feeding, soiling and wetting, diapering, dressing, bathing, responses to people, and responses to new situations. Figure 3-3a shows some questionnaire items and responses.

Once the mother has completed the basic questionnaire, she is asked to give her general impressions of the infant's temperament, including his activity level, positive and negative moods, and distractibility. See Figure 3-3b for this portion of the questionnaire.

The completion of the scoring process yields one of five diagnostic clusters for the infant: difficult, slow to warm up, intermediate high and low, or easy. Difficult infants are arrhythmical, withdrawing, low in adaptability, intense, and negative. Easy infants are rhythmical, approaching, adaptable, mild, and positive. Slow-to-warm-up infants are inactive, low in approach and adaptability, and negative but mild. The assignment of one of these clusters gives the examiner an overall impression of the difficulty of the infant. In addition, the examiner can help the parents to solve problems on the basis of the various category ratings. Infants with different temperaments develop at different rates; for example, active infants walk earlier. Parents can be apprised of this information and can plan accordingly, but use of diagnostic labels should be avoided.

A sample copy of the Questionnaire, scoring Sheet, and Profile Sheet can be obtained by writing to William Carey, M.D., 319 West Front St., Media, Pa. 19063. Please include a check for $5 to help cover expenses.

Usefulness with High-Risk Children. One of the primary values of this tool is its ability to detect to what extent problems in maternal-infant interaction are contributed to by the infant's temperament. By assessing the temperamental qualities of the infant, the nurse can individualize his care and help parents to understand that some "difficult" behaviors may not be a result of their care techniques. This reassurance to high-risk parents could be of the utmost importance.

The benefit of having the section of the questionnaire where the mother globally rates her infants herself, after she completes the initial 95 items, is that, if the mother's impression of her infant is at great variance with the way she answered the questionnaire, there may be a problem in maternal perception of her infant. The nurse may wish to counsel the mother to enable her to realize this discrepancy.

For example, an exhausted 21-year-old primiparous mother described her five-month-old infant as being a "horrible" baby who cried continuously and did not like her. The nurse decided to give the

Figure 3-3a. Carey-McDevitt Infant Temperament Questionnaire—
A Sample of the Questions

Using the following scale, please circle the number that indicates how often the infant's recent and current behavior has been like that described by each item.

Almost never 1	Rarely 2	Variable, usually does not 3	Variable, usually does 4	Frequently 5	Almost always 6

1. The infant eats about the same amount of solid food (within 1 oz.) from day to day.	almost never	1	2	3	4	5	6	almost always
2. The infant is fussy on waking up and going to sleep (frowns, cries).	almost never	1	2	3	4	5	6	almost always
3. The infant plays with a toy for under a minute and then looks for another toy or activity.	almost never	1	2	3	4	5	6	almost always
4. The infant sits still while watching TV or other nearby activity.	almost never	1	2	3	4	5	6	almost always
5. The infant accepts right away any change in place or position of feeding or person giving it.	almost never	1	2	3	4	5	6	almost always
6. The infant accepts nail cutting without protest.	almost never	1	2	3	4	5	6	almost always
7. The infant's hunger cry can be stopped for over a minute by picking up, pacifier, putting on bib, etc.	almost never	1	2	3	4	5	6	almost always
8. The infant plays continuously for more than 10 min. at a time with a favorite toy.	almost never	1	2	3	4	5	6	almost always
9. The infant accepts his/her bath any time of the day without resisting it.	almost never	1	2	3	4	5	6	almost always
10. The infant takes feedings quietly with mild expression of likes and dislikes.	almost never	1	2	3	4	5	6	almost always
11. The infant indicates discomfort (fusses or squirms) when diaper is soiled with bowel movement.	almost never	1	2	3	4	5	6	almost always
12. The infant lies quietly in the bath.	almost never	1	2	3	4	5	6	almost always
13. The infant wants and takes milk feedings at about the same times (within one hour) from day to day.	almost never	1	2	3	4	5	6	almost always
14. The infant is shy (turns away or clings to mother) on meeting another child for the first time.	almost never	1	2	3	4	5	6	almost always

95. There are a total of 95 Items.

mother a temperament questionnaire. From this test, the nurse determined that the child was rather negative in mood, but that he did show signs of rhythmicity in his activities, was easily distractible, and seemed quite adaptable to new situations. The nurse discussed with the mother, that, while her baby did seem to have some difficult behavior patterns, he did have many more easy aspects to his temperament. The nurse counseled the mother on ways she might help alleviate the periods of crying, such as using distraction to help the infant stop crying.

Figure 3-3b.* Carey-McDevitt Infant Temperament Questionnaire—
Mother's General Impression

Mother's general impressions of infant's temperament

A. How would you describe your baby's temperament in your own words?

B. In comparison with what you know of other babies of the same age, how would you rate your baby as to the following criteria? (Circle one)

I. Activity level—the amount of physical activity during sleep, feeding, play, dressing, etc.

(1) high (2) medium (3) low

II. Regularity—of bodily functioning in sleep, hunger, bowel movements, etc.

(1) fairly regular (2) variable (3) fairly irregular

III. Adaptability to change in routine—the ease or difficulty with which initial response can be modified in socially desirable way.

(1) generally adaptable (2) variable (3) generally slow at adaptation

IV. Response to new situations—initial reaction to new stimuli, to food, people, places, toys, or procedures:

(1) approach (2) variable (3) withdrawal

V. Level of sensory threshold—the amount of external stimulation, such as sounds or changes in food or people, necessary to produce a response in the baby.

(1) high threshold (much stimulation needed) (2) medium
(3) low threshold (little stimulation)

VI. Intensity of response—the energy content of responses regardless of their quality.

(1) generally intense (2) variable (3) generally mild

VII. Positive or negative mood—amount of pleasant or unpleasant behavior throughout day.

(1) generally positive · (2) variable (3) generally negative

VIII. Distractibility—the effectiveness of external stimuli (sounds, toys, people, etc.) in interfering with ongoing behavior.

(1) easily distractible (2) variable (3) non-distractible

XI. Persistence and attention span—duration of maintaining specific activities with or without external obstacles.

(1) persistent (2) variable (3) non-persistent

C. How has the baby's temperament been a problem for you?

D. In general, temperament of baby is:

(a) about average
(b) more difficult than average
(c) easier than average

*Figures 3-3a and 3-3b are reproduced with permission from Infant Temperament Questionnaire (revised 1977) by William B. Carey, M.D., and Sean C. McDevitt, Ph.D.

In addition, Drs. Carey, McDevitt, and associates are also developing an instrument for children from one to three years and have recently developed a Behavioral Style Questionnaire for three- to seven-year-old children. These instruments may also be useful for the nurse working with high-risk families.

Vineland Social Maturity Scale

The Vineland Social Maturity Scale is applicable for infants through adolescence and shows a progression of the child's ability to care for his own needs as well as participate in activities which lead to independence. It provides a scale of normal behavior as well as a measure of individual differences which may signal mental deficits or emotional disturbances. The scale may also be used to measure improvement following treatment or therapy.[8]

This scale does not attempt to measure intelligence or personality directly. Rather, it specifically samples levels of functioning and self-direction in areas of self-help activities (activities of daily living), locomotion, communication, and socialization skills. It also helps to detect situations in which lack of opportunity or other limiting factors cause the child to perform poorly.

Nursing Application. While it is possible to derive numerical "social quotients" from the information gathered, in actual clinical practice it is perhaps more fruitfully used as an interviewing device. When creatively used, the Vineland Social Maturity Scale helps to uncover in a natural, relaxed atmosphere much additional meaningful information about the child. For example, in questioning about the child's level of proficiency in self-feeding skills, it is easy to digress briefly to learn if he is a finicky eater or demonstrates pronounced likes or dislikes which may be troublesome to cater to in a family setting or even reflect underlying physical problems, such as a history or pica leading to lead intoxication.

When using the scale the nurse may interview both parents to assess how they "see" the child differently. This interview may identify conflicts between the parents and foster communication between them on their view of the child's ability and need for encouragement toward independent behavior.

During interviews using this scale, mothers often express concern about some aspect of their child's development which they forget or are reluctant to bring up in a more purely medical contact with their pediatrician. One example of this is that of a mother whose five-year-old son was reliably toilet trained, but insisted on removing all articles of clothing each time he went to the bathroom and then presented the clothing to his mother for assistance in redressing. The problems which this would create in a nursery school or kindergarten setting are obvious, but the mother had never discussed it with her pediatrician.

Administration of the Scale. The nurse administering this test keeps a scoring sheet, and does not give one to the subject (or his parent if she is asking the parent for the information). She begins asking questions about activities well below the anticipated scoring level, and does not ask them in order as they appear on the scoring sheet. It frequently works well to start with one basic area, such as eating, explore it fully, and then go on to another area. The nurse should use a sympathetic tone and manner in asking for information, rather than a stilted, formal approach.

After the seemingly casual, but actually systematic, coverage of the basic areas, the nurse may find it useful to inquire about the child's play interests and activities and to elicit information regarding any fears the child may have, how much temper he displays, and under what precipitating conditions. Finally, the nurse should routinely ask the parents to give their own independent estimate of the age level at which they believe their child is functioning.

The Vineland Social Maturity Scale can be obtained from the American Guidance Service, Inc., Publishers' Building, Circle Pines, Minnesota 55014.

Usefulness with High-Risk Children. There are many types of problems which might be detected

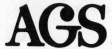

Vineland Social Maturity Scale

BY EDGAR A. DOLL, Ph.D.

NAME.. SEX............ Grade......... Date...............
　　　Last　　　　　　　　　　　　First　　　　　　　　　　　　　　　　　　　Year　　Month　　Day

Residence.. School.............. Born...............
　　　　　　　　　　　　　　　　　　　　　　　　　　　　　　　　　　　　Year　　Month　　Day

M.A............... I.Q......... Test Used................. When........ Age..............
　　　　　　　　　　　　　　　　　　　　　　　　　　　　　　　　　　Years　　Months　　Days

Occupation.. Class........... Years Exp............. Schooling..........

Father's Occupation........................... Class........... Years Exp............. Schooling..........

Mother's Occupation.......................... Class........... Years Exp............. Schooling..........

Informant............................... Relationship............ Recorder..........

Informant's est.. Basal Score*.............

Handicaps... Additional pts...........

REMARKS: .... Total score..............

.... Age equivalent..............

.... Social quotient..............

Age Periods

Category†	Score*	Items	O - I	LA Mean
C	....	1. "Crows"; laughs	....	.25
SHG	....	2. Balances head	....	.25
SHG	....	3. Grasps objects within reach	....	.30
S	....	4. Reaches for familiar persons	....	.30
SHG	....	5. Rolls over	....	.30
SHG	....	6. Reaches for nearby objects	....	.35
O	....	7. Occupies self unattended	....	.43
SHG	....	8. Sits unsupported	....	.45
SHG	....	9. Pulls self upright	....	.55
C	....	10. "Talks"; imitates sounds	....	.55
SHE	....	11. Drinks from cup or glass assisted	....	.55
L	....	12. Moves about on floor	....	.63
SHG	....	13. Grasps with thumb and finger	....	.65
S	....	14. Demands personal attention	....	.70
SHG	....	15. Stands alone	....	.85
SHE	....	16. Does not drool	....	.90
C	....	17. Follows simple instructions	....	.93

† Key to categorical arrangement of items:
S H G — Self-help general　　　　C — Communication　　L — Locomotion
S H D — Self-help dressing　　　　S D — Self-direction　　O — Occupation
S H E — Self-help eating　　　　　S — Socialization
* For method of scoring see "The Measurement of Social Competence."

AMERICAN GUIDANCE SERVICE, INC.
PUBLISHERS' BUILDING, CIRCLE PINES, MINNESOTA 55014

Figure 3-4. Vineland Social Maturity Scale. Reprinted by special permission of American Guidance Service, Inc., Vineland Social Maturity Scale by Edgar A. Doll, Ph.D.

I - II

L	....	18. Walks about room unattended	1.03
O	....	19. Marks with pencil or crayon	1.10
SHE	....	20. Masticates food	1.10
SHD	....	21. Pulls off socks	1.13
O	....	22. Transfers objects	1.20
SHG	....	23. Overcomes simple obstacles	1.30
O	....	24. Fetches or carries familiar objects	1.38
SHE	....	25. Drinks from cup or glass unassisted	1.40
SHG	....	26. Gives up baby carriage	1.43
S	....	27. Plays with other children	1.50
SHE	....	28. Eats with spoon	1.53
L	....	29. Goes about house or yard	1.63
SHE	....	30. Discriminates edible substances	1.65
C	....	31. Uses names of familiar objects	1.70
L	....	32. Walks upstairs unassisted	1.75
SHE	....	33. Unwraps candy	1.85
C	....	34. Talks in short sentences	1.95

II - III

SHG	....	35. Asks to go to toilet	1.98
O	....	36. Initiates own play activities	2.03
SHD	....	37. Removes coat or dress	2.05
SHE	....	38. Eats with fork	2.35
SHE	....	39. Gets drink unassisted	2.43
SHD	....	40. Dries own hands	2.60
SHG	....	41. Avoids simple hazards	2.85
SHD	....	42. Puts on coat or dress unassisted	2.85
O	....	43. Cuts with scissors	2.88
C	....	44. Relates experiences	3.15

III - IV

L	....	45. Walks downstairs one step per tread	3.23
S	....	46. Plays cooperatively at kindergarten level	3.28
SHD	....	47. Buttons coat or dress	3.35
O	....	48. Helps at little household tasks	3.55
S	....	49. "Performs" for others	3.75
SHD	....	50. Washes hands unaided	3.83

IV - V

SHG	....	51. Cares for self at toilet	3.83
SHD	....	52. Washes face unassisted	4.65
L	....	53. Goes about neighborhood unattended	4.70
SHD	....	54. Dresses self except tying	4.80
O	....	55. Uses pencil or crayon for drawing	5.13
S	....	56. Plays competitive exercise games	5.13

73

V - VI

O	57. Uses skates, sled, wagon	5.13
C	58. Prints simple words	5.23
S	59. Plays simple table games	5.63
SD	60. Is trusted with money	5.83
L	61. Goes to school unattended	5.83

VI - VII

SHE	62. Uses table knife for spreading	6.03
C	63. Uses pencil for writing	6.15
SHD	64. Bathes self assisted	6.23
SHD	65. Goes to bed unassisted	6.75

VII - VIII

SHG	66. Tells time to quarter hour	7.28
SHE	67. Uses table knife for cutting	8.05
S	68. Disavows literal Santa Claus	8.28
S	69. Participates in pre-adolescent play	8.28
SHD	70. Combs or brushes hair	8.45

VIII - IX

O	71. Uses tools or utensils	8.50
O	72. Does routine household tasks	8.53
C	73. Reads on own initiative	8.55
SHD	74. Bathes self unaided	8.85

COPY

IX - X

SHE	75. Cares for self at table	9.03
SD	76. Makes minor purchases	9.38
L	77. Goes about home town freely	9.43

X - XI

C	78. Writes occasional short letters	9.63
C	79. Makes telephone calls	10.30
O	80. Does small remunerative work	10.90
C	81. Answers ads; purchases by mail	11.20

XI - XII

O	82. Does simple creative work	11.25
SD	83. Is left to care for self or others	11.45
C	84. Enjoys books, newspapers, magazines	11.58

XII - XV

S	85. Plays difficult games	12.30
SHD	86. Exercises complete care of dress	12.38
SD	87. Buys own clothing accessories	13.00
S	88. Engages in adolescent group activities	14.10
O	89. Performs responsible routine chores	14.65

XV - XVIII

C	....	90. Communicates by letter	14.95
C	....	91. Follows current events	15.35
L	....	92. Goes to nearby places alone	15.85
SD	....	93. Goes out unsupervised daytime	16.13
SD	....	94. Has own spending money	16.53
SD	....	95. Buys all own clothing	17.37

XVIII - XX

L	....	96. Goes to distant points alone	18.05
SD	....	97. Looks after own health	18.48
O	....	98. Has a job or continues schooling	18.53
SD	....	99. Goes out nights unrestricted	18.70
SD	....	100. Controls own major expenditures	19.68
SD	....	101. Assumes personal responsibility	20.53

XX - XXV

SD	....	102. Uses money providently	21.5+
S	....	103. Assumes responsibility beyond own needs	21.5+
S	....	104. Contributes to social welfare	25+
SD	....	105. Provides for future	25+

XXV+

O	....	106. Performs skilled work	25+
O	....	107. Engages in beneficial recreation	25+
O	....	108. Systematizes own work	25+
S	....	109. Inspires confidence	25+
S	....	110. Promotes civic progress	25+
O	....	111. Supervises occupational pursuits	25+
SD	....	112. Purchases for others	25+
O	....	113. Directs or manages affairs of others	25+
O	....	114. Performs expert or professional work	25+
S	....	115. Shares community responsibility	25+
O	....	116. Creates own opportunities	25+
S	....	117. Advances general welfare	25+

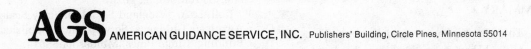

AGS AMERICAN GUIDANCE SERVICE, INC. Publishers' Building, Circle Pines, Minnesota 55014

through the use of the Vineland Scale. A child suffering from deprivation will be unable to perform skills appropriate for his age level due to lack of opportunity. A child who is mentally retarded will also be unable to perform. An overprotective mother who does not allow her child to do things which he should be doing for his age may stifle his development, and this could be detected by using a Vineland Scale in conjunction with some other scales.

For example, the parents of a five-year-old child hospitalized for hernia repair but who also presented with delayed speech and language development were concerned with the child's expressive communication difficulties and the problems these might present in kindergarten. However, they maintained that otherwise the child was bright and understood everything that was said to him. They felt that the older children in the family speaking up for the child was the primary reason for his delay in talking. Clinically, however, it appeared that the child's delay in talking was probably secondary to some degree of mental retardation, which the parents either had not recognized or were unable to admit. Through use of the Vineland, it became apparent to the nurse that the child was delayed in other areas as well. When the parents were asked to estimate at what age the older siblings had been most like the patient, they unerringly agreed on the age range of three and a half to four years, almost precisely where the information which they had given in response to the Vineland had placed the child. This paved the way to a discussion of the advisability of enrolling the child in a preschool rather than kindergarten and led to their acceptance of a referral to a Child Development Clinic for a more intensive study of the child and appraisal of his needs.

SUMMARY

This chapter has stressed the importance of the child's behavior on the parental relationship and has presented the nurse with general information on the use of assessment tools and specific information on various assessment tools. The nurse who works with high-risk families is often in a position to screen for particular problems, assess the severity of other problems, determine individual abilities, and refer the child and his parents for further help if she discovers a need for this type of intervention. The nurse may discover difficulties in the manner in which high-risk family members interact with each other by determining a problem in a child's performance on an assessment tool. A nurse who is able to assess mothering behavior, fathering behavior, and the performance of their child, can administer improved nursing care to the entire family.

REFERENCES

1.   Babson, S. G. and R. C. Benson. *Management of High-Risk Pregnancy and Intensive Care of the Neonate.* St. Louis: C. V. Mosby Co., 1971.
2.   Bayley. *Bayley Scales of Infant Development* (Mental Scale Record Form, Motor Scale Record Form, Infant Behavior Record). The Psychological Corporation, 304 E. 45th St., New York, New York, 10017.
3.   Brazelton, T. B. *Neonatal Behavioral Assessment Scale.* London: S.I.M.P./Heinemann Medical Books; Philadelphia: J. B. Lippincott Co., 1973.
4.   Carey, W. B. "A Simplified Method for Measuring Infant Temperament." Journal of Pediatrics, 77 #2, August 1970, 188–194.
5.   Carey, W. B. "Clinical Applications of Infant Temperament Measurements." *The Journal of Pediatrics,* October 1972, 823–828.
6.   Cattell, P. *Infant Intelligence Scale.* The Psychological Corporation, 304 E. 45th St., New York, New York, 10017.
7.   Cromwell, R. L. and D. Davis." "Behavior Classification of Emotionally Disturbed Children." Paper read at Council for Exceptional Children, Portland, Oregon, April 1965. Source for Tool: Rue L. Cromwell, Lafayette Clinic, 951 E. Lafayette, Detroit, Mich., 48207.
8.   Doll, E. A. "Vineland Social Maturity Scale," American Guidance Service, Inc., Publisher's Building, Circle Pines, Minnesota 55014.
9.   Frankenburg, W. K., A. D. Goldstein, and B. W. Camp. "The Revised Denver Developmental Screening Test: Its Accuracy as a Screening In-

strument." *Journal of Pediatrics*, 79 #6, December 1971, 988–995.

10. Frankenburg, W. K. and B. W. Camp. *Pediatric Screening Tests*. Springfield, Ill.: Charles C Thomas Publisher, 1975.

11. Haar, E. et al. "Personality Differentiation of Neonates. A Nurse Rating Scale Method." *American Academy of Child Psychiatry*, 3, 1964, 330–342.

12. Klein, M. and L. Stein." "Low Birth Weight and the Battered Child Syndrome." *American Journal of Diseases in Children*, 122, July 1971, 15–18.

13. Knobloch, H., B. Pasamanick, and E. S. Sherard. *A Developmental Screening Inventory*. The Division of Child Development, Ohio State University College of Medicine, Columbus, Ohio.

14. Koppitz, E. M. *Psychological Evaluation of Human Figure Drawings*. New York: Grune & Stratton, 1967.

15. Kron, R. E. and M. Stein. "Newborn Sucking Behavior Affected by Obstetric Sedation." *Pediatrics*, 37, 1966, 1012–1016.

16. Kurtz, R. A. "Comparative Evaluation of Suspected Retardates." *American Journal of Diseases in Children*, 109, January 1965, 58–65.

17. Lester, B. M. et al. "A Multivariate Study of the Effects of High Risk Factors on Performance on the Brazelton Neonatal Assessment Scale." *Child Development*, 47, 1976, 515–517.

18. Roy, H. L., J. D. Schein, and D. R. Frisina. *Picture Vocabulary Test for Deaf Children*. Washington, D. C.: Gallaudet College, Cooperative Research Project No. 1383, 1964.

19. Sameroff, A. "Psychological Needs of the Mother in Early Mother-Infant Interactions." In Avery, G. B. (ed.). *Neonatology Pathophysiology and Management of the Newborn*. Philadelphia: J. B. Lippincott Co., 1975, 1023–1045.

20. Sandler, L. et al. "Responses of Urban Preschool Children to a Developmental Screening Test." *Journal of Pediatrics*, 77 #5, November 1970, 775–781.

21. Thomas, A., S. Chess, and H. Birch. *Temperament and Behavior Disorders in Children*. New York: New York University Press, and London: University of London Press, 1968.

The Family at Risk Due to a High-Risk Child
PART TWO

A child who is at risk creates many difficulties for the other family members, including crises, grief, and other reactions. Regardless of its timing—at birth, early or late childhood—any child-related risk situation results in a family at risk.

The following chapters will describe the family difficulties resulting from many specific child risk situations and suggest nursing approaches. The specific child risk situations chosen are representative of the problems but are not intended to be exhaustive.

The High-Risk Pregnancy

Mary Brewer Jones, R.N., B.A.

CHAPTER FOUR

Normal pregnancy is an alteration of the normal health state of the mother rather than an illness. The high-risk pregnancy, however, presents a risk to the health or the normal development of the child or mother. In addition, the emotional effects of the risk pregnancy, the stress of additional medical procedures, and the potential loss of the child may drastically affect the psychological development of the family itself. The nurse is in an ideal position to provide care during the high-risk pregnancy, since she interacts with the mother and the family in both inpatient and outpatient settings throughout pregnancy, delivery, and the postpartum period.

Although there are no firm figures available on the number of high-risk pregnancies occurring each year in the United States, mortality and morbidity statistics and specific disease statistics reflect a part of the severity of the problem. In 1974, the perinatal death rate was approximately 14.5 for each 1,000 live births and the maternal death rate was one for each 4,800 births.[4] Many of the pathological processes which can result in perinatal death also produce disorders of the special senses and adversely affect later development of the child. One or more of the factors which place the mother or child at risk will be present in approximately 20 percent of all pregnancies.

PRESENT CONCEPTS

Pregnancy is classified as high-risk if there is a likelihood that the infant will not be liveborn or if the mother or infant is in danger of physical or psychological impairment as a result of the pregnancy. High-risk characteristics are summarized in Figure 4-1. Obviously, not all of these characteristics are equally hazardous for mother or fetus. Some, such as maternal obesity, may require only careful watchfulness throughout pregnancy while others, such as chronic illness, require both observation and medical intervention. Assessment and evaluation must continue throughout pregnancy, since a high-risk condition can develop prior to conception, at any time during pregnancy, or during labor and delivery.

There are very few risk conditions which affect only the mother or only the fetus. More often, the mother has the risk characteristic, the physical effect is felt by

Figure 4-1. Pregnancy Risk Characteristics

Prepregnancy Characteristics
    Age (below 16 or above 35 years of age)
    Stature and weight (height below 60 inches, prepregnant weight greater than 20 percent under or over standard weight and
        height)
    Nutritional deficiency (unable or unwilling to maintain a balanced dietary intake)
    Multiple pregnancies (more than 5)
    Difficulties with previous pregnancies (any delivery other than spontaneous or low forceps, 24 hour or longer labor, two fetal
        losses before 28 weeks, any fetal loss after 28 weeks, a neonatal death, premature labor)
    Maternal chronic illness (diabetes, chronic hypertension, heart disease, thyroid disorders)

Prenatal Characteristics
    Maternal infection
    Maternal medication and addiction (use of over-the-counter medications on a prolonged basis, drug addiction, alcoholism,
        smoking, use of prescription medications on a long-term basis)
    Exposure to radiation
    Intrauterine growth retardation
    Postmaturity (pregnancy longer than 42 documented weeks)
    Multiple gestation
    Pre-eclampsia/eclampsia
    Rh sensitization
    Hemorrhagic complications (placenta previa, abruption)
    Polyhydramnios or oligohydramnios (can indicate fetal malformations)

Labor and Delivery Characteristics
    Abnormal presentation
    Fever
    Premature onset of labor
    Premature rupture of membranes
    Fetal distress
    Prolonged labor and/or delivery
    Precipitous delivery
    Complicated delivery
    Cord accident
    Placental abruption

the fetus, and the psychosocial aspects affect the entire family. Hyperthyroidism is an example of a risk characteristic of the mother. The fetus may be growth retarded because of the mother's illness and the medicines she must take. The entire family may be anxious and concerned about both the mother's health and its effect on the expected child.

Maternal Risk Characteristics

Those problems which affect primarily the mother are often chronic conditions which were present before pregnancy. Chronic illnesses such as diabetes, hypertension, or heart disease may be made worse by pregnancy, further taxing the mother's physical reserves and increasing the stress on the family unit. Family disorder caused by the mother's addiction to drugs or alcohol may also increase during pregnancy. Mothers and families with

chronic risk conditions require care before, during, and after pregnancy.

Acute maternal problems more often occur in the latter stages of pregnancy or during labor and delivery and may present a risk to both mother and baby. These problems are sudden and unexpected and may require immediate care to prevent harm to the child or the mother. The family has little time to prepare itself emotionally for such unexpected events as placenta previa, a prolapsed cord, or even for the arrival of more than one baby. In addition, the family may feel isolated by the intense physical activity of the staff if emergency care is required. Acute problems tend to create more family panic but over a shorter period of time than do chronic problems.

Maternal Age. Neonatal mortality is lowest in women between 20 and 30 years of age. The adolescent is at risk because she is not biologically mature herself and is less apt to be psychologically prepared to care for an infant. The infant death rate and the incidence of low birth weight infants is highest in teenage pregnancy. At a time when the birth rate in other groups is declining, the birth rate among unmarried teenagers is rising.[6] Unmarried adolescents are less likely to go to traditional health care facilities for early prenatal care, thus lessening the chances for intervention if a risk condition is present.

Women over the age of 35 have a higher incidence of infants with chromosomal abnormalities. For example, the risk of Down's syndrome is less than 1 in 1,000 for women up to the age of 30 but approximately 1 in 100 for women who are 40 and 1 in 40 for the 45 year old.[4]

Hemorrhage. Bleeding disorders prior to delivery threaten both the mother and baby. Hemorrhage after delivery remains as a threat to the mother. One-fourth of the maternal deaths from hemorrhage in 1974 were due to postpartum hemorrhage.[4] Other risk conditions such as infection, multiple birth, complicated delivery, and polyhydramnios increase the risk of postpartum hemorrhage. Observation of the high-risk patient should not end with delivery but must continue into the postpartum period.

Fetal Risk Characteristics

Fetal development can be compromised if conditions exist which interfere with normal fetal growth or if toxic substances are introduced into the fetal circulation.

Physiologic Implications. Deviations from normal growth occur when the mother's circulation delivers too much or too little of the essential nutrients and oxygen to the fetus. The infant of the diabetic mother, for example, receives more than the needed amount of glucose from the maternal circulation. Physical or emotional stress in the diabetic mother activates her endocrine and nervous systems, resulting in a release of glucocorticoids from the adrenals and of glucose from the liver.

Since the diabetic mother cannot metabolize all of this additional glucose, the excess is transferred via the placenta to the fetus where it is used to create additional fetal tissue. Prolonged maternal hyperglycemia is associated with an increased incidence of congenital anomalies in the fetus and with an increased incidence of difficult deliveries as a result of excessive fetal size.

Fetal growth is retarded when insufficient oxygen or nutrients reach the fetal circulation. The amount of blood (and therefore the amount of nutrients and oxygen) reaching the fetus is diminished when there is constriction of the placental blood vessels. Vasoconstriction is a problem in the mother who suffers from hypertension or who smokes. Some types of maternal heart disease can also cause growth retardation. If the pumping ability of the mother's heart is overtaxed by the increase in blood volume which occurs normally in pregnancy, the volume of blood reaching the placenta is reduced even though the blood vessels themselves are not constricted.

Abnormal development of the fetus can be caused by a variety of toxic substances which are passed from the maternal to the fetal circulation without being filtered out by the placenta. Some of these substances, such as the organisms which cause cytomegalovirus, toxoplasmosis, herpes, syphillis and rubella, can be harmful to both the mother and fetus. Others, including many prescription and nonprescription drugs, are not dangerous and are often beneficial to the mother but cause a variety of fetal anomalies when introduced into the fetal circulation. The intake of more than a modest amount of alcohol by the mother has recently been identified as a cause of retarded fetal development. Substances toxic to the fetus can cause congenital malformation and mental retardation. The risk to the fetus is greatest during the early months of pregnancy when fetal growth and organ formation are most rapid.

The Rh positive fetus of the Rh negative mother is at risk if a previous Rh positive pregnancy or blood transfusion has sensitized the mother. The sensitized mother produces antibodies which attack fetal red blood cells, causing fetal anemia. Although the incidence of Rh isoimmunization has dropped dramatically since the introduction of RhoGam, the Rh positive fetus of an Rh negative mother is still at risk of anemia if the mother was sensitized prior to the present pregnancy.

Antepartum Assessment. Within the past decade, several tests which aid in assessing the status of the fetus prior to delivery have been developed. Ultrasonography, when used to monitor fetal growth, and serial estriol determinations are useful adjuncts in determining the ability of the placenta to adequately nourish the fetus. Many genetic defects can be identified through cell cultures grown from amniotic fluid obtained by amniocentesis during the first trimester. Amniocentesis is also used in the later stages of pregnancy to monitor the bilirubin level of the fetus suffering from Rh isoimmunization and to assess fetal lung maturity prior to elective delivery. Electronic fetal monitoring prior to labor aids in identifying the fetus who is being overly stressed by a poor uterine environment.[3] During labor, monitoring provides a continuous record of both fetal heart activity and uterine contractions. Early detection of fetal distress during labor, whether by electronic monitoring or a knowledgeable labor room staff, permits early treatment and decreases the risk of permanent neurologic damage.

Many of these tests can be reassuring to the family during a high-risk pregnancy. A normal amniotic cell culture can relieve the family with a history of Tay-Sachs disease. Normal fetal heart activity during labor can relieve the parents of some of their anxiety during this stressful period. However, assessment procedures can also add to the family's anxiety. Some procedures are uncomfortable or intrusive and can disrupt family life if they must be done outside the home community. Most tests increase the cost of pregnancy. It is important for the family to be supported by the health care team when assessment procedures are needed and especially if the results of any of these tests are not normal.

FAMILY DIFFICULTIES

Family stress often occurs when pregnancy is normal, and this stress is amplified in the high-risk pregnancy. Fear for the health of the mother or the expected child can lead to long-term emotional problems for the family if family members do not cope well with their problems during pregnancy. For example, if the mother's health is impaired by the pregnancy, the family may blame the child and cause him to suffer for the loss of his mother's health. The nurse helps the family avoid such long-term psychological consequences by helping the family deal with problems as they occur during pregnancy. Figure 4-2 concisely lists family problems related to high-risk pregnancy.

Psychological Effects of the High-Risk Pregnancy

The high-risk pregnancy may cause a variety of psychological problems for the family. Emotions such as blame, guilt, or feelings of failure can disrupt family equilibrium and make the pregnancy even more difficult.

Denial. The family's initial reaction to the news that a high-risk situation exists may be denial. It may be especially hard for the family to believe that the mother or baby is at risk during this pregnancy if the family has had other normal pregnancies or if the mother does not feel sick. Denial can be used as a mechanism for coping with the stress of a high-risk pregnancy or as a defense against becoming attached to an infant who may not survive. Denial may be expressed as failure to seek prenatal care, to

Figure 4-2. Family Difficulties Related to High-Risk Pregnancy

Psychological Effects of the High-Risk Pregnancy
   Denial
   Blame and guilt
   Feelings of failure
   Ambivalence

Grief and Mourning
   Anticipatory grief
   Loss of the expected child
   Fetal and infant death
   Maternal disability or death

acknowledge that a risk situation exists, to keep appointments, or to follow instructions.

For example, an Rh negative mother, sensitized by her last pregnancy ten years ago, failed to keep her next two appointments after a rising antibody titer was discovered on her third prenatal visit. The family could not accept the fact that this baby was at risk since their other two children were perfectly normal. The family was referred to a visiting public health nurse who was able to work with them, explaining the physiology of what had happened and why close observation throughout pregnancy was necessary. Through her help, the family was able to acknowledge that a risk existed and returned to the clinic for the needed care. The status of the fetus was followed by antibody titers and then by periodic amniocentesis. The baby was delivered at 38 weeks of gestation, required only phototherapy in the nursery, and went home with the mother.

Blame and Guilt. Because pregnancy is thought of as a normal physiologic process, the presence of risk conditions or the failure to conclude pregnancy with a normal delivery can lead to feelings of guilt and failure in one or both parents. The mother may feel guilty if her health is the cause of the risk situation. The father may experience guilt if he feels responsible for the pregnancy which is jeopardizing the health of his wife or child. It is not unusual for one parent to blame the other for the problem or for one parent to feel that it is all his or her fault. Even if the pregnancy ends with the delivery of a normal infant, such feelings of guilt can persist, resulting in a poor pattern of parenting.

The problem of maternal guilt can be particularly difficult to deal with if the mother views her situation as punishment for something she or someone else did. The mother who expects the "punishment" is usually not willing to take any action herself to improve her condition or to cooperate with others in ameliorating the risk situation.

For example, a 17-year-old diabetic patient had run away from home to live with a young man of whom her parents disapproved. She neglected her own care and sought medical help only in the last trimester of her first pregnancy when she was hospitalized for uncontrolled diabetes. During hospitalization, she would repeatedly inject her daily insulin dose into the mattress and refuse to eat the hospital diet. She stated that her parents hated her and she was being punished for running away. The mother left the hospital several days after cesarean section delivery without visiting or inquiring about her baby. The baby died of multiple congenital anomalies several days later.

Feelings of Failure. The high-risk pregnancy is extremely threatening to the family if either the father or mother associates successful childbearing with success as a man or woman. In this situation, the woman who has problems with pregnancy may feel that she is a failure as a woman.

A difficult family situation developed in one case when a young husband came to the recovery room to see his wife, who had just delivered a stillborn infant during the sixth month of pregnancy. His first statement to her concerned the fact that all three of his sisters had succeeded in giving birth during the previous year. The wife later remarked to a nurse that her sister had been divorced when she had not been able to carry a child to term. The husband's blame and the mother's feelings of failure for the death of the child created difficult parental relationships.

Since much of the nursing and medical care given during pregnancy is directed toward delivery of a healthy baby, the mother may lose her sense of her own self-worth. Many women, when pregnant, improve their own health care in order to assure the best outcome possible for their babies, and in a high-risk situation the mother will often endure painful procedures or prolonged hospitalization because she wants the best for her baby. However, if the mother feels that she is being cared for only because others are concerned for her baby, she may feel that she is not important or is a failure and consequently neglect her own care during and after the pregnancy. The risk is greatest if the mother is not sure that she wants either the pregnancy or the baby.

For example, an unmarried adolescent girl

with pre-eclampsia who had not yet decided to keep her baby repeatedly ignored decisions made for her about the food she should eat and the amount of rest she should get. When the girl was included in talks with the nurses and dieticians and when the emphasis was changed from concern over the baby to a personal concern for the patient, she started to participate in and assume responsibility for her own care.[2]

The mother's needs are also important following birth. Problems from one pregnancy can recur in the next if the mother feels that she does not have to continue caring for herself.

For example, a pediatric outreach nurse visiting in the home of a hypertensive mother discovered that the mother had not returned to the clinic for follow-up although she had kept all the appointments made for the baby. The mother stated that the nurses had emphasized only the importance of the baby's follow-up care. She felt that the baby was the only one who mattered. This was a woman who, because of her hypertension, needed to be in a continuing health care program, both for her current needs and for pre-pregnancy counseling if another pregnancy were desired.

Ambivalence. Even in normal pregnancy, there are times when both the mother and father have alternating feelings about the pregnancy and the arrival of the new baby. The parents, realizing that the baby is going to cause changes in their lifestyle, can have the feeling of both wanting and not wanting the child. These feelings can be accentuated if pregnancy results in unforeseen complications and disruptions of the normal pattern of daily living.

Both the mother and father may have alternating feelings of love and concern, fear and anger toward the fetus and toward each other. The parents, while hoping that the pregnancy will end successfully, can still have some negative feelings about the baby if the mother's health is endangered by the pregnancy. The mother may feel resentment toward her husband if he desired the pregnancy more than she did or if she feels that he "got her into this." The mother may also resent having to give up her job or reduce her level of activity, par-

ticularly if previous pregnancies did not noticeably change her lifestyle. The father may resent the mother's increased need for physical and emotional support.

Such ambivalence often makes it difficult for the parents to communicate with each other. If either partner is afraid to express dissatisfaction, anger, fear, or resentment, the partners may not be able to give each other the emotional support needed to cope with the problem pregnancy. Failure to communicate openly about both the positive and negative emotions of pregnancy may set a pattern of noncommunication which continues after the arrival of the baby. Because she may feel it is unacceptable to express negative feelings about pregnancy, the mother may express her hostility in more subtle ways—eating improperly, smoking or drinking excessively, or overusing tranquilizers or other medications. The father may come home later after work, drink more, or spend more time in activities outside of the home.

In one case, a woman hospitalized because of placenta previa expressed alternating feelings of concern, fear, and resentment for her unborn baby. She had remarried after several years of widowhood and her husband had adopted her children from her first marriage. Although she was not anxious to become pregnant, she wanted to give her husband a child of his own. When she required hospitalization, some family disorganization resulted. Friction developed in the home when the children had to give up some of their after-school activities to help with the housework. The hospitalized mother felt that she was no good either to her husband or to her children. Although she expressed hope that the baby would live, she reluctantly commented on how much family trouble the baby was causing. In this case, the family was able to cope with the stresses they had to face. The mother was hospitalized for eight weeks, delivered by cesarean section, and took home a well child. Although the situation had been stressful for all the family, they had been able to work together and felt that the successful outcome of the pregnancy was a result of all of their efforts.

Children in the family can also have ambivalent feelings toward the expected child. The young child may want a brother or sister and yet may see the baby as the cause of his separation from his mother or of increased friction between his parents. If he is reprimanded for stating these less-than-loving feelings, he may find some other means of expressing them. If this takes the form of disturbing behavior, the strain on the family is increased. If this resentment is not dealt with before the new baby comes home, jealousy and resentment may continue to be acted out in disruptive ways.

Grief and Mourning

Unfortunately, the high-risk pregnancy does not always end with the birth of a living or normal child. Even if the parents were aware of this possibility, they will still mourn the child they have lost.

Grief and mourning in the high-risk pregnancy is not restricted to those families whose newborns die or are abnormal. Grief can occur at any time during pregnancy if the parents feel loss of the child or of the mother's health is possible.

Anticipatory Grief. Anticipatory grief is a mechanism which allows one to prepare for a potential loss. Some steps in grief work take place during the period before the loss actually occurs.

If the high-risk parents feel that they are going to lose their baby before birth, grief can begin while the fetus is still alive. If the fetus does die, the parents' anticipatory grief helps them resolve the loss. However, if the baby is born alive, the parents must initiate the process of relating to their child. If they cannot make this transition, the child will suffer continued emotional deprivation after birth. Nurses should be aware that parents who react to the birth of a well baby with disbelief or lack of emotion may need help in developing an affectional relationship with their child.

For example, several forms of mothering disorders are seen more frequently following a high-risk pregnancy. A mild disorder is persistent concern over a minor abnormality or a minor acute illness in the child. More serious is the "vulnerable child syndrome" in which the parents continue to expect the child to die during childhood because of the previously resolved risk situation. This attitude can lead to severe emotional disturbances in the child.

Loss of the Expected Child. If a child is born prematurely or with a mental or physical disability, the parents will need to grieve for the normal child they were expecting before they can begin the process of relating to the child they have. The parents may also feel they have failed because they did not produce a full-term healthy child. The family's grief may be particularly severe if there was little or no advance warning that the child would not be normal or if the family had continued to deny that there was ever a risk situation.

Fetal and Infant Death. Much has been written about the grieving process and the steps a family must go through when a child is lost. A family goes through this grieving process after the loss of a stillborn or newborn infant just as after the death of an older child.[5] The grieving may be made more difficult for the mother of a stillborn infant if other family members or members of the hospital staff encourage the parents to forget about the stillborn as quickly as possible and to look forward to another pregnancy. This attitude may be enforced by a routine which removes any evidence of the infant's existence as quickly as possible and discourages the parents' attempts to express grief over the outcome of the pregnancy.

The parents must terminate this pregnancy and break their ties to the infant they have lost. If the parents are not supported by other family members or by hospital personnel, they may fear that their reactions to the infant's death are abnormal or that they are emotionally unstable. Since the parents are often reluctant to communicate these seemingly abnormal worries to each other, there can be a lack of husband-wife support.

Maternal Disability or Death. The maternal death rate has fallen from 1 per 1,200 live births in 1950 to 1 per 4,800 births in 1974. Hemorrhage, hypertension, and infection still account for approximately half of the maternal deaths in the United States.[4] Death of the mother completely disrupts the family structure and often leaves the father with the care of a baby at a time when his emotional reserves are lowest. The father and other children in the family may find it difficult to care for the new baby if they feel he is somehow responsible for the mother's death. If the mother contributed to the family income, her loss will also create economic problems for the family. Nursing intervention following a mother's death can include referrals to community agencies which furnish family counseling and help with child care.

The mother may also be physically or emotionally disabled as a result of pregnancy. Aggravation of a preexisting medical condition, such as heart disease, may limit her activity after pregnancy and increase her need for medical care. Young children may not receive sufficient supervision if the mother's activity is limited and if the family cannot afford outside help. Again, loss of the mother's income if she was working prior to pregnancy is a further stress on the family. The family may need help in planning for the mother's medical care and for child care as well as in dealing with emotional problems, such as feelings of guilt and failure.

The parents can suffer emotionally if complications of pregnancy result in the mother's inability to have other children. The unexpected loss of reproductive ability as a result of hemorrhage or infection can be particularly devastating if the mother derives her sense of self-worth primarily from her ability to bear children. Exacerbation of preexisting psychiatric disorders or development of severe depression after childbirth are also causes of emotional disability which affect both the mother and the family.

CLINICAL APPROACHES

Nurses can play an active and important role in helping families make satisfactory adjustments to the stresses created by the high-risk pregnancy. Continuity of nursing care, from the first visit until after the postpartum period, is important in identifying or preventing additional problems during pregnancy and in helping the family readjust following pregnancy.

Providing Family Care

In addition to providing care for the high-risk mother, the nurse must also consider the needs of the father and siblings. The family is strengthened if all members have a chance to express their fears and concerns openly and if they can work together in dealing with these stresses. The family will also be able to cooperate better in providing special care for the mother if all were included in developing the care plan.

A variety of nursing techniques can be used to involve the family in the care being provided for the mother and baby. For example, family members can be encouraged to come to the clinic and stay with the mother whenever possible. This gives the parents a chance to ask questions and participate jointly in planning the mother's care. Providing opportunities for both parents and children to visit the clinic or hospital and ask questions helps decrease the fearfulness related to an unknown medical condition or treatment. If antenatal testing is done, the family can be given a picture from the ultrasound exam or a strip showing the baby's heart beat from a normal oxytocin challenge test. This makes the coming baby more of a reality and gives the parents something tangible to associate with their baby.

Early Nursing Care

There are benefits to both the patient and the nurse if the patient enters a health care system early in pregnancy. Routine care, including assessment of the mother's physical status, development of a nutritional program and assessment of the emotional needs of the mother and other family members should begin as early in pregnancy as possible. Early access permits early identification of potential or existing risk factors, intervention for genetic abnormalities, and early treatment of developing maternal medical problems.

The woman who has a family physician will

be more likely to receive health care early in pregnancy. The clinic patient may find early prenatal care less available or not easily accessible. Families may not come in for care if they feel that obstetrical care is impersonalized, have difficulty finding transportation, or encounter a language barrier.

Having experienced or especially trained obstetrical nurses make the initial contact with the family is one method of making care more easily accessible. For example, at the Bexar County Hospital, San Antonio, Texas, anyone with a problem relating to reproduction is seen on the first visit by an obstetric nurse clinician, who takes the initial history and sees that all routine laboratory work is done. Women receive immediate medical attention if needed on the first visit. Mothers needing routine obstetrical care are given later clinic appointments. Patient education classes are conducted by the nurses and a small play area is provided for children who must come to the hospital with their mothers.

Nurses also encourage early entrance into a prenatal program by supporting or developing local educational programs which help community members become aware of available obstetric resources and the benefits of early prenatal care. Since illegitimacy and teenage pregnancy are associated with a higher rate of obstetric complications, educational programs for young people are particularly beneficial.

For example, the staff nurses in our labor room have prepared a slide presentation on labor and delivery which they take on request to community groups. This program has been particularly well received by high schools which have special classes for pregnant students. These young girls not only have a chance to discuss labor and delivery with the nurses but also can ask questions about family planning, prenatal care, and the reproductive process.

Providing Continuous Care

Adequate follow-up can best be achieved by having the same personnel see the parent(s) at each visit. Having a previously established relationship with the mother helps the nurse identify new problems, supervise existing problems, and assess the patient's understanding of her particular situation. Although continuity of care is most easily achieved in a private medical practice, it is essential for high-risk pregnant parents in any setting. Whether the clinic is publicly funded, a part of a military medical system, or a health maintenance organization, patients are more apt to keep their appointments and discuss their family difficulties if they know they will be seen by someone they know who cares about them.

The benefits of continuity of care include better communication of information, coordination of special laboratory procedures, more accurate evaluation of the patient's ability to follow her care plan, and a closer sharing and helping relationship with the family members.

One method of maintaining continuity of care is a problem-oriented medical record system. The Maternity and Infant Care Project of Erie County, New York, uses such a system, which summarizes risk factors and the status of current problems. Their personnel have found the system valuable in improving communication among members of the health care team and quality of care to their high-risk population.[1]

Patient teaching should also be continued in the coordinated program of health care. The high-risk pregnant mother needs the opportunity to discuss routine care during pregnancy, infant care, and the process of labor and delivery in addition to specific counseling about her risk situation and the family changes. Relaxation and breathing techniques can be taught prior to labor. A tour of the labor suite will help the parents prepare for hospital admission when labor begins.

Reducing the Stress of Hospitalization

Hospitalization prior to labor may be necessary for management of medical problems such as pre-eclampsia, diabetes, or placenta previa. Family separation, unfamiliarity of hospital routine, and association of pain with hospitalization may make a woman reluctant to enter or remain in the hospital. Bed rest and hospitalization also require the mother to assume a dependent role. Although she may not feel ill or think of herself as being ill, she loses much control over what she may or may not do and must depend on others to supply many of her physical needs. This dependent role may be particularly disturbing to her if she is used to leading an active life.

In spite of the stress produced, hospitalization can, in many cases, improve the outcome for both the mother and the baby. If hospitalization permits the mother to carry her baby to term, the risks of prematurity and mother-family-infant separation can be avoided. Hospitalization prior to delivery is also financially advantageous to the family if prenatal hospitalization makes long-term care of the baby in an expensive neonatal intensive care unit unnecessary.

When hospitalization is necessary, the nurse can make it more palatable for both the woman and her family. For example, feelings of dependency can be reduced by encouraging ambulation instead of bed rest whenever possible. Activity is to be encouraged in the diabetic patient, as physical activity uses up some of the excess blood sugar. The patient whose insulin dosage is regulated in the hospital may develop an insulin reaction at home when she resumes her more active daily routine unless she was encouraged to remain active while in the hospital.

A team approach to hospitalization, with the patient participating in plans for her care, can also reduce the stress of hospitalization. The physical therapy department can provide an exercise program when needed. The dietician can work with the mother to plan a diet which is medically advantageous and socially acceptable. A hospital chaplain can provide spiritual guidance. Occupational therapists, volunteers, or Red Cross workers can provide projects which help pass the time or develop a new skill. The mother who learns a new hand skill and enjoys making handcrafted items for her family

or for the baby continues to feel that she is contributing to her family.

Labor and delivery will be a particularly stressful time for the high-risk family. Care during this period should continue to include both parents. Questions should be answered honestly and nurses should neither raise false hopes nor exaggerate problems which arise during labor. Both parents should be kept informed of the mother's progress.

Nursing Care after Delivery

Nursing care continues to be important after delivery. If the high-risk pregnancy ends with the birth of a well child, the parents may need help in readjusting from the risk state. If stillbirth occurs or the child is born disabled, nursing help can be invaluable in getting the parents through a difficult period. Parents will often feel less emotionally isolated if they are supported by the health care team as they work through their grief reaction.

Well-Child Care after a High-Risk Pregnancy. After the extremely stressful situation that made the pregnancy high risk, it may be difficult for the family to return to normal. The parents may become anxious because of normal variations in infant behavior (for instance, worrying if the baby is slow to nurse or if the stool is soft). The parents may ask endless questions in an effort to reassure themselves that the mother and baby are really well.

The parents should become more secure in handling their baby and begin to realize that all has ended well within a week or so after birth. If this does not happen, the risk of developing the vulnerable child syndrome or other maladaptive behavior is increased. Nurses dealing with such behavior in an older child may find the roots of the problem in the high-risk pregnancy.

Nursing care during the postpartum period should include a continuing assessment of the parents' reaction to their baby. This assessment should note how the parents touch the baby, if the parents seek eye contact with the baby, and if the baby is cuddled and watched during feedings. Increasing eye and body contact between parents and child indicates normal bonding is taking place. Both obstetrical and nursery nurses should emphasize the normal outcome of the pregnancy, pointing out the normal aspects of the newborn's appearance and behavior. The parents may not have been receptive to teaching about child care during the prenatal period if they feared that their child would not live, and will need that teaching after delivery.

Stillbirth. One of the first questions after a stillbirth is, "Should the parents see the baby?" There is no definitive answer to this question. Each situation must be evaluated individually before a decision is made.

There are several advantages to letting the family see the baby. The family may terminate this pregnancy and complete the grief process more quickly if they see their baby. If the baby suffered from congenital anomalies, the parents may build up an image of the baby in their minds that is far worse than reality. A family counselor who works with our patients describes this process as taking tragedy and turning it into horror. It is interesting to note that, even if the infant is previable or deformed in some manner, parents usually remember the positive aspects of the baby. They often will point out some familial characteristic or emphasize the baby's normal features.

Some families will be more comfortable not seeing their baby. Others will want to explore their own feelings with family and staff before making a decision. Neither the decision to see or not to see the baby is wrong. The final decision should not be based on what is easiest physically or emotionally for the hospital staff but rather on the decision made by the parents. The staff, however, can help the family reach a decision which the family finds most comfortable.

In one case, a husband and wife lost their first child after a pregnancy of five and a half months. The physician and both sets of grandparents encouraged the couple to resume their daily routines as quickly as possible, feeling that this would help them put this pregnancy out of their minds. The couple, not knowing what else to do, had the hospital dispose of the fetus and both parents returned to their jobs. Over the next six months, the wife became increasingly despondent with periods of weeping and an increasing inability to concentrate. She sought psychiatric help and, after a period of counseling, she and her husband were advised to give a name to the baby they had lost, to conduct memorial services, and in other ways to acknowledge the existence of the child and their grief over the loss. These actions resulted in a period of intense grief for the parents, during which they were supported by family and friends. Recovery from their grief was not prolonged and both parents felt a great relief from dealing openly with their feelings about the child they had lost. The delay in working through this grief may have been prevented by seeing and acknowledging the stillborn infant immediately after birth.

The nurse can also help the family by encouraging the parents to talk honestly with each other. The nurse can make it easier for parents to express the emotions they are feeling by using such comments as, "Many parents who have lost a child in situations like yours have told me that they felt bewildered and depressed. I wonder if you have had similar feelings." If the parents feel that their fears and worries are not abnormal, they will be more willing to share these feelings with each other and with other supportive people.

The nurse can offer emotional support through touching and listening. Nurses, like everyone else, often feel that they do not know the right thing to say or the helpful thing to do in a grief situation and, therefore, simply avoid the situation. However, a nurse's presence, sometimes more than words, helps the mother feel less isolated and more cared about.

Nurses can also be emotionally affected when a stillbirth occurs. If the mother has been hospitalized prior to the birth or is a long-time patient in the clinic or office, the members of the health care team will share her grief at the loss of her child. Sharing in the parents' grief through touching, listening, and even crying can be helpful not only to the family but to the nurse as well.

Developing Specialized Clinics

Special clinics that focus on specific risk pregnancy problems are helpful in bringing parents with similar problems together and in focusing on the effects of the problem on the family. Nurses not only actively participate in the nursing care in the clinic but also help plan and develop the clinic services.

Special clinics for diabetic and pre-eclamptic women have been established by the Bexar County Hospital. These clinics are located in the existing clinic area and are staffed by qualified nurses from the labor and delivery room. Because they make use of existing facilities and personnel, the clinics require no additional financial backing. Both undergraduate and graduate nursing students gain experience in the care of the high-risk family by spending time in these clinics.

Nurse-run Diabetic Clinic. Diabetic management presents a particular challenge during pregnancy. Women with preexisting diabetes find their diabetes more difficult to manage during pregnancy. A woman can also develop diabetes during pregnancy, the diabetes disappearing again shortly after delivery. The older, multiparous patient who develops diabetes during pregnancy may find it particularly difficult to manage diet restrictions and insulin injections. If she has not had problems with previous pregnancies and is feeling well, she may not appreciate the value of maintaining a normal blood glucose.

Because of the difficulties and frustrations felt by so many diabetic patients, a special clinic was established for this group of women. Care is coordinated by a nurse clinician with physician supervision. The special clinic provides an opportunity for education, close medical supervision, and a one-to-one nurse-patient relationship. The patient is able to air her frustrations and feelings and receive care relating specifically to her needs.

Nurse-run Toxemia Clinic. This clinic provides continuity of care to young women in their first pregnancies who are at risk of developing pre-eclampsia. The benefits of this clinic are much the same as for the diabetic clinic. The one-to-one relationship gives the mother a chance to ask the many questions related to her risk pregnancy. Since the clinic nurse performs the ultrasonography examinations and oxytocin challenge tests and assists with amniocentesis, she is better able to prepare the mother for the tests and reduce anxieties over the treatment.

SUMMARY

The patient and her family are central in the management of the high-risk pregnancy. Education, support, and assistance in the maintenance of family integrity are appropriate areas for nursing assistance. Care of the high-risk family during pregnancy should focus not only on medical intervention but also on emotional and psychological support for all members of the family unit.

REFERENCES

1. Ademowore, A. and E. Myers. "Use of the Problem-Oriented Medical Record by Nurses Caring for High-Risk Antepartum Patients." *JOGN Nursing*, 6, 1977, 17–22.
2. Anderson, C. "The Lengthening Shadow: a Case Study in Adolescent, Out-of-Wedlock Pregnancy." *JOGN Nursing*, 5, 1976, 19–22.
3. Jones, M. "Antepartum Assessment in High-Risk Pregnancy." *JOGN Nursing*, 4, 1975, 23–27.
4. Pritchard, J. and P. MacDonald. *Williams Obstetrics*, 15th Ed. New York: Appleton-Century-Crofts, 1976, 4–5, 787.
5. Saylor, D. E. "Nursing Response to Mothers of Stillborn Infants." *JOGN Nursing*, July/August 1977, 39–42.
6. Schwartz, B. "Rock and 'Bye, Baby." *JOGN Nursing*, 4, 1975, 27–30.

ADDITIONAL READINGS

1. Donnelly, E. "The Real of Her." *JOGN Nursing*, 3, 1974, 48–52.

2. Juhasz, J. and R. Kilker. "High-Risk Pregnancy." In *Maternity Nursing Today*. J. Clausen et al. (eds.). New York: McGraw-Hill, 1973, 727–763.

PERTINENT ORGANIZATIONS

NATIONAL

*   *National Foundation—March of Dimes*
    Box 2000

White Plains, New York 10602
Local chapters will be listed in telephone directories. Have films, booklets on high-risk pregnancy. Can often furnish help with educational projects in local areas.

LOCAL

*   Family counseling can often be found locally through community-supported United Way and similar organizations.

The Premature Infant

Suzanne Hall Johnson, R.N., M.N.

CHAPTER FIVE

Recent advances in transportation of ill infants to regional centers and in treatments by the specialized neonatal team have reduced the complications of infants born prematurely. Reducing the complications for the infant and saving his life are of course the first priority for the health team, however, a close second priority is preventing complications and reducing problems for the family. Unfortunately many of the treatments aimed at keeping the premature infant healthy create some of the problems for the family. Premature birth causes numerous family difficulties that place the family at risk of abnormal development, but sensitive, observant, and creative nursing care can prevent or reduce the problems for the family while still maintaining the health of the infant.

Returning the premature infant to a family that is able to provide a nurturing environment is essential, since parents influence the future development of their child with the environment they provide. For the premature infant, the family environment may be particularly critical to future development. Arthur Parmelee, M.D., suggests that the premature infant is even more sensitive to his environment than the full-term infant.[9] It is not enough for the health team to save the life of the child and prevent physical difficulties if the child returns to a family that is unable to provide an optimum environment for his future development.

BASIC CONCEPTS OF PREMATURITY

Any infant of less that 2,500 grams is considered a *low birth weight* infant. Within the low birth weight group there are two types of infants based on length of gestation. The *premature infant* is one born with less than 37 weeks gestation, while the *small for gestational age* infant commonly has had 37 to 42 weeks of gestation but weighs less than expected.[5]

The premature infant and small for gestational age infant are distinguished because of the differences in their medical problems. The premature infant who is appropriate for gestational age is basically immature and has difficulties based on the extent of his development before birth. Respiratory distress, apneas, nutritional problems, and other possible complications are related to his immature lungs, nerves, stomach, and other organs. The small for gestation infant has had the normal gestation period with development of most organs and is basically an undernourished term infant. His difficulties are related to the type and length of undernourishment and include pneumothorax, hypoglycemia, and congenital malformations.[5] The complications for the low birth weight infants lead to about half the infant deaths in the first month following birth and may lead to continuing neurological or other problems.

Families' reactions to both premature and small for gestational age birth include grieving, fears, and guilt. The main differences for the two families are related to the different amount of time for preparation for the birth; the small for dates infant is born near the expected due date while the premature infant is often born unexpectedly. Although the difficulties for the family with the premature infant will be described in the following section, the potential problems are frequently applicable to families of small for dates infants.

Premature birth most frequently refers to the birth of a preterm live infant. Birth that occurs before the period of viability for the infant (20 to 22 weeks of gestation or 500 grams) is termed a spontaneous abortion. Previously most of these infants were stillborn or died soon after birth. The family difficulties related to stillbirth are discussed in other chapters. The recent advances in treatment for very small premature infants has increased their chances of survival. Premature infants' survival chances increase and length of treatment decreases as the infants' length of gestation increases. In one study the death rate was 3 percent for infants born weighing between 2,000 and 2,500 grams, 13 percent for those between 1,500 and 2,000 grams, and 40 percent for those between 1,000 to 1,500 grams. Fortunately most low birth weight infants are near 2,500 grams with decreasing percentages in each lower weight group. Approximately 7 percent of births are of low birth weight, with over 4 percent in the 2,000 to 2,500 group, 1 percent in the 1,500 to 2,000 group, and .5 percent in the 1,000 to 1,500 group.[1] The length of treatment for premature infants ranges

from a few days for the premature near term and close to 2,500 grams without complications to several months for the very early or small infant with complications.

Since both the survival chances and length of treatment influence the family reactions, the premature infant's gestational age before birth affects the family difficulties. Generally the family of an infant born near term with excellent chances of survival and short treatment period has initial difficulties similar to, but of shorter duration than those of the parents of an infant of shorter gestation with possibly more complications and longer treatment.

The cause of most premature births is unknown. It is probably a combination of several factors: maternal, paternal, fetal, and environmental. Some maternal physical factors which may lead to prematurity are hypertensive disease, toxemia, placenta previa, premature separation of the placenta, and cervical incompetence. Maternal personal factors that may lead to prematurity are cigarette smoking, very young or old age, history of other premature births, absence of prenatal care, and malnutrition. Paternal factors include older age and genetic endowment. Some fetal factors that may precipitate premature birth include congenital anomaly, fetal diseases, and multiple birth. Environmental factors include foods, stress, and falls. It is often difficult to predict premature birth, since other presently unknown factors influence premature labor.

The nurse's goal in working with the family of a premature infant is to return the infant in excellent health to parents who are excited and ready to incorporate him as an individual family member. If this is not possible due to the death of a severely ill infant, the nurse's goal is to help the family to cope with the death of their infant. These goals are met by preventing or reducing the family difficulties presented in the next section.

FAMILY DIFFICULTIES

Although there are several potential and common difficulties for the family with a premature infant, the exact degree and manifestation of the difficulty depends on the individual families' reaction to the situation. Parents already confident of their parenting abilities from previous children are less susceptible to feelings of inadequacy than "first-time" parents. Parents who previously reacted to stressful situations by blaming their spouses are likely to have greater problems with blame following the premature birth situation.

The following families demonstrate how individual family reactions and abilities influence the type and extent of problems they have following a premature birth. Two families gave birth to premature infants who were 30 weeks gestational age, were approximately the same size, had similar temperature and breathing difficulties, and were transported from the home hospitals to a regional medical center for intensive care. The father of one family asked to accompany the child to the regional center where he asked to meet all of the physicians and nurses responsible for his child, touched and held his infant, photographed the child, and immediately called to tell his wife about the infant to make arrangements for her to visit the medical center. This couple visited the child often, stroked and talked to him in the isolette, and cuddled him out of the isolette. Although this couple feared for the future of their infant, they felt close to their child and were satisfied in their parenting. The second set of parents did not contact the medical staff, ask about the baby, or otherwise follow the baby after he was transferred. They were more withdrawn and waited for the medical team to call them. This family not only feared the child's death, but they also felt unsuccessful at parenting and frustrated in not knowing what to do for their child.

Socioeconomic status, age, previous experiences, and family relationship factors all influence the parents' reactions to the premature birth situation.

Since prematurity has a high incidence among low socioeconomic families (14 percent for non-white while 7 percent of births for whites) the environmental factors related to poverty or near-poverty may influence the family's reaction to the prema-

ture birth.[11] Some socioeconomic factors which may lead to the premature birth, such as nonuse of medical services and poor nutrition, can also influence a family's reactions to their premature infant. A mistrust of health care professionals makes it difficult for the parents of a premature infant to establish a trust relationship and to ask for help in the crisis. A lack of finances can make the required medical care difficult unless community assistance can be found. A lack of personal transportation makes it difficult for parents to visit their infants in their own hospital and especially in a distant regional center. Fathers who are paid an hourly wage and are faced with additional financial burdens may find it difficult to leave work to visit the infant. The family whose first language is different from that of the professional team has an additional difficulty in communicating fears and problems.

The age of the parents may contribute to prematurity and parental reactions. A 16-year-old mother has a greater chance of prematurity than the 20-year-old, yet most adolescents have not developed a wide range of coping abilities with which to face the premature infant crisis. Also, for the adolescent mother the premature infant is usually the first child, which adds the fears of learning new mothering behaviors to the crisis of the premature birth. The adolescent single mother may have no support during the crisis stage or in parenting when the infant returns home. The nurse can help the adolescent mother by providing extra teaching of the mothering tasks and extra counseling to foster adolescent attachment and plans for the future with her infant.

The family's previous experiences with birth influence the way they react to premature birth. Parents with several other children may find that mothering and fathering behaviors develop quite easily, however they are often concerned that the premature infant is smaller and behaves differently from their previous infants. The parents who have had no children will be learning the new parenting behaviors during the crisis of the premature birth. The parents who have had previous positive experiences with a premature infant will probably experience a milder crisis, while those who have had a previous grief experience with the death or illness of a child will probably experience an extreme crisis even if the infant is developing well. Nurses must assess the family's previous experiences with full-term and premature infants. For the family who has had negative experiences, the nurse should stress that this premature infant is an individual with his own individual abilities and difficulties.

The family that greatly desires a child but has found it difficult to conceive or has had experiences with spontaneous abortions and stillbirths will probably find the premature birth a greater crisis than the family without these experiences. The nurse should help the parents to express their grief at the previous loss of pregnancies and their grave concern about the outcome of this pregnancy. The waiting period before knowing if the infant survived may be difficult for them.

Family relationships greatly influence the parents' reactions to the premature birth. The family's ingenuity at solving problems, such as how to become close to the new infant or how to get transportation to the referral center, is important to their reactions. The family's flexibility of roles influences how well its members will support each other during the crisis of a premature infant. Those who support each other during the crisis and learn new ways of coping with the stresses strengthen their relationship. Inflexibility in family roles can lead to blaming one another for the premature birth, lack of assistance for planning visits to the referral center, and family disunity.

Many of the following difficulties are related. For example, the parents with a fear of the child's death may also feel that they are not involved with the child and have difficulty establishing a reciprocal parenting relationship.

When prevention of the premature birth is not possible, the nurse's goals are to assess the family's reactions, prevent the family difficulties, decrease the magnitude of the problems, and reduce the stress on the family caused by the premature birth. Since the nurse may not be able to prevent or solve all of the family problems because many are di-

rectly related to presently unchangeable premature birth experiences, the nurse must develop interventions that help the parents cope with the problems.

The potential family problems described in the next section were identified through the author's interviews and experiences with families following premature birth. The assessment, causes, and nursing interventions for each problem will be discussed. The family difficulties are concisely listed in Figure 5-1.

Grief

The difference in the appearance and behaviors of the expected full-term infant and the actual premature infant creates disappointment for the parents. The parents' grief for the loss of their anticipated full-term infant is similar to other parents' grief for the loss of a terminally ill child.

The premature infant's characteristic thin body and uncoordinated behaviors are unlike what the parents pictured for their infant. The premature infant lacks fat pads under his skin, and thus looks slightly "emaciated." The infant's appearance greatly influences the family's initial reactions and grief. They often think that he is very frail and that touching him might break something. Although it is impossible to change the physical characteristics of the infant, the nurse can help the family's reaction by helping them recognize that although the infant is small he is completely formed, will not

Figure 5-1. Family Difficulties for the Family with a Premature Infant

Grief

Fears
  fear of the unknown
  fear of death
  fear of abnormal development

Guilt

Parental attachment
  physical separation
  mechanical separation
  emotional separation

Dissatisfaction with parenting

Reshifting of family roles

Inability to express their emotional needs

break with touch, and will fill out with continued development.

The behaviors of the premature infant are somewhat different from the behaviors of the full-term because of the immature reflexes and neurological development. Although premature infants move their arms and legs quite well, they seem to have less control in their movements than full-term infants. The premature infant has a weak grasp, and the parents are discouraged when the child does not grasp their finger as they would expect a normal newborn to do. Since the premature infant has a very sensitive Moro reflex, he often startles and cries at the opening of the isolette door or on a first touch, which often makes the parents feel their touch hurts him. These uncoordinated movements and unexpected behaviors may frighten some parents and prevent them from being comfortable interacting with their child.[2] The nurse can help parents understand that these behaviors are normal for the premature infant and that he will continue to develop new abilities.

Although the chances of survival for most premature infants are good, the very small premature infant or one with serious complications may die. Anticipation of the possible death or the actual death of their premature infant increases the parent's grief.

The nurse can help the family to deal with their grief by helping them recognize that their reactions are normal and necessary in dealing with their loss. The nurse must support the family in their present stage and help them deal with the fears and problems of that stage without forcing them prematurely to another stage. The nurse should not scold the family in denial that they have a very sick child, but should support the parents by telling them the honest information about the child's condition. For parents who blame each other, the nurse allows the expression of their feelings of blame while giving them accurate information on the possible causes for the premature birth. The nurse must not get drawn into the parents' feelings by also denying the premature birth or becoming angry with the parents when they are angry. The best way to help the parents through the grief process is to help them identify their reactions at each stage, associate their feelings with the stress of the premature birth, recognize that their reactions are normal, and gather information about their individual infant.

Although it is normal for the parents of a premature infant to grieve, it may become pathological. Parents who are in an early stage an unreasonably long time are having difficulty resolving the grief. Examples are parents who are in denial for weeks, where the parents will not go in to see the baby, or are angry for weeks at the partner or hospital staff. In addition, when parents' grief reactions greatly interfere with their ability to meet the needs of their family, there is a need for additional assistance in resolving their grief. For instance, if in the depression stage a mother and father would like to stay with the infant continuously for several days but fail to make effective arrangements for their children at home, this is a pathological response needing immediate attention.

Fears

The parents have many fears following a premature delivery. Fear of the unknown and fear of the infant's death or abnormal development are common. The presence of a fear is not abnormal when it is based on real, unknown, or dangerous situations for the infant. It is unrealistic if the fears continue when the situation is clarified and danger has passed.

Fear of the Unknown. Since a premature birth occurs before the expected delivery date, it is essentially an unexpected delivery with unknown experiences and fears for the parents. The tasks associated with the last months of pregnancy, such as preparing the baby's room and final explanation to the siblings about the arrival of the new child have often not been done at the time of a premature birth. In addition, for families who wanted to share this experience with prepared childbirth techniques, the early birth often comes before the completion of the special childbirth classes. Although the amount of unpreparedness of the family depends upon the degree of prematurity and the parents' advance planning, premature birth almost always results in the parents being unprepared for the birth.

Although the unexpected characteristic of the birth can rarely be prevented, the nurse can increase the parents' ability to control the situation. The nurse teaching prenatal classes should encourage participation in class early enough in pregnancy to conclude preparation for childbirth several weeks before the due date. The family can arrange for babysitters for other children and transportation to the hospital many weeks before the delivery date. It is of special importance that anticipatory guidance be provided to the childbearing couple who are at increased risk for delivering a premature infant. By taking a thorough history from the couple and establishing a data base, the nurse could identify predisposing factors and initiate early childbirth teaching.

In addition, parents with premature infants often experience fear of the unknown future of their infant. The period of uncertainty includes the time before and during the medical team's examination and assessment of the difficulties and abilities for the individual infant and the frequent critical period of the first days when new difficulties may arise. Even after the medical team has assessed the infant's present condition, they have difficulty predicting the future. Some infants who are expected to do well develop unexpected difficulties, while some who are expected to do poorly do very well.

The author has found that parents can tolerate the unknown if the medical team is honest with them about changes in the child's condition and acknowledges the difficult waiting period. Medical staff or nursing staff who are not yet sure about the prognosis of the child often avoid the parents because they have nothing certain to report. The parents handle the fear of the unknown best when the nurse describes the uncertain period, expresses that one of the hardest things for parents is to "not know" what will happen, and gives the parents an idea of when the uncertain and critical period for the infant will probably be over.

For example, a family with a recently born premature infant found it difficult to get a clear message from the medical staff about whether the child could live normally or die. Some of the neonatal staff avoided any commitment and avoided the family, while others gave their best guess but had conflicting answers. When one primary nurse worked with the family and explained that premature infants frequently have an uncertain period the first few days when difficulties may resolve or become more serious, the parents became more trusting of the medical staff. The family found it especially helpful to express to the nurse that the unknown seemed worse than knowing of actual difficulties. The primary nurse arranged for another family who had parented a premature infant to help this family wait through the critical period by acknowledging the difficulty of not knowing the future for their child and accompanying them to the cafeteria to eat while leaving word with the nurses where they could be paged.

Fear of Death. Fear that their premature infant will die is a major difficulty for the parents. This fear often comes from the medical team's reactions. Although today, with the development of the specialized intensive care procedures and staff, premature infants' survival rate is good, many physicians and nurses still remember the days when premature infants often died. In order to "spare" the parents from the hurt of the child's death, some professionals still routinely tell the parents that the child will probably not survive. Messages from a medical team such as "your baby is awfully small" or "I doubt if he will make it" increase the parents' fears that the baby will die. Preparing parents "for the worst" and discouraging closeness with their child does not reduce the grief at the child's death and interferes with parents' early attachment with their infant that lives.

Professionals should base their judgment and their explanations about the survival of the premature infant on each individual infant's condition, including statements about the child's specific difficulties, abilities, and length of the critical "uncertain" period. Nurses caring for a premature infant should discuss the baby's change of condition as well as his abilities, with statements like, "We increased the oxygen 5 percent to help him breathe easier," "His breaths are full and rhythmic now," and "He is moving his arms and legs actively between naps."

The parents also often fear for the survival of their child because he has been admitted to an intensive care center. Explanations by the medical team frequently relate hospitalization or transportation of the infant to the infant's need for continuous observation and specialized medical care. Although only critical adults are admitted to adult intensive care units, many infants with only minor difficulties are admitted to neonatal intensive care units for observation and routine treatments. When an infant is admitted only to prevent problems or for minor observation, the nurse should tell the parents about their child's abilities and that although the nursery is called an "Intensive Care Nursery," many babies are admitted as a preventative measure for observation or extra warmth in an isolette. Fortunately, nurses in normal newborn nurseries are being trained to care for the less severe infants and fewer less critical infants are being placed in intensive care nurseries.

One family was fearful for the survival of their child when the child was whisked away quickly from the delivery room and the nurse told the father that the infant would probably "not live." Although the medical team later explained to the parents that the small premature infant was rushed away to be observed, suctioned, and warmed and that he had no major difficulties, the parents were very fearful for the child's life. The mother was afraid to hear the telephone ring, as she thought the hospital would be calling to say the child had died, while the husband called home every two hours from work fearing the infant's death. The parents did not tell their friends or neighbors about the birth of the child because they felt the child would probably die. When they visited the infant in the hospital, they were so frightened that they did not look closely at the child, did not relax when holding the child, and frequently misinterpreted explanations of the child's condition. Although a primary nurse worked very closely with this family throughout and after the hospitalization of their premature infant, their initial fear of the death recurred during minor incidences such as a scrape or cold.

Unfortunately, once developed, the parent's fear of death of the premature infant often continues long after he is out of danger. The parents reexperience the fear that their child may die whenever they observe changes in the child. Neonatal professionals who focus more on problems than abilities do not describe the infant's new abilities and strength but generally state that the child is now "out of danger." Such general comments frequently do not completely relieve the parents after possibly weeks of specific comments on the child's difficulties. Many parents of premature infants have their infant sleep beside their bed for up to a year or two, for fear something would happen to the baby and they would not be able to hear him. Some mothers explained that during the night they rolled over and touched the baby to make sure he was still alive. Some parents express that they are very tense at a sign of a cold, the child's first trip to school, or other stressful times.

It is most reassuring to the parents if the nurse describes and shows them their infant's new developments as he matures. For example, one set of parents whose child was apneic, were very concerned that the child would stop breathing and die. The mother had continuous fears that she would come to the hospital and find the isolette empty. When the premature infant began to breathe in a more normal pattern without apnea, the parents were told their child was "out of danger." Although this greatly relieved the parents, the mother continued to dream of an empty crib. The nurse described and had both parents observe their infant's normal breathing pattern. They noticed that although the child's breathing was slightly arrhythmic there was never a long pause, and they learned this was normal. This explicit information about their baby and his new abilities helped to relieve this family's fear of death for their premature infant.

The nurse must prevent the parents' unnecessary fear of death of the premature infant or help them to reduce this fear as soon as the child is out of danger. By describing the individual child's actual condition and abilities, the nurse helps the parents respond with the appropriate fears for their child and cope with realistic fears of his death.

Fear of Abnormal Development. Along with or after the fear of death for their premature infant, the parents often fear that if the child lives he will not develop normally. They are often concerned that the baby's brain, extremities, or other organs have not developed normally.

The parents of a premature infant who was transported very quickly after delivery to a regional center were fearful to visit their child to see him "partly developed." The parents told the home hospital nurse that since the baby was not due for four weeks, the child must not be completely formed. The mother had terrible visions about what parts of the baby might not have been formed. This nurse explained that the baby's organs and extremities were all developed before the time of birth, had the neonatal nurse who cared for the child before transport describe the appearance of the baby, called the regional center to have a picture sent to the mother, and arranged for the father to visit the child immediately. The parents were soon showing the picture of their well-formed infant to friends.

The parents also often fear that the child's experiences soon after birth will lead to abnormal development. For example, one family felt that the child would not develop normally because he had not had any oxygen in the first six hours after delivery, but by the evening, the nursing staff had added oxygen to the baby's isolette. The parents were concerned because that baby did not get oxygen right after birth and felt that his brain might have been damaged. The nurse explained to the family that it is very common for the premature infant to breathe normally in regular air for many hours and six to 12 hours later need extra oxygen. In addition, the nurse explained the blood oxygen level tests and the baby's color characteristics during the first six hours to show that the child had fine oxygenation during that early period.

Another frequent fear of parents is that various medical procedures may lead to abnormal development and retardation of the child. Parents often fear that oxygen will cause abnormal development, if they do not understand that the amount of oxygen is sensitively regulated to supply exactly the amount he needs—no more or less. Frequently monitoring and maintenance of blood oxygen levels has prevented the past retinal problems. Blood transfusions may cause great fears in parents whose religion associates blood transfusion with evil or damaging consequences.

One family with a premature infant had close contact with their infant while he was in the hospital. The parents came in almost daily to care for their infant. The baby was being fed intravenously through a scalp vein and, therefore, had a small needle taped to his head. The nurses explained to the family that the baby was being fed additional food and nutrients through the intravenous tube in his head. These parents, at an interview eight months later, stated that they were concerned about the child's mental abilities since he had "fluid introduced into his brain." After the nurse explained that the IV fluid went under the skin and not through the bone or into the brain, the parents were relieved and wished they had known that before so they would not have continually worried about their child's mental abilities.

The author has found that many families express their fears of abnormal development reluctantly and very seldom during the time of treatment. The nurse not only explains any treatments and their purposes, but asks for feedback from the parents about their thoughts on the meaning of the treatment, and follows up the parents at a later time when it is easier for them to express their continuing fears of abnormal development.

Parents of premature infants continue to be very concerned about their child's development. They focus on weight gain more than the normal full-term infant's parents, and they are often more concerned about the child's developmental stage than are parents of full-term infants. These parents very astutely observe how their infant compares to friends' children of approximately the same age. They are often very upset if their child sleeps through the night, walks, sits, or performs any behavior later than another child. Although parents of full-term infants are often greatly reassured by a summary statement that the child is doing well or developing normally, most parents of premature infants need more explicit explanations to be comforted. The nurse not only states that the child is doing well and developing normally, but also shows the parents the child's actual normal behaviors. An effective approach for reassuring parents of the normal development of their child is for the nurse to perform a physical or behavioral assessment of the child in front of the parents while emphasizing the normal physical appearance of the child, the behavior such as a strong suck and strong muscles, and normal responses such as rooting or stepping. The Brazelton Neonatal Tool, Denver Developmental Test, and other childhood assessment guides described in the "Assessment of Children's Behavior" chapter are useful assessment tools for demonstrating the child's abilities. In addition, the nurse explains to the parents that the number of weeks premature should be subtracted from the child's age when determining his developmental age. It is not fair to expect two one-month-old infants of 30 weeks and 42 weeks gestation, respectively, to be at the same developmental level. Using the age of the child starting with the "due dates" is the most realistic easy way to determine the child's expected developmental level. The nurse must also stress the individuality of each child's development. Parents who have had other children can be reminded that just as those children developed their abilities faster or slower than others at their own individual rates, the premature infant has his own individual rate and pattern that is normal for him.

Guilt

Parents often experience guilt feelings following the premature birth of their infant. Mothers frequently review their experiences in the weeks preceding delivery to identify any of their own actions which they think may have contributed to the premature birth, such as a fall, unusual physical activity, or even a trip or other fairly common experience. The mother has the greatest trouble with guilt if she has had any other abnormal births or did something during the pregnancy that was against the advice of her physician. Unfortunately, most mothers are unaware of the probable causes of prematurity and associate the birth with many probably unrelated experiences.

Fathers usually experience less guilt than the mothers. However, fathers may experience guilt if they encouraged the mother to do something during pregnancy that they later associate with the premature birth, such as taking medication. The father's reaction may increase the mother's guilt. If the father blames the mother for something that she did which may have caused the premature birth, this blame increases the mother's guilt feelings and increases the difficulty between the two parents.

For example, one mother with a premature infant stated that she felt the premature birth was due to an airline trip she had taken during the first trimester of her pregnancy. She stated that she should not have gone on the airplane because the altitude and atmosphere caused the later premature birth. Although the nurses and physicians explained to the mother that the atmosphere in the plane is maintained at a normal level and probably could not cause the early birth several months later, the mother's guilt continued.

It is very difficult for the nurse to help reduce the mother's guilt feelings. The many probable and many unknown factors make it difficult to say absolutely if the mother's experiences did nor did not precipitate the premature delivery. However, it is well accepted that such normal daily behaviors as housecleaning or recreation would probably not precipitate the premature birth of a normal infant from a normal pregnancy. When the premature birth can be associated with one of the known factors such as a birth of twins, teaching the mother about the cause can reduce her anxiety and guilt. When a major cause can not be identified, the nurse can help the parents at least to reduce their focus on the situation they suspect by describing the many other factors which may have contributed to the premature birth.

Parental Attachment

Parental attachment problems due to the parents' feeling of distance and uninvolvement with their premature infant are among the saddest difficulties. Since infants born prematurely often have mild to severe difficulties with respiratory distress, temperature regulation, and other medical problems, the infants require specialized nursing observation and intervention. Since external heat, suctioning, oxygen, and other treatments must be started at first signs of difficulty to prevent additional complications, the premature infant is often rushed away from the parents immediately after delivery. This immediate and rushed separation is described by one mother, who stated, "All I saw was a fast blur. I did not know he was a baby at all." The parents often do not have the opportunity to visually examine, or cuddle, their infant. The immediate separation not only delays the parents' attachment to their child, but often leaves them bewildered and numb as well. Physical, mechanical, and emotional separation are frequent and interfere with the parental attachment process.

Physical Separation. Physical separation is the separation of parent and premature infant by distance. Premature infants are usually taken to an intensive care nursery, often off the obstetrical unit from the mother, or transported to a regional medical center in another city. This separation of parent and premature infant by distance decreases the parents' opportunity for frequent visits and involvement with their child. In a comparative research study, the author has found that parents with transported premature infants have significantly greater interactional deprivation and significantly less chance for involvement with their infants than those with premature infants who remain in their home hospital.[3]

For example, one family described their feelings of lack of closeness with their hospitalized premature infant very explicitly. In an interview with the author, the mother stated, "I do not feel like a mother. I have no baby to show or care for." In a later interview, three months after the infant's return home, the mother still commented, "I am holding my child, but I often wonder where he came from." This child was taken away from the mother for respiratory distress treatment immediately after birth and was quickly transferred to a regional center before she could touch him. Although the father went with the baby to the regional center, the mother felt a complete lack of involvement with the child for the first weeks after birth.

The development of new regional neonatal intensive care centers has increased the ability to provide up-to-date services to the premature infant. However, it also requires that the infants be transported away from the original hospitals to the referral centers, which often creates a separation of great distances and places the infant in a location often unfamiliar to the parents.

There are some ways to decrease the distance between the parent and transported infant. Parents of transported or home hospital infants should be allowed to visit their infants at any time. The distance of separation can be reduced by having one parent go to the premature nursery with the premature infant, although the father is then unable to support his wife during this difficult time. When the mother with a high-risk pregnancy is directly admitted to the regional center for the birth of her infant, the mother and child remain in the same hospital although they may be many miles from their home-town and other family members.

Other means for reducing separation are to provide the parents with facilities that help them stay longer at each visit, such as comfortable chairs in the nursery and private rooms for interacting with the baby, or facilities near the hospital to promote frequent visits, such as a dorm or special arrangements for motel housing. Parent care units where the parent stays with the infant and provides the nurturing care are being developed in many intensive care nurseries, although some units find space difficult to provide.

The nurse can reduce the feeling of separation between parents and child even if there is distance between them by giving something to the parents of the child to help them remember and picture him. A color picture of the child with as little mechanical apparatus in view as possible and the child's eyes open, in an active state, helps to remind the parents of their child. Preferably the picture is taken at the home hospital and left with the parent that remains if the child is transferred. One nurse gave the parents a duplicate of the baby's name band and found that the mother enjoyed showing it to other people to tell them about her baby. The nurse can receive tremendous satisfaction thinking of new ways to remind the parents of their child.

Parents who believe in prayer, meditation, extrasensory perception, or other means of communicating will benefit by nursing actions that help to use their beliefs. The author has found that the parents of premature infants experience tremendous feelings of involvement and helping if they can transfer their feelings of love to their separated infant through prayer or other methods. Although there is no guarantee of success, there is also no risk in using these methods, so the author has tried using techniques to help parents express love and closeness to their infant if they felt useless and were unable to stay with their child at the referral center. The nurse must first determine what type of words she should use in describing the strategy to the parents. For religious parents the nurse may use the word "praying"; for parents who have undergone meditation training, the nurse may call it "meditation"; for parents without these experiences the nurse may call it a "feeling of love." The nurse explains that each parent should find a time without noise and interference when he can lie down and picture the child in his mind. He should lie in a comfortable, relaxed position, breathe slowly, and think about sending "love," "prayers," "good feelings," or other comforting thoughts to his infant. Although the author recommends that the family members do this once or twice a day for approximately ten minutes, many families stated that this relaxed them so much they did it more frequently. Even when they could not visit every day, some parents said they had pictured and felt close to their child this way each day. Although initially some families were upset thinking about the child, they soon began to feel that they were helping and be-

came more relaxed or even fell asleep, feeling comforted. Additional information is needed on the effects of prayer, meditation, and other methods on the premature infant's condition and the parents' feeling of closeness and involvement. Initial experiences show that it is a promising strategy for some families.

Mechanical Separation. Another kind of separation that occurs even when the parents are within arms range of the baby is a mechanical separation. Most premature infants are in an isolette, many may have a special oxygen hood over their heads, and some have eye patches to protect the baby's eyes from a bilirubin light. The mechanical equipment separates the parent and infant as it interferes with visual and cuddling interactions. Less obvious, the mechanical separation also frequently causes a sound overload when the noise in the nursery from the apnea monitors, cardiac monitors, or other machines make it difficult for the parents to hear the normal cooing, sucking, or crying sounds of their infant and to feel comfortable in talking to him.

Some mechanical separation can be decreased. The nurse first determines what mechanical equipment may interfere with the parents' interaction with their infant. She then determines if this equipment is necessary at all times, or if it can be safely removed or altered for the parents' visit. For example, an isolette that is used just for additional external heat for the child is usually not necessary every minute, so the child can be wrapped warmly and held by the parents. However, if the infant is in the isolette for oxygen, he cannot be removed since the oxygen must be maintained at the precise level to keep his blood oxygen at the desired level. An apnea monitor which monitors respiratory rate may be removed while the infant is being held or bathed by the parents, provided a nurse is near to observe the child for any cessation of respiration. A cardiac monitor should sometimes be left in place since it is difficult for the nurse to assess precise cardiac function without interfering with the parents by listening with a stethoscope, however the noise level of the beat indicator may be reduced or turned off if the heart rate alarm is set for the critical heart rates or the nurse can observe the lighted indicator. Safety of the baby is the first concern in removal of mechanical equipment, however, mechanical equipment often can be temporarily removed or altered to help the parents to interact with the child while not endangering him.

Emotional Separation. Emotional separation occurs even when the parents are near the infant and mechanical interference is reduced. Emotional separation occurs when the parents are afraid to interact with the child. Some parents' fears that decrease their interaction include thinking they may hurt the child or that the child may die.

The nurse can help reduce the emotional separation between the parents and the premature infant by including the parents early in the care of the premature infant. The nurse should help the parents develop comforting, feeding, bathing, and diapering behaviors as soon as the infant and parents show readiness. Even the child on a respirator can have the parents diaper and, more important perhaps, soothe the child by stroking his head and arms. Nurses' stroking and parents' recorded talking have been shown to decrease the premature infant's apneas and improve his development.[4,6] Sensitive neonatal nurses admit they often plan their care to include extra touching and stroking of the infants. Montagu describes the infant's need for touching. Labor is "the beginning caressing which should be continued in very special ways in the period immediately following birth and considerable time thereafter."[8] In a controlled study, Dolores Krieger found that therapeutic touch significantly affected the blood hemoglobin in the group of adult patients.[7] When the parents are encouraged to touch and handle their own infant, the infant benefits from the stroking, while the parents benefit from doing something to help the infant. The parents should be encouraged to relax, think about helping the infant, stroke the infant on several surfaces, and notice his reactions. Infants react individually to different pressure touches on different surfaces of their body. The parents will soon learn how to relax and comfort their infant by stroking and enjoy the closeness with him, as shown in Figure 5-2.

The nurse not only includes the parents in participating but also in planning the caretaking behaviors. For example, when a premature infant is weak at sucking he is often intermittently fed with gavage and nipple feedings. Certainly the parents should be involved in planning the schedule of when the infant will be nipple-fed or even breast fed by the mother. Mothers can be instructed in safe procedures for expressing breast milk to leave for the baby when they are home.[10] This not only benefits the baby but also increases the mother's involvement and ensures her milk production when the baby does return home. In addition, before discharge, the parents should not only be involved in the caretaking, but should actually plan when the bath should be given, whether the child will be on demand feedings, when the last feeding before night will be, or other decisions that will develop the child's caretaking pattern similar to the home routine and environment. Without this involvement, parents frequently complain that they were uncomfortable in caring for the child, were not prepared for the change in their home routines, and that their infant had difficulty fitting into their wake, sleep, and eating patterns at home.

Dissatisfaction with Parenting

The parents of a premature infant often feel dissatisfied with their parenting and lack confidence in themselves as parents. Since confidence and satisfaction in parenting come when an infant responds positively to the parents' caretaking actions, it is easy to understand how the parents of the premature infant have great difficulties. The parents' experiences at the birth, their separation following the birth, and their fears of the child's death increase their stress, reduce their perceptiveness of the child's needs and responses, and result in dissatisfaction in their own parenting.

The parents with a premature infant often find it difficult to identify the child's unique behaviors and abilities. The nurse is in a valuable position to help the parents identify the individual characteristics of their child because she has cared for the infant and is sensitive to his reactions to touch and

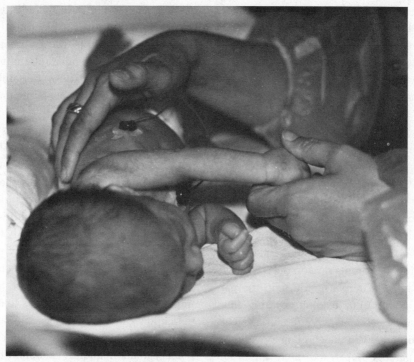

Figure 5-2. When the mother softly strokes her premature infant, the infant relaxes and the mother is pleased with her mothering ability.

caretaking. While the nurse and parents observe the actions of the child, the nurse can comment on their infant's individual behaviors with such words as, "See how he moves his lips to suck, he does that before a feeding as if to tell us he is hungry."

After the parents begin to identify the individual characteristics of their child, they must adopt caretaking behaviors based on these individual traits. For example, premature infants who are overstimulated by quick, rushed, touch motions resulting in the child's uncoordinated extremity movements, need their parents to gently stroke and relax them. One father developed a caretaking behavior based on the individual characteristics of his premature infant when he learned to periodically move the nipple of the bottle in his infant's mouth to stimulate a suck when his infant stopped sucking before receiving adequate nutrition.

Once the parents have identified the individual needs of their premature infant and have developed caretaking behaviors that fill these needs, the parents must notice the child's positive change in behavior in response to their caretaking behaviors. Many parents of premature infants adopt effective parenting behaviors for feeding, cuddling, and bathing the child, however many have difficulty recognizing their infants' reactions and receiving positive feedback. Although the nurse can temporarily reassure the parents that their behaviors in caretaking are good by telling them they are doing a caretaking procedure correctly, this reassurance does not have as strong an impact on the parents as does the feedback and reassurance that comes from the infant himself.

One mother of a prematurely born six-month-old child consistently returned to the outpatient clinic with complaints about the feeding of the child. She complained that the child was eating slowly, not taking enough formula, and was regurgitating some milk. Although in the previous visits the health team tried to reassure the mother by telling her that the baby was healthy and in a normal weight range, the mother was not reassured and returned with the same complaints. Although her feeding behavior seemed adequate to meet the nutritional needs of the child, the mother lacked confidence in it. When the nurse visited the mother to observe the feeding, the mother again complained that the child fell asleep during the feeding and regurgitated a small amount of formula. The nurse not only explained that this was a normal response for any infant but also commented on the baby's behaviors showing satisfaction and comfort during and following the feeding: the good amount of formula that the child drank with his initial quick strong sucking, the baby's very comforted, relaxed sleep after the feeding, and the adequate length of time that the child waited before waking to initiate another feeding. While discussing the positive characteristics and behaviors of the baby that showed adequate feeding and comforting, this mother began noticing and mentioning other behaviors, such as the baby's alertness before feeding and response to the mother's voice. As this mother began to recognize her infant's responses that demonstrated excellent mothering and caretaking behaviors, the mother's feeding complaints were eliminated and her statements showing satisfaction and confidence increased.

Reshifting of Family Roles

The experiences and difficulties related to the premature birth affect the interaction and role of each family member. A denial reaction from one parent can anger the other parent in bargaining or other steps of grief. An anger reaction of one partner also frequently pushes the other partner away and reduces sharing support. Honest sharing of concerns and fears between parents can fortunately lead to closeness and positive feelings.

The parents of a premature infant stated they initially were fairly independent of each other. Following the premature birth, both parents expressed sadness and concern for their child. They started doing more things together, including sharing the household chores and cooking dinner. Working together and having the partner near helped com-

fort each partner. The couple visited their child together each evening. Although the family wished they did not have this stressful experience, they stated that they had become close and learned how to support each other because of it.

Reactions to the premature birth also may change the relationship between the parents and their other children. So much of the parents attention and fears are directed toward the premature infant that the other children often feel unloved. This is especially true of younger children who do not understand where the parent is and that they are loved even when the parent is absent and for infants who miss the consistent touch and voice of their parents. The parents with a premature infant should recognize the needs of the other children and plan their schedule to meet some of their needs as well. Although joint visiting of parents to the premature infant helps them support each other, it leaves the other children alone without a parent for possibly long periods of time, if their infant is in a distant regional center. If there is no consistent caretaker, such as a relative or friend who had cared for the children numerous times before, the parents may need to alternate their visiting so that one parent remains home with the other children.

For example, a couple visited their transported premature infant and stayed overnight at the regional center so they could support each other and see the child frequently during those few days. They left their seven-year-old son at home with neighbors during the weekends. Although the parents spent some extra time with their son during the week and explained to him that the new baby was sick and needed them to visit on the weekends, the child increasingly misbehaved when they were away. During the fourth weekend when the parents visited their premature infant in the hospital, the son set fire to the barn resulting in the desired return of his parents. When the parents talked to their son and rearranged the schedule for the mother to visit during the week and father on the weekends, the mischievous behavior of their son decreased.

The nurse should help the parents to identify

the unique needs of themselves and all family members, generate alternative actions to meet the needs, and select the coping patterns and relationships that would help their family. The nurse can do this by asking the parents about their work and recreation needs and about any young or elderly family members, their ages, and what sort of arrangements were made for them during their visits to the premature nursery. It is important for the nurse to communicate the parents' plan for visiting with the other nurses in the intensive care unit so all nurses will support the parents' decisions and plan for visiting. Although nurses rightfully encourage parents to visit frequently to foster the parental attachment to the child, they must recognize the family's childrearing, working, or other needs. If the parents cannot visit as frequently as the nursing staff expects, instead of assuming the parents are unconcerned the nurse identifies whether the cause for the infrequent visits is one of the parental difficulties, such as fear of death, or appropriate coping to meet other family needs.

Inability to Express Their Emotional Needs

Many parents of premature infants have difficulty expressing their emotional needs and fears. Since the premature birth situation is new and very stressful for most families, their reactions are often unique for them. A woman who is often optimistic may suddenly be sad and depressed. Parents who usually communicate freely may find it hard to share their sad feelings. Fairly independent family members may find that each wants more companionship to avoid the depression of being alone. Whatever reaction occurs for the family, most families find that it is hard to identify and express their emotional needs and fears and therefore find it difficult to seek the needed assistance.

For example, the father of the premature infant, mentioned earlier, who had been fed intravenously through the scalp vein was usually verbal and assertive in his job in a computer firm. However, in the crisis of the premature birth, this father

was unable to express his fear that the IV fluid was going into the child's brain and causing brain damage. This fear continued until the author's interview with the family six months after the baby's discharge. The father stated that because he was not a "professional father" he did not have much experience, did not know what was occurring with the child, and did not know what to ask. His inability to express his fears resulted in prolonged stress for the family.

Many families have difficulty expressing when they need information or when they have been overloaded with information. Some parents listen to the nurse's explanation of the baby's condition and their treatment in the nursery and nod, smile, and state they understand, although many times they need additional information on a very basic level, such as how the baby will be fed or diapered. Just as some families find it difficult to express their need for more information, many parents find it difficult to express that they are getting too much information. Too much information at one time about the child and treatments can lead to confusion and greater anxiety for the parents.

For example, parents who visited their premature infant for the first time after his transportation to the regional center were told about the baby's difficulties with digestion and respirations, the treatments like the suctioning and respirator assistance, the baby's care such as feeding schedule, and the finances such as insurance coverage. As a result of receiving all of the information at once without help to arrange priorities for action, the parents had difficulty acting on any of the information. They were afraid to visit the baby, did not check on their insurance policy, and did not follow any of the suggestions they were given. Unfortunately, this family was unable to express that they were overloaded with information and needed very simple instructions on what they could do to help the infant and family.

Although the family with a premature infant often has great difficulty expressing emotional needs and fears, the nurse can provide the environment and the relationship to help the family members identify their need, express what difficulties they are having, and directly ask for the support and help they need.

For the nurse to help the family express their emotional needs and fears, the nurse must evaluate the impact of explanations on the family members and use this evaluation to determine what other information and explanations are needed. Although explanations are most effective at the baby's bedside, where the nurse can show the family members the baby's characteristics or the equipment being discussed, the family members are often very distracted in the nursery environment. One very effective means of evaluating the family's response to explanations is for the nurse to accompany the family to a quieter area, such as a cafeteria or parent room, for a cup of coffee. This provides a more informal and less distracting environment where the parents can think about their infant, their needs, and their concerns. A consistent primary nurse is able to build on past explanations and help the family identify and express their own needs.

The nurse helps the family set priorities for their actions. This includes not only a description of the child and difficulties, but also of what the parents can do to help. A list of actions for the parents put in the form of priorities is most valuable in helping the parents to focus on their most important needs and to act in the most productive way.

Trained parents of past premature infants are very valuable in helping the new parents to identify and express their emotional needs. Past parents that share the type of reactions which they experienced while still listening for the individual reactions of the new family help the new parents identify their concerns and questions. The new parents feel relieved to know that other parents have experienced similar difficulties that are not unusual or signs of mental illness.

Past parents of premature infants may provide excellent support for present parents and help them identify their emotional needs. In helping families to set up a self-help organization, the nurse helps to train the parents in the essential aspects of counseling. The nurse trains the previous parent "counselor" to:

1. Identify and describe to the present parents their concern for the family's reactions and difficulties related to premature birth and their role as family advocate.
2. Support the present parents by phone, at the hospital, or home contact as needed by the present family.
3. Recognize the uniqueness of families' experiences following premature births, with no two families experiencing it exactly the same.
4. Focus on the family difficulties, such as uncertainty, while avoiding forecasting the future of the infant.
5. Help the present parents identify their family problems and generate their own alternatives of action.

NURSING APPROACHES

The specific nursing actions described below apply many basic nursing approaches that are discussed in later chapters. Assessment, counseling, teaching, role theory, family involvement, financial, and primary nursing strategies are all essential to the nurse working with the family of a premature infant and used in the following critical periods.

Critical Periods

There are specific critical periods for the family in the premature birth experience which are important times for nursing intervention to prevent or reduce the family problems. These critical periods are very stress-producing and often result in a crisis for the family if their usual coping behaviors do not adequately reduce the stress. The author has found in practice with many families with premature infants that the following experiences tend to be critical times frequently resulting in crises.

The Start of Labor. The initiation of labor can be a crisis-producing event for many families. The family is often unprepared for the onset of premature labor, with no arrangements for transportation or child care. The primigravida mother may be uncertain that her symptoms are labor and may find it difficult to convince others. This unpreparedness and disbelief leads the family to uncertainty and stress.

For example, one mother explained that she started labor at 28 weeks gestation. She knew that labor was beginning when she lost fluid from the bag of waters, similar to her previous labor and delivery several years earlier. She called to her husband who was at home, but he did not believe her because it "wasn't time." As she explained in a frightened tone of voice he also became concerned because they had just moved to the town and he did not know the way to the hospital. When the mother called the physician to say that labor had started, the office nurse would not let her talk to the physician and said that she was probably having a few abdominal cramps. Later at the hospital, the mother had a short labor and was assisted by her husband who had remembered some of the Lamaze techniques from the previous child. Fortunately, this family's neighbor watched for the family's son to return home from school and explained to him that the parents had gone to the hospital because the new baby was about to arrive. This family experienced a crisis at the unexpected labor, but fortunately had a neighbor to help with some of their concerns.

Delivery. At the time of a premature delivery the nurses and physicians are preparing for the birth of an infant who may be in critical condition. Their focus is on the survival of the infant. When a risk infant is delivered, he is usually rushed to an area where neonatal specialists can assess him and provide warmth, suctioning, and other preventive interventions. If the neonatal team is not actually present in a delivery room, the child may be rushed to an intensive care nursery. Since the child is the center of focus, especially if he has any difficulties, the mother and father are often forgotten by the medical team. This is a time of great stress for them.

For example, in one family who gave birth to a premature infant of 26 weeks gestation, the mother commented that she had not seen her baby for he

was rushed out of the delivery room. The father said he saw a baby, two nurses and a doctor rushing past him to the intensive care nursery. He continued to wait in the father's waiting room; he thought that it was his baby but was afraid to ask. He finally went to the nurses' station and asked about the baby. The infant had been rushed away and no one had informed him of the sex, weight, or other vital statistics.

Although the nurse certainly will not impede the infant's care, she can reduce the effect of these events on the family. Experienced delivery room or neonatal nurses who are well prepared for the birth of a high-risk infant with prearranged training and equipment will be less tense and have less need to rush in the last minutes when delivery is imminent. Having a special neonatal team prepared and in close contact with the delivery room allows the team to arrive in time to prepare for a risk delivery, to carry out special treatments effectively and confidently, and to give the obstetrical team time to care for the parents at this critical time. Some professionals feel that fathers should be encouraged to attend the birth of a premature infant as well as any other infant, for the uncertainty of the situation may be worse than the actual risk delivery. One primary nurse from the clinic, obstetric, or neonatal department should take responsibility for working with the parents during this critical period while others work with the infant.

Explanations about the Infant. Explanations about the infant can be stressful for the parents, but no explanations or conflicting explanations are even more stressful. For example, when the father in the previous example went to the nurses' station, the nurse did not know if it was his baby that rushed by. She told him to remain in the waiting room and someone would come and talk to him, however, no one came. Although he was very concerned about his wife, he did not want to leave the waiting room because he wanted to hear about the baby. The father was left alone with tremendous uncertainties—as was his wife. He asked everyone that went by about his baby and when he asked one nurse who was present at the delivery, he was finally told that the baby was a one-and-a-half-pound male and that boys of that size have little chance for survival. That is the only information he received at that time. The parents' period of uncertainty was a very critical time for them. Even when they were informed many weeks later that the child was ready for discharge, they were still very concerned because of the initial statement by the nurse that a child of that size had very little chance.

Nurses can lessen the critical aspects of this event by talking with the family immediately after delivery, even if it is just to say that the child is being seen by the neonatal team and they just do not know about the infant's condition as yet. Parents can handle the waiting much better with each other's and staff support than when they are left alone and ignored.

Information given the parents should be honest and based on their individual child's abilities and potential problems. Information about percentages of other infants the size of their child is sometimes helpful, but only in conjunction with a detailed individual assessment of their own child. Along with discussing the potential difficulties, it is important to tell the parents what is being done to prevent or watch for those difficulties. The nurse should also explain that the child's difficulties are related to early birth and will decrease as the child continues to grow and develop, as he would have during the same time in the uterus, to decrease the parents' fear that the problems will remain through his life. If there is a likelihood that the child will need additional specialized care that the home hospital cannot provide, this would be the best time to tell them that although the child is getting the care he needs at this time, he may need some special care and equipment at a regional center. Information on the length of time the child will be at risk can be important to the family, so they will know how long the uncertainty of the crisis will last and when to feel relief that most of the danger has passed. An infant's worsening condition or imminent death must be reported to the parents immediately and honestly.

In addition, it is very important for the nurses and physicians to give coordinated information to the parents about their child. The degree and type of difficulties should be expressed similarly by both. A problem which is mentioned must be discussed until its resolution can be explained. Very often the family is told about the difficulty but not about the resolution of the problem, therefore the parents think the problem is continuing. One way to have a consistent story and to continue it over time is to assign a neonatal primary nurse to work with the family to plan explanations, coordinate approach with the medical staff, and design individual interventions for the family. The unit Kardex reports and weekly meetings are excellent opportunities for nurses to coordinate their specific messages and plans for each family. Frequently the physician gives the most detail about the medical difficulties while the nurse gives information on the changing condition, caretaking, and individuality of the child. The nurse talks to the family about the infant's abilities, how well formed he is, and some of the very individual characteristics which are important in the development of maternal and paternal attachment. This consistent individualized information reduces the parents' stress.

The Postpartum Unit. The mother's return to the postpartum unit can be a critical event for the family. When she returns to the postpartum unit without her baby, she often sees many other mothers smiling at and cuddling their normal full-term infants. Although the mother of the premature infant finds it emotionally difficult to be with other mothers with their normal, actively feeding babies, many prefer the company of other mothers to being alone. Many mothers of premature infants have stated that the other mothers in their room comforted them and became close to them during their time of crisis. They also stated, though, that the most depressing time was when the full-term babies were brought out to the other mothers for feeding, because they "had no baby."

For example, one mother who delivered her premature infant by cesarean section was placed with three other mothers with normal newborns in a postpartum room. This mother had great difficulty at first when the normal newborns were brought to all the other mothers, but the concern and interest of the other mothers demonstrated by even sharing some of the bathing and diapering routine helped her. This mother stated that although it was hard to be in the room with other mothers, she preferred it to being alone in her room or with a mother who had experienced the same loss as she. Unfortunately, the crisis for this mother was actually increased due to the lack of understanding by the nursing staff. Several times a nurse came to the mother of the premature infant, who had then been transported to another hospital, and scolded her for not being ready to feed her baby. Understandably, this lack of recognition and understanding from the nursing staff greatly upset the mother.

Nurses can help reduce the stresses at this time by discussing the options of room placement with the mother. Some of the mothers do prefer being in a room alone, if financially possible, in order to privately grieve with the family over the premature birth. Other mothers prefer having company. If the mother is placed in a room with other mothers, the nurse must teach the mothers with the full-term infants to develop a supportive relationship of understanding rather than overprotectiveness. Some of these roommate mothers have greatly helped mothers with premature infants in many ways, including going with the mother to visit her child, letting the mother with the premature infant help to dress or diaper their babies, and just understanding the concern of the mother over the health of her baby.

Some professionals advocate that the premature mother should be returned to a unit with other mothers while others believe that she should be returned to a private room. Either absolute position can be harmful. Individual arrangement of the postpartum environment will meet the parents' individual needs best.

The Parents' First Visit to the Nursery. For the numerous families who did not touch or have eye-to-eye contact with the infant after delivery, the parents' first visit to their premature infant in the nursery is a very critical period. They see their premature infant who is slightly smaller and scrawnier than their imagined full-term infant, with tubes and strange equipment, and possibly in a nursery far from home.

For example, one mother with a premature infant was afraid to see the infant. Although the grandparents and father had all visited the intensive care nursery and touched the child, the mother was very apprehensive about going to see her baby. She was unable to express any definite fears at that time, however, later she mentioned that she was afraid that her child would look horrifying and that she had had many dreams about his terrible and bloody appearance. Her fears about the appearance of the child were worse than the reality. When the mother did see the child, with the nurse's help to see clearly through the porthole of the isolette to her child's beautiful face and movements, her fears about his appearance were reduced.

The nurse can help reduce the stress during the parents' first visit to the premature infant by setting up an environment that highlights the individual infant and reduces the other distracting elements in the environment. The nurse should encourage the parents to visit the child as soon as possible by offering to be with them during the visit, helping the mother to get to the nursery if she needs assistance, and telling the mother that her fears of the baby's appearance are normal and can be alleviated by seeing the child. The nurse should reduce distractions by turning down the monitor beat volume, while visually monitoring the baby, wiping the sides of the isolette of moisture to aid vision, putting tubings of the child under a blanket, and removing unnecessary equipment. In addition, the nurse helps relax the mother and increase interaction with her child by providing a chair near the child at a height that permits eye-to-eye contact and stroking the infant to show that it does not hurt the child.

Transport to a Regional Neonatal Intensive Care Center. If the baby is transported from place of delivery to a regional center for intensive care, this is an extremely stressful time for the parents because of the potentially critical condition requiring transport of the infant and the removal of the infant from them. The parents' visit and contact with their baby before transport fosters their attachment and prevents imagined fears of their child's appearance. There is often a short time before transport when the child has been stabilized and the parents may see the infant. The familiar medical team from the home hospital and new medical team from the regional center jointly talk to the parents to explain where the child is going, who will be responsible for his care, the specialty experience of the personnel, the phone number and people to contact at the center, and the primary nurse at the home hospital or public health nurse who will support them during this crisis. It is explained that the parents are welcome at any time to visit the child in the medical center, and if possible a relative can accompany the team by ambulance or car to the medical center. As soon as the child arrives at the medical center, the neonatal primary nurse calls the parents and notifies them of the condition in which he arrived. A picture of the baby may be sent to the parents so they will have something to remind them of the baby. A nurse at the home hospital or in the community also works closely with the family to help them collect and understand information about their infant and cope with the stresses.

The criticalness of this transportation period is shown in the following example. One mother of a transported premature infant was consulted by the medical team from the regional center when they came to get the child. She stated that seeing the child, talking to the medical team, and knowing where the child was going comforted her. In addition, the husband went with the child to the regional center so that he could stay up-to-date on the child's condition and do whatever he could for him. After the infant and her husband left, the mother suddenly realized the critical situation. The child she had just delivered was being rushed to a medical center along with her husband. She felt very alone and became hysterical. Between her sobs she stated that she just could not handle the situation alone, that too much was happening, and that

everything was going wrong. Unfortunately, the nurses in the postpartum unit avoided her, apparently because they did not know what to say and had no way to cheer her. However, another mother on the unit heard her and sat with her during part of the evening until the phone call came from her husband that the infant had arrived safely at the regional center. This other mother knew that she could not reassure the mother that the child would be fine, but did support her in her difficulty of being alone and worried about the child. This crisis intervention role can often be taken by other mothers, relatives, or the nurse. The nurse must assess who is capable and willing to provide this support to reduce the stress during transfer of the infant.

The Mother's Return Home Without Her Baby. The mother's return home without her child is a very critical event. The mother normally returns home alone while her premature infant remains in a nursery for additional observation and treatment. The mother often finds this a very sad time. She is no longer pregnant yet often feels she does not have a baby either. She feels very alone and her home seems very quiet. The mother often does not know what to do with herself and her anxiety and fears for the child increase along with the loneliness. She is also often at a loss of what to tell friends, fearful about sending out birth announcements, and uncertain what to tell her other young children who were prepared for the arrival of a new child and are now confused about the parents' lone return and sadness.

For example, one father described his wife's reaction when she returned home without her child. She spent most of the day walking up and down the hall looking in the baby's room as if hoping that the child would be there. Although he came home from work early and the eldest son helped with the housekeeping chores, the mother seemed very lonely without their baby. They were very disturbed at the physician's suggestion that they not announce the birth of their child in the local newspaper since the child might not live, because the announcement of the birth to other people was very important to them. Although the baby spent nine weeks in the intensive care unit, he developed normally and returned home. In an interview three months after discharge, the family still expressed concern about the child's birth announcement. After the nurse encouraged them to personally contact the local papers, the announcement was printed in the next week and the parents proudly sent announcements to relatives, friends, and even the nurse.

The nurse can greatly help reduce the stresses at the mother's return home without her infant. Explaining that the reaction of loneliness and looking for the child are normal can reduce the mother's fears about her loneliness. The neonatal nurse who will follow the infant and family calls the mother before and on the day she returns home to establish a pattern of visiting and communication between the nurse and parents. The community health nurse talks with the mother about plans for the infant's return and explanations to friends and relatives. This preparation for the mother's return home without the baby begins before her discharge from the hospital and continues after her return home. Something the mother can take home to remind her of the baby, such as a picture or duplicate baby bracelet from the child, can increase her feeling of closeness with the child. The nurse must individualize her nursing actions to determine what reminder of the baby will work best for each parent.

The Baby's Homecoming. Although the parents are pleased that they will have their infant home, they often continue to feel the child needs special care and are very concerned whether they can give that care at home. Many parents state they cannot stay awake all night to watch the infant.

Parents who have not taken care of any other children before have additional anxieties related to caring for an infant; parents who have had other children are anxious about caring for this one who was very small and required continued observation and care; while parents who have cared for a previous premature infant may have little anxiety if the child developed normally or great anxiety if developmental problems, crib death, or childhood deaths occurred. It is often near the time of discharge that parents, who previously had hoped for an early discharge of the child, start to express the hope that the infant can stay longer.

For example, one mother with a premature infant who had been hospitalized for four weeks and subsequently developed normally was very hesitant to take her infant home, even though she had fed, bathed, and cared for him during his stay in the hospital. During several interviews about her fears of taking the infant home, the mother expressed her fear that the baby would stop breathing as she had seen him do in the hospital, and she stated that she had no apnea monitor or other means to continuously watch the child. Unfortunately, no one had told the mother that the baby's reflexes, breathing patterns, and physiological states were all developing so that he did not need the intensive care he had initially. After the primary nurse guided the mother's observations to the baby's abilities and the staff nurses stated the baby did not need close watching, she became excited about the infant's homecoming.

The nurse has a very important role in reducing the crisis related to the child's return home to the family. She includes the family in the care of the child as soon as possible. It is often possible for the family to stroke and feed the child in an isolette. The nurse explains to the parents in the very beginning that the premature infant's difficulties such as temperature regulation and breathing are related to his early birth and that as he develops, his temperature regulation and breathing pattern will develop normally. The nurse expresses that uncomplicated problems related to prematurity are temporary and stresses that the child is continuing to develop normally although out of the womb. The nurse describes how the baby is developing as he reaches milestones, such as gaining sucking strength to suck some formula, regulating his breathing to need no reminding, and maintaining his temperature with blankets and no extra external heat. The parents recognize their infant's progress if changes in nursing care such as removal of the monitor or removal from the isolette are explained with emphasis on the child's new abilities. By the time of discharge the parents who have recognized the infant's development are less fearful of accepting the responsibility for his care. As in any discharge planning, the nursing assessment and plan are developed early with collaboration between parents, physician, community nurse, and neonatal nurse. The transition of nursing care of the infant and parents from the hospital setting to the community setting should be coordinated. The community health nurse visits and communicates with the hospital nurse, and the primary hospital nurse visits the mother and public health nurse in the community.

Changes in the Child. Any change in the infant can be a very critical event for the new parents who fear the worst and assume any change is bad. Even positive changes based on the child's new abilities are critical times for the family. A premature infant who develops normally needs progressively less intensive care and is often moved from the initial location of intensive care to a less acute location in the nursery. Although this change is a positive one based on the child's continued development, parents who come to visit their child see an empty isolette or another baby in their infant's place and panic that their child has died. Certainly any changes indicating additional complications in the child's condition, such as starting of apnea, administering of oxygen, or use of respirator, are crisis-producing for the parents.

Even after the child has developed normally and returns home, the parents find that changes can produce panic. Any behavioral changes such as the infant's first sleeping through the night or arching his back to roll over, can cause fear reactions for the family. Some parents fear when their infant first sleeps through the night that he may have suffocated and shake him to be certain he is alive, while others fear their child is having seizures when he is just arching his back to learn to roll over.

The nurse greatly reduces the parents' stress reactions to normal developmental changes by immediately describing the positive aspects in their child and teaching the parents to anticipate the expected developmental changes. Explanations about the new behaviors the infant is developing and the treatment changes to expect help prevent the parents' crisis reaction to change. The nurse calls the parents to tell them of any positive treatment change, such as movement of the child from the nursery or removal from the isolette to crib. The community health nurse teaches the parents about expected developmental changes in the growing child and normal childhood difficulties such as minor injuries and illnesses to prevent their panic.

SUMMARY

The parents' experiences surrounding the premature birth cause numerous serious difficulties for the family. The nurse's ability to care for the premature infant, consistency in being available to talk with the parents, practice in various family settings, and concern for sending the infant into an optimal family environment place her in a unique and valuable position to help the family with a premature infant. By recognizing the parents' potential problems, she can prevent or reduce the effects on the family and move toward her goal of returning a healthy infant to a healthy family.

REFERENCES

1. Babson, S. G. and R. Benson. *Management of High-Risk Pregnancy and Intensive Care of the Neonate.* St. Louis: C. V. Mosby Co., 1971.
2. Johnson, S. H. and J. Grubbs. "The Premature Infant's Reflex Behaviors: Effect on the Maternal-Child Relationship." *JOGN Nursing,* 4 #3, May/June 1975, 15–20.
3. Johnson, S. H. "The Extent of Interactional Deprivation of the Mother with a Transported Premature Infant." San Jose State Foundation Grant, 1977.
4. Katz, V. "Auditory Stimulation and Developmental Behavior of the Premature Infant." *Nursing Research,* 20 #3, 1971, 196.
5. Klaus, M. H. and A. A. Fanaroff. *Care of the High-Risk Neonate.* Philadelphia: W. B. Saunders, 1973.
6. Kramer, M. et al. "Extra Tactile Stimulation of the Premature Infant." *Nursing Research,* 24, September/October 1975, 324–334.

7. Krieger, D. "Therapeutic Touch: The Imprimatur of Nursing." *American Journal of Nursing,* May 1975, 784–787.
8. Montagu, M. F. A. *Touching: The Human Significance of the Skin.* New York: Columbia University Press, 1971, 63.
9. Parmelee, A. H. and L. Liverman. *Prematurity.* Los Angeles: Department of Pediatrics, University of California, 1971.
10. ——. "Maintaining a Milk Supply While Separated from the Infant." Menlo Park, Calif.: Nursing Mothers Counsel, Inc., 1977.
11. ——. "Lowering Infant Mortality—How Far Have We Come?" Stanford Medical Alumni Association, *Stanford M. D.,* 13 #2, 1974, 2–6.

ADDITIONAL READINGS

1. Beckwith, L. "Caregiver—Infant Interaction and the Development of the High Risk Infant." In *Intervention Strategies for High Risk Infants and Young Children.* Baltimore, Md.: University Park Press, 1976, 119–139.
2. Choi, M. W. "A Comparison of Maternal Psychological Reactions to Premature and Full-Size Newborns." *Maternal-Child Nursing Journal,* 2 #1, Spring 1973, 1–12.
3. Christensen, A. Z. "Coping with the Crisis of a Premature Birth—One Couple's Story." *MCN,* January/February 1977, 33–37.
4. Kennell, J. and M. Klaus. "Care of the Mother of the High-Risk Infant." *Clinical Obstetrics and Gynecology,* 14 #3, 1971, 926.
5. Slade, C. I. et al. "Working with Parents of High-Risk Newborns." *JOGN Nursing,* 6 #2, March/April 1977, 21–25.

PERTINENT ORGANIZATIONS

NATIONAL
- *LaLeche League International*
9616 Minneapolis Ave
Franklin Park, Illinois, 60131
Provides support and help resolving problems for mothers who are breast feeding. Will help mothers with premature infants.

LOCAL
- Families with difficulties related to premature birth may receive help from local religious groups or premature infant family groups established in some communities.

The Physically Disabled Child

Selcuk T. Sahin, R.N. Ed.D.

CHAPTER SIX

The physically disabled child is a child whose growth and development differs significantly from the majority of children because of a physiological-physical difficulty. This child's needs and pattern of life are similar to those of the normal child. However, the norms have to be altered in order to promote his maximum potential. Viewed in this way, the family and the nurse can aid the child's self-actualization and thus ameliorate the disabling nature of his deviation. Self-actualization includes becoming what he can become and being satisfied with it.

Understanding the full impact of a physically disabled child on the family members and the family unit requires a review of the family functions and responsibilities. Family difficulties usually arise because the family members and family unit either fail or are at risk of failing to accomplish tasks expected of them by the society.

The present trends in our society point to inclusion of physically disabled persons at all levels of social life. Many special education laws in the country, for instance, are designed to welcome such children to the mainstreams of education. Such mainstreaming at a young age and social inclusion at various ages of the physically disabled person can help make life easier for his family and their perceived failure less crippling. The nurse can capitalize on such new trends in her counseling of the families of the physically disabled child. More important, the nurse can link herself with existing and newly developing institutions and groups to make herself available to a large population of families through various media. These new trends open many doors to nursing while at the same time placing challenging demands on the nurse. It is an opportune time to develop a nursing model—to develop a much needed role to fill a painful gap.

BASIC CONCEPTS

A physical disability is a physiologically based deviation from the norm that negatively affects the family's pattern of daily living. Such a condition has the potential to arrest the maximum growth and development and self-actualization of the family and of the disabled child. A physical disability may or may not be associated with mental disability. The next chapter will discuss specific family problems related to a mentally disabled child, while this chapter focuses on the family with a physically disabled child.

There are many types of physical disabilities and their characteristics will greatly influence the family. The most influential factors are: 1) present at birth (myelodysplasia) versus later diagnosed or later occurring (juvenile myasthenia gravis, rheumatic heart disease); 2) life-threatening (congenital heart disease) versus not life-threatening (congenital hip dislocation); 3) long-term and potentially permanently handicapping (cerebral palsy) versus short-term and often treatable (cleft lip and palate); 4) substantially interfering with daily routines (deaf-mutism) versus not substantially interfering with daily routines (syndactyly); 5) outwardly observable (phocomelia) versus not outwardly observable (psychomotor epilepsy).

The impact on the family of having a physically disabled child is more intense if the physical disability is life-threatening, potentially permanently handicapping, substantially interfering with daily routines, and outwardly observable, and the presence of physical disabilities at birth makes bonding difficult.

Impact on the Family. The functions of the family are closely related to the expectations of the society of which it is a part. The family is a system of dynamic relationships among its members and with the community. As such, the family provides means of meeting the needs of its own members and of society. The main family responsibilities that correspond to the societal expectations of the family functions are: 1) procreation (of a normal child), 2) provision of safe environment, 3) promotion of growth and development potential, and 4) socialization of the young.

When a family procreates a new member who is potentially less than what the society requires for *its* survival—such as a physically disabled child —the family is at risk of being a failure. The birth constitutes a crisis and brings about grief because the birth of a potentially unacceptable member of society means that the family has failed its procrea-

tion function. All other functions of the family are at risk, and this calls for exceptional parenting.

Nurse's Role. The challenge for the nurse is to help the family meet its societal obligations in the best ways possible under the circumstances: to help the family ameliorate the impact of perceived failure and to promote the growth and development potential of this new member. A positive way is to work with what is available—strengths of the family and of the child—so that this event does not become a handicap for the family and the child. The nurse can help the family to see that this child can meet the societal expectations to a degree and can try to increase this degree. To be effective the nurse needs to show honesty and courage, respect for the family, competence in her knowledge and skills, and unquestionable caring.

Although various nursing functions, such as teaching, counseling, and advocacy, need to be carried out in the nursing management of the family with a physically disabled child, a crucial nursing approach is that of a case-manager. Depending upon the nature of the physical disability, the child and family are probably being seen by various specialists: geneticist, orthopedist, urologist, neurologist, and so on. The family who is faced with a sometimes splintered health care delivery system is often confused by at times conflicting opinions and usually overwhelmed by the demands made by the various specialists. Each specialist may suggest a plan of action and daily routine to the family which is reasonable on its own but, when combined with expectations of other specialists, may be quite unreasonable. The nurse can play the role of a "case-manager" or "coordinator of services" and keep an overall perspective on what is expected of the family. Furthermore, in such a role, the nurse can act as the translator in specialist-family contacts. She can be the helping professional who assists the family to "make sense of it all," makes plans, and mobilizes to activate such plans.

Present Trends. Present trends in the management of special-needs children include mainstreaming, parental involvement, and individualized programs. *Mainstreaming* means the inclusion of the special-needs child within the larger order of social and educational programs. The special needs must be met within the confines of regular programs as much as possible.[3] The special-needs children must *not* be separated out. *Parental involvement* has as its premises that parents are important, knowledgeable, and work to actualize what is best for their children. *Individualized health and education programs* are designed to meet the needs of the special-needs children without stigmatizing labels and with the objective of providing equal opportunity for all children.

Overlapping all three main trends is the developmental approach embellished by a normalization concept. Since all children are different, differences are normal and all children are therefore normal.[4] As such, the special-needs children need not conform to the usual programs, but the programs must be altered to promote the maximum potential of the children.

The family is the central unit of society and is influenced by the community of which it is a part. The family unit, therefore, can obtain help from and has responsibilities to the community. The family as a unit is in fact larger than the sum of its parts; it has a life of its own which is directly related to societal expectations. The family is our client and we nurse the family coping with the physically disabled child.

Family Difficulties. The birth of a physically disabled child is usually an unexpected traumatic event in a family's life. It brings about crisis, grief, and chronic sorrow. The extent of such family reactions differs from family to family. Some influential factors that determine the extent of family difficulties are: 1) family preparation before birth, 2) family economic status, 3) the extent of anomaly, 4) family's previous knowledge and feelings regarding others with such anomalies, 5) attitudes of health personnel and other helping professionals involved, 6) family cultural background, 7) styles of family living, 8) family connectedness which will define their support group, 9) family dynamics and

role differentiation, 10) age of the family and its members and corresponding family tasks, and 11) sex of the child. What are considered to be major problems with one family may not be perceived as a problem with another. Parenting is difficult in any circumstances, but parenting of a high-risk child requires exceptional qualities.

The family unit itself has special needs and faces major difficulties which mainly arise from potential failure to meet societal expectations. The family difficulties so experienced are many, depend on many factors, may change over time, and require special knowledge and skills from the nurse. Above all, the nurse must be aware of this family-needs variance and be flexible enough to adjust her nursing approaches to the particular family make-up and specific problems. This skill is probably the most crucial one and usually is built over time, with experience. A prerequisite to such expertise is the acquiring of knowledge regarding some common family difficulties and some appropriate nursing strategies.

The following section will elaborate on some common difficulties experienced by the families of physically disabled children and mention some nursing strategies which can aid the family to reach self-actualization despite such difficulties. These difficulties, concisely shown in Figure 6-1, will be discussed under three major headings: 1) the birth of a physically disabled child, 2) as the child grows, and 3) future children.

FAMILY DIFFICULTIES RELATING TO THE BIRTH OF A PHYSICALLY DISABLED CHILD

Birth of a physically disabled child refers to either the time of biological birth or the period in which the child is diagnosed as being physically disabled. For instance, a child with meningomyelocele is diagnosed at birth; a child with moderate or minor cerebral palsy might be diagnosed at several months or years of age; a juvenile diabetic or epileptic may be diagnosed at school age.

Figure 6-1. Difficulties Experienced by Families of Physically Disabled Children

Difficulties Relating to the Birth
  Being told
    grief
    shock
    disbelief
    anger, fear, guilt
    bonding

Difficulties Experienced as the Child Grows
  Searching for causes
    learning to differentiate between useful and not-so-useful
      professional advice
    need for receiving an honest diagnosis and prognosis
  Long-term management
    finances
    family dynamics
    self-actualization of family members
    inadequate servicing or over-servicing
    peer acceptance of the child and the family
    long-term care of the child

Difficulties Related to Future Children
  Genetic couseling
  Amniocentesis and abortion

Although both the birth and the diagnosis seem to bring about similar familial reactions and family difficulties, there is a basic difference in bonding. While bonding may be difficult with a child with a congenital deformity, this may not be a factor for the child who is diagnosed to have a physical disability at age two or four or eight. On the other hand, feelings of guilt may be more intense when the physical disability is diagnosed later in life, especially in those instances where the particular disability was not actually congenital or genetic, such as rheumatic heart disease or encephalopathy pursuant to a severe viral infection.

Difficulties Relating to Being Informed

How and what the family is told about the physical defect greatly influences their grief and initial bonding to the child.

Grief. Most families display feelings of shock, disbelief, and anger when they learn the diagnosis and the possible prognosis. All individuals and families wish to procreate a perfect offspring, but the family with a disabled child has failed in its procreation function by bringing into life a less than perfect new member.

One mother of a cleft-lip baby said that the room started blurring and buzzing when she heard about the defect. She could not believe it. The new father also said that he felt as though someone hit him hard in the belly; he felt dizzy. Both parents were shocked by the news.

There is a period of disbelief in an unexpected and unwanted event—a bad dream. An observable physical defect is immediately noticed. The only pertinent denial is the family's denial of the *impact* of the problem on the child or the family. A nonobservable defect may allow a longer period of disbelief. In most instances this is a short (one to six days), self-limiting time-dependent phase.[7] As one couple put it, "we thought we were having a bad dream, we'd wake up and everything would be all right. We thought maybe the pediatrician mistook our baby for another, or someone changed the baby. But this was for only a short time."

Parents experience anger at professionals, the rest of the family, but rarely at the child. Fear of the infant's death, the secret wish of death (of the defective child), and the parental guilt feeling compound into an overriding sadness characterized by feelings of helplessness. Another characteristic of this stage is the theological conflicts that arise. How could a merciful God allow this to happen? Although some religious people seem to display less guilt initially because it is the will of God, later they seem to have more difficulties with the feeling that, if God punished them, they must have been "bad" or "sinned."[5]

Grief is even more difficult for the family with a "borderline child" who seems normal at one point, but not normal at another, several times a day. Problems of acceptance are amplified for this child and the family. Parents of such children report reliving the birth crisis frequently throughout their lives.

How the family is told contributes significantly to the degree of shock and the pursuant grief. Although families differ in the way they would like to be told, there are some general desired approaches, honest, correct, caring, and gracious being most often mentioned by families. Most nurses who have been faced with such situations grope for words, do not know what to say, and therefore stay away. It is the nonverbal communication that affects the families more significantly —not what the nurse says, but what she does *not* say; what she does and what she does *not* do: frequency and duration of the nurse's visit to the patient bed, eye-contact, talking about infant care, baby pictures, and so on. Many parents say that the delivery room and nursery staff made them feel that they should be ashamed, not by the words they uttered, but by their behavior.

For example, Mrs. H. had delivered her first baby. The baby had multiple, non-life threatening, not easily observable, but potentially handicapping anomalies. Mrs. H. was ushered out of the delivery room with an unclear excuse. Quickly the baby was taken down to the nursery. Nobody told the parents. The obstetrician told the parents that the baby was a 5 pound 8 ounce boy and was OK. The delivery room nurses disappeared. Later, the recovery room nurse did not know anything about the baby. The parents asked the postpartum floor nurses about the baby, and they were told the baby was doing OK. They were expecting rooming-in, but the baby was not brought in. When the parents walked down to the nursery to look in, the baby's bassinet was placed away from the window and the nursery nurses did not bring the baby close up and were unavailable for questions. The pediatrician was around but was busy. The parents observed nurses busily running about and their own name being mentioned in whispers. Upon parental insistence, the pediatrician came over and said that the baby was a little small and tired, therefore he was being kept at the nursery for a while, and he told the parents not to worry. Nurses came in to take the mother's temperature but rushed out of the room. The next day the obstetrician checked the mother but disclaimed any knowledge of the baby and told the mother to ask the pediatrician. The pediatrician

was busy but sent the message that the baby had to be kept at the nursery for a little longer. The parents were told not to worry. That evening, the pediatrician's associate stopped in for a minute and said that there was a minor problem with the baby, and it was best for the baby to stay in the nursery but not to worry and get some rest. The pediatrician was not available on the phone. The third day, postpartum, the pediatrician sent the message that the baby should not be circumcised and the floor nurse said Mrs. H. did not have to attend the baby bath and feeding class. The photographer said that he was not given permission to snap a picture of Mrs. H.'s baby.

Unfortunately, the professionals' behaviors expressed something was wrong. This fear of unknown problems may be worse than the fear of known problems. Most parents say that they would like to be "told" as soon as possible. From families' perspective, being told means more than just hearing a diagnosis in medical terms. Parents want information on the total management of the situation. But how can professionals tell when they are not sure themselves? "Just be honest with us," say the parents. Honesty must be combined with caring and graciousness. The nurse must understand the impact on the family of the birth of a potentially handicapped child and show honesty, courage, and caring in dealing with the family during these times. Probably the attending physician will give the "bad news" to the family. This is the initial step of "being told." But what follows is an even more important part of being told, through the nurse's attitudes and behavior toward the family.

Difficulties Relating to Bonding. The difficulties related to being told create problems with bonding. Bonding is particularly difficult when the offspring has a life-threatening physical disability such as congenital heart disease. Mr. and Mrs. T. said, "We weren't sure if Jane would live or die. We tried not to get too attached to her, fearing that we would be crushed if she died."

Bonding requires crisis resolution. The crisis was precipitated by being told; its resolution is facilitated by successful grief-work. The nurse is in an optimum position to continue with the telling process started by the physician, be with the family through the grief process, and help them resolve the crisis.

Difficulties with bonding do not stem solely from the attitudes and behaviors of the mother or family. The child is an equal partner to this, since infants differ substantially in their responsiveness to caretakers and determine interaction. There are mothers, parents, and families who make every effort to communicate with an infant, but the infant does not respond. This precipitates a decrease in parental attempts at communication.[2] Factors such as separation of infant and mother for health care measures and intrusive measures are usually considered in terms of how they affect the family's response to the infant and the nature of their subsequent parenting; however, the role of the physically disabled infant must also be kept in mind. Helping the family members to continue to interact with a possibly poorly responding infant may result in a positive child response and facilitate bonding.

Others' reactions to the baby constitute an important difficulty. New parents watch nurses, doctors, and visitors very carefully to see their reactions. The parents, especially the mother, interprets others' reactions in terms of their acceptance of the infant. Evasion of the topic, not visiting or not holding the baby, not talking about future plans, and not taking pictures may be interpreted as rejection, revulsion, and shame.

Assessment of one's own abilities to take care and parent this child is another source of difficulty. This is a period when the parents may reassess their capabilities in other realms and find inadequacies. Appropriate health teaching and home care for parents and families are crucial. The nurse must engage in this teaching to increase parental self-confidence. The nurse can impart necessary skills to the parents so that they can say, "I can do it."

Identifying the family support system is another important potential family difficulty. The grief the parents are experiencing may make it difficult for them to feel the support significant others are showing. It is difficult to accept help from others, especially when one is not sure of his or her capabilities, or is experiencing failure. The nurse can help the parents identify and use supportive people.

When the parents are able to see that many significant others are not repelled by the infant; feel they have the capacity and skill to take care of this baby; and can see and hear significant others' offer of support, they will be able to accept help. Then there is hope, because the infant is living and will go on living, the professionals care, parents are capable, the family support system will help, and there are several alternatives to helping the baby reach his or her maximum potential.

With hope, attachment and, therefore, bonding are easier. The families can now emphasize the normality and strengths of the baby while realizing his or her limitations. The birth crisis is over and its resolution is marked by reorganization plans for the family's future.

FAMILY DIFFICULTIES EXPERIENCED AS THE CHILD GROWS

The birth crisis may be over but the scar is there to stay. Having a physically disabled child is a life-long process and requires skills of coping at various junctures. Families of normal children experience the usual developmental crises. The family with a physically disabled child also experiences these, but more intensely; furthermore, they experience additional crises resulting from the physically disabled child. These difficulties are many and generally stem from the family's potential risk of not meeting their own or societal expectations. Perhaps the basic problem is to learn to live with the emotional tension and sorrow precipitated by having produced a less than perfect offspring. Family difficulties include not only incorporating the physically defective child into the family, but planning for future children as well. At various junctures, this sorrow surfaces and periods of disequilibrium follow. During such periods the family needs a buffer system and some professional help to move into an extended period of equilibrium.

Difficulties Relating to Searching for Causes

Searching for a definite diagnosis, prognosis, and treatment possibilities is a natural activity for parents of a physically disabled child. Families need guidance regarding where to go and who to believe. There have been numerous situations in which diagnoses were inaccurate. The families want and need an accurate diagnosis. They do not want to overlook any condition which might be corrected if caught early, but they do not want to expose the child to unnecessary traumatic intrusive measures. Should they allow surgery? Should they allow countless tests? The fear of death they had experienced at the time of the child's birth resurfaces when different surgical procedures and repeated hospitalizations are recommended by specialists. So the families keep going to different specialists for second, third, and fourth opinions.

The family's urge to secure various expert opinions is reinforced by the specialists themselves, who refer the family to other specialists. The referrals are made but the family is often not thoroughly informed of the results. The nurse must keep in mind that many families may be justified in this doctor-shopping behavior. It is much more beneficial to help the family receive all the opinions and explanations they need than to dismiss the behavior as a sign of nonacceptance of the child or denial of the disability. The nurse can help the family select a balanced mix of well-respected specialists who can provide the family with reasonably accurate diagnostic and prognostic information. There is a great need for coordination of services or case-management in order to help the family sort out conflicting professional advice which may result from such an endeavor. The nurse can fulfill this function by interpreting results of specialists' professional opinions and helping the family incorporate the necessary programs and procedures suggested by the specialists into the family routine.

Difficulties Relating to Long-Term Management

The family needs to reorder its style of living in order to accommodate the physically disabled child and reach a new state of equilibrium. Long-term plans must be made. Specific family difficulties commonly arise in relation to finances, support systems, family dynamics, long-term care for the affected child, promoting self-actualization of the family members, and peer acceptance of the child and the family.

Finances. Family financial difficulties are manifold, since the physically disabled child frequently needs many services. The family has to make decisions about allocation of family financial resources in order not to compromise the self-actualization of the rest of the family members. The nurse can help the family identify their financial needs and resources. Helping the family remain in charge of their financial decisions allows the family members to retain their self-respect and self-sufficiency. However, it would be useful to alert the family to the existence of agencies which can be contacted if they need and desire outside financial support.

Family Dynamics. The family support system needs to be further identified. This might consist of relatives, neighbors, friends, helping professionals, parent groups, and clergy. The nurse can help the family identify the support group and the ways in which they can be supportive. It is important to assist the family to "hear" how such people are trying to be helpful and accept their help without losing self-control or self-esteem. "I don't want pity" is a sentiment shared by many families.

Family dynamics must be considered with caution and care. Role differentiation, division of labor, sibling rivalry, sibling grief and burden, sibling socialization, and authority must be considered. One family with a cerebral palsy child reported: "We had clear-cut roles before Andy was born. We have now decided to be more flexible.

Sometimes my husband vacuums the kitchen and I do the exercises with Andy. David and Mary (sibs) had to take on extra chores although they are only 5 and 7. Sometimes David and Mary are jealous of Andy; other times they seem to be feeling bad. We try not to go places where we cannot take Andy. Mary and David resent this sometimes."

Another mother expressed her concerns: "The other day my 8-year-old boy came home crying and muddy. Some of his friends called him names and said that his sister had "no legs." They called him nurse maid because he pushes my daughter's wheelchair. He was furious and got into a fight. He was *hurt*, in more ways than one! The next day he didn't want to go to a neighbor's halloween party."

The nurse can help the family identify the difficulties and possible solutions to the changes in the family relationships. The parents of a physically disabled child may also be parents of a normal child. They should be encouraged to enjoy their other children and at times have a chance to be without the physically disabled child. While the families should be encouraged to include their physically disabled child in the family and community activities, they should also be encouraged to engage in some activities without him.

Self-Actualization. Self-actualization of family members is an important concern. How can the family care for the physically disabled child and promote his maximum potential and still promote the self-actualization of the rest of the family? Cultural and social events, recreation, swim lessons, and neighbor's birthday parties pose problems. Allocation of time and attention is difficult. Should the physically disabled child dominate the family?

The nurse can help the family expand their support system to include outside agencies which might be able to provide some relief to the family. Sometimes a nurse-facilitated parent discussion group is most helpful to the family in this regard. The family may hear other parents who have resolved not to let the physically disabled child's needs dominate the family. When this decision is also reinforced by the nurse, the parents usually feel comfort through approval. Other families can follow suit without extreme feelings of guilt. "Finally we decided that although Mary has a heart defect she is only one-fifth of this family. We have two other children also. So now we can spend time and money on the other children without guilt." Attitudes such as this on the parents' part can also help facilitate appropriate disciplining of the physically disabled child without guilt.

Health Servicing Difficulties. Family difficulties with inadequate servicing or over-servicing can be equally serious. Several families mention that their physically disabled child was "abandoned" by the professionals. "I feel intimidated when I need to see the pediatrician. He doesn't want to be bothered with Seth." "They wanted to experiment with my April; since she had cerebral palsy they were willing to risk her life." "The orthopedist said Paul was institutional material and refused to correct his scoliosis."

On the other hand, some families are overserviced by various federal, state, and educational agencies. Each of these agencies seems to want to study the family and the child and make recommendations. Although good intentioned, such suggestions may be perceived as overloading demands by the family. "Everyone wants to come and look us over. We are supposed to do what they suggest. They each have programs that we have to follow. We love to help Jane, but then there's no time for just living and having fun." "All the programs I have to follow for Bob, exercises I have to do, diets I have to cook! I don't have any time for Suzy and Dave. I can't go and see a friend." The nurse must help the parents in sorting out such demands and devising a reasonable program without compromising necessary care.

Peer Acceptance. Peer acceptance of the child and the family poses important and long-term difficulties which are very painful. Peer acceptance problems start at birth with difficulties in visiting hours, baby gifts, home visits of neighbors to see the baby (the absence of, in this case) and continue with problems of family invitations to social events, school problems involving inadequate social inclusion and possible scapegoating, further complicated with inappropriate teacher attitudes. The sibling(s) of the affected child also can suffer problems of social inclusion or guilt for being popular, for he might go to neighbors' birthday parties without the affected sibling.

The school nurse can play a vital role in fostering peer acceptance of the physically disabled child at school. She might plan age-appropriate health teaching classes where she can discuss the disabilities in question. These classes can at times involve the physically disabled child to demonstrate his knowledge and skills and apparatus such as wheelchairs, braces, and prostheses. Especially if the class presentation is coupled with a special talent show of this child (music, paintings), this type of child-involvement can be very rewarding. However, this has to be planned for and executed very carefully. The main objectives are to provide the physically disabled child with a chance 1) to demonstrate his strengths and achievements to his peers, 2) to acknowledge that he has some differences which is OK, and 3) to reveal to his peers that he has common interests with them.

Encouraging the inclusion of the physically disabled child in clubs and special interest groups can also be very useful. The family's social inclusion can also be facilitated by such club-type community participation.

Long-Term Care. Difficulties relating to long-term care of the affected child can be all-consuming. For instance, should institutionalization be considered? putting the child up for adoption? giving him up to the state? What does this do to the family? If the child is kept at home, from where and how does the family obtain sufficient information regarding his home care? Who will take care of him when the parents die? Can the parents raise and save enough money to assure the care of this child after they die? Can they assure a spot in society for him? Fathers worry about this even more than the mothers do, especially if the affected child is male.

The education of the physically disabled child is a major issue. Developing special skills and talents and not overemphasizing remediation of weaknesses is a sound approach. But care must be

taken also not to overemphasize achievement in these children, thereby increasing the pressure. Problems with the child's acceptance into regular nursery schools[1] and public schools can be alleviated by taking advantage of laws advocating mainstreaming where possible. The nurse can serve an advocacy role in this regard. The school nurse is in an important position to interface the medical and educational approaches to this problem.

Body-image problems of the physically disabled child and the perceptions of the family are important issues.[10] The families need help in dealing with this. How can they explain it to the child? How can the family help the child to capitalize on strengths and beauties without shrinking under negative perceptions? And how about the child's peers who call him names and rough him up? How can the parents protect the child without loss of his autonomy and self-respect? The nurse can help the family deal with such issues and devise some courses of action.

Various degrees of rejection of the physically disabled child and his family by relatives, significant others, and peers are not very unusual. How can the family deal with this? How can they explain this to the child without ruining his self-confidence and self-worth? The nurse can assist the family in dealing with the family's own feelings first, and then support the family in their efforts to educate other people in their environment. As the child grows and becomes more keenly aware of rejection by some others, the family will need further support from the nurse to help the child deal with this.

Long-term "acceptance" of a child's limitations and potential is an issue much discussed in the literature. Often prognostic capabilities are questionable and the predictive value of present-day assessment tools is poor. Therefore, it is often unfair and unrealistic to expect the family to "accept" unquestioningly. Furthermore, this type of total acceptance signifies lack of hope to many people. Perhaps we need to redefine acceptance as resolution of birth crisis and mobilization to "do something" to help the child realize his best potential; his best potential need not be defined. Then the family is not robbed of hope but also realizes that this child's growth and development may differ from that of the majority of children.

The multifaceted nature of the problems precipitated by having a physically disabled child and the resultant family difficulties define a range of normality in family coping. The healthy chronic sorrow experienced by the families must be accepted as normal by professionals as long as it does not immobilize or disintegrate the family.

FAMILY DIFFICULTIES RELATED TO FUTURE CHILDREN

Difficulties Relating to Genetic Counseling

When parents begin to consider expanding their family, they wish to assess their chances of having "a normal child." Therefore, the need for genetic counseling is great, as it might provide an answer to the cause of the past defect and also identify the possibilities of the recurrence of the defect in the future children.

During this period, the crisis and grief experienced at the birth of the affected child surfaces in the minds of the family members. The chronic sorrow is present, and they might have to make serious decisions regarding future children. They must decide whether or not they should bear more children. The choice is rarely clear-cut, so the parents must weigh the risks of the effects of another defective child against their desire for more children. The families need much guidance and support while they make such decisions. Although the actual diagnosis is often the responsibility of the geneticist-physician, the nurse can help in obtaining accurate family history and pedigree and can counsel the family to identify the meaning of the risks and benefits.

When the parents find out, often from the geneticist, that there is a genetic problem, this new shock may cause them to relive the birth crisis they had experienced with the physically disabled child. It is almost like a double grief, one for history and one for future.

The guilt feeling this family had resolved

earlier surfaces because finally they have learned that they are really responsible for the defect. One mother said, "The doctor told me that something I have in my body is responsible for Johnny's problem—genes he called it. I feel so guilty and ashamed. So it is my fault!" Several conferences later, the mother understood that in fact she was not responsible for acquiring these genes—she had no choice. Also parents grieve for the future, yet unborn children and feel guilty about their genetic liability.

The parents may blame each other or themselves and have an overwhelming sense of guilt. The nurse should make herself available to the family and provide support in order to facilitate their coping. Of course, the nurse must have accurate knowledge of the genetic defect in question. One of the most important concepts to discuss with parents during genetic counseling is that of probability. Acquiring this concept will help parents understand why this traumatic event happened to them. It will also aid them in reaching decisions about having more children.[8] The family can be apprised of the availability of antenatal diagnosis of some genetic defects—amniocentesis. The pros and cons of the procedure must be discussed with the family.

Difficulties Relating to Amniocentesis and Abortion

If the parents decide to have another child, amniocentesis and abortion difficulties are added to the difficulties of incorporating a physically disabled child into the family. The nurse must help the family decide on the meaning for them of the risks and advantages of amniocentesis and abortion.

Advancements in the techniques of amniocentesis have increased the scope of antenatal diagnosis of genetic defects. Over 60 genetically transmitted conditions can be detected by studies of the amniotic fluid and cells obtained through amniocentesis. This number is growing quickly.[9] However, a negative result of amniocentesis study does not guarantee a perfect child.

Promises and limitations of amniocentesis pose an anxiety-provoking difficulty for families.

Families should be reminded that negative results will not guarantee a perfect baby. However, certain specific malformations can be ruled out, and this is valuable information. The parents must be warned that the amniocentesis may have to be repeated if, for some reason, the fluid and cells obtained do not culture well.

Fear of harm to the baby is a common family difficulty. Before the procedure is done, the family must be informed again of the possible complications of amniocentesis. Among these are feto-maternal hemorrhage, fetal harm and subsequent abortion, placental injury and resultant bloody fluid and maternal abdominal pain. However, with the technological advances and refinements of the technique, the risks of such complications are reported to be under 1 percent.[11] Many parents feel that the advantages of amniocentesis outweigh the risks.

Waiting for the results of amniocentesis is a difficult time for the family. This is a period of intense reminiscence of their first experience with the birth of a physically disabled child. Also during the waiting period, parental ambivalence about possible abortion is heightened. It would be advisable to make a home visit during this time, when a postamniocentesis maternal blood sample can be obtained and parental anxieties and fears can be discussed in the home environment.

When normal amniocentesis results come and the pregnancy is not to be terminated, most parents are overjoyed and can enjoy the pregnancy. A few parents remain somewhat anxious until they can hold their normal baby. If, however, the amniocentesis results are positive for a defect, the family is contacted for a conference. This conference includes crisis intervention and starts possible abortion counseling.

Family difficulties relating to abortion of the assumed malformed fetus are quite intense. Some of these difficulties and concerns are similar to those experienced by having an abortion for any reason. In addition, a complicating factor is that the mother actually wants a baby, but a normal one. Furthermore, she is not absolutely sure that this baby is "abnormal." This feeling is particularly heightened if the abortion is decided upon because of a sex-linked transmission where it is often not possible to determine if the fetus is affected, but all male fetuses are aborted. For this reason, it would be good to check the aborted fetus carefully, and if it is indeed affected to assure and, if desired, show the family that this is so.

Prior to abortion, the duration, pain, and labor type experience involved in the procedure must be explained to the mother.[6] One important point to remember is that the aborted fetus is not going to look like a glob but will look more like a baby since amniocentesis is usually done between 17 and 20 weeks of gestation.[11] The parents must be told about this if they are planning on seeing the aborted fetus. It is psychologically sound to abort the fetus soon after the positive amniocentesis results are received. Waiting longer might postpone the procedure until after the baby starts kicking, which can magnify the postabortion trauma and grief. This is why it is so crucial to discuss abortion prior to amniocentesis.

The families need postabortion instructions regarding the physical care of the mother, sexual activity, and contraception as well as continued genetic counseling.

Clearly, the family preparation and support through the amniocentesis and possible abortion period requires good teaching and counseling skills from the nurse. The nurse's attitudes and behaviors throughout the process are crucial.

NURSING APPROACHES

The main strategy for caring for the family with a physically disabled child is the normalization focus with a developmental approach. This means facilitating self-actualization of the family by capitalizing on its strengths and nurturing its weaknesses.

Since having a physically disabled child results in the family being at-risk of not fulfilling the universal family functions, the major nursing objective is to assist the family in carrying out its functions. Therefore, the basic nursing approaches pertinent to the management of the family with a physically disabled child are to help the family meet its universal family functions of procreation, provide a safe environment for family members, and promote the maximum potential of family members and the socialization of the young. A chart of the family functions with basic nursing goals and approaches is in Table 6-1.

Procreation. In some ways the family has failed in its function this time. Will this failure be repeated? Whose fault is it? Can the family succeed in this function at another time? Should they in fact abort their subsequent efforts and adopt a child? With the main goals of prevention of environmentally determined physical disabilities and amelioration of present disabilities, the nurse can utilize her skills in counseling and teaching to aid the family in finding some answers to these questions and in making pertinent family decisions.

Provision of Safe Environment. The nurse can help the family nurture the physically disabled child. The objectives mutually set with the family would be mainly biologic in nature. Depending on the nature of the physical disability, health teaching should include considerations on the physical set-up, nutrition, hygiene, immunizations, and rest-exercise balance. Also important is the provision of a physical environment that will assure biologic safety and growth for the rest of the family. The actual physical care of the physically disabled child is part of the nurse's teaching plan. The goals of increasing the family competence and confidence as well as preventing additional disabilities without overloading the family can guide the nurse in her health-teaching efforts tailored to the needs of the particular family.

Promotion of Growth and Development Poten-

Table 6-1. Basic Nursing Goals and Approaches Related to Family Functions

Family Function	Nursing Goals	Nursing Approaches
Procreation	1. prevention of environmental genetic defects 2. amelioration of present disabilities	1. counseling—genetic, amniocentesis, abortion 2. teaching—family planning, health teaching, formal and informal techniques
Provision of safe environment	1. increasing the family competence 2. prevention of other disabilities and of overloading the family	1. teaching—general health, specific skills
Promotion of growth and development potential	1. prevention of secondary handicaps 2. promotion of maximum potential	1. counseling—anticipatory guidance in growth and developmental crises 2. early identification—screening, assessment, case-finding 3. early intervention—home care and agency programs 4. advocacy—helping family obtain services and control 5. case-management—integration of multidisciplinary team
Socialization of the young	1. increasing social inclusion of the child and the family 2. facilitating proper care and education of the child	1. teaching—the family, school personnel, peers 2. advocacy—for mainstreaming and proper education 3. consulting—the various agencies to provide nursing input 4. referring—agencies, parent or sibling groups

tial. Promotion of growth and development potential of any child is a complex task. This complexity is intensified when the child is physically disabled. Helping families see the specific positive results of their efforts reinforces their constructive behavior and increases their self-confidence. Equally important is the concern for self-actualization of *all* family members. The physically disabled child need not dominate the family resources and lifestyles. The nurse can help the family obtain necessary supplementary resources as well as aid the family to allocate its resources to all members.

With the main goals of prevention of secondary handicaps and promotion of the maximum potential of the child and the family, the nurse can utilize her skills to provide anticipatory guidance in growth and developmental crises, early identification and early intervention, and assume family advocacy focus in coordinating the professional care and services the family is in contact with.

Socialization of the Young. The family with a physically disabled child needs to bring the child up to have socially acceptable virtues so he can function as an effective member of the society. The family is expected to provide for a "spot" or "status" for this child in the larger order of things. That is, the family must ready its young for the society physically, culturally, and materially.

The socialization function is the major societal expectation of the family. The family with a physically disabled child needs much support and guidance in rearing the child to share common norms, conform to shared rules, and hold a job and earn a living doing socially acceptable things.

The cultural concern represents a composite of biological and psychosocial responsibilities for the family and involves family interaction with many institutions of social living. The nurse can contribute to the family efforts to raise a culturally acceptable physically disabled child by assisting the family in increasing social inclusion of the child and the family and facilitating the provision of proper care and education for the child.

For instance, the nurse can help to assure the child's mainstreaming through an advocacy ap-

proach. Nurse-initiated referrals of the family to the appropriate agencies and groups may actualize some of the advocacy attempts. In addition, linking the family with parent discussion support groups can aid the family to enlarge their support system and increase the family's social inclusion. It would be useful for the nurse to consult various professionals and agencies regarding the physically disabled child's regimen in order to assure nursing input and adequate follow through.

Parent-Desired Qualities of the Nurse. What do the parents and families of physically disabled children think the helping professional should *be* like and *act* like? Families are different, with different needs and wants. But there are quite a few commonalities in what attributes the families think the helping professional, in this case the nurse, should possess. Among those often mentioned are: 1) accurate knowledge, 2) good working relationship with colleagues, 3) a contact network for useful referral, 4) understanding that chronic sorrow is normal for these families, 5) willingness to identify and nurture family strengths and to teach the parents how to care for the physically disabled child, 6) an attitude and behavior which suggest that the parents are important and they are respected, 7) honesty and courage regarding the child's potentials and limitations. This should be balanced with graciousness to decrease the sting and, above all, 8) caring.

By caring most parents mean having an understanding heart, empathy. They would like to deal with a professional who can really understand how it is for the parents. It is not pity or a patronizing attitude, but being able to put oneself in the parents' position, however momentarily, and really understanding. The nursing approaches must be carried through with this type of understanding. One father said that he would like the nurse to "be with" him when he crosses the bridge over the tumultuous river, when he has to deal with the sorrow, and when he is trying to make sense of what the numerous specialists say.

The nurse's role so defined is difficult to play and is very demanding, for it requires knowledge, skills, and much strength. In order to feel and display the kind of caring the parents desire, the nurse has to share their pain. Sharing the pain brings about nursing difficulties—hence, the need for a support system for the nurse.

The nurse is the helping professional best suited for the job; still she should not try to rely on her own resources and strengths alone. Drawing upon what other related professionals might be able to offer can provide the nurse with additional strengths and competencies, thereby increasing her effectiveness. It is crucial to increase the opportunities for the nurse to play her role for which she is potentially so fit and for which the family needs are so great.

SUMMARY

The birth of a physically disabled child precipitates a crisis in the family and brings about grief and chronic sorrow. As parents go through stages of grief work, they resolve the crisis and bond with the child. Yet, at various junctures this chronic sorrow surfaces and periods of disequilibrium follow. During such periods many families need professional help to resolve the problems. The nurse can help in this process by assessing, preventing, and ameliorating the family difficulties.

Family difficulties are many and generally stem from the family's potential risk of not being able to carry out its functions. The nursing role in the management of the family with a physically disabled child is to work with all family members so they experience satisfaction from working together to meet their goals.

REFERENCES

1. Abelson, G. "Measuring Preschool's Readiness to Mainstreaming Handicapped Children." *Child Welfare*, March 1976, 219.
2. Brazelton, B. T. "Importance of New Techniques of Neonatal Assessment." Paper presented 2/22/1977, Denver meetings of the American Association for the Advancement of Science.
3. Commonwealth of Massachusetts. "An Act Further Regulating Programs for Children Requiring Special Education and Providing Reimbursement Therefore." Acts 1972—Chapter 766.
4. Commonwealth of Massachusetts Department of Education. *Core Evaluation Manual, Chapter 766.* Bedford: The Institute for Educational Services, Inc., 1974.
5. Drotar, D. et al. "The Adaptation of Parents to the Birth of an Infant with a Congenital Malformation: A Hypothetical Model." Reprint, Department of Pediatrics, Case-Western Reserve University School of Medicine, Cleveland, Ohio, 1975.
6. Keller, C. and P. Copeland. "Counseling the Abortion Patient Is More than Talk." *American Journal of Nursing.* January 1972, 102–104.
7. Mercer, P. T. "Responses of Mothers to the Birth of an Infant with a Defect." *A.N.A. Clinical Sessions,* 1974, 340–348.
8. Sahin, S. T. "The Multifaceted Role of the Nurse as Genetic Counselor." *The American Journal of Maternal Child Nursing,* 1 #4, July–August 1976, 211–216.
9. Swinyard, C. A. "Counseling Parents of Children with Birth Defects." *Consultant,* April 1976, 208–210.
10. Waechter, E. H. "Developmental Consequences of Congenital Abnormalities." *Nursing Forum,* XIV #2, 1975, 109–129.
11. Watt, M. "Management of Patients At-Risk for Fetal Malformations." *Nursing Mirror,* May 6, 1976, 61–63.

ADDITIONAL READINGS

1. Ballard, R. "Sharing the Pain—Help for Parents with a Handicapped Child. *Health Visitor,* December 1976, 395–396.
2. Butani, P. "Reactions of Mothers to the Birth of an Anomalous Infant: A Review of the Literature." *Maternal-Child Nursing Journal,* 3, Spring 1974, 59–75.

PERTINENT ORGANIZATIONS

NATIONAL
- *American Association of University Affiliated Programs for the Developmentally Disabled*
  110 17th Street, N.W.
  Washington, D.C.

- *American Foundation for the Blind*
  15 West 16th Street
  New York, New York 10011
- *American Speech and Hearing Association*
  9030 Old Georgetown Road
  Bethesda, Maryland 20014
- *Child Welfare Resource Information Exchange*
  2011 Eye Street
  Suite 501
  Washington, D.C. 20006
- *Closer Look: National Information Center for the Handicapped*
  Box 1492
  Washington, D.C. 20013
- *Epilepsy Foundation of America*
  1828 L. Street, N.W.
  Washington, D.C. 20014
- *International Association of Parents of the Deaf*
  814 Thayer Avenue
  Silver Spring, Maryland 20910
- *Muscular Dystrophy Associations of America*
  810 7th Avenue
  New York, New York 10019

- *National Center for Child Advocacy*
  U.S. Department of Health, Education, and Welfare
  Office of Child Development
  P.O. Box 1182
  Washington, D.C. 20013
- *Office for Handicapped Individuals*
  330 Independence Avenue, S.W.
  Washington, D.C. 20201
- *Parenting Materials Information Center*
  Southwest Educational Development Laboratory
  211 East 7th Street
  Austin, Texas 78701
- *United Cerebral Palsy Association*
  66 East 34th Street
  New York, New York 10016

LOCAL
- Many local church, hospital, health, and community groups are helpful to these families.

The Mentally Disabled Child

Marie A. Wacht, R.N., B.S.N.

CHAPTER SEVEN

Advances in family planning for women at risk of having an abnormal infant and prenatal diagnosis of fetal disabling conditions have led to a greater ability to prevent mental disabilities. Increasing understanding of family relationships that involve the mentally disabled child in the family and the community have led to optimal developmental attainment for these children. The family is essential in providing the environment for maximum achievement of the child's potential. However, the difficulties related to rearing a mentally disabled child can disrupt family functioning and result in serious problems for both the child and the family. The nurse plays a central role in helping the child and the family deal with these problems and reach their highest level of individual and family development.

BASIC CONCEPTS OF MENTAL DISABILITY AND THE FAMILY

Although 15 percent of the newborn population are at risk of mental disability due to prenatal or birth conditions, fortunately many of these infants do develop normally. Only 3 percent are eventually diagnosed as mentally retarded.[1,4] Mental disabilities occur among all ethnic or socioeconomic groups. However, there may be a higher risk among the impoverished since poor nutrition, lack of health care, and other factors influence mental development.

Mental disabilities are difficult to diagnose. There are some children who are believed to be retarded, but actually have normal intellectual ability. These functional disabilities are caused by the discrepancy between the accepted behavior in their environment and the majority standards by which they are tested. There are also some children whose actual mental delay is not recognized because their behaviors demonstrating mental delay are misinterpreted as culturally determined.

Mental disability is a developmental delay caused by an impairment in mental development. These developmental delays may influence more types of behaviors than those caused by physical difficulties since the mind controls all complex behaviors. Both the child's intellectual functioning and his daily adaptive behaviors are impaired. The child may have speech, fine motor, and gross motor delays such as difficulty communicating, using a spoon, or walking.

Some mental disabilities are present at birth such as Down's syndrome, severe meningomyelocele with hydrocephalus, or birth trauma resulting in severe cerebral anoxia. Other mental disabilities may not become apparent until later; for example, some metabolic disorders may first become symptomatic in the preschool years and autism may not be recognized until late infancy. Some other mental disabilities can occur at any time during a child's developmental years as a result of trauma, infectious diseases, neoplasms, or accidents such as suffocation which cause cerebral anoxia. Mental disabilities may occur alone or in association with physical disabilities such as severe cerebral palsy, or with syndromes like the Cornelia de Lange's syndrome.

Mental disabilities span a large range of disabilities. The profoundly disabled child must have all his basic needs met by others. A mildly disabled child might lack intellectual capacity for abstract thought but adapt well socially to his family and assume major responsibility for meeting his own needs. The borderline mentally disabled child may be able to meet all his own needs, but may be labeled as mentally retarded because of imperfections of intelligence testing.

Although additional categories for mentally retarded children have been used to identify the expectations for the child, categorizing children in this way prevents treating each one as an individual with individual abilities and potential to achieve more. Using a planned assessment, the nurse can describe the child's actual difficulties rather than use a general category description.

Cause and Prevention of Mental Disabilities. As with other high-risk situations, there are many suspected causes of mental disabilities. These are:

1. Health practice factors, such as poor communicable disease control, causing diseases like rubella which result in sensory deficits and mental impairment in the unborn child.
2. Nutritional factors, such as poor prenatal nutrition, which causes low birth weight infants, or poor infant nutrition, which results in poor brain development. Both produce increased risk for mental disability.
3. Genetic influences, such as recessive traits carried by parents, which cause diseases like Tay-Sachs or Hurler's syndrome, a metabolic disorder.
4. Lifestyle factors such as drug use or abuse associated with the birth of a defective infant, or alcohol abuse often related to the birth of an infant with microcephaly.
5. Environmental influences such as ingestion of toxic levels of lead by a child, causing neurologic damage, or safety hazards like near-drowning accidents causing cerebral anoxia.
6. Behavioral factors such as child abuse resulting in cerebral trauma and possible developmental and emotional handicap.

To prevent mental disabilities the nurse works to reduce these factors by providing optimal health care services, nutrition, health education, genetic counseling, and prenatal diagnosis.

Integration of Mental Disability Concepts. There are three models of mental disability: developmental, normalization, and interaction models. Together these three influence the strategies used by health professionals to help the disabled child and his family.

The developmental model is the most desirable and least dehumanizing approach to mental disability.[5] This model involves three assumptions concerning helping the mentally disabled child. First, continued development is always possible. Second, the next developmental step is based on present developmental and maturational abilities. And third, reducing unfavorable environmental conditions modifies disability. In the developmental model the mentally disabled child is consequently viewed as an individual who is capable of growth, learning, and development with the rate and direction influenced by the care and services he receives.

The normalization model stresses that the mentally disabled child must be viewed as normal and human, not as a deviant or object of pity.[6] He is given experiences that allow him to develop and relate to his family and community in as normal a way as possible. This principle is the basis for the trend toward the disabled child living at home with his family, attending schools in the community, and having social and recreational experiences. The principle of normalization should be applied to all aspects of a child's life and used in conjunction with the developmental model, creating an individual plan for each child to most effectively foster his normal growth and development.

The interaction model emphasizes the importance of the family. The child's ability to thrive and the potential quality of his life depends on the physical, psychological, intellectual, and social well-being he develops from interacting with his family members. The family's attitudes toward, acceptance of, and expectations for the mentally disabled child can have more influence on his life than other environmental experiences he will have. The presence of a mentally disabled child within a family is a unique experience. It is a crisis that gives the child and other family members the opportunity for family closeness or disintegration.

Mental disabilities can be approached from an integration of these three concepts. The possibility of development from the developmental model, the importance of normal daily behaviors from the normalization principle, and the value of family relationships from the interaction concept take into account both the value of interventions and the importance of working with the family of the mentally disabled child.

FAMILY DIFFICULTIES

Having a mentally disabled child is a crisis which requires special changes and coping abilities to include the child in the family. Identification and acceptance of mental disabilities are difficult for many families; developing ways to promote optimal development and to include the child in the family requires joint adaptation by all of the family members. The family's difficulties and reactions determine the amount of family disruption.

Potential family difficulties extend through any developmental period or are specific to one period. The child's developmental needs and the families' potential problems are shown in Figures 7-1 and 7-2.

Any Time Period

Family members experience intermittent problems of grief, guilt, relationships, and finances during any of the developmental periods for the child.

Grief. Families experience the process of grieving when they are faced with caring for a mentally disabled child. This process is not unlike the mourning that is experienced at the loss of someone through death, as described in the chapter on the "Terminally Ill Child." In fact, the anticipated child is lost to these parents. When the parents' dreams and hopes for this child are not met, a feeling of hopelessness results. The parents' movement through the grieving process helps them develop realistic hopes and expectations for the child. Since individual family members differ in the exact problems and timing for each stage, each member will grieve in an individual way and need individualized help.

Postpartum depression may be increased by the grief of having a mentally disabled newborn. Separation of the mother and risk child, early caretaking by professionals, and concerns about the ability to care for the newborn at home increase the mother's grief and depression.[3]

The mother of a newborn son with Down's syndrome affectionately cared for him at home, but because of her worries about her abilities to care for her child, she spent her first two weeks crying, which was distressing to the father. With positive and supportive information from the pediatrician and follow-up home visits by the public health nurse, the mother was able to cope with her grief, become comfortable in her son's care, and begin planning, with the father, for their son's future developmental needs.

Figure 7-1. Needs of the Mentally Disabled
Child and the Family

Infancy Period
Child needs:
1. care, nurturance
2. acceptance
3. developmental opportunities
4. socialization
Family needs:
1. emotional support
2. opportunity for attachment
3. early, accurate information
4. developmental guidance
5. assistance in planning and coordinating the child's care

Early Childhood Period
Child needs:
1. care
2. developmental opportunities
3. socialization
4. discipline
Family needs:
1. positive relationship with child
2. information about teaching and discipline
3. genetic counseling
4. support from other parents
5. independence from child

School Age Period
Child needs:
1. developmental opportunities
2. socialization
3. acceptance for academic abilities
Family needs:
1. understanding of child's abilities
2. participation in child's programs
3. awareness of child's effect on family

Adolescent Period
Child needs:
1. developmental opportunities
2. socialization
3. independence and responsibility
4. value of his increasing abilities
5. coping with puberty
Family needs:
1. awareness of child's need for independence and responsibility
2. understanding child's changes of puberty
3. participation in child's socialization
4. sensitivity to the child's realization of his limitations

Adulthood
Child needs:
1. developmental opportunities
2. socialization
3. independence and responsibility
4. basic human rights
Family needs:
1. acceptance of the child as an adult
2. assistance in planning for the child's care after their death

Figure 7-2. Potential Family Difficulties

Any Time
Grief
Guilt and blame
Relationship difficulties
Finances

Infancy
Attachment and expectations

Early Childhood
Family planning

School Age
Parents' participation at school
Placement decision

Adolescence
Social difficulties
Sibling childbearing fear

Adulthood
Independence

Brothers and sisters also grieve the loss of their idea of the perfect brother or sister and of what they feel is their parents' love, since more parent time is directed away from them to the care of and concern for their disabled child. The siblings need simple, honest, supportive explanations of the child's condition and the parents' reactions.

For example, two-year-old Jeffrey's normal sibling rivalry was compounded by regressive behavior when his parents were preoccupied with their own grieving and overwhelming care of their mentally and physically disabled infant daughter. After his parents arranged for occasional homecare for their daughter to spend more time alone with Jeffrey, and after special outings with his grandparents, Jeffrey resumed his developmental abilities and affectionately "helped" with his sister's care.

Grandparents, friends, and neighbors may also be experiencing grief, for they too have had good wishes and expectations for the parents and the infant. Friends and relatives may have difficulties with their own grief, blaming the parents and interfering in the family's decisions. Counseling may help them develop ways to support the family.

These feelings of grief are normal and show a valuable process of including the child in the family. Supportive friends, extended family, and professionals can all help the family by accepting their feelings and changes as normal and supporting their individual progression through the stages.

Guilt and Blame. The parents of a mentally disabled child look for causes and often associate something they did with the child's disability. Guilt feelings are common, as is blame of the other parent, both leading to devastating feelings and interactions.

For example, one family contemplated divorce because the father's family accused the mother's family of having "bad genes." The mother herself felt guilt because she used a medication during her pregnancy. Genetic counseling, including discussion of the parents' fears, clarified both concerns for these parents and reduced their blaming of each other and themselves.

Relationships. Parents must accept and treat the disabled child as one member of the family and not make the child its center or omit him from the family. Brothers and sisters need to be allowed to play with the mentally disabled child and develop a personal relationship with him without frequent avoidance or blaming.

The growing child needs direct, consistent, and nurturing discipline. A child with mental disability often cannot understand subtle cues about his inappropriate behavior. He needs clearly stated, consistent, and direct messages. For example, although scolding a child may be used to eliminate undesired behaviors, positively reinforcing his desirable behaviors by showing affection and approval is necessary to foster continuance of those behaviors. Use of reinforcers and avoidance of punishment is discussed in the "Behavior Modification Strategies" chapter.

All parents need respite from their children for rest, relaxation, and recreation. The parents of a mentally disabled child may have difficulty finding babysitters who are willing to care for children with special needs and problems. Community centers, home care services, local schools, or other programs may have services to care for children with medical, learning, and behavioral limitations. Fear of ridicule or rejection by these persons and the realistic difficulty of finding persons qualified to care for a child with many needs reduces the parents' ability to have some independence from their child and continue other adult friendships.

Finances. While the financial responsibilities for raising a normal child are great, they are often even greater for the mentally disabled child who has special needs. Special schooling, recreation programs, and medical care are important to the child's optimal development but can be costly. Parents need help using resources such as Crippled Children Services, Supplemental Security Income through the Social Security System, and the many other public and private agencies which serve families with special needs. Nursing approaches to reduce financial problems are discussed in the "Financial Strategies" chapter.

Infancy

Infancy and early childhood is a period of rapid growth and development. The infant needs care, nurturance, and stimulating opportunities to foster growth and development because the experiences in these first few years have lasting and pervasive effects on the child's future growth and development. Special caretaking and learning approaches frequently require extra parental time and energy.

In addition to special care, the infant also needs acceptance for his uniqueness, being viewed only secondarily as a mentally disabled infant. He needs recognition for his abilities, not only his limitations. A young mother gave birth at home to an infant daughter with Cornelia de Lange's syndrome, a condition delaying growth. From supportive friends at home, and later from professionals in the hospital and community, she was able to enjoy Robin's affection and sensory awareness, rather than focus all of her attention on her daughter's deformed limbs and delayed growth.

Attachment and Expectations. Immediately following the birth of a mentally disabled infant each parent needs the opportunity to develop an attachment with the infant. The crisis atmosphere often communicated by medical personnel following the birth of a possibly disabled infant and the common separation of the infant from the parents reduces the opportunity for attachment. Nurses should encourage parents to see, hold, and interact with their mentally disabled infant shortly after birth.

After parents experience the initial shock of hearing that their child is disabled, they have difficulty readjusting their expectations for their child. For example, they may ask, "Will he live?" or "Will he grow?" Parents need early, accurate information in order to effectively care and plan for their child. Learning to carry out their child's special physical care and developmental stimulation helps the parents to understand the child's abilities and unique characteristics, as well as his limitations.

Early Childhood

The mentally disabled child in early childhood needs opportunities for the development of physical, language, cognitive, and psychosocial skills. Since "a year's intensive stimulation at age two or three may be worth two or three years at age eight, or a lifetime at age twelve,"[6] learning programs must begin as soon as mental disability is recognized. Parents must decide on their involvement and plan additional learning experiences.

For a family whose child's disability is just starting to show, early childhood is the time of major stress. Since many mental disabilities may not affect the infant's appearance or behavior, the first signs of the disability occur in the early childhood period. The parents often compare their child to other children at a similar age and are distressed at differences. They need to develop a new hope for this child and face a new reality.

Family Planning. The early childhood years may be when the parents are planning to have more children. Genetic and personal counseling may help them make responsible decisions about future pregnancies. For example, when the parents of a child with severe neurologic disability and mental retardation learned that they were possibly carriers of this disorder, they chose sterilization and adoption as an option to having another child of their own.

If a new baby is planned, the parents are often anxious about the normality of this pregnancy and are often faced with many of the difficulties discussed in the chapter on the "High-Risk Pregnancy." When the new baby is born, the family must develop a way of dividing their attention and time between the new baby and their child with special needs. If the younger sibling develops more rapidly than the mentally disabled child, the family is again faced with the overt reality of their child's disabilities.

School Age

During the school years, the mentally disabled child needs continuing developmental opportunities through his school and home experiences. With the philosophy of normalization, today's school programs share the common goal of bringing these children back to the regular classroom rather than isolating them. Since traditional teaching methods are not as effective with some mentally disabled children, reading, writing, and arithmetic may need to be presented in smaller study groups, with greater repetition before mastery, more concrete examples, and more relevance to usual daily activities.

In family and school, the mentally disabled child needs to learn and constantly practice social skills such as manners and grooming, using the schoolbus, crossing the street, identifying and avoiding physical dangers, and interacting with friends. The mentally disabled child needs friends with which to share experiences and groups in which to participate in recreational and athletic activities. Summer camping, scouting groups, and the Special Olympics which is sponsored by the Joseph P. Kennedy Foundation provide valuable experiences.

Parents' Participation at School. Placement in classes at school is a recognized stress period for parents of all children because they must confront their expectations for their child. Their views of the child's abilities may differ from those of the teachers who compare the child's performance with that of his peers. Parents may be discouraged with the child's slow progress and will need assistance in understanding that their child, despite limitations, has potential for growth and development. For some children, academic learning may not be possible, nor as valuable as learning social skills to function effectively in everyday life.

Since parents have the closest and longest contacts with their child, and the mentally disabled child needs reinforcement of learning, the parents must be involved from the beginning in their child's education. Parents must be encouraged to participate in observing, problem-solving, planning, and decision-making that affects their child's education. The feeling of success that they experience when their child learns a new skill is important in developing a positive and close relationship between them.

Paul is a nine-year-old whose progress at school seemed at a standstill until his mother was able to alter her work hours and meet regularly with his teacher to review his school program. Her assistance with his homework and her awareness of his acquired knowledge resulted in his developmental progress, his mother's greater appreciation of his abilities, and her satisfaction in helping him.

Placement Decision. A child who is severely disabled may become too difficult for the family to care for at home. At this time the parents may consider out-of-home placement if this was not considered before. Such a decision is difficult, complex, and will affect the whole family. Consideration must be given to all possible alternatives, such as extra help at home, day care centers, and residential programs as well as the quality, cost, and nearness of programs.

The choice of out-of-home placement may result in normal feelings of ambivalence, inadequacy, and guilt for the parents, and confusion and loneliness for the child. Eleven-year-old Karen tells us, "When I was in the second grade, my brother was getting hard to handle and scaring all my friends away. It made people uncomfortable, so we had to take him to a different place to live. We hated giving him up in the first place and we all had a very hard time, including him. He needs more love because of not being able to live with us."

Adolescence

Adolescence is a difficult time for normal children, and even more difficult for those with developmental delay. The adolescent often wants the experiences without the responsibilities of an adult. The mentally disabled child will desire independence, yet the more seriously disabled adolescents still need to rely on others for essential needs.

A mentally disabled adolescent also needs to develop additional social and work skills to develop as an independent adult. Experiences that will enable him to develop initiative and responsibility to carry out a task, skill to complete the task, and then receive fulfillment from completing a task are important for the continued development of the mentally disabled adolescent.

As do all adolescents, the disabled need opportunity to develop responsibilities within their families and independence away from their families, so that they can grow in self-esteem and responsibility for themselves. They need carefully planned situations for assuming independence through experiences that are safe and progressive. When the adolescent succeeds at this, he needs his family to value him for his successes, abilities, and contributions to his own development and to the family.

When Christine entered junior high school she resented taking the bus to school while other students walked, and she resented having a "babysitter" after school before her mother returned from work. To cope with this, a progressive plan for increased independence and responsibility was developed with the participation of Christine, her mother, and a public health nurse. During the school year Christine learned to walk to and from school and spent two hours alone before her mother's return by setting the table for dinner, washing dishes, and vacuuming carpets. This resulted in Christine's pride in her accomplishments, opportunity for her to socialize with classmates while walking to school, and her mother's pride and realization of her daughter's abilities to accomplish these behaviors.

Social Difficulties. The physical and emotional changes of puberty may be more difficult for mentally disabled children to understand. Coping with the physical changes and developing new grooming and appearance skills are important for the adolescent. Though sex education is needed even earlier, it can now be reviewed in a clear, patient, and acceptant manner for the adolescent through special family planning and sexuality clinics planned to meet the learning abilities and needs of the mentally disabled. For the higher functioning adolescent with an inheritable disorder, genetic counseling for the adolescent may be needed to identify possible disability in his future offspring and teach him about this risk.

With the changes of puberty, there is an increased interest in socialization with the opposite sex. Adolescents with disabilities need the help of adults to plan and successfully carry out social activities that can provide experiences and develop appropriate skills in showing affection for others in a mature and acceptable manner.

For example, parents and professionals can assist adolescents to arrange group activities like dances or picnics that provide interaction between adolescents but with the guidance of adults who can assist them in their interactions and with whom they can feel free to discuss personal concerns about these interactions.

During adolescence the mentally disabled child must realize his own limitations while building on his strengths. The child's friends, both disabled and normal, may also be developing at varying rates, and the adolescent who is mentally disabled may feel "left out" of situations where he may have been welcome before. The mentally disabled adolescent sees siblings and friends, not much older than himself, moving away from home, going away to school, getting married. He sees them leaving their families to be "on their own," but he may not be capable of living away from home yet.

The common parental difficulties of allowing the adolescent to choose his own lifestyle, work, and living location are especially difficult for the parent of the mentally disabled child. Adolescence may be an especially difficult time for the parents of mentally disabled children because they sometimes have a tendency to view their disabled child as an "eternal child" and a "special child." They may need support in facing their child's desire, need, and ability for independence. The nurse helps the family identify realistic alternatives based on the adolescent's individual abilities.

Sibling Childbearing Fear. Adolescent brothers and sisters of a child with a mental disability may need genetic counseling for themselves. The family should anticipate that they will be worried about also having children with mental disabilities, even if they are not expressing this to their parents or asking questions. Information should not be forced on them, but opportunities for genetic counseling must be available when they are ready. Brothers and sisters need to hear that they are normal and have the potential of having normal children. If they are carriers of disorders, this situation needs to be clearly and sensitively explained, and often repeated, to prevent them from making unrealistic commitments to never having children or confusing the highly emotional information provided.

Adulthood

The mentally disabled individual who has reached his adult years may be in the dilemma of being legally an adult yet not having the intellectual skills and behavioral characteristics for complete independence and adequate adult functioning. He wishes to drive a car, cook his own meals, select his own clothes, manage his own money, and marry. Although many mentally disabled people become independent, many always need some help with daily living.

The mentally disabled adult needs continued opportunities for intellectual, psychological, social, and physical development. He needs an environment that continues to foster opportunities for learning, becoming independent, and socializing. He needs, with support and direction of advocates, opportunities to make choices, take risks, and assume responsibilities in his living situation, his work, and his relationships with others. Various kinds of jobs or workshops, group homes in the community, and participation in the community's leisure and recreational activities can provide this.

Independence. The family must accept their child as an adult who is capable of a degree of independent functioning based on his abilities. The parents can receive satisfaction when helping their mentally disabled adult family member cope with and use his desires and abilities to be sexually active, to marry, to live independently, and to make an income.

Just as the parents may have difficulty accepting their adult son's or daughter's abilities to be mature and independent, they may also have difficulty identifying when and how he or she needs additional help. Less disabled adults may need only the usual parental help of love and support, while more severely mentally disabled adults may need help with finances, transportation, care of their surroundings, meal planning, and clothing selection and care.

Parents must arrange for continuation of this needed help after their deaths. They often ask, "What will happen when I die?" They need to arrange for financial assistance and guardianship from relatives and friends, or through private and government programs.

NURSING APPROACHES

Nursing action is influential in determining whether the family will overcome the difficulties of having a mentally disabled child and continue their growth toward acceptance and satisfaction or whether they will continue with frustration, anger, guilt, and chronic sorrow. The goal of nursing action is to reduce the potential difficulties and promote the child's and family's development. Nurses in many settings provide the prevention, case-finding, developmental testing, early intervention teaching, counseling, planning, and evaluation approaches essential to the family with a mentally retarded member.

Prevention. Nursing action in mental disabilities services begins prior to the birth of the child.

Specially trained nurses provide genetic counseling for the prevention of mental disabilities. Genetic counseling includes an accurate diagnosis whenever possible, an explanation of patterns of inheritance and the interpretation of the chances of offspring having the disability, and discussion of childbearing options available to the parents, with the focus on the individual family's desires and needs. Decisions are never made for families, but the families are given information, alternatives, and the objective guidance and support for their decision-making process. Follow-up counseling and referral for additional services are also included in genetic counseling. A multidisciplinary team of nurses, physicians, social workers, and other health professionals provide the most comprehensive genetic counseling service.

The obstetric, pediatric, or community nurse is often the first member of the health care team to assess the family's need and make the referral for genetic counseling. The nurse's knowledge of the family's medical and social history, the family's expectations from genetic counseling, their specific questions related to the cause of their child's disability, their cultural or religious beliefs about why birth defects occur, and their coping abilities need to be shared with the team to individualize the genetic counseling.

The nurse in family planning and prenatal services plays a valuable role in identification of the family at risk of having a mentally disabled infant. The nurse assesses the family for the presence of the several causative factors mentioned earlier.

Public health nurses in the community have been involved for many years in the prevention of mental disabilities. In home visiting, health education, and school activities, nurses teach families about good nutrition and control of infectious diseases. They also plan and provide community child care centers, child abuse prevention programs, child developmental programs, and educational programs for teenage mothers which all contribute to prevention and identification of disabled children.

Case-Finding. The nurse in the well-baby clinic,

school, or community may first recognize the delay in a child's growth and development and refer the family for more comprehensive evaluation. Often the nurse has already established a relationship with the family and is a valuable supportive person to the family during this uncertain time when they question, "What is wrong with my child?" This community nurse is very important in initial case-finding and in supporting the family if the child does have mental disabilities.

Developmental Testing. The nurse in the community well-baby clinic, the home, the newborn nursery, the pediatric unit, or the child development center is often the first person to combine observations with a screening test to assess developmental progress. Continued developmental assessment for advances or changes during the child's growth may be needed. Developmental assessment includes the observation of a child's physical growth and skills, ability to learn and to relate to others, responses to his environment, and the comparison of these with other children of similar background. Many standardized tests are now available which not only facilitate screening and provide a comparison but also make it easier to record this information so that sequential screening can be done to measure a child's progress or lag in his rate of development. Denver Development and other screening tools are described in the chapter on "Assessment of Children's Behavior."

Early Intervention. Nurses are involved in the intensive care for seriously injured or defective neonates. Accompanying the provision of intense physical care is intervention to meet the family's emotional needs. Specific approaches that help the family through grieving and with their attachment to their child are the provision of:

1. Opportunities to get to know and feel close to their child by helping in his care;
2. Communication of concern for the family's as well as for the child's welfare;
3. Discussion of their child's abilities as well as his disabilities;
4. Counseling about their feelings and their plans to include their child in their family;

5. Inclusion of the family in the child's early developmental stimulation program;
6. Opportunities to participate in the coordination of needed services for his special needs.

Since the birth of a disabled infant is also emotionally stressful for health care professionals, identifying their own feelings about caring for a disabled child and developing support from each other are essential to providing sensitive and comprehensive services to these children and their families.

Teaching. Nurses today are providing consultation and education that will improve the provision of services to mentally disabled individuals and their families. The goal of teaching is to explain the child's difficulties, abilities, and needs so that the parents can identify their own value in participating in their child's developmental program. Developmental education programs now strongly encourage family participation by combining "at school" activities with "at home" experiences. School hours are often extended to evenings and Saturdays to accommodate and include both parents. From this involvement the family learns to incorporate developmental principles into their caring for and playing with their child and to develop confidence in their ability to foster their child's learning.

Nurses are teaching prenatal, child development, and genetics classes to high school and college students and to families, educators, and other professionals. This community education is essential for its members to prevent mental disabilities, to plan services to meet the needs of its disabled members, to help neighbors with these difficulties, and to help themselves when mental disabilities occur in their own families.

Counseling. Counseling is the main strategy of all nursing interventions with families of mentally disabled children. Acceptance of the family's difficulty in making and continually reviewing their decision on their role in caring for their child and assistance with sharing their feelings with all family members are important counseling considerations for the nurse. Nursing counseling helps the family identify the developing abilities and disabilities of their child and their complementary roles.

The primary nurse in the hospital, clinic, developmental education center, or the home is in an excellent position to counsel families. With her comprehensive view of past family events and coping abilities, the primary nurse is best able to identify and assist the family at risk who is not constructively coping, resolving their grief, or making future plans.

Planning and Evaluating. All family members must be included in evaluation and planning for the mentally disabled child. The parents know the child intimately and see the minute signs of progress that he makes. Parents "have a thousand clues which help the professional better reach and evaluate their exceptional child."[2] The older and less disabled child is also a member of the team that is evaluating him and planning with him. In accordance with normalization, the disabled individual deserves the opportunity to assert himself, make choices, and take risks concerning his own future.

Nurses are becoming dynamically involved in evaluating the needs of the mentally disabled in their communities and assuming greater responsibility for helping to plan and implement new policy and programs. Nurses not only work in programs, but they help determine the need, design programs, and evaluate the services and effects of developmental education programs. Nurses are involved in political planning bodies and in administrative capacities that can foster higher quality and comprehensive care to mentally disabled children and their families.

SUMMARY

The presence of a mentally disabled child within a family is a unique experience. It is a risk experience that can lead to family disintegration or to optimal growth and closeness for all family members. Through planning and providing services that prevent or reduce the difficulties for these families, the nurse plays a vital role.

REFERENCES

1. Barnard, K. "Trends in the Care and Prevention of Developmental Disabilities." *American Journal of Nursing*, 75 #10, October 1975, 1700–1704.
2. Buscaglia, L. *The Disabled and Their Parents: A Counseling Challenge.* Thorofare, N.J.: Charles B. Slack, 1975, 269.
3. Klaus, M. and J. Kennell. *Maternal-Infant Bonding.* St. Louis: C. V. Mosby Co., 1976, 41–46, 93–94.
4. Richmond, J. B., G. Tarjan, and R. S. Mendelsohn. *Mental Retardation: A Handbook for the Primary Physician.* Chicago: American Medical Association, 1974, 1–4.
5. Wolfensberger, W. "The Origin and Nature of Our Institutional Models." In *Changing Patterns in Residential Services for the Mentally Retarded.* Washington, D.C.: President's Committee on Mental Retardation Monograph, 1969, 63–143.
6. ———. *The Principle of Normalization in Human Services.* Toronto, Ca.: National Institute on Mental Retardation, 1972, 26–29, 130.

ADDITIONAL READINGS

1. Barnard, K. and M. Erickson. *Teaching Children with Developmental Problems: A Family Care Approach.* St. Louis: C. V. Mosby Co., 1976.
2. Chinn, P. C., C. Drew, and D. R. Logan. *Mental Retardation: A Life Cycle Approach.* St. Louis: C. V. Mosby Co., 1975.
3. Grossman, F. K. *Brothers and Sisters of Retarded Children.* New York: Syracuse University Press, 1972.
4. O'Neill, S. M., B. N. McLaughlin, and M. B. Knapp. *Behavioral Approaches to Children with Developmental Delays.* St. Louis: C. V. Mosby Co., 1977.
5. Smith, D. and A. Wilson. *The Child with Down's Syndrome.* Philadelphia: W. B. Saunders Co., 1973.

PERTINENT ORGANIZATIONS

NATIONAL
- *American Association on Mental Deficiency*
  5201 Connecticut Avenue, N.W.
  Washington, D.C. 20015
  Provides information on local resources, educational programs.

- *Association for Children with Learning Disabilities*
  5225 Grace Street
  Pittsburgh, Pennsylvania 15236
  Provides referral for service, educational programs.
- *Epilepsy Foundation of America*
  1828 "L" Street N.W., Suite 406
  Washington, D. C. 20036
  Provides information and referral services, educational programs.
- *National Association for Retarded Citizens*
  2709 Avenue E East
  Arlington, Texas 76011
  Provides referral for service, educational programs, treatment programs.
- *National Easter Seal Society*
  2023 West Ogden Avenue
  Chicago, Illinois 60612
  Provides information on local resources, treatment programs.

- *National Society for Autistic Children*
  169 Tampa Avenue
  Albany, New York 12208
  Provides information and referral for services for autistic children.
- *United Cerebral Palsy Association*
  66 East 34th Street
  New York, New York 10016
  Provides information on local resources, educational programs, and treatment programs.

LOCAL
- Health Department
    Community Mental Health Services
    Crippled Children Services
    Public Health Nursing
- Department or Social Services
- Social Security Administration
    Supplemental Security Income

The Failure to Thrive Child

Lynda Harrison, R.N., M.S.N.

CHAPTER EIGHT

The term "failure to thrive" has been used to characterize infants and children whose weight and often height fall below expected standards. The term refers to symptoms and not to a specific cause of the problem. There is considerable variation in its definition in the literature, but there seem to be two general classes of definitions.

The first class of definitions views failure to thrive as *physical growth failure* stemming from a variety of causes, including environmental factors, metabolic disease, defects in a major organ system, or genetic defects. The second class of definitions involves *psychosocial failure to thrive* or growth failure for which there is no organic explanation. There are both general and specific criteria of failure to thrive within this class. Some writers state that the child's weight must be below the third percentile on a standard growth chart, some specify that improvement must take place in a nurturing environment, and others identify behaviors which must be present in order to make the diagnosis.

For the purpose of this chapter, the term failure to thrive is defined as growth failure below the third percentile on a standard growth chart for which no organic cause can be found. Although failure to thrive children are generally referred to in this chapter as infants, it is recognized that the problem is not limited to the first 12 months of life.

Because studies have used different definitions of failure to thrive, the incidence of the problem is difficult to determine. In retrospective analyses of hospital records, 2 percent of admissions at Philadelphia Children's Hospital and 5 percent of pediatric admissions at Missouri Hospital were found to be failure to thrive.[1,12] The incidence in the community is probably higher than is revealed by hospital records.

There seems to be an equal distribution of the problem among both sexes and among different races.[7] The syndrome is usually discovered in very young children. One study found, for example, that half of the failure to thrive children had been hospitalized by the age of six months.[6]

BASIC CONCEPTS OF FAILURE TO THRIVE

Failure to thrive is usually a result of some problem in the relationship between the child and his primary caretaker. Because the mother has been viewed as the child's primary caretaker in our society, most of the literature on causes of failure to thrive focuses on the mother-infant relationship. Additional information on the dynamics of the father-infant and mother-father relationships in failure to thrive families is needed.

Three basic causes of the child's growth failure can be identified in the literature. Disturbances in the neuro-endocrine system, resulting from inadequate parent-child relationships, have been postulated by several researchers to be responsible for growth failure in the nonthriving child. Emotionally engendered hyperactivity of the adrenal cortex may suppress growth.[3] Emotionally deprived environments resulting in abnormal patterns of sleep may inhibit the secretion of pituitary hormones including the growth hormone.[5]

Inadequate food intake is one causative factor of children's growth failure. One study concluded that mothers of failure to thrive infants were offering their children less food than they had reported to their physicians. When the researchers provided the infants with an increased amount of food, all gained weight.[13] Another researcher has suggested that food deprivation causes endocrine abnormalities which may result initially in pituitary hyperfunction and later in hypothalamic insensitivity and pituitary hypofunction.[9]

Inadequate nurturing, also described as maladaptive mothering or maternal deprivation, is frequently cited as a factor contributing to an infant's failure to thrive.[2] Maternal attachment and mothering behaviors as discussed in the "Assessment of Mothering Behavior" chapter are important to assess in the failure to thrive situation. Some of the factors which have been identified as contributing to maladaptive mothering include prenatal or postnatal problems, early parental separation, physical difficulties in the infant, parents inadequately nurtured in their own childhoods, adolescent parents, and socioeconomic or psychosocial strains on the family. In addition, the infant's failure to develop normally undermines the parent's confidence in his or her parenting ability, resulting in a reciprocal process in which both parent and infant fail to thrive.

Treatment of Failure to Thrive. While most studies suggest the need for long-term supportive care for the failure to thrive family, some research suggests that even short-term intervention can stimulate a reversal in the maladaptive parent-child relationships which are associated with the syndrome.

Providing the infant with sufficient nutrients and positive interactions is the basis for treatment. The failure to thrive infant should receive 140 calories per kilogram of ideal weight for height each day in order to stimulate weight gain.[13] Meeting the infant's psychosocial needs for oral gratification, trust, and stimulation is as important as providing for his nutritional needs. The hospitalized failure to thrive infant needs a consistent caretaker who can attend to his needs for rocking, cuddling, and stimulation as well as to other aspects of physical care.

A key aspect of treatment is to support the parents, helping them to mobilize their love for their children and to find satisfaction with parenthood. Since many of the parents were deprived in their own childhood, they may need extra nurturing and support. Failure to thrive parents often demonstrate hostile and threatening behavior toward helping persons, perhaps in an attempt to relieve their own guilt. Acceptance of the parents despite such behavior is considered of primary importance in the treatment approach. Collaboration with the parents in planning the infant's care while avoiding an authority role helps the parents share in the child's improvement.

What Makes Failure to Thrive a Risk to the Family? There may be critical periods during which a child is at greater risk for the long-term sequelae of early malnutrition and emotional deprivation. At least one study has suggested that the effects of failure to thrive may be reversible; while some children remain below average in physical and intellectual development, others later develop normally.[6]

Due to the reciprocal relationship between parent and infant, the infant's failure to grow and develop as expected may undermine the parent's confidence and lead to a cycle of maladaptive parent-child interaction patterns. Parents often perceive early problems with their infants (both prenatally and postnatally) as forerunners of things to come, and it is often at this point that interactional problems begin.[11] A child's early failure to thrive, therefore, can become a self-fulfilling prophecy if the parents interpret this as indicative of other long-term problems. One mother illustrated this phenomenon when she stated that she had had pneumonia during her pregnancy and thought this was the start of her infant's feeding problems.

Early and unanticipated problems with an infant can tax a parent's already overburdened reserves. In families with marginal coping abilities, the infant's failure to thrive may precipitate major parenting disorders. For example, Laurie was an 18-year-old unmarried mother who was ambivalent during her pregnancy about whether to keep her baby or place it for adoption. When the baby was born, Laurie decided that she would keep her. The public health nurse visited frequently during the first few weeks following the birth, and observed that the mother and baby seemed to be developing a close and adaptive relationship. When the baby began having feeding problems and was hospitalized at age three weeks, however, Laurie found it increasingly difficult to fulfill her mothering role. When she visited her baby in the hospital Laurie preferred not to hold or feed her. Shortly after the baby's discharge from the hospital, Laurie asked that her baby be placed for adoption.

CHARACTERISTICS OF FAILURE TO THRIVE FAMILIES

Identifying characteristics of the failure to thrive family is useful in alerting health professionals to potential high-risk situations, however not all of these characteristics are found in every failure to thrive family. Figure 8-1 briefly lists these characteristics.

Infant Characteristics. The most commonly identified physical and behavioral characteristics of failure to thrive infants include:

• Failure to grow and gain weight;

Figure 8-1. Characteristics of the Failure to Thrive Family

Infant Characteristics
  Physical characteristics—failure to grow and gain weight
  Behavioral characteristics—developmental slowness

Characteristics of Mothers
  Low self-esteem and feelings of inadequacy
  Desire to be taken care of
  Literal concrete thinking patterns
  Use of denial, isolation, and projection defense mechanisms
  Predisposition to acting out rather than thinking
  Inaccessibility and suspicion of helping persons
  Difficulty in accurately perceiving the infant's needs

Characteristics of Fathers
  Ineffectual in childrearing behaviors
  Often absent from home

Characteristics of Siblings
  Poor physical health

Family Stability and Socioeconomic Characteristics
  Marital problems
  Low socioeconomic class

Other Family Difficulties
  Guilt
  Grief
  Child abuse

• Developmental slowness;
• Gastrointestinal difficulties and feeding problems;
• Unusual watchfulness;
• Minimal smiling;
• Decreased vocalizations;
• Lack of cuddliness;
• Position of tonic immobility;
• Sleep disturbances;
• Lack of interest in environmental stimuli or toys.

Based on her work with failure to thrive families the author has developed a tool with which to assess adaptive or maladaptive infant behaviors (Table 8-1). Infant behaviors which are conducive to physical development and the acquisition of a sense of trust are considered adaptive. Behaviors which may inhibit physical development and the acquisition of a sense of trust are maladaptive. By using such a tool, nurses might identify specific problem areas for intervention, as well as evaluate changes in infant behavior over the course of the nurse-family relationship.[8]

Table 8-1. Categories of Adaptive and Maladaptive Infant Behaviors

Critical Period	Adaptive	Maladaptive
Sleeping	Receives adequate sleep for normal growth —at least 16 hours per day—without restless sleep patterns or prolonged crying at nap or bedtime after other needs have been met	Receives inadequate sleep for normal growth—less than 16 hours per day—and shows restless sleep patterns or prolonged crying at nap or bedtime
Feeding	Actively seeks food offered	Resists food offered
	Effectively sucks and swallows food	Does not suck effectively
	Demonstrates pleasurable relief after eating	Remains fussy after adequate amount of feeding—no pleasurable relief
Response to Environment	Demonstrates active response to environment by exploring or reaching-out behavior	Seems apathetic to environment
Vocalizing	Demonstrates vocalizations when alert, if developmentally ready	Makes infrequent or no vocalizations during visit although developmentally ready
Smiling	Demonstrates smiling behavior if older than two months	Does not demonstrate smiling behavior during visit
Cuddling	Cuddles when held	Resists being held or stiffens when held

Modified from Harrison, L. "Nursing Intervention with the Failure to Thrive Family." Copyright March/April 1976, the American Journal of Nursing Company. Reproduced with permission from *MCN*, The American Journal of Maternal Child Nursing, Vol. 1 No. 2, p. 113.

A case example illustrates the range of adaptive and maladaptive behaviors which might be encountered with an individual failure to thrive infant. Brian was 11 months old at the time of the public health nurse's first visit, and well below the third percentile in weight. He was noted to lie placidly in the middle of the bed throughout the hour-long visit. He did not attempt to roll over or reach out for objects, though he did follow stimuli with his eyes, and cooed in response to his sister's talking to him. On subsequent visits a more complete assessment revealed the following observations: his sleep behavior was adaptive (Brian's mother reported that he slept 14 hours per day); he demonstrated maladaptive feeding behavior by resisting food offered to him, although he could effectively suck and swallow his food; he continued to remain passive in response to environmental stimuli, though he did demonstrate smiling and vocalizing behavior on every home visit; and his response to being held remained maladaptive, for he would stiffen, rather than cuddle, in his mother's arms.

Mother's Characteristics. Frequently mentioned characteristics of nonthriving mothers include unplanned or unwanted pregnancies, a high incidence of complications during their pregnancies, and a history of inadequate nurturing in their own childhoods. The following psychological characteristics have been described in nonthriving mothers:

1. Low self-esteem and feelings of inadequacy. This may be reflected in such comments as "I can never do anything right." The appearance of the mother, or even of her home, may also reflect the mother's self-image.
2. Desire for an anaclitic relationship and a need to be taken care of. If the mother has been deprived of adequate parenting as a child, she may demonstrate excessively dependent behavior as an adult. This de-

pendency might be reflected in the mother's relationship with the nurse, if, for example, she relies on the nurse to make her plans and arrangements rather than carry them out independently in order to ensure the nurse's ongoing support and attention.

3. Literal, concrete thinking patterns. These mothers may respond best to teaching by direct example since it may be difficult for them to apply abstract principles to their own situations.

4. Major defense mechanisms of denial, isolation, and projection. Many failure to thrive mothers deny that their child has a growth problem and frequently seem to be isolated from the community, having few supportive relationships with friends or relatives.

5. Predisposition toward acting out rather than thinking. This characteristic may be seen in behavior which seems to reflect poor judgment, such as spending all of the monthly income on a new piece of furniture and having no money left for food.

6. Inaccessibility and suspicion of helping persons. Professionals can be particularly threatening to persons with low self-concepts, and it may take great patience and persistence to develop a trusting relationship with a failure to thrive mother.

7. Difficulty in accurately perceiving the infant's needs. This characteristic is illustrated by the mother who becomes extremely frustrated with her infant's crying and claims she has tried everything to comfort him, but may have overlooked hunger, one of the most common causes of the behavior.[4]

Adaptive parenting behaviors are those which demonstrate a realistic perception of the infant's needs, abilities, and characteristics, and which promote his optimum growth and development. Maladaptive parenting behaviors, on the other hand, demonstrate an unrealistic perception of the infant or a lack of attachment between the infant and parent. A tool assessing adaptive and maladaptive behaviors of the primary caretakers of failure to thrive children is shown in Table 8-2.

The following case history illustrates the value of this tool in assessing the feeding behaviors of one failure to thrive mother. Over the course of eight home visits to Carolyn and her 12-month-old son, Jason, the public health nurse was able to observe Jason's feeding only twice. Visits were scheduled to coincide with the baby's mealtimes, however Carolyn often reported that she had already fed the child before the nurse arrived. The nurse noted that Carolyn adequately prepared the appropriate amounts and types of food for Jason. Her maladaptive feeding behaviors were in the area of feeding technique. When Carolyn became impatient with Jason's efforts to feed himself, she restrained his hands. Jason responded by closing his mouth and refusing to take more food. This mother did not seem to understand the importance of allowing an infant to participate in and enjoy his feedings.

Father's Characteristics. The fact that little has been written about fathers of failure to thrive infants illustrates the need for more family-centered research into this problem. Failure to thrive fathers are frequently absent from the home, or when present are often ineffectual in childrearing behaviors.[10] For example, one father was present during most of the public health nurse's home visits, although he was not always willing to actively participate in the discussions. When he did participate, he deferred questions regarding the infant to his wife, stating, "She's the one who takes care of the baby." Nor did he hold, cuddle, or feed the baby during the nurse's visits.

Siblings' Characteristics. There is also little information on the siblings in the failure to thrive family. Siblings are usually close in age and tend to have poor physical and emotional health. Since failure to thrive of one child is often precipitated by difficulties in mothering, the other children are probably also affected although the symptoms may be slightly different.

Family Characteristics. Marital problems are common in failure to thrive families, which are frequently described as disorganized, multiproblem families. Since failure to thrive families are often from lower socioeconomic classes, marital difficulties related to low social status and lack of money are common. In addition, parents of the failure to

Table 8-2. Categories of Adaptive and Maladaptive Parenting Behaviors

Critical Period	Adaptive	Maladaptive
Feeding behaviors	Offers appropriate amounts and/or types of food to infant	Provides inadequate types or amounts of food for infant
	Holds infant in comfortable position during feeding	Does not hold infant, or holds in uncomfortable position during feeding
	Burps baby during and/or after feeding	Does not burp infant
	Prepares food appropriately	Prepares food inappropriately
	Offers food at comfortable pace for infant	Offers food at pace too rapid for infant's comfort
Infant stimulation	Provides appropriate verbal stimulation for infant during visit	Provides no or only aggressive verbal stimulation for infant during visit
	Provides tactile stimulation for infant at times other than during feeding or moving infant away from danger	Does not provide tactile stimulation or only that of aggressive handling of infant
	Provides age-appropriate toys	No evidence of age-appropriate toys
	Interacts with infant in a way that provides for infant's satisfaction	Frustrates infant during interactions
Infant rest	Provides quiet or relaxed environment for infant's rest, including scheduled rest periods	Does not provide quiet environment or consistent schedule for rest periods
	Ensures that infant's needs for food, warmth, and/or dryness are met before sleep	Does not attend to infant's needs for food, warmth, and/or dryness before sleep
Perception	Demonstrates realistic perception of infant's condition in accordance with medical and/or nursing diagnoses	Shows unrealistic perception of infant's condition
	Has realistic expectations of infant	Demonstrates unrealistic expectations of infant
	Recognizes infant's unfolding skills or behavior	Has no awareness of infant's development
	Shows realistic perception of own mothering behavior	Shows unrealistic perception of own mothering
Initiative	Shows initiative in attempts to manage infant's problems, including actively seeking information about infant	Shows no initiative in attempts to meet infant's needs or to manage problems. Does not follow through with plans
Recreation	Provides positive outlets for own recreation or relaxation	Does not provide positive outlets for own recreation or relaxation
Interaction with other children	Demonstrates positive interaction with other children in the home	Demonstrates hostile-aggressive interactions with other children in the home
Mothering role	Expresses satisfaction with mothering	Expresses dissatisfaction with mothering

Adapted from Harrison, L. "Nursing Intervention with the Failure to Thrive Family." Copyright March/April 1976, the American Journal of Nursing Company. Reproduced with permission from *MCN*, The American Journal of Maternal Child Nursing, Vol. 1 No. 2, p. 112.

thrive infant often experience guilt over poor parenting and feelings of inadequacy in providing for the child's needs. They may also experience grief for their loss of a normal infant, or fear of loss if their infant is physically ill. Also, failure to thrive based on parental neglect may be a sign or a precursor of child abuse.

NURSING APPROACHES

Given the present belief that the cause of failure to thrive is related to maladaptive parenting, most treatment is aimed at promoting positive parent-child relationships and enabling parents to meet their child's physical and emotional needs. Nurses in a variety of settings are in positions to promote adaptive parent-child relationships.

There are two important issues to consider in any attempt to help a failure to thrive family. The first involves the need to exercise caution in defining "positive" parent-child relationships. It is extremely important to acknowledge and accept cultural and individual variations in styles of parenting. The tool for assessing parenting behaviors which was presented earlier (Table 8-2) is a beginning effort to differentiate maladaptive and adaptive parenting behaviors, however, further research is needed in a variety of settings in order to determine its validity.

The second issue concerns the importance of differentiating between manipulation of the parent-child relationship by the nurse and helping the parents to change their interaction patterns by choice. Any treatment approach which does not allow the helped person to make an active choice to change is unlikely to result in any long-term change in behavior. The most important actions include prevention, assessment, teaching, counseling, and evaluation.

Prevention

Nurses working in schools, public health agencies, and primary health care facilities are in key positions to prevent the problem or to identify high-risk cases before maladaptive interaction patterns have become firmly established. There are several preventive approaches.

Family life education programs are valuable in preparing youngsters for the realities of parenthood. These programs should promote an understanding of child and family development, provide for experience in child care, and allow an exploration of feelings about having children. Discussion of alternative family patterns might suggest options for those who do not want to be parents.

Adolescent parent child-care classes provide an opportunity for young parents to learn specific nurturing skills and offer a supportive environment in which mutual problems can be shared and resolved. One high school in an urban area, for example, provides day care for children of adolescent students. Each day the adolescent parent spends time in the nursery where trained child-care staff provide teaching and support to promote the development of positive parent-child relationships.

Prenatal counseling should include anticipatory guidance regarding infant behavior and the common feelings and problems which accompany parenthood. "Statements showing acceptance of stresses related to parenthood, such as "A new baby's crying can really be frustrating for the parents," are helpful. Emotional support and nurturing of the expectant couple are important components of prenatal counseling.

Early parent-infant contact has been found to promote bonding, attachment, and engrossment between the parent and child. Providing rooming-in facilities and unlimited visiting privileges for fathers in obstetric units helps to encourage this early contact.

Early identification of high-risk families and referral to a public health nurse or primary care nurse is another aspect of prevention. Nurses in all settings working with families in the childbearing cycle should establish programs to assess the behaviors and interaction patterns of parents and infants, being alert to the characteristics of failure to thrive families discussed previously.

Assessment

A thorough and accurate assessment of the family's situation and problems is imperative. The importance of starting where the family is and directing helping efforts to the individual needs of the parent and child cannot be too strongly emphasized. One failure to thrive family, for example, may identify their greatest problem as inadequate housing. In this case, the nurse's first goal should be to help them find an adequate home.

Clarifying the Nurse's Role. Identifying how the nurse may be of help to the family is an important first step in establishing a working relationship. Negotiation of the nursing-family relationship is done using counseling techniques. The parent and nurse mutually identify the problems to be addressed in the relationship. Some families may appear apathetic and find it difficult to make choices and establish mutual goals with the nurse. Allowing such families to make small choices at first, such as when the nurse should visit, may be useful.

This first step is unfortunately often difficult for nurses who may be uncertain about their role with failure to thrive families. The problem is compounded when other helping persons such as social workers or physicians are also involved with the family and all roles must be clarified. For example, one mother, Sharon, was already working with a child protective worker when the public health nurse began visiting her. Sharon's initial greeting to the nurse was, "I guess you're here to tell me how to take care of my baby, too." The nurse responded that because of her nursing background she might be able to help the family with health concerns and with questions about child care and development. The nurse clarified that she did not have a legal mandate to visit and that Sharon could choose whether or not she wanted the nurse's services. An agreement was made for the nurse to make three home visits to the family to work on resolving the baby's feeding problems, and then to evaluate whether to continue the relationship.

Assessing the family's perception of the problem and their plans to resolve it should be done early in the nurse-family relationship. Many failure to thrive parents focus their concern on minor systemic symptoms which the child may exhibit and seem unaware of the child's growth failure, which may be frightening and threatening to the parents. Since most children get colds, parents frequently focus on this more minor problem. The nurse establishes her relationship and goals around the parents' main concern while teaching them about the difficulties of poor development. Some families may actively resent the nurse's help. It is best to accept the parents' choice while assuring them of the nurse's ongoing availability to help with any health problems that occur. Many parents will accept help during an acute illness.

Assessment of the Infant. Observation of the infant provides an opportunity to evaluate his status and also offers an entry point for the nurse working with the failure to thrive family. Parents often find it easier to relate to the physical aspects of the nurse's role until they establish a trusting and working relationship with her.

Measuring the infant's height and weight is a valuable part of the initial physical exam, and should be repeated periodically to assess the child's progress. The interval between these measurements should not be so short as to overemphasize the child's growth problem and further undermine the parents' self-confidence. One mother, for example, stated that she perceived the scale as a measure of her mothering ability.

Other aspects of the physical exam which assume particular importance with the failure to thrive infant include assessment of vision and hearing to rule out physical reasons for possible developmental delays; attention to the condition of the skin for evidence of vitamin nutritional deficiency, dehydration, or trauma; and evaluation of muscle tone and movement, again to rule out possible organic problems.

If the infant is acutely ill, the nurse should obtain a full history of the problem from the parent.

While performing a more thorough physical assessment of the infant including assessment of the temperature, ears, throat, chest, abdomen, and lymph nodes, the nurse might teach the parent to observe for signs of serious illness. Empathizing with the parent about the stresses and difficulties imposed on parents by a child's illness is also helpful.

Behavioral assessment of the infant can be accomplished by means of direct observation by the nurse and eliciting the parents' description of the infant's behaviors and activities. Sleeping, feeding, response to environment, vocalizing, smiling, and cuddling behaviors should be identified as described in the tool "Categories of Adaptive and Maladaptive Infant Behavior," Table 8-1. Direct observation of the infant's feeding behavior is especially important to determine specific nutritional difficulties and interaction that occurs during feeding.

Tools such as the Denver Developmental Screening Test and others discussed in the chapter on Assessment of Children's Behavior are useful in assessing the infant's behaviors and provide a valuable opportunity for the nurse to teach the parents about growth and development. For example, one mother told the nurse that she feared her eight-month-old baby, Anne, was retarded because she could not stand up. The nurse administered the Denver Developmental Screening Test to Anne in Paula's presence, discussed the child's abilities, and showed Paula that Anne's developmental level was normal for her age.

Assessment of Family Interactions. Assessment of parenting behaviors may require many contacts with the family. The presence of the nurse may affect the way the parent interacts with the child, and thus the behavior observed during a prearranged home visit may not be characteristic of the usual parent-child interactions. For example, a father may respond to a baby's crying by picking him up and comforting him in the nurse's presence, while the mother may report that he will sometimes hit the infant.

Assessment of family interaction patterns should include attention to the interaction between mother and father, parents and other children, and parents and extended family. What are the communication patterns between the mother and father? Do the parents share responsibility for the care of the children? Do they seem to respect one another? Is there evidence of physical violence between the parents? Do the parents relate with their other children differently from the failure to thrive child? Are there relatives or extended family members in geographic proximity and are they supportive to the nonthriving family? Relationships with extended family members can be extremely significant to the failure to thrive family. For example, one failure to thrive mother, Kathy, was living with her aunt who exerted great pressure for Kathy to divorce her husband. When Kathy moved away from the aunt's house and criticism, her infant began to gain weight immediately.

Assessment of family health, social, and financial status may lead to the discovery of problems which make it difficult for the parents to cope with their parenting responsibilities. If the family does not have enough money for food, providing the children with adequate nutrition becomes extremely difficult. Similarly, a parent's poor health hinders his ability to care for the children.

Teaching

There are three general principles of particular importance in teaching the failure to thrive family. The first relates to the need for *collaboration* with the parents in developing and implementing a teaching program. Assuming an authority role implies a superior-inferior relationship and may only further decrease the parents' self-esteem.

The second principle is to *include pertinent others* in the teaching program. Implementing this principle is sometimes difficult in situations where there are many people responsible for the care of the failure to thrive child, however the nurse can plan visits when all family members are present and ask questions to include all in the discussion.

The third principle involves the need to *clarify the relevance of the problem* in order to increase the parents' motivation to learn. The tendency of failure to thrive parents to be unaware of the problem of the child's low weight has been discussed previously. In attempting to help the family to recognize the growth problem, it is important that the nurse not frighten or threaten them in the process. One failure to thrive father told the nurse that he thought his child was small because both he and his wife were small, and he saw no need for concern. The nurse agreed that the parents' size may be a contributing factor, but explained the physician's concern that the child's nutritional needs be adequately met in order to ensure the optimum development of the child. Although weight gain was only one of several ways to assess the child's nutritional status, it was the only one which had been assessed thus far. The nurse asked the parents whether she might visit them several more times in order to more closely evaluate the child's nutrition and to determine whether there might be other factors contributing to the child's low weight.

Teaching Normal Infant Care. Teaching related to infant feeding is a frequently needed nursing intervention for failure to thrive families. The types of food required by the infant as well as specific amounts and preparation techniques may need to be demonstrated to the failure to thrive parent. It is most helpful to consult a nutrition reference which specifies exact amounts of food needed by infants of various ages. If this information is not available, the nurse might calculate the infant's dietary needs by employing the formula given earlier (140 calories per kilogram of ideal weight for height per day).[13]

A common problem encountered with nonthriving families, particularly where there are several children in the household, is a lack of cleanliness in the child's eating utensils and bottles. The need for adequate washing is especially important if the child has a gastrointestinal upset such as vomiting or diarrhea. It is sometimes difficult to suggest better washing practices without further decreasing the parent's self-esteem. Again, an empathetic approach, perhaps mentioning how tiring chores are when raising an infant, can help.

In addition, many parents may need basic information or demonstrations on the treatment of common infant feeding problems such as regurgitation after meals. For example, one mother reported that her five-month-old infant spit up after almost every meal. On further discussion she stated that she usually put the infant on his abdomen in the crib immediately after he finished eating. The nurse suggested that the mother place the baby in an upright position for ten minutes after his meals. On the following visit, the mother stated that the problem was resolved.

Failure to thrive parents often need teaching of normal child behavior and development. The nurse might explain, for example, that crying and fussing when the mother leaves the room is normal behavior for an eight-month-old, so that a parent will better understand that the child is not spoiled or demanding undue attention. Discussing the importance of verbal and tactile stimulation can also be a therapeutic teaching tool. Statements such as "Sarah sure looks at you closely when you talk to her like that. She must really enjoy it!" reinforces the parents' interaction with the infant.

Some parents need encouragement to have fun with and enjoy their children. The nurse might ask what they really enjoy the most about their child. Home health aides have been employed in some locales to act as role models for the parents and teach them how to play with their children.

Teaching ways to provide for the infant's rest is especially important in view of the postulation that the growth problems of failure to thrive children may be the result of inadequate sleep.[5] Does the child have a quiet and consistent place for sleeping? Is he fed, dry, and warm when placed in bed? Does he have some type of a routine for sleeping-wakefulness established? Sleep needs of infants vary: some need 16 hours per day, while others seem to need no more than 10 to 12 hours per day. Does the parent know how to determine whether the child is tired? For example, one failure to thrive father reported that his infant would cry when placed in his crib, but would not settle with feeding, holding, rocking, or changing. He finally discovered that the infant would fall asleep if left alone crying in his crib for five or ten minutes. Parents need support in such situations and reassurance that often it is necessary to try several approaches before discovering what works best for a particular child.

Teaching Family Health Care. Teaching related to specific health problems of the infant is important for the failure to thrive family. Vomiting and diarrhea are perhaps the most common systemic problems encountered in failure to thrive infants. After assessing the infant and ruling out a pathologic cause for the vomiting or diarrhea, the nurse might instruct the parents to place the infant on a clear liquid diet and observe for signs of dehydration. Infantile colic is another frequently encountered problem. The nurse should teach the parents that colic usually results from a cycle of crying, air-swallowing, distention, pain, and then crying again, and that treatment is aimed at interrupting this cycle. Measures such as proper burping techniques, size of nipple holes, and occasionally a mild tranquilizer are commonly employed treatment methods.

Teaching related to family health matters may be important since parents often need to meet their own needs before they can focus on the infant's problem. In some cases, the illness of a family member may pose a direct threat to the health of the child. For example, one failure to thrive father was found to have a positive tine test, but continually failed to report to the clinic for a chest x-ray. A great deal of teaching and support was done by the public health nurse before he finally had the chest x-ray showing possible tuberculosis lesions and started treatment. Meanwhile the failure to thrive infant and other members had been exposed to the illness.

Counseling

Counseling assists the family in identifying their individual difficulties and planning ways to deal with them.

Promoting Satisfaction with Parenthood. The aim of intervention within this category is to reverse what might previously have been a frustrating and unrewarding relationship between a parent and failure to thrive child. Three specific ways in which nurses might accomplish this goal are increasing the parents' awareness of the skills and positive aspects of their infant's behavior, recognizing and supporting positive parenting behaviors, and working with parents to help them develop appropriate ways to handle their own frustrations, such as helping them find satisfying recreational outlets. During one home visit, for example, Mary mentioned that she was tired of being "cooped up" all day with her seven-month-old infant, but she was reluctant to attend the mothers' group because her husband Steve thought that her "place" was in the home. The nurse supported Mary to discuss her need for contact with other mothers so she could enjoy her mothering more.

Helping the parents to identify and meet their own personal goals may indirectly help them to find increased satisfaction with their parenting roles. It is generally accepted that a person must feel fulfilled as an individual to be able to give of himself to another. If the child's birth has interfered with the parent's life goals it is important for the nurse to help the parent grieve the loss of these goals and establish new ones that can be attained and lead to satisfaction.

Promoting Insight. The findings discussed earlier that nonthriving mothers tend to use denial as a major defense, to have literal thinking patterns, and to have difficulty in perceiving their infants' needs suggest that promoting insight into their own and the infant's behavior may be a helpful process. Encouraging the parents to verbalize their feelings regarding child care and about the infant's behavior may help them to clarify and to deal with their negative feelings.

The nurse helps the family see the effect of their conflict on the infant's health to increase the parents' motivation to provide needed parenting behaviors. For example, Carl and Ellen were living apart when the nurse first started visiting the family to help resolve the infant's feeding problems. Following the parents' reunion the infant's condition improved dramatically. When the nurse shared this observation with Ellen, she commented, "I guess all the trouble Carl and I were having got passed on to the baby."

Promoting the Use of Community Resources. The nurse is in a key position to acquaint the family with community resources such as health care resources, day care facilities, parent education groups, mothers' clubs, and family counseling agencies. Information alone is often not sufficient, however. At times parents may resist utilizing resources. Encouraging the parents to express their feelings regarding the use of the particular resource may provide a clue to the reason behind the resistance. For example, one mother of a failure to thrive infant refused to pick up food vouchers to buy milk for her infant. On exploring Debbie's feelings regarding going to the center to obtain the vouchers, Debbie revealed that she was afraid of a particular social worker at the center who had a reputation for "taking your kids away." With this information the nurse could inform Debbie that she would not have contact with the social worker while obtaining her vouchers and explore the basis for Debbie's concern that Tammy would be taken from her.

Evaluation

In addition to considering infant weight gain, change in the parent-child relationship must be considered as a criterion in evaluating the effectiveness of intervention with the failure to thrive family. The tools which have been presented to assess infant and parent behaviors provide one means to measure the change. Following each contact with the family the nurse might tally the number of adaptive and maladaptive parenting and infant behaviors observed in the various categories identified in the tools. After four or five visits it should be possible to determine whether there has been a change in specific parenting or infant behaviors. The nurse might observe, for instance, an increase in the number of adaptive parenting behaviors in the area of infant feeding, but a continuing problem in the parents' infant-stimulation behaviors. Such an observation would assist the nurse in

evaluating her interventions and in planning future goals with the family.

Evaluation may need to be continued for many months or years. The length of time required for effective treatment of the failure to thrive family depends on the individual situation. Some families may respond to short-term (six to eight weeks) nursing care, while others may require support over a longer period of time. Making a consistent helping person available (such as a nursing specialist in a clinic setting, or a public health nurse in the community) is one way to provide the failure to thrive family with such long-term support.

Once the acute problems identified in the nonthriving family have been resolved, the family may no longer perceive a need for nursing intervention. Long-term evaluation is important in such instances not only to allow for ongoing nursing assessment of the family situation, but also to assure the family of the nurse's continuing availability. This type of follow-up might be ensured by the nurse arranging bi-monthly visits or telephone calls to maintain contact with the family.

SUMMARY

Failure to thrive is not only an infant's problem but is a major problem placing the family at risk. The failure to thrive infant is often a symptom of other family difficulties. Nursing actions of prevention, assessment, teaching, counseling, and evaluation are focused on all family members.

REFERENCES

1. Barbero, G. "Failure to Thrive." In M. Klaus, T. Leger, and M. Trause (eds.). *Maternal Attachment and Mothering Disorders: A Round Table.* Johnson and Johnson Baby Products Company, 1975.
2. Barnard, M. and L. Wolf. "Psychosocial Failure to Thrive—Nursing Assessment and Intervention." *Nursing Clinics of North America,* 8, 1973, 557–565.
3. Blodgett, F. "Growth Retardation Related to

Maternal Deprivation." In A. Solnit and S. Provence (eds.). *Modern Perspectives in Child Development.* New York: International Universities Press, 1963.

4.   Fischhoff, J., C. Whitten, and M. Pettit. "A Psychiatric Study of Mothers of Infants with Growth Failure Secondary to Maternal Deprivation." *Journal of Pediatrics,* 79, 1971, 209–215.

5.   Gardner, L. "Deprivation Dwarfism." *Scientific American,* 227, 1972, 76–82.

6.   Glaser, H., M. Heagarty, D. Bullard, and E. Pivchik. "Physical and Psychological Development of Children with Early Failure to Thrive." *Journal of Pediatrics,* 73, 1968, 690–698.

7.   Hannaway, P. "Failure to Thrive—A Study of 100 Infants and Children." *Clinical Pediatrics,* 9, 1970, 96–99.

8.   Harrison, L. "Nursing Intervention with the Failure to Thrive Family." *MCN—The American Journal of Maternal-Child Nursing,* 1, 1976, 111–116.

9.   Krieger, I. and R. Mellinger. "Pituitary Function in the Deprivation Syndrome." *Journal of Pediatrics,* 79, 1971, 216–225.

10. Leonard, M., J. Rhymes, and A. Solnit. "Failure to Thrive in Infants—A Family Problem." *American Journal of Diseases of Children,* 113, 1966, 600–612.

11. Rhymes, J. "Working with Mothers and Babies Who Fail to Thrive." *American Journal of Nursing,* 66, 1966, 1972–1976.

12. Shaheen, E., D. Alexander, M. Truskowsky, and G. Barbero. Failure to Thrive—A Retrospective Profile. *Clinical Pediatrics,* 7, 1968, 255–261.

13. Whitten, C., M. Pettit, and J. Fischhoff. "Evidence that Growth Failure from Maternal Deprivation Is Secondary to Undereating." *The Journal of the American Medical Association,* 209, 1969, 1675–1682.

PERTINENT ORGANIZATIONS

NATIONAL

*   *International Childbirth Education Association (ICEA)*
    P.O. Box 9316
    Midtown Plaza
    Rochester, New York, 14604
    A service organization of providers and consumers to explore new aspects of family-centered maternity care.

LOCAL

*   Local parent education and support groups sponsored by churches, hospitals, mental health clinics, or community health agencies are all resources which may promote positive parent-child relationships and prevent failure to thrive.

The Hyperactive Child

Suzanne Hall Johnson, R.N., M.N.

CHAPTER NINE

While parenting a fairly normal child places the stress of normal developmental crises on the family, parenting the hyperactive child who is overactive, impulsive, excitable, and has a short attention span frequently stresses the family to its limits. Since the family with a hyperactive child must face a great deal of stress, there is danger of child abuse, marital discord, social isolation, and great difficulty in the relationship between the family members. In addition to the family being at risk, the hyperactive child is also at risk for learning disabilities, developmental disabilities, and psychosocial problems that may remain even after the actual symptoms of hyperactivity disappear in adolescence.

The family with a hyperactive child is a significant problem to both the family and the community. Although hyperactivity has only been described as an actual syndrome for about ten years, it is prevalent. Approximately 10 percent of all school children are considered hyperactive.[3] About half of the children seen for psychological problems are also considered hyperactive, and boys are more likely to be affected than girls.[3] It is apparent that, with the significant prevalence of hyperactivity and with the amount of aggression and behavioral disturbance the children produce in the schools, hyperactivity is not only the child's problem but the family's and the community's problem as well.

The nurse's role with a family with a hyperactive child includes identifying children who are at risk of hyperactivity and helping the family to reduce the hyperactive behaviors or cope with the present behaviors. Although much of the prevention, case findings, and treatment by the nurse occurs in community settings such as the school and community mental health centers, the hospital nurse also frequently sees hyperactive children. Since hyperactive children may be admitted because of their frequent accidental injuries or other childhood illnesses, the hospital based nurse is instrumental in case finding, preventing hyperactive behavior, and initiating or continuing treatment for the family.

BASIC CONCEPTS OF THE HYPERACTIVE SYNDROME

The hyperactive syndrome is referred to by many different names. Minimal brain injury, minimal neurological impairment, or hyperkinesis are terms reflecting the cause of or the behavior common to this syndrome. The term "hyperactive syndrome," chosen by the World Health Organization because it suggests the behaviors without implying the cause, will be used in this chapter.[3]

The hyperactive syndrome is a child's behavior pattern which includes continuous overactivity, short attention span, impulsiveness, and excitability. The hyperactive child is therefore a child with hyperactive behaviors regardless of the cause. This behavioral diagnosis is useful in implying the behaviors which cause difficulties for the family.

Common Characteristics of the Hyperactive Child

It is often difficult to identify the hyperactive child because his behaviors are actually similar to the behaviors of any child. The main difference between the hyperactive child and the more normally behaved child is that the hyperactive child displays very active behaviors with more intensity and frequency than the typical child. The hyperactive child responds with great activity to even minimal stimulus and is unable to filter or ignore stimuli; he is therefore hyperactive at home, school, and in other settings. The child may know the correct behavior but is frequently unable to control his reactions and activity. There are five major categories of characteristics for the hyperactive child: overactivity, distractibility, impulsiveness, excitability, and concomitant emotional difficulties.

Overactivity. The hyperactive child frequently responds with extreme activity to even minimal stimuli. Most hyperactive children have difficulty going to sleep, staying asleep, and wake up very early in the morning. He wears out his crib, playpen, eating chair, and clothes before he has outgrown them.[7] He very seldom walks, but runs instead, even in inappropriate settings such as a church wedding or a funeral. The hyperactive child climbs anything he can find, pokes his fingers in electrical outlets and other holes, tastes anything he can get into his mouth, and tears apart toys before he tires of them. The child is unable to sit for very long and responds by actively thrashing about in his eating chair or in the car, before the end of a short meal or a short drive.

Most parents find this activity enjoyable to watch when it is channeled in correct settings such as sports or yelling and running outside; however, they find it very frustrating when the child cannot inhibit his actions in a more quiet setting when the parents are talking, doing their normal chores, or visiting neighbors and friends. The parents feel that they are *always* having to say "no" and stopping the child from getting into difficulty. This overactivity inclines a hyperactive child to greater accidental injuries than the more typically behaved child of his age.

Distractibility. The hyperactive child is frequently very distractible and has an extremely short attention span. He may not be able to concentrate on an interesting project for more than ten seconds and frequently answers the first one or two questions on a test accurately but then answers the rest of the questions rapidly and haphazardly.[3] The hyperactive child frequently loses his toys and clothes because his attention has turned to other matters. Unlike many more normally behaved children, the hyperactive child may not be able to concentrate on a single television show but instead turns it on, watches for ten minutes, and then runs off to do something more active.

The parents find this distractibility distressing, for whenever they sit to talk with the child about his school work, appropriate behavior, or to include him in a family conversation he is quickly distracted by something else. The parents frequently feel that they cannot get or hold his attention. This short attention span creates great difficulties at school because the hyperactive child who concentrates on spelling, reading, or mathematics for only a few minutes has great difficulty in learning and even greater difficulty in showing these skills in a test situation. This distractibility which leads him to being a poor student plus his overactivity which may be shown in aggressiveness toward other children makes this child difficult for the teacher to handle and unliked by his classmates.

Impulsiveness. The hyperactive child is frequently impulsive. He acts before he thinks on almost all occasions. He seems fearless, uninhibited, and defiant. The hyperactive child is often unable to put off any project or wish for even a minute. He seems unable to delay gratification and requires immediate attention.

The parents find this impulsiveness very frustrating. Not only does he change his interests and projects and physical activities very quickly, but the hyperactive child's emotional level may change just as quickly. The parents are frequently bewildered and frustrated, not knowing what to do when the child may switch quickly from laughter and happy excitement into tears and expressions of agony. This impulsiveness frequently results in the hyperactive child interfering with the activities of other children and being considered a pest by them. It also leads to clumsy behavior and accident proneness.

Excitability. The hyperactive child is usually very excitable. It takes very little stimulus to provoke very active, show-off behavior. Even small discouragements or reprimands may lead to active temper tantrums. He is very excitable when interacting with other people and frequently fights with siblings, classmates, and neighbors. Changing rules or complex rules for his behavior are confusing and may excite him to either a temper tantrum or a loud argument.

This excitability makes it difficult for the parents to find some quiet time for their own emotional fulfillment. The many temper tantrums, fights, and show-off behaviors cause great frustration for them and lead to angry neighbors and friends and possible social isolation of the family.

Concomitant Emotional Difficulties. The hyperactive child frequently has additional emotional difficulties related to his behaviors and how other people react to these behaviors. Some hyperactive children are angry at other classmates, siblings, and the parents and display great hostility and dangerous aggression toward others. The hyperactive child frequently has a poor self-concept and feels that he is a "bad" child. He may even state, "I'm not right inside."[3]

Since the emotional difficulties include the child's discouragement with himself and disturbances in interacting with other people, the parents are frequently frustrated in not knowing what to do to make the child feel better and to behave in a more socially acceptable manner. Along with the overactive behavior, these emotional difficulties push friends and helping adults away, often leaving the child alone though he needs great emotional support. Although the overactive behaviors frequently diminish in adolescence anywhere between the ages of 12 and 20, the resulting emotional difficulties frequently continue.[3]

Hyperactive Versus Typical Behaviors. Although many of these characteristics can be observed in the normal behavior of any child, the hyperactive child displays them consistently over a period of time. These active behaviors are rarely mixed with the more quiet relaxful loving behaviors that the more normal child can display. The more normally behaved child has a repertoire of behavior that he can choose from to react to any kind of situation or stimulus, while the hyperactive child tends to react in the hyperactive manner on most occasions. This inability to discriminate among stimuli and react with different behaviors is the main difference between the hyperactive and the more typical child.

Causes of Hyperactivity

Like most high-risk situations the causes of hyperactive behavior are multiple and often unknown. Often, a known cause for hyperactivity in one child does not cause this same behavior in another. It is also true that for many hyperactive behaviors no known cause has been identified. Hyperactivity is probably a behavior pattern that results from one of many difficulties or from a combination of several difficulties. There are two basic types of factors that are believed to be related to hyperactivity: organic factors and psychogenic factors.

Organic factors that may lead to hyperactivity include prenatal factors such as genetic traits. Hyperactive behavior seems to recur in families, since a hyperactive child is more likely to have relatives who have had hyperactive behaviors then the normal child.[3] Prenatal diseases or conditions such as toxemia, cerebral anoxia, prematurity, and jaundice with kernicterus are also possible causes of hyperactivity. Some postnatal difficulties such as trauma, encephalitis meningitis, lead encephalopathy, and cerebral tumors may also affect the neurological system and encourage hyperactive reactions.[6] Nutritional factors such as artificial food coloring, flavoring, and sugars have recently become suspected causes of or aggravating factors in hyperactivity.[1,5]

Psychogenic and sociological factors may also encourage hyperactive behaviors. Continual parental loss of patience and aggressive discipline may encourage hyperactive behaviors in the child. It is likely that these psychogenic factors are actually the parental reaction to the hyperactive behaviors already displayed in the child. In effect, the psychogenic factors and the organic factors probably work together in causing or increasing the hyperactive behaviors of the child. Freeman describes the multiple cause concisely when he says, "The behavior manifested by these children seems to be the final common pathway for the expression of diverse pathologies."[3]

Diagnosis

The nurse is instrumental in helping to diagnose the hyperactive child. Through observations of a child's behavior over periods of time in the school or community health settings, the nurse can help to identify children with potential hyperactive difficulties. This early recognition of the child's difficulties is important in implementing treatment and then reducing the child's emotional difficulties related to the hyperactive behaviors and in preventing and reducing the family's difficulties in coping with the hyperactive child.

The medical diagnosis of hyperactivity is difficult because of the multiple causes and lack of definite signs that suggest hyperactivity and rule out other conditions. Since it is thought that the main mechanisms behind hyperactivity are biochemical abnormalities in the frontal areas of the brain, hypothalamus, and reticular activating system, the diagnosis involves looking for signs of abnormality in these areas. However only 30 to 50 percent of hyperactive patients show an abnormal electroencephalogram.[14] There are sometimes soft neurological signs found on a neurological examination, such as coordination deficits, disorders of attention, impulsiveness, and disorders in hearing and speech.[3] Psychological tests may show some visual perception difficulties and performance difficulties. Although the hyperactive child frequently has a normal or slightly above normal intelligence quotient, his actual performance in school does not reflect this. His psychiatric examination may show the use of many aggressive defense mechanisms and conflicts with hostile feelings.[3]

FAMILY DIFFICULTIES

The family with a hyperactive child is truly at risk. The parents find it difficult to control their child and wonder what they are doing wrong to create this problem. The siblings are frequently angry at their hyperactive brother or sister who continually interferes with their own play and school work. Initially, family members may blame each other for what they consider poor discipline of the child. The aggressive behavior of the child may overtax the parents' patience and encourage abusive discipline measures and fighting between the parents. Figure 9-1 concisely lists the difficulties for this family.

This family greatly needs successes and closeness, yet many find the cycle of the child's aggressiveness and the parents' frustrations difficult to change. By helping to decrease the hyperactive activity and increase the family's ability to cope with these behaviors and see the positive aspects in their child, the nurse can help turn the difficulties into family strengths and greatly benefit the family with the hyperactive child.

Parent-Infant Bonding Difficulty

Many hyperactive children show overactive reactions or unusual sensitivity to stimuli even during infancy. They stiffened when they were

Figure 9-1. Family Difficulties for the Family
with a Hyperactive Child

Parent-Infant Bonding Difficulty

Guilt and Blame Difficulties

Relationship Difficulties
  Parent-to-child difficulties
  Parent-to-parent difficulties
  Child-to-child difficulties
  Child-to-peer difficulties
  Family-to-friend, -relative, or -neighbor difficulties

Decision Difficulties
  Education decision
  Nutrition decision
  Medication decision

Physical and Emotional Exhaustion

held, arched their backs squalled and thrashed about when they were picked up. This type of behavior often leads the mother to feel frantic and rejected at not being able to enjoy a quiet relaxation response of the child from being held or fed. Frequently these infants sleep very little and continue to cry past the three-month normal colicky period. Similar to the mother with a premature infant who has difficulty bonding to her infant and who experiences unexpected responses to her mothering, the mother with a hyperactive child often has difficulty establishing a mutually satisfying interaction with her newborn infant. For example, one mother stated that her hyperactive child had been very fussy as an infant. When she held him for breast feeding, he would tightly arch his back and move away from the nipple. Fortunately, this mother felt adequate in her parenting and instead of being discouraged tried other approaches with the child. She found that if she did not cuddle or change the position of the child or provide any other stimulation that he would then begin to root and suck at the nipple.

The nurse through her behavioral assessment of the newborn infant can identify infants who react with activity and tenseness to even minimal stimulation. Behavioral assessment tools such as those described in the chapter "Assessment of Children's Behavior" are valuable. When the nurse identifies a child who is more active than normal during the regular feeding, diapering, and caretaking activities, the nurse can help the parents to recognize these individual behaviors of their child and to

adapt their parenting to elicit more positive reactions. The nurse can assure the parents that the child's reactions are not a result of bad parenting but are the child's individual type of reacting. In the example above, the mother did not blame herself for being a bad parent but instead changed her behaviors so that the child would quiet and establish normal feeding patterns. The nurse recognizes that greater than normal activity for an infant is a possible warning but does not necessarily lead to continued hyperactive difficulty in childhood. For greatly abnormal behaviors on stimulation, the nurse refers the child to the physician or psychologist with her observations for further assessment.

Guilt and Blame Difficulties

The hyperactive child himself frequently feels guilty and is often blamed by his parents and teachers for his disruptive behavior. He is frequently getting into trouble where most communication to him involves the word "no" and punishment. Although many hyperactive children can tell you the correct behavior in a situation, they still find it very difficult to respond and behave in that manner. With the many negative reactions of others toward him and the lack of positive reinforcement, the hyperactive child frequently has very low self-esteem. He feels that he is a "bad" boy and often shows depression.

The parents, also, often feel guilty and blame themselves for the active and aggressive behavior of the child. Many parents ask themselves "what have I done" to cause my child to act this way. The large amount of literature for laymen describing parenting techniques and how discipline and punishment affect a child's behavior reinforces the parents' feeling of guilt as the cause of their child's uncontrolled behavior. Since it is common for parents to have different feelings about specific discipline techniques, this guilt feeling may turn into blame of the spouse for using poor disciplining techniques. It is not uncommon to hear the husband say to the wife, "you are just too lenient—he acts this way because you let him do anything," or for the wife to say to the husband, "You are too strict, you punish him too often." This guilt and blaming of the other spouse leads to poor self-esteem and fighting between the parents rather than to satisfaction in parenting and mutual support.

The nurse can help the family members to cope with their guilt and blaming of each other. First she discusses the probable organic causes for the hyperactivity, describing any known possible cause for that child. She emphasizes that hyperactivity is very common, using any local statistics such as that 10 percent of children in schools have similar hyperactive tendencies. She acknowledges that guilt is a very common feeling. When something occurs with an unknown cause, it is common for parents to place the blame on themselves rather than to look for a multitude of sources. The nurse also helps the family recognize that regardless of the cause they need to learn to cope with the hyperactive child. She therefore turns their attention to identifying specific problems and generating solutions to them while taking their focus off blaming themselves.

Since the parents' guilt is based on their feeling that they have a "bad" child, one of the nurse's most important approaches is to help them to view the positive aspects of their child and set realistic expectations for his behavior.[4] The parents first need to accept that their child may not be a "model child" but that he has some very positive individual qualities of his own. The nurse lists with the family the child's hyperactive behaviors and helps them to recognize that these types of behavior are actually normal for most children, but their child behaves hyperactively more frequently and consistently than other children. The nurse stresses that children are not all good or bad or all normal or hyperactive. The hyperactive child just tends more toward the active end of the continuum from the extremes of a very active child to a very quiet child. The nurse helps the family to identify where the very active behaviors of the child are very appropriate and actually positive traits. For example, she may emphasize that the child does very well in sports and has very many interests. During one hour he may be able to work on many projects while some children will still be working on one. The

nurse can help to identify for the family some of the traits of the hyperactive child that can be viewed positively.

After recognizing the positive aspects of the child, the parents can begin to recognize that they may not be able to completely reduce all the active behavior of the child even if they would want to. With the parents' acceptance that the child will be active, they can help form realistic expectations for their parenting which will help guide the child into appropriate use of his active behavior rather than try to stop his activity. Taking these steps will help to reduce the parents' own guilt and blame, and they will be better able to help the child form a more realistic and positive image of himself.

For example, the parents of a hyperactive child who was the second born child felt very guilty about their inability to control the child in the same way they could control their more quiet first born child. Although their first born child was doing very well in school, was well-liked by her classmates, and enjoyed cooking and doing quiet activities with the family, the hyperactive child was failing in school, the parents of schoolmates were calling to complain about his fighting with the other children, and the parents were constantly frustrated when trying to include him in their own household projects. With the help of the community health nurse, these parents began to recognize the very different positive traits of their active child, including his ability in sports and tremendous energy and willingness to do active projects. Setting more realistic expectations for themselves, the parents realized that they could not and did not want to make the child conform to the typical more quiet child. Instead of trying to discipline the child into doing quiet chores around the house, the whole family considered the problem and found that the hyperactive child was very interested in doing the more active and strenuous chores such as helping the father to dig the garden, cut the grass, and take out the trash. When these realistic activities were established for the child, instead of being blamed for dropping and breaking a dish in doing dishwashing, he was supported for doing the more strenuous work around the house. The guilt of being or having a "bad" child was reduced for the child and the parents.

Relationship Difficulties

The child's hyperactive behavior influences the parents, the other children, and friends, relatives, and neighbors. The different types of relationship difficulties are described in the following sections.

Parent-Child Relationship. The hyperactive child disrupts the family and makes parenting difficult. The child's overactivity, distractibility, impulsiveness, and excitability tax the parents' patience and lead to frustration and frequently anger. This uncontrolled behavior is especially disruptive when the parent is trying to accomplish something, such as shop in the store, prepare dinner, drive to a store, or complete necessary family projects. If family disruption becomes too great, divorce may result, or a parent may become so angry that he resorts to the extreme physical violence of child or spouse abuse.

The nurse's main role in helping the parents with the disruptive behavior of the child is to help them, first, to decrease the child's disruptive behaviors and, second, to learn how to cope with the remaining overactive behaviors. Although treatment for the hyperactive child including medications and behavior modification programs may limit some overactive behaviors, in most cases it is not possible to or desirable to completely reduce the child's overactivity. The nurse helps the family to cope with these behaviors so that instead of being disruptive to the family life the child actually makes his unique contribution to the family. The nursing interventions that help to decrease the overactive behavior include use of medications, correct nutrition, and behavior modification plans. Nursing interventions that help the family to cope with the overactive behaviors include counseling and teaching. These teaching approaches will be discussed in more detail in the nursing approaches section of this chapter.

Parent-to-Parent Difficulties. The parents' in-creased frustration and need to look for a cause for the child's overactive behavior often result in their blaming each other. Disagreements are very frequent, with each parent blaming the other for their unsuccessful discipline actions. The parental relationship is also threatened because each parent has already lost patience and become frustrated and angry in trying to deal with the child's behavior. For example, in one family the wife explains she always looks forward to her husband returning in the evening from work because she is tired from having to control the child all day. The husband explains that he is always anxious to get home from work because of the stresses at work. The parents relate that they often have very heated arguments soon after the husband returns home from work. It appeared that each parent was looking forward to support and help from the other when they got together at the end of the day; however, each seemed unable to provide the caring or support for the other. This need for help and support from the other parent and lack of energy to provide it seems to be a common difficulty in the relationship between the parents.

The nurse can help the parents to identify the reasons for the difficulty in their interactions and to suggest new approaches for supporting each other. Most parents readily identify their disagreements over ways to discipline a child. The nurse can help the parents to discuss plans for rules and discipline of the child so that they have a mutually agreeable plan. They can then support each other to carry out this consistent plan rather than spend more energy in disagreement. When the parents agree on limits for the child and for disciplinary action when a child breaks the rules, they will be acting in a consistent manner that helps the child identify and follow the rules and increases the closeness between the parents.

If there are major problems with a parent's style of discipline, such as the parent who has no limits at all or the parent who is abusive, then the nurse can help the parents to develop a more effective style of discipline. The hyperactive child seems to react poorly to either extreme of discipline—

with uncontrolled behavior when there are very few limits and with aggressive behavior when abuse is used in punishing. The nurse helps the family to recognize the importance of and to develop consistent and simple rules for the behavior of the child.

Child-to-Child Difficulties. The overactive behavior of the child also affects the other children in the family. Although it is normal for brothers and sisters to be selfish with food or to steal and ruin toys, the hyperactive child seems to more consistently and aggressively interfere with the play and life of his brothers and sisters. As in other high-risk situations, the parents' attention is frequently on the hyperactive or unusual child, thus leaving the other siblings feeling less loved or wanted. One mother expressed that when she is holding and caressing her quieter child, the hyperactive child will climb in her lap or push and pull until the mother reacts and no longer can enjoy the time with the quieter child. The quiet child frequently has nightmares in which his brother is killed in a very traumatic accident. Sometimes the quieter child will take on active behaviors similar to the hyperactive child to gain more parental attention.

The nurse reinforces the family's recognition that all of their children are important and helps them recognize that the quieter children have similar needs for love and discipline, although they are often less aggressive in getting the parents attention. Through showing recognition of individual traits and love for the child, the parents can support the more normal child without making it necessary for him to be aggressive in return to the hyperactive child or aggressive to the parents to get attention. One mother who took her hyperactive child out of school to a psychiatrist once a week found the other child starting to complain about going to school. When she started taking this child out for lunch once a week during his lunch period, the complaints about school and his hyperactive brother subsided.

The nurse can help the quieter child to find ways of behaving to avoid the interference of his hyperactive brother or sister. Each child can de-velop his "own" place where his parents or brother or sister are not allowed to interfere with him. If the family has enough room, each child could have his own room which may be off limits to the others. In a family with less living space, each child could have a bed of his own where he could play which is off limits to the other child. When the quieter child is old enough to understand that behavior is often a response to what someone else does, the nurse or the parent can explain to the child that yelling, pushing, or otherwise goading the hyperactive child will only increase his overactivity. Through experience, the quieter child will very quickly learn to know what behaviors will increase or decrease the aggression of his brother or sister. Standard rules of no hitting, pushing, or calling names may be important for the safety of both the hyperactive and the quiet child.

Child-to-Peer Difficulty. The hyperactive child frequently has difficulties with his schoolmates and other peers. Young school age children may make fun of the hyperactive child who frequently appears clumsy, has more difficulty speaking, and does poorly in school. Overactivity and aggressive behaviors may make him a "bully" in the class. Frequently, the short attention span of the hyperactive child makes it difficult for him to play in the normal childhood games because he becomes frustrated with the rules and loses interest in the game before the other children.

As in other high-risk situations where the child appears different and is made fun of by his peers, the nurse and especially the school nurse can help the teacher explain to the class about the differences in people's behaviors and can help the classmates pick games with more activity and less complex rules to play with the hyperactive child.

Family-to-Friend, -Relative, or -Neighbor Difficulties. When the school children return home and tell their own parents about the aggressiveness of the hyperactive child or when the hyperactive child visits friends and relatives and smashes or ruins some of their treasured possessions, the child becomes a less than desirable friend, relative, or neighbor. These people frequently will avoid inviting the hyperactive child or his family to their houses. Very often the relatives or neighbors blame the overactivity on the parents' poor discipline or parenting. This hurts the parents, who are already sensitive about their parenting and causes them to defend their actions and avoid these otherwise greatly needed friends.

The nurse can help to reduce the parents' social isolation from friends by helping them to explain the child's behaviors and needs and to share their concerns with others. The parents may ask friends or relatives if they would mind removing their valuable possessions from the reach of a child so that there is no risk of damage while they visit. If this is not possible, the parents can arrange to visit friends and relatives while leaving their children at home with a babysitter.

One family with a hyperactive child enjoys taking the child with them to friends houses, however they have made a rule for themselves to stay no longer than a half an hour when their hyperactive child becomes more unruly and unable to sit through a conversation. They have explained this to their friends and find that they visit friends more often and have a better relationship than if they tried to force longer visits. When they have parties where children are invited, they will have a picnic on a playground where the children are allowed to run and yell, so that the parents can have a quiet talk without the distraction of the active children in the house. When the parents explain their difficulties to other friends, relatives, and neighbors, although they may get more suggestions of how to cope with the problems than they need, they will often get understanding and support from these very important people.

The family may frequently have difficulty with babysitters. The babysitter will find the child, even more than the typical child, is very unruly and does not obey. Many families with hyperactive children find that they go from babysitter to babysitter because their child becomes known as unruly. Unfortunately the child needing a consistent babysitter is least likely to have babysitters return. As with their friends, relatives, and neighbors, the parents need to be honest with the babysitter about the child's activities and responses to stimuli. The family needs to communicate to the babysitter the same simple, firm rules about bedtime, eating, bathing, and other routines. In addition, telling the babysitter what she can do when the child becomes overly active and unruly, such as placing the child in his bedroom and closing the door until he is quiet, will help the babysitter know how to react to a temper tantrum situation. In any babysitting situation the babysitter should know the phone number where she can reach the parents, doctor, or other necessary people. When the babysitter is new or especially young, the parents may leave her for only a short time and not go very far away until she has learned how to react effectively to the hyperactive child.

Decision Difficulties

The parents with a hyperactive child have several decisions to make on education, nutrition, and medication approaches that they would like to take with the child. The nurse can help them to look at the advantages and disadvantages of different approaches.

Education Decision. Most hyperactive children do poorly in the school situation because of their inability to sit for very long or to concentrate on a project such as reading, spelling, or mathematics. In most of the school settings there are additional distracting stimuli, such as other children getting out of their seats and walking around, or other noises. This is especially true in the team-teaching or open type of environment that is used to stimulate children. This increased stimulation, although helpful to many of the normal and quiet children, is very disruptive to the hyperactive child and makes it difficult for him to concentrate on any task for very long. Therefore, the hyperactive child frequently needs a different learning environment from that provided in a normal classroom.

The family along with the nurse, physician, psychologist, and teacher can identify the different possibilities for the learning environment of the child. For example, private tutoring, special education classes, private schools, and other types of special education settings may be helpful to the hyperactive child. The nurse helps the parents gather all the information about their child's abilities and needs and about the possible resources and costs. She helps them to consider the recommendations of the different professionals and to decide on the educational setting which would be the most beneficial for them.

The school nurse can help the teachers in the different settings to understand the child and his individual difficulties. She can also help the family to learn teaching approaches that they can use in counseling the child in their school work. For example, the parents may be able to help the hyperactive child with his homework if they set up a quiet time and place where other stimulation is decreased. They may work with the child in short intervals, such as 10-minute periods right after school, before dinner, after dinner, and before bed, when the school work is done rather than in a longer period requiring a greater attention span.

Nutrition Decisions. The family with a hyperactive child needs to decide on their beliefs in the role of nutrition in the activity of the child and then decide on the extent to which they would be willing to change their own food habits. There has been some recent evidence that food additives such as food coloring and flavoring and possibly sugar may increase the child's hyperactivity.[1,5] In one family the child's hyperactive behaviors were almost completely controlled by elimination of food additives and sugar from the child's diet. The mother explains that when she does allow the child to have sweets and food additives, such as the ice cream at a birthday party, the child becomes very active and difficult to control within an hour or two. Realizing what increases the activity of her child, this mother makes decisions on when she can tolerate the overactivity and when not. In many cases she will avoid food colorings and sugars because the amount of time it takes for her to cook more natural foods is well compensated by the time it saves her in trying to control the child. This mother does allow the child to have sweets on special occasions and she prepares herself to have more energy, patience, and

set limits for the child when the hyperactivity begins. Fortunately she has found a way to control the overactivity of her child and is able to make decisions about when she can and cannot tolerate this type of behavior.

The nurse can help the family to recognize if nutrition changes do help to reduce the overactivity of their child. The nurse encourages the family to read labels on all foods before serving them and to eliminate foods with any preservatives, food coloring, flavor additives, or sugar. If the family finds that this is helpful after several months on the natural diet, then the parents can add some of the sugars or other foods slowly to see how the child reacts. This is very similar to the way that food is originally added to a baby's diet to see if he has any unwanted reaction.

If the child does benefit from reducing food colorings, additives, and sugars, the nurse teaches the parents that most childhood medications are dispersed in a red colored syrup which would be likely to increase the child's activity. If the child is ill and requires medication, the parents should request that it not be diluted in this kind of syrup base but in another type of liquid or powder form without added coloring or sugar.

Medication Decision. The decision to medicate the child to help reduce the overactive behaviors is a difficult one. Contrary to what would be expected, the medications that help reduce the overactivity in many children are stimulants such as amphetemines.[2] Although these drugs do help to reduce the overactivity in many hyperactive children, they are not miracle drugs which solve all the problems. The hyperactive child does not suddenly become a docile and quiet child. The medication does help control some of the overactivity so that the child can pay more attention at school, learn more, and be less disruptive to other people.

Although the physician is very helpful in suggesting the type and amount of medication for the child, it is truly the parents' decision whether to use medication in controlling the child. The nurse helps the family to collect the important information, such as the exact behaviors of the child, his learning difficulties, and the amount of difficulty and frustration they have in controlling him. The nurse can help the family to realize the decision is not irreversible. They may decide at any time to take the child off the medication and it need not be a continuous form of treatment.

Physical and Emotional Exhaustion

Understandably the parents of a hyperactive child are frequently physically and emotionally exhausted from trying to control the overactive child. These parents need time to meet their own needs for physical relaxation and emotional support. The nurse can help them to recognize that their own physical and emotional needs are very important and must be met if they are to help the hyperactive child. The nurse helps the parents to plan for their own physical activities, such as swimming or running for exercise, and physical relaxation, such as a strict "quiet time" once a day when each family member goes to his own room and must play quietly. The nurse helps the parents to plan time where they can provide each other with emotional support. Helping the parents to choose day-care centers where the child will have the needed care and they will have additional time for rest or their own growth is important. The parents might consider separating, with one parent taking care of the children while the other parent has some quiet time of his own. One family has arranged for the husband to babysit the children every Tuesday night while the wife goes to a sewing class. Every Thursday night the wife babysits so the husband can go out for a drink and some cards with his friends.

The nurse emphasizes that all family members, including the hyperactive child, the other siblings, and both parents, must have their own needs met. This assures each family member that he is important to the whole family and creates a feeling of dealing with the problem and growing together.

NURSING APPROACHES

The nurse works with all family members so that the family has the strength to help the child and cope with his behaviors. When the family works together to identify their needs and solve their difficulties, positive family relationships grow.

The nurse has two main goals in working with the family of a hyperactive child. First she reduces the hyperactive behavior of the child by either reducing the cause or stimulation leading to the hyperactive behavior. The second goal is to help the family to cope with any remaining hyperactive behavior.

An additional difficulty for the nurse working with a family with a hyperactive child is her own reaction to the child. The nurse, as others, responds with frustration and anger to the overactive child who is aggressive and has a short attention span. By recognizing her own reactions to the child, the nurse is better able to empathize with the family about their reactions and difficulties and is less likely to get angry with the parents. When the hyperactive child has to be hospitalized due to an accidental injury or other childhood illness, the nurse is very aware of the aggressive, frustrating, and demanding activities of the hyperactive child who frequently fights his treatments and interferes with the hospital routine. The nurse working with the family of the hyperactive child must recognize and deal with her own problems and reactions to the child as well as help the family with their difficulties.

Approaches that Decrease Hyperactive Behavior

The main approaches that reduce the child's overactive behaviors are environmental control, behavior modification, medication, and nutrition. By identifying the problem behaviors and reevaluating changes using a specific assessment tool like the one in Figure 9-2, the nurse and family can determine the success of the approaches to decrease the hyperactivity.

Environmental Control. By controlling the child's environment the nurse or the parent can decrease the amount of stimulation which creates the overactivity in the child. The room of the hyperactive child should be furnished simply with plain walls and curtains, and toys should be put

Figure 9-2. Questionnaire to Determine Target Hyperactive Behavior

Parent's Questionnaire

Name of Child _____ **Date** _____

Please answer all questions. Beside *each* item below, indicate the degree of the problem by a check mark (✔)	Not at all	Just a little	Pretty much	Very much
1. Picks at things (nails, fingers, hair, clothing).				
2. Sassy to grown-ups.				
3. Problems with making or keeping friends.				
4. Excitable, Impulsive.				
5. Wants to run things.				
6. Sucks or chews (thumb; clothing; blankets).				
7. Cries easily or often.				
8. Carries a chip on his shoulder.				
9. Daydreams.				
10. Difficulty in learning.				
11. Restless in the "squirmy" sense.				
12. Fearful (of new situations; new people or places; going to school).				
13. Restless, always up and on the go.				
14. Destructive.				
15. Tells lies or stories that aren't true.				
16. Shy.				
17. Gets into more trouble than others same age.				
18. Speaks differently from others same age (baby talk; stuttering; hard to understand).				
19. Denies mistakes or blames others.				
20. Quarrelsome.				
21. Pouts and sulks.				
22. Steals.				
23. Disobedient or obeys but resentfully.				
24. Worries more than others (about being alone; illness or death).				
25. Fails to finish things.				
26. Feelings easily hurt.				
27. Bullies others.				
28. Unable to stop a repetitive activity.				
29. Cruel.				
30. Childish or immature (wants help he shouldn't need; clings; needs constant reassurance).				
31. Distractibility or attention span a problem.				
32. Headaches.				
33. Mood changes quickly and drastically.				
34. Doesn't like or doesn't follow rules or restrictions.				
35. Fights constantly.				
36. Doesn't get along well with brothers or sisters.				
37. Easily frustrated in efforts.				
38. Disturbs other children.				
39. Basically an unhappy child.				
40. Problems with eating (poor appetite; up between bites).				
41. Stomach aches.				
42. Problems with sleep (can't fall asleep; up too early; up in the night).				

Figure 9-2. Questionnaire to Determine Target Hyperactive Behavior (continued)

	Not at all	Just a little	Pretty much	Very much
43. Other aches and pains.				
44. Vomiting or nausea.				
45. Feels cheated in family circle.				
46. Boasts and brags.				
47. Lets self be pushed around.				
48. Bowel problems (frequently loose; irregular habits; constipation).				

Teacher's Questionnaire

Name of Child _____ Grade _____

Date of Evaluation _____

Please answer all questions. Beside *each* **item, indicate the degree of the problem by a check mark (✔)**

	Not at all	Just a little	Pretty much	Very much
1. Restless in the "squirmy" sense.				
2. Makes inappropriate noises when he shouldn't.				
3. Demands must be met immediately.				
4. Acts "smart" (impudent or sassy).				
5. Temper outbursts and unpredictable behavior.				
6. Overly sensitive to criticism.				
7. Distractibility or attention span a problem.				

	Not at all	Just a little	Pretty much	Very much
8. Disturbs other children.				
9. Daydreams.				
10. Pouts and sulks.				
11. Mood changes quickly and drastically.				
12. Quarrelsome.				
13. Submissive attitude toward authority.				
14. Restless, always "up and on the go."				

	Not at all	Just a little	Pretty much	Very much
15. Excitable, impulsive.				
16. Excessive demands for teacher's attention.				
17. Appears to be unaccepted by group.				
18. Appears to be easily led by other children.				
19. No sense of fair play.				
20. Appears to lack leadership.				
21. Fails to finish things that he starts.				

Figure 9-2. Questionnaire to Determine Target Hyperactive Behavior (continued)

	Not at all	Just a little	Pretty much	Very much
22. Childish and immature.				
23. Denies mistakes or blames others.				
24. Does not get along well with other children.				
25. Uncooperative with classmates.				
26. Easily frustrated in efforts.				
27. Uncooperative with teacher.				
28. Difficulty in learning.				

The Hyperkinesis Index is based on a questionnaire developed by C. Keith Conners, Ph.D., and distributed by Abbott Laboratories. Reproduced with permission of Abbott Laboratories.

away in a toy chest out of sight of the child. The periods for homework should be short, quiet periods at a location where other distracting toys or equipment are limited. The child should be encouraged to use his energy and activity in appropriate places, such as the playground and during recreation breaks at school. This child needs to go outside and use his energy even on wet or snowy days so he must be dressed appropriately whether at home or at school to enjoy the outside environment. A yard near the home should be cleared for the child to play aggressively without injury. Since these children are more susceptible to accidents and injuries, potentially hazardous settings such as near a street should be prohibited and a safer environment supplied.

In the hospital setting environmental control is very important for the hyperactive child. Room assignment and roommate assignment should be carefully evaluated to ensure a quiet room with the least amount of personnel coming and going as possible. The number of medical staff who take care of the child should be limited, although such important members as the physician, social worker, schoolteacher, nurse, and speech therapist should be included. The primary nurse helps limit the number of medical people interacting with the child by limiting medical rounds and different types of students if necessary. Although important for all children, it is especially important for the hyperactive child to have the hospital environment as much like the home environment as possible.

Before surgery, for example, it would be best to allow the child to fall asleep on the mother's lap in his room after a preoperative shot than to be sedated near the operating room. This may be the time for a parent to be permitted in the recovery room near her child during the recovery phase.

The nurse can help the parents to plan the home environment to reduce some of the child's overactivity and provide a safe environment for him. Most parents are very perceptive of the changes in the child as they alter the environment around him. One family stated that the most important environmental control they have is the child's room. His room is equipped very simply and when he misbehaves, is very active, and the rest of the family cannot tolerate it, the child only needs a reminder to go to his room. There he rocks on the bed or kicks a large bean bag until he is in better control of his aggressive behavior and able to return to the family. The family stated that the few times this does not work they actively restrain the child, tightly holding him on their laps so that he cannot move and thrash around, and gradually let go as he regains control over himself.

Behavior Modification. Behavior modification is another important strategy for the family to help reduce the child's overactive behavior that disrupts the family. The nurse helps the family to identify behaviors that are very disruptive and ones that are desirable. Since each family is different and identifies different behaviors as being disruptive or desirable, this list is individualized with every family.

Basically the family rewards the desirable behavior and removes a reward, ignores, or punishes an undesirable behavior. Since it is frequently difficult for a child or anyone to learn several behaviors at once, the family is encouraged to pick one or two behaviors to focus on at a time. Other behavior modification approaches are discussed in the chapter "Behavior Modification Strategies."

Rewarding a desirable behavior is quite easy. Through praise, hugs, and other actions, a desired behavior is easily rewarded and both the parents and the child are satisfied. The parents are encouraged to continue to reward desirable behavior even after it becomes a pattern so the behavior will continue and to provide opportunities for expression of love between the parents and the child.

Discouraging undesirable behavior is more difficult. Effective discouragement of the behavior includes six basic factors. The discipline should be:

1. Firm—definite and not negotiable.
2. Clear—the exact discipline, punishment, or taking away of reward is well known.
3. Consistent—the same discipline every time a negative behavior is seen.
4. Simple—common single rule without a lot of complex variations.
5. Immediate—occurs directly after the undesired behavior.
6. Nonaggressive—placing in a quiet location or using verbal displeasure or physical restraint without hitting or violence.

The behavior modification plan, including undesired behaviors, should be agreed upon by all family members so that it will be used consistently. In addition, any friends, relatives, schoolteachers, babysitters, or hospital nurses need to know the plan when a child is in another environment. When a child is hospitalized, the hospital primary nurse works with the parents and the nurses on a behavior modification plan that will be used by all medical personnel, using rewards and punishment very similar to those used at home. In the hospital environment the nurse also uses clear and simple limits, firmly and immediately applied for intolerable behavior and rewards activity channeled in acceptable ways.

The nurse helps the family to evaluate and change the behavior modification plan by assessing the changes and frequency of the desirable or undesirable behavior. As the child begins to control his actions, the family very slowly allows more freedom and self-control. New stimulation and experiences are added gradually while the child continues to learn control and are reduced when the child is overwhelmed with a new situation. Fortunately, the hyperactive behaviors decrease as the child grows older and more self-control is possible by adolescence.

Medication Approaches. As mentioned, stimulant medications may be used to reduce some of the overactivity of the hyperactive child. After helping the family to make a decision on whether or not they will use medication, the nurse helps any family who has chosen to try medication. She helps the family to assess the changes in the child's behavior caused by the medication, which helps the physician to decide the strength of medication necessary for that child. A few hyperactive children may respond to medication with increased overactive behaviors, so the nurse and family must observe for the positive effects and side effects of the medication. Since the child may react differently to the medication as he grows older, the nurse helps to observe for recurrence of aggressive behaviors. In coordination with the physician and the school, the family may decide to take the child off the medication periodically to see how he reacts without it. Fortunately, families are becoming more strict on giving medication to their children and seriously consider the benefits and the risks in making the original and continuing decision to use medication with the children.

Although the medication's control of overactive behavior benefits the child by helping him to learn more, succeed in school, and make friends, the control of his overactive behavior also helps the teacher and the family by relieving them from the stress of dealing with a hyperactive child. Therefore, medication should not be the only answer but the nurse, physician, schoolteacher, and family need to work together to learn how to cope with the child's natural reactions. Medication may be used intermittently at particularly stressful times, such as during hospitalization or a terminal illness of one of the family members.

Nutrition. As already mentioned, decreasing the amount of food additives, food coloring, and sugar may decrease the child's overactive behaviors. The nurse helps the family identify what foods may cause the problem, how to cook for the whole family nutritiously without the food additives, counsels the mother on nutrition, and refers to the dietician when necessary.

Approaches that Help the Family Cope with Hyperactive Behavior

Through teaching and counseling the family can learn new ways to cope with the child's hyperactive behaviors.

Teaching. The nurse teaches the family with a hyperactive child about possible causes, how stimulation increases overactive behavior, how to use behavior modification, what kind of medication may help, and what foods may increase overactive behavior. Being knowledgeable about the condition of the child, what causes the problem, and how they can prevent it helps the family to cope with the hyperactive child.

The nurse also educates the community to the problems and needs of the family with a hyperactive child, working with teachers and other parents to prevent labeling the parents of hyperactive children as bad parents and to foster understanding of the possible causes of and needed approaches to hyperactivity.

Counseling. The main strategy for working with the family of a hyperactive child is counseling. Counseling helps the family to identify and reduce their guilt, set realistic goals for themselves and the child, identify their own family difficulties, and generate and select possible solutions. Counseling stresses the importance of all family members planning and working together to reduce the family difficulties and hyperactivity of the child. Specific

strategies for counseling the high-risk family are described in the chapter on "Counseling Strategies."

It is frequently helpful for families with hyperactive children to share difficulties and successful approaches with each other. In one group with several parents of hyperactive children, the families have been very supportive of each other, offering to babysit for each other as they already know the problems and the approaches to use with the hyperactive child.

Since many health professionals are involved in teaching and counseling the family, they work in a coordinated team. Physicians, dieticians, psychologists, school nurses, hospital nurses, school teachers, nurse practitioners, and others are involved in the counseling with the family. Rather than each professional identifying different problems and approaches which may conflict with each other, all health professionals help develop a common family care plan with coordinated approaches.

Evaluation and Follow-up

The nurse continues to evaluate the child and family problems as they deal with the hyperactive child. As in other high-risk situations, evaluation and follow-up are essential since the hyperactive problem may continue until the child is an adolescent and some emotional difficulties may continue beyond that time. Although the child may be under control, at certain times, intermittent crises may cause the child to become hyperactive again. As the nurse works with the family over time, she helps them to recognize and cope with the up and down progress of the child as he gains control of his own behaviors. As the family requires more or less help as the child grows, the nurse changes her role accordingly.

SUMMARY

The hyperactive child presents a challenge to both the family and the nurse. The child's overactivity, distractibility, impulsiveness, excitability, and resulting emotional difficulties make him very disruptive to the members of the family, school, hospital, or other settings. The hyperactive behavior has a potential to completely disrupt the family, which may lead to abuse or divorce, but has an equal potential to stimulate the parents' coping abilities and closeness. The nurse helps the family to reduce hyperactive behaviors through environmental control, behavior modification, medication, and nutrition and to cope with the remaining hyperactive behaviors through teaching and counseling.

REFERENCES

1. Burns, A. "The Role of Food Colorings and Flavors in Producing Hyperkinesis with Learning Disabilities in Children." *Journal of the New York State School Nurse-Teacher Association*, 7, Spring 1976, 29–30.
2. Cline, F. W. "Stimulants and Their Use with Hyperactive Children." *Nurse Practitioner*, 2, November/December 1976, 33–34.
3. Freedman, A. M. et al. *Comprehensive Textbook of Psychiatry.* Vol. 2, 2nd Ed. Baltimore: Williams and Wilkins Co., 1975, 2201–2203.
4. Schmitt, B. "Guidelines for Living with a Hyperactive Child." *Pediatrics*, 60 #3, September 1977, 387.
5. Stine, J. J. "Symptom Alleviation in the Hyperactive Child by Dietary Modification." *American Journal of Orthopsychiatry*, 46 #4, October 1976, 637–645.
6. Tachdjian, M. *Pediatric Orthopedics.* Philadelphia: W. B. Saunders, 1973.
7. Woodard, P. B. and B. Brodie. "The Hyperactive Child: Who Is He?" *Nursing Clinics of North America*, 9, December 1974, 727–745.

ADDITIONAL READINGS

1. Davids, A. "An Objective Instrument for Assessing Hyperkinesis in Children." *Journal of Learning Disabilities*, 4, November 1971, 35–37.
2. Johnson, C. F. and R. Prinz. "Hyperactivity Is in the Eyes of the Beholder." *Clinical Pediatrics*, 15 #3, March 1976, 222–238.
3. Lucas, B. et al. "Nutrient Intake and Stimulant Drugs in Hyperactive Children." *Journal of the American Dietetic Association*, 70 #4, April 1977, 373–377.
4. Stewart, M. A. and S. W. Olds. *Raising a Hyperactive Child.* New York: Harper & Row, 1973.

PERTINENT ORGANIZATIONS

NATIONAL
* *Association for Children with Learning Disabilities*
  4156 Library Road
  Pittsburgh, Pennsylvania 15234
  National office and local chapters provide information for helping children with learning disabilities including the hyperactive child.

* *California Association for Neurologically Handicapped Children*
  645 Odin Drive
  Pleasant Hill, California 94523
  Provides publications pertaining to learning disabilities and hyperactive difficulties. List of publications and price list available.

LOCAL
* Local groups helping with parenting problems, abuse, and learning disabilities are helpful to the family with a hyperactive child.

The Terminally Ill Child

Donna Lee Wong, R.N., M.N., P.N.A./P

CHAPTER TEN

Tremendous grief accompanies any child's death. Although every person who knows that child is in some way affected by the loss, the loss is greatest for the child and his family. The care of a child who has died unexpectedly or whose death is anticipated includes caring for all members of his family.

Incidence. The neonate is most vulnerable to the risks against survival. For example, two-thirds of all the deaths which take place during the first year of life occur during the perinatal period. The number of deaths during these four weeks is greater than the combined number of deaths from all other causes among individuals less than 65 years of age.[1]

Following the perinatal period, crib death or sudden infant death syndrome (SIDS) is the number one cause of infant mortality. As the term implies, SIDS is sudden, unexpected, unexplained, and a special kind of tragedy because there is no warning or known prevention. Accidents, the leading cause of death in children over one year of age, also occur with no warning, but in most instances, are preventable.

Cancer annually claims the lives of approximately 3,000 children under the age of 15 years in the United States.[4] The recent chemotherapeutic and radiologic advances in the treatment of leukemia and other childhood malignant diseases have transformed these previously short-term fatal illnesses into long-term chronic, but potentially terminal conditions. However, terminal illness among children still remains a significant problem.

BASIC CONCEPTS OF GRIEF AND DYING

Grief Symptoms. Erich Lindemann found many symptoms to be common among all persons in acute grief.[3] One of the most important implications in the recognition of such responses is that they are normal, usual, and expected.

1. *Sensations of somatic distress,* such as a need for sighing, an empty feeling in the stomach, loss of appetite, a tightness in the throat, and a feeling of exhaustion from any physical or emotional exertion;
2. *An intense preoccupation* with the image of the deceased;
3. *Feelings of guilt,* particularly surrounding their actions before the death in terms of how they might have averted the tragedy;

4. *Hostile reactions,* such as loss of warmth toward others, a tendency toward irritability and anger, or a wish not to be bothered by friends or relatives; and

5. *Loss of the usual pattern of conduct,* with a tendency to move aimlessly about looking for something to do or what they think they ought to do.

Stages in Dying. Elisabeth Kübler-Ross describes typical stages that many people progress through during their final stage of life.[2]

In the stage of *denial* and isolation, the person responds with, "No, not me," regardless of whether or not the person was explicitly told his diagnosis. Doctor shopping, delaying agreement to treatment, acting very happy and optimistic in spite of the news, and refusing to tell or talk to anyone about the diagnosis are common examples of denial during the initial phase. All of these reactions are healthy ways of dealing with a most difficult and painful situation. They allow people time to collect their thoughts and mobilize their energies toward goal-directed, adaptive behaviors. Partial denial is used by people at times throughout the dying process. Without this protective mechanism, few people could survive the constant emotional burden of anticipating their death. The denial allows them the opportunity to live out the remaining time with hope, peace, and possibly acceptance.

The *anger* stage includes rage, hostility, envy, and resentment directed at oneself or others. Everything of life that the person loves, worked for, and hoped to achieve is suddenly snatched from him. He is angry toward those who are physically strong, who do not have to endure the painful treatments, and who can realize their dreams. He is not angry at the persons themselves, but at the things they represent: health, vitality, hope, optimism, and an undiminished joy of life.

The *bargaining* stage is frequently difficult to identify, because the bargaining for extra time is often silent. As the anger subsides, the person may explore ways of delaying the inevitable through wishful thinking. As a ten-year-old child told his mother, "Do you know what I wished for on my last birthday? Another birthday."

If the person has a religious orientation, much of the bargaining is done with God. This may be seen in such activities as praying frequently, attending church services more regularly, requesting visits from a minister, priest, or rabbi, or asking others to beseech God's help.

The fourth stage is *depression.* There are two types of depression: the one experienced for past losses and the one experienced for anticipated or impending losses.

Depression related to past losses occurs frequently for a child with a chronic terminal illness. Loss of hair from the treatment, restriction in physical activity, loss of a body part or function, and change in daily routine constitute past losses. Guilt or shame may accompany this depression.

The second type of depression is a method of preparing for the impending loss of all love objects. Unlike the survivors who are saying good-bye to one person, the dying person is saying good-bye to everything and everyone he loves. His loss is so great that no one really knows the intensity of that person's feelings unless he is also experiencing it.

The final stage of dying is *acceptance.* At this point, the dying person is no longer angry or depressed. The denial has lost its protective function, and whatever bargaining does occur is usually for a quick, painless death rather than a prolongation of life. It is not a happy period, but is simply devoid of negative emotions. The person is disinterested in the news of the world, may prefer to be left alone except for the most important people in his life, and wants peace and solitude. Such behavior usually signifies to others that the end is near. It is often a time when family members and health professionals need more help and support than the dying person, if they have not progressed to a similar level of acceptance.

For example, one family whose teenage son was dying knew that his death was very near and requested that all chemotherapy and painful procedures be stopped. They prayed that their son would die soon, in comfort and peace. When the child's respirations became labored, the nurse began oxygen via nasal cannula, but the child resisted. The father calmly told the nurse, "Take the tube away. We are ready. It is time for our son to die in peace and with dignity." In a few moments, the breathing stopped. The nursing staff, who had all gathered in the room to say their last good-byes to the child, cried with the parents, but it was the parents who consoled them.

The progression through the stages from denial to acceptance is the usual sequence but is in no way inflexible, or absolute. Each stage or behavior is fluid and may be present or recurrent throughout the dying process. It is not unusual for someone to verbally proceed through each stage during a conversation.

For example, one mother expressed the following thoughts, which are representative of each stage, from denial to beginning acceptance: "When I look at my son, I really can't believe he has leukemia. He is so healthy, happy, active—just so alive. I pray that I never hear the word relapse. The doctor told me that if he remains in this remission for three years, he is probably cured. I count the days and pray he enters high school—that's when the three years are up. . . . I get so angry when I hear about these delinquents killing people. I think to myself, why should my son have this terrible disease when those rotten kids are healthy? What did we ever do to deserve this? . . . But sometimes the reality of what leukemia means really hits home. Did you hear that Johnny relapsed and the drugs aren't working? When I heard that I cried all day, because inside I know it could be my child. I started to think what it must be like to see your child die. I felt so sad and empty inside. But at the same time, I realize that I have other children and my husband. We would have to survive, for all of us would still be living. I am so grateful to have a wonderful husband. I know we can go through this, no matter what happens to our child, because we have each other."

Dr. Ross feels that the helping person's role is one of support through active listening. The goal is not to push the dying person through each stage,

but to support him while he is in that stage. However, it is usually through such intervention that the person is able to cope with the denial, anger, and depression, and hopefully reach acceptance. Professionals need to appreciate the importance of accepting each person where he is in his process of dealing with death rather than judge him as "in stage II, but should be in stage IV." When one respects the function that stage of behavior plays in helping the person accept his mortality, and accepts the behavior as a normal and healthy consequence of dying, then active, empathetic support can be offered.

The Risk Situation

The risk situation for the terminally ill child includes the child's risk of death and the family's risk of disintegration as a reaction to the death. On the scale of stressful life events, death of a close family member, such as a child, has tremendous psychological impact on the individual. Several factors influence the dying child's and the other family members' ability to cope with the crisis of impending loss.

One of the purposes of identifying the risk situation is to delineate those variables which influence the resolution of the crisis. The author has found that several factors help determine those families who are more or less likely to cope successfully with the crisis.

Status of the Marital Relationship. There seems to be a positive correlation between the strength of the marital relationship and the ability of the parents to adjust to the impending or actual loss. Where husband and wife have a pattern of discussing their positive and negative feelings, there tends to be much less guilt, indecision, blame, denial, and anger. Although there are still crises and disruptions in their usual behavior, sharing partners tend to deal with each crisis successfully, experience less overlapping and accummulation of crises, and have less overwhelming and destructive experiences than nonsharing partners.

In the moderately adjusted or disturbed family there are no major difficulties in everyday functioning. Minor differences or problems tend to be avoided or ignored rather than resolved. However, major crises expose the areas of contention. In the poorly adjusted family, during a crisis parents place blame on each other, emphasize past misdeeds, and search for reasons which enhance the guilt in the other partner. They may seek ineffective patterns of coping, such as excessive drinking, promiscuous behavior, and physical aggression. The weaker the family relationship, the greater is the family risk in a major crisis such as terminal illness.

Ability to Communicate with Significant Others Outside the Family. Some individuals who do not communicate effectively with their spouses, or who may not have a spouse, gain emotional support from others. When there is no support from a significant other within the individual's own social milieu, the nurse may be a supporting person.

Ability to Communicate with the Child. Occasionally, the parents can communicate effectively with each other but are unable to deal with the child's feelings or questions. This is particularly true in the case of young children, where verbal communication is the least useful method, and adolescents, whose attitude toward parental authority may inhibit their willingness to talk or listen. Nurses can facilitate communication between parents and child by helping parents understand how each age child views the life-threatening illness and how they can support the child verbally and nonverbally.

Ability to Use Verbal Communication. Almost all methods of psychological intervention, including active listening, counseling, crisis intervention, and psychotherapy, require verbal communication between two individuals. The ability to ventilate feelings, such as anger, fear, guilt, anxiety, and sadness, helps people cope with the emotion. It also allows validation of feelings and thoughts.

For example, one mother told the nurse counselor that before her son had become ill, she had dreams of his dying. After she learned of his fatal illness, she wondered if such thoughts had "caused him to get sick." Her guilt over this was so great that she had never told anyone about the dreams

until now. Through verbalizing the fear and realistically discussing the effects of dreams on future events, the mother was able to logically dispel her thoughts about "causing the illness."

Ability to Use Approach Coping Mechanisms. Coping mechanisms are behaviors which are directed at reducing tension but may or may not be effective. Coping behaviors which result in movement toward adjustment are called approach behaviors and those which result in movement away from adjustment are avoidance behaviors. Figure 10-1 lists several approach and avoidance behaviors.

None of the indices from the table is sufficient by itself to assess the possible success or failure of the resolution of a crisis. Rather, each behavior must be seen in the context of the total assessment of the family system and of each of its members. The observation of several avoidance behaviors in the emotionally healthy family will denote much less risk than an equal number of avoidance behaviors in a poorly adjusted family.

GENERAL FAMILY DIFFICULTIES

There are many general family difficulties for the family of a terminally ill child as listed in Figure 10-2.

Anticipatory Grief of Expected Death. When death is expected, anticipatory grieving begins before the death. The loss does not hurt less and it may not even be shortened, for in long-term, potentially fatal illnesses, the grief becomes chronic rather than acute. The parents mourn the loss of their child long before he is gone. They may mourn the pain they see their child enduring, the uncertainty of the future, and the loss of a family life unburdened by emotional, physical, and financial crisis. Unlike the parents who experience a sudden loss, these fathers and mothers are unable to resolve their grief until the child is "cured" or dead. In another sense, when death is expected, time is on the family's side. Parents are able to complete "unfinished business" before the end, work through

Figure 10-1. Assessment of Coping Behaviors

Approach Behavior (directed toward acceptance and successful resolution of the crisis)	Avoidance Behavior (directed toward denial and avoidance of the crisis)
Asks for information regarding diagnosis and child's present condition	Fails to recognize the seriousness of the child's condition despite physical evidence
Seeks help and support from others	Refuses to agree to treatment
Anticipates future problems; actively seeks guidance and answers	Intellectualizes about the illness, but in areas unrelated to the child's condition
Talks about the process of dying and death, either of own child's or others'	Angry and hostile to staff, regardless of their attitude or behavior
Plans realistically for the future	Avoids staff, family members, or child
Acknowledges and accepts child's awareness of diagnosis and prognosis	Entertains unrealistic future plans for child, with little emphasis on the present
Expresses feelings, such as sorrow, depression, anger, and realizes reason for the emotional reaction	Unable to adjust to or accept a change in progression of disease
Realistically perceives the child's condition, adjusts to changes (such as remission to relapse)	Continually looks for new cures with no perspective toward possible benefit
Recognizes own growth through passage of time, such as earlier denial and nonacceptance of diagnosis	Refuses to acknowledge child's understanding of disease and prognosis
Expresses feelings openly	Uses magical thinking and fantasy, may seek "occult" help
Experiences somatic distress when fear of loss or actual loss is greatest	Places complete faith in religion to point of relinquishing own responsibility
	Withdraws from outside world
	Punishes self because of guilt and blame
	Makes no change in lifestyle to meet needs of other family members
	Unable to discuss death on any level, such as previous experience with loss

initial grief stages, and help the child and other siblings cope with their reactions.

Sudden Grief of Unexpected Death. In sudden unexpected death, there is no preliminary chance to deal with the loss, only the cruel reality that nothing remains of their child except their memories. Because of this lack of time to prepare, many parents feel great guilt and remorse for not having done something different or more with the child. They may berate themselves for disciplining the child too harshly or refusing him special favors. They repeatedly say to themselves and others, "Oh,

if only I had known, I would have _____ differently." Parents of sudden infant death children experience great guilt feelings. It is important to listen to statements about such feelings to help parents deal with the guilt to progress through the resolution of grief.

Infant and Toddler: Separation Difficulties. For the infant or toddler who does not grasp the external meaning of death, separation from their parents and home is the most difficult crisis situation. Such separation is tremendously difficult for the child, who usually responds with angry protest, passive despair, and eventually, interpersonal detachment.

Parents may stay away for many reasons: denial of the seriousness of the illness, guilt over previous life events, unresolved grief for another loss in their lives, or anger toward the child for bringing them such sorrow and tragedy. Unless helped to deal with such feelings, they will not be able to continue their effective parenting with their child during his hospitalization.

Preschool Child: Punishment, Fear of Bodily Harm, and Guilt Feelings. Young children realize

Figure 10-2. General Family Difficulties for the Family with a Terminally Ill Child

Anticipatory Grief of Expected Death
Sudden Grief of Unexpected Death
Infant and Toddler: Separation Difficulties
Preschool Child: Punishment, Fear of Bodily Harm, and Guilt Feelings
School-Age Child: Evil Will, Fear of Mutilation, and Guilt Feelings
Adolescent Child: Altered Body Image and Loss of Identity and Independence
Parental Guilt

that death exists, but they do not see death as irreversible or inevitable. Most of their concepts regarding death are learned from the attitudes of their parents and other significant people. If parents act upset when their children ask about death, funerals, or other aspects of the subject, children quickly learn to keep such questions to themselves. They also deduce that death must be something terrible and frightening, since others refuse to talk about it, whisper behind their backs, or become visibly anxious about that topic. Since children in the oedipal period normally have aggressive feelings toward their parents, these children may see their illness as a punishment and proof of their "badness."

Preschool-age siblings are also victims of the developmental processes of this period. Because of magical thinking, or the feeling that their thoughts cause events, they may fear that they caused their brother or sister to become ill as a result of previous jealous thoughts. If that sibling dies, the surviving child's guilt is great.

Such feelings of guilt are particularly significant in unexpected death, such as sudden infant death, when sibling rivalry is great between the young child and the newly introduced child. When the parent has no logical answer for the infant's death, the older sibling is certain that his thoughts caused it. The surviving siblings need an explanation of the death, reassurance of their innocence in the event, and provision for their grief.

School-Age Child: Evil Will, Fear of Mutilation, and Guilt Feelings. These children come to realize that death is irreversible, universal, and inevitable. Children between six and nine years of age tend to personify death, as the devil, a witch, or a ghost. These children associate illness and death with evil and punishment and fear the mutilation and body injury that may occur with catastrophic death.

School-age children also have the understanding necessary to separate fact from fantasy or cause from effect, provided they are given appropriate explanations concerning the nature of the illness and its treatment. With this higher level of comprehension comes the fear of communicability of disease, questions on why they are sick when

others are not, cause of the illness, contemplation of the consequences of disease on their physical and social functioning, and wonderment about dying and death itself.

One example of guilt was related by a preadolescent who told the nurse counselor that her illness was a punishment from God. She explained it in this way: "In our religion, God has two books. In one book, he writes down all the good things you do, and on the other side, all the bad things. At the end of the year, he adds up each side. If you have done more bad things, he punishes you. I guess I have done more bad things; that is why he sent me this illness." The nurse asked: "What do you think you did to deserve this?" The child answered: "That's what is so terrible. I don't know. I am trying to do good things so he won't make the disease come back, but if I don't know what I did that was wrong, it is hard to make up for it." In further sessions, this child reasoned that her siblings had not gotten the illness because in the "book" they had more good deeds. In an early drawing, she demonstrated her feelings of inferiority and isolation by drawing herself last in a group picture of the family, with only her back and head showing. Part of the nurse's intervention was to help her realize what control she had over her destiny, to improve her self-image and feelings of self-esteem, and to clarify the religious versus the literal meaning of God's two books.

Adolescent: Altered Body Image and Loss of Self-Identity and Independence. It is adolescents who must deal with the most stresses, of all the risks inherent in each age group. When a potentially terminal illness befalls them, they must deal with additional body changes and functions which greatly hinder their already critical feelings of group identity and self-image. For the child with cancer, loss of hair, increased fatigue, side effects of drugs, or periods of hospitalization interfere with the successful realization of their developmental goals. The regression and loss of self-control often accompanying painful illnesses devastate their sense of independence.

They are in particular jeopardy because they

no longer have the protective defenses of childhood or the alternate coping mechanisms of adulthood to help them deal with the thought of finality. They need adult trust and companionship more than ever, yet they may be most resistant to establishing deeper relationships with their parents or other significant people. Although they desire the cohesiveness and camaraderie of their peer group, they resent the vitality and strength of other adolescents who are well. For example, the terminally ill adolescent may be depressed because of his enforced separation from peers, yet strenuously object to any suggestion that his friends be encouraged to visit.

Adolescents may be the most lonely, isolated group of dying people, and one of the most difficult to reach and understand. Nurses are in an exceptional position to meet the needs of dying adolescents because of their extended contact with them during hospitalization. Nurses must be willing to communicate with adolescents on their age level, as with all other age groups, and be patient enough to wait for acceptance from them.

Parental Guilt. Almost all parents experience guilt upon learning of their child's diagnosis. Parents may blame themselves for many probably unrelated behaviors. Although guilt is a normal reaction to any loss, guilt that prevents individuals from dealing effectively with the present crisis is a greater risk.

For example, one mother whose child was dying from aplastic anemia was unable to discuss her feelings regarding the child's approaching death. Although she was physically present with the child, she could give little emotional support. She usually sat quietly in the room, asking no questions and offering no conversation. However, one day after learning that none of the siblings were possible donors for a bone marrow transplant (the last hope for recovery), the mother told the nurse counselor that she wondered if God was punishing her for her daughter's birth. She explained that this child, the oldest of four children, was born out of wedlock, of a father who then abandoned the mother. After the birth, the mother and infant had moved to a new location, where she had met her

present husband. He had accepted the child and fathered the three other children, however, none of the children knew of their different parentage.

The mother felt certain in her heart that God had chosen this child, not one of the other siblings who could have been a compatible donor sibling, to punish the mother for her previous misdeeds. The guilt was so tremendous that it prevented her from dealing with the present loss of her child. Following the child's death, the mother was unable to tell the other children the truth (she told them their sister went away to get better) and she behaved as if her daughter was still at home (she set a place at the table and kept her bedroom and possessions unchanged). Although the nurse counselor and other members of the nursing staff tried to help this woman, she denied the crisis and refused to talk about the death.

FAMILY DIFFICULTIES AT SPECIFIC TERMINAL ILLNESS STAGES

Many illnesses, such as leukemia, are now chronic disorders, and death, although anticipated, is uncertain. The family's adjustment is extended over an indefinite period of time with several phases: discovery of diagnosis, remission therapy, maintenance therapy, relapse, terminal stage, post-death, or for long-term survivors, cessation of therapy. Within these stages many of the general difficulties already discussed and additional specific difficulties occur (Figure 10-3). Although similar stages are present in most chronic life-threatening illnesses, a leukemia case will be used to describe the family reactions.

Phase I—Discovery of the Diagnosis

Shock. The onset of childhood leukemia is usually insidious, and before the diagnosis is confirmed, the symptoms may be attributed to common problems, such as a cold, virus, or flu. Therefore, when parents learn of the diagnosis of leukemia, they usually react with stunned disbelief.

For example, as one mother stated: "I sat and calmly listened to the doctor. However, once he

Figure 10-3. Family Difficulties at Specific Terminal Illness Stages

Phase I—Discovery of the Diagnosis
  Shock
  What to tell the child

Phase II—Remission Therapy
  Depression and bargaining
  Parents' anger
  Child's anger
  Sibling anger
  Discipline
  Altered body image

Phase III—Maintenance Therapy
  School
  Hope and fear

Phase IV—Relapse
  Recurring grief
  Cessation of therapy

Phase V—Terminal Stage
  Acceptance
  Including all significant people

Phase VI—Postdeath
  Review of the relationship
  Subsequent children

said the word 'leukemia' I heard everything else as if I wasn't really there. When I left his office, I closed the door and hit the wall, screaming inside myself, 'No, it can't be true.' I cried but the real impact of that day didn't materialize until I had a chance to calm down." To parents, the words leukemia and cancer are synonymous with death. The "survival statistics," the chemotherapy, and the possible side effects of the drugs are only words, with little meaning. At that moment, there is no hope, no chance for recovery, only the death sentence imposed by the diagnosis.

Once the shock and disbelief have worn off, the reality of the news has an overwhelming impact. At this point someone must be available to assess the parents' understanding of the disease, its treatment, and potential prognosis, or the parents will prepare themselves for the child's death and be unable to face many of the other important issues surrounding the illness.

What to Tell the Child. One of the most significant dilemmas that arises shortly after learning of the diagnosis is the issue of how to treat the ill child and what to tell him. Initially, many parents react

by overprotecting and overattending to the hospitalized child. At the same time, they may have told the child nothing of the seriousness of the condition, except that he will be well. The child soon perceives the opposing messages.

For example, as one eight-year-old boy said to his mother, "If I only have anemia and the medicine will cure it, why are you always sad? I can see that you have been crying after you leave to talk to the doctor or nurse. If I am so well, how come you stay here every night? When my sister was in the hospital for her tonsil operation, you visited during the day."

The question of "to tell or not to tell" a child the truth is a difficult one. Some parents elect to keep the truth from the child and other siblings in the hope of sparing them the emotional burden of coping with such serious news. However, the strengths of this decision are short-lived. A child who is not told his diagnosis quickly becomes aware of its seriousness, yet he also knows that he cannot talk to anyone about it and, therefore, is deprived of the opportunity to discuss his fears and questions.

Exactly what and how to tell children about their diagnosis is a very individual matter. The author has found several principles to be useful guidelines.

1. The explanation must be based on the child's cognitive ability related to his developmental age.
2. The explanation must build on what the child is thinking. Asking children such questions as "What do you think is wrong with you?" or "What have you heard others say?" provides information on which to base an answer.
3. The explanation must be honest.

Although the truth may be difficult to say, in the long run, it will make answering new questions easier. As one parent stated, "I don't know what we would have done if we had not told our son (10 years old) the truth. How would we have explained the hair loss, the blood tests every week, the medicine that makes him vomit? Sometimes it's very hard because he knows he has leukemia and he hears that people can die from it. But at least we know what he is thinking and we talk about it. It's rare that he asks questions. He treats his illness as something of the past. I only wish I could adjust so well. But he actually helps us, because we see his physical and emotional strength, and I know it sounds silly, but he gives us hope!''

Phase II—Remission Therapy

Depression and Bargaining. Immediately following the confirmation of the diagnosis, the child begins therapy. For many long-term illnesses, such as leukemia, therapy can arrest or eradicate the disease and induce a remission. During this time, parents commonly react with depression and bargaining. The depression is a reaction to observing the side effects of the drugs at a time when they expect initial improvement from the chemotherapy. They are anxious about the known effects of the therapeutic agents and fearful of the possible hazards, such as overwhelming infection or hemorrhage.

There is usually a great deal of bargaining for time for the drugs to work, the body to make its own cells, and the bone marrow results to show a remission. Much psychic energy is directed at waiting for the confirmation of a remission.

Parents' Anger. Anger is very common, and is frequently directed at the hospital staff. Parents, mothers in particular, complain about the nursing care, that the doctor never spends enough time explaining the child's progress, or that the laboratory technicians are not skillful. The anger is not against specific people but against the injustice of what is happening to their child and to themselves. Allowing parents to participate in their child's care as much as possible and encouraging them to verbalize their complaints helps them work through the anger.

For example, one family, who realized the necessity of the protective isolation, literally stood guard outside their child's door. At first the hospital staff resented their behavior, regarding it as a

direct afront to their ability. However, once they understood the parents' need to feel in control and that they were doing everything they could for their son, the staff respected their "guard duty" and made a concerted effort to practice scrupulous reverse isolation technique. Unfortunately, this child died within two weeks of the diagnosis from a rare complication. The parents expressed their relief that the cause of death was not infection, and attributed that fact to their protection of their child from all harmful germs.

Child's Anger. Children also feel angry during this time, particularly because of all the traumatic procedures they are subjected to. For the leukemic child, bone marrow aspiration, lumbar punctures, intravenous injections and blood tests are common painful intrusive procedures. Once they begin to feel better it is not unlikely for them to express their anger by becoming uncooperative for the most minor request. Needle play, dramatic doctor-nurse play, and aggression outlets such as punching bags, dart sets, or water guns help children ventilate such feelings. Since parents may receive the brunt of this anger, the nurse should discuss the reasons for the child's behavior with them.

For example, one mother thought that the child's aggressive behavior was a reaction to the medicine, and wondered how she could ever cope with this side effect once the child was discharged. The nurse counselor discussed with the parents the possible causes of the child's anger and suggested appropriate outlets. One that was especially effective involved hanging a large punching balloon over the bed. It worked very well *after* the child drew the doctor's face on the balloon!

Sibling Anger. The siblings experience feelings of anger and resentment during their brother's or sister's long hospitalization. Separation from their parents, the disrupted family life, and lack of "rewards" for their good behavior fuel the anger. Some children misbehave because negative behavior elicits a parental response, such as a stern reprimand or a spanking. Techniques that tend to help the other siblings cope with the sudden change in family life are continued phone or visiting contact with the child and parents, and alternation of each parent during prolonged visits or rooming-in.

As the ill child improves or the illness progresses, the parents must refocus their responsibilities for themselves and all the children. The marital relationship needs reevaluation so that both parents share in the emotional crisis and support. If the mother constantly stays with the ill child, she may be emotionally drained and in need of an opportunity for a night's rest at home. Encouraging both parents to "take a night off," while another family member stays with the child, can be invaluable in helping some parents recoup their emotional energies.

Discipline. Parents frequently comment on their insecurity in disciplining their child, even in simple disagreements over eating, dressing, or bathing. Discipline or limit setting is an essential component of childhood security. Being overprotected and treated as "special" increases children's fear that something is wrong.

For example, when the nurse counselor asked one child how he knew he was better, he stated: "I know I am well because I have to do all my chores and I get spanked when I do something wrong."

Without limits and controls, these children are prone to the same behavior problems of any other healthy child. If he is given everything he wants when he is well, he will be a most frustrated, unhappy, and demanding child during the terminal phase of the illness when it is impossible to meet his requests.

Altered Body Image. One side effect of therapy is hair loss, which has particular psychological significance for different age groups and for parents. For young children, particularly those under five years, the hair loss is usually inconsequential. The parents have the more difficult adjustment, and especially fear the reactions of others to the baldness. One way of helping parents deal with the likely questions is to prepare them for this beforehand by asking them what they think they could say and how they might react to embarrassment if a specific situation occurred.

Reactions of school-age children depend a great deal on how they have been prepared for the hair loss and how they see their parents adjusting to it. Much of their anxiety relates to the anticipation of the loss, rather than the actual baldness. Many of the children prefer to wear a wig, particularly when in the company of peers. Others may feel comfortable wearing a scarf, bandana, or hat. The important thing is to tell children about the expected loss *before* it occurs and to stress that it is temporary. New hair growth usually occurs within three months, although for girls, it may be longer before they wish to discard the wig.

It is important to distinguish between the parents' or the child's concern for the baldness. Most children seem to adjust fairly easily to the baldness once they know how to camouflage it. Parents, on the other hand, may be so anxious over the baldness that they overprotect and isolate the child from feared embarrassment and ridicule.

For example, one mother related the following story which illustrates her concern and the child's adjustment: "The first day Peter was home on a weekend pass a terrible incident occurred. His friends came over to see him, but I feared he would get germs from them, so I sent them away. However, Peter heard me and instead, he went upstairs to his room and stuck his bald head out the window to talk with them! I heard them call him 'Baldy.' I was so upset that I ran upstairs and yanked him inside. He started crying. I told him not to worry about the bad names they called him. He looked up at me and angrily told me that I had made him cry by sending them away. He didn't care if they said 'Baldy'; he only wanted to play." With this example to work with, the nurse counselor helped the mother see that the fear and anxiety over the hair loss was hers, not the child's.

Adolescents have the most difficult time adjusting to the hair loss because it occurs at a time when peer acceptance and group conformity is most important. They need time to express their anger and fears of rejection. The author has found that actively involving the adolescent in purchasing a wig *before* the hair begins to fall out is very beneficial. It provides adolescents with a feeling of participation and self-control before they must face the actual loss and allows them to secure a wig which is as similar to their own hair as possible.

For example, one 13-year-old girl, whose wig was styled exactly like her own hair, commented, "I think I like my wig a little better than my hair!" To convince herself that no one could detect the difference, she periodically wore the wig to school. Because no one could tell the difference between her hair or the wig, she was very comfortable about wearing it when her own hair was gone.

Phase III—Maintenance Therapy

Many life-threatening illnesses progress through several cycles of remissions and exacerbations. During this time daily living must continue along with therapy.

School. Specific arrangements should be made for continuation of school in the hospital and reentrance to school after discharge. Discussing the child's needs with the principal, teacher, and school nurse is essential. Part of this preparation is reeducating others to the more favorable prognosis for these children. One fear of school personnel is that a catastrophic event will occur in the classroom, most significantly, that the child will suddenly die. Reassuring them that this is extremely unlikely is important, even if such fears are not verbalized. Other areas for guidance include talking to the class about the reason for the child's absence and expected body changes, such as hair loss and weight gain, and answering questions from other parents, such as the prevalent fear of the communicability of the disease.

One incident which illustrates the necessity of informing school personnel about the child's condition occurred during a routine physical examination of the school children. All the youngsters were told to remove their shirts. John, who was wearing a wig, refused to take off his turtleneck sweater. The school nurse insisted and while forcing the child to comply, accidently removed his wig. Of course, he was greatly embarrassed and ran into the lavatory. The nurse felt extremely guilty, especially since she had been informed previously of the child's diag-

nosis. She realized her lack of judgment and explained to the class the reason for John's baldness (which they already knew because of the teacher's earlier discussion). She immediately went to the child and apologized, then accompanied him back to class. The incident had positive benefits in that John had been worrying about his wig falling off and now saw that he could survive the ordeal. He also realized that he could have prevented the situation by calmly explaining who he was and why he could not remove his sweater.

Hope and Fear. Even under the best of circumstances the "waiting out" period is difficult. There is a constant need for reevaluation of the child's progress, reconfirmation that some children do survive, and reassurance that minor ailments are just minor.

Many parents find that the best times are the hardest. As one father explained, "When I see my daughter so happy, so well, so alive, I deeply fear the loss of these moments. Sometimes I watch her; I know I should be happy for how well she is doing, yet a great depression falls upon me because I realize the tremendous loss in our lives if she dies."

Phase IV—Relapse

Recurring Grief. If the remission ends in a relapse, there is an exacerbation of all previous fears of death, although most of the stages, such as denial, are shortened. One of the most difficult realizations for parents is the knowledge that with each relapse, the chances for eventual recovery are diminished. Several parents have told the author that after the primary remission ended, they never felt as hopeful again, even if another remission was induced. Repeated hospitalizations for any reason during a long-term illness constitute recurring crises because they represent the potential seriousness of the disease.

Cessation of Therapy. Recurrent grief is also present when therapy is terminated in the hope of a permanent remission. Parents demonstrate tremendous ambivalence over "giving up the drugs," which have been the reason for the favorable prognosis. Parents show behaviors of overprotectiveness toward the child, fanatic scrutiny for any sign of pathology, and great insecurity in the decision to terminate therapy.

Many professionals fail to realize the special needs of these "liberated" families and erroneously label their fears and anxieties as "dependence on the illness." If parents perceive such judgments, they feel very guilty and begin to question their motivations for their behavior. It is important to stress to them that feeling depressed upon learning such good news is normal and expected. After living with the dread of relapse and the ever-present fear of losing one's child, they must progress through a transitional period before they can again reorganize their lives.

Phase V—Terminal Stage

Acceptance. After a series of remissions and exacerbations in some illnesses, there comes a time when no more new drugs exist, and the chance for inducing another remission is highly unlikely. Occasionally, parents are allowed the opportunity of choosing the way they want their child to live out his remaining life. Health professionals must provide the support and information necessary for parents to make an "informed consent" for the use of extraordinary measures, termination of all treatment, or home care.

During the terminal phase, the family's reactions are influenced by their previous acceptance or denial of the child's illness. Frequently, parents wish for death to come quickly once they know the treatment is ineffective. One universal parental wish is for the death to be peaceful. Although parents often worry about how death will occur, they often fear asking questions because of their expectation that others will think badly of them for inquiring. As a result, they usually fantasize much worse possibilities of what happens when death is imminent than if they had been told the actual circumstances. Encouraging parents to ask about the final stages, to ventilate their feelings of wishing all of this misery to end, and to prepare for funeral arrangements before the death helps them

deal with many unresolved guilt feelings and fantasies of the unknown.

Including All Significant People. It is also important to discuss with parents how to tell the other siblings that their sister or brother may die soon, and to explore some of the usual reactions of children to death.

For example, one family, who had not told their ten-year-old son of his older brother's serious illness and impending death, realized how poorly prepared he was when he expressed anger at his brother for refusing to talk with him over the telephone. He interpreted this negative response as indicative of the ill brother's loss of love and interest in his younger sibling. When the brother did die, this child became hysterical, refusing to believe his parents. He would not attend any funeral services and was very angry at his parents and surviving older brother, who did expect the death. The parents felt very guilty because they realized that they should not have kept the truth from the child.

Siblings and fathers seem to need extra help during the terminal phase, most likely as a result of inadequate support during the previous phases. The nurse must *always* include the entire family in counseling sessions. Sometimes this involves seeing the children and the parents separately, but it has proved to be essential in helping everyone deal with the crisis of an impending loss. In those families where the parents fail to reach the same degree of acceptance or to use similar coping mechanisms, it is important to assist each in accepting the other's behavior.

For instance, many mothers view their husbands' stoicism as a cold, uncaring attitude toward the child's condition and the mothering responsibilities. However, upon talking to these fathers, it is apparent some must cope by suppressing their emotions in order to maintain control. One father stated, "If I cry I fear that I will never stop."

Phase VI—Postdeath

Review of the Relationship. Families can prepare themselves for the expected loss, but when it occurs, the grief is acute. There is a tendency at this time to review the events of the child's life during the time of his illness and to evaluate the effectiveness of their efforts. It is very important that they see their relationship with their child as positive. Unresolved guilt feelings delay the resolution of mourning. During this time, nurses should encourage parents to verbalize their memories of their child.

For example, one father expressed his thoughts in this way: "I don't regret anything we did for our son. He was happy for a long time. I am very proud of our close relationship. He died peacefully and with those he loved nearby him. I am not bitter anymore about 'why *my* son?' Now my thoughts turn to 'Why *any* child?' I want to help others who are going through this, if I can."

Subsequent Children. One common problem after the child's death is the parents' decision to have additional children. Many, if not all, fear the recurrence of the illness in the subsequent child. Others try to replace the lost child by having another one as soon as possible or attributing to a sibling the characteristics of the dead child. With support and counseling, parents usually can work through grief and make such decisions when they are psychologically ready. Any sudden decision for change, such as moving to a new location, may be a clue that the family needs additional intervention.

NURSING APPROACHES

Some general nursing approaches are described here, while more specific strategies are discussed in later chapters.

Crisis Intervention

Since death is both a maturational and a situational crisis, it seems appropriate to employ crisis intervention. However, one possible shortcoming of this technique is that the difficulties seen in a family with a terminally ill child engender multiple crises. The concentrated approach in crisis intervention may be insufficient over a long-term situational crisis, unless the professional is aware of the need for flexibility and modification of his or her

approach. For example, the resolution of the crisis may not occur for years, since the chronic grief work cannot be completed until the child dies or is "cured."

Counseling

Counseling, which employs the art of listening, empathetic support, appropriate crisis intervention when needed, and brief therapy for previous unresolved conflicts, meets more of the emotional needs of these families than the use of any other strategy alone.

The specific techniques used in counseling are communication, both verbal and nonverbal, play, and drawing. With children, nonverbal communication, such as body movement, eye contact, and space can be much more informative than verbalization. Dramatic play and drawing are tools for assessment, intervention, and evaluation. Dramatic, or imaginative, make-believe play allows the child freedom of conscious and unconscious expression. For the terminally ill child, fantasy play with needles or other medical equipment, nurse-doctor dolls in a hospital, and family doll house settings is particularly valuable to help uncover fears, hidden thoughts, and misconceptions.

Spontaneous and directed art are also natural forms of self-expression for children, because what they draw is closely interwoven with their self-concept. Whether one uses art or play, it is preferable to direct the activity away from identification with the child. For example, asking children to draw "what it's like for *someone* to be in a hospital" is less anxiety-producing than requesting them to draw "how it was for *them* to be in the hospital."

Counseling can occur through work on an individual and/or group basis. Family sessions, which include all or some of the members as dictated by the nature of the discussion, are essential to the overall success of helping a family adjust to the death of a child. Having group sessions of dying children, siblings, or parents is also an effective method of counseling, and meets the needs of larger numbers of people than individual or family sessions.

Assessment

Assessment leads to the identification of the problem. There are several important areas to assess for the family of a potentially terminally ill child.

Knowledge of Other Children with a Similar Diagnosis. If parents respond affirmatively, it is important to explore the events of the other child's illness and the parents' perception of that knowledge. There is a strong tendency to compare their child's symptoms, treatments, response to therapy, and so on with the other child's. Frequently, this causes many problems and misconceptions.

For example, one mother who resisted agreeing to chemotherapy was labeled as "hostile and dumb" by the medical staff. During the first session with the nurse counselor, the mother stated that her friend's daughter died of the same illness a year ago. This friend visited the mother as soon as she had learned of the diagnosis and related all the events of her own child's illness, including her death. After listening to all the side effects of the drugs, which eventually failed, the mother was understandably ambivalent in her feelings about agreeing to treatment. However, after exploring her thoughts of refusing chemotherapy, the mother realized she could not live with her guilt if the child died untreated, and therefore she had to do everything possible. But as she stated, "I understand this in my head, but it still bothers me in my heart."

Past Experiences with Death. Almost all parents and many children are able to relate some previous experience with death of a person or pet. How they relate that experience yields valuable information about their future ability to talk about dying and death. It also helps the nurse assess their comfort in talking to the children about death, funerals, and so on.

For example, one family, who elected to have their child at home for the remainder of the terminal phase, was able to prepare the other siblings and arrange for funeral services fairly comfortably. When asked about their ability to deal with such subjects openly, the mother responded that both her parents had died at home after long illnesses. As a child, she was never shielded from death, but allowed to attend funeral and wake services. She felt that her religion and belief in an afterlife were a support to her. The father gained no comfort from religious associations and had had few experiences with death, but was able to share his wife's strength. His most motivating influence for bringing his son home was, "I want him to die with his boots on." In other words, he wanted dignity and respect for his son.

Influence of Religion. For some people, religion and faith are a blessing at a time of crisis, while for others, it is a shackling burden because of the guilt it signifies. Questions such as, "Has your religion been of help to you?" or "Why do you think God sent this illness to you?" uncover feelings of shame, guilt, bitterness, and anger. Frequently, it is advisable to have a priest, minister, or rabbi talk to the family, especially when they feel as if God is punishing them for a previous misdeed. Receiving confession, praying to God for forgiveness, or some other penitence may relieve them of their guilt, or at least, allow them to deal with it.

Marital Relationship and Support System. The importance of identifying this has been discussed under the risk situation. One question which focuses on a specific answer to assessing the individual's support system is "Who do you go to when you need to talk about something?"

Coping Behaviors in Previous Crises. Exploring the way a family dealt with a previous crisis identifies their possible strengths and weaknesses in adjusting to this situation.

Effect of Child's Illness on Marriage and Life. Asking how the child's illness has affected their lives helps uncover areas of possible denial, inability to express feelings, ability to openly identify feelings, or reactions of blame, anger, and resentment.

Feelings about "Real" Cause of Disease. Although the etiology of many expected and unexpected causes of death are unknown, parents frequently supply their own explanation. Asking them, "I know the doctor said there is no known cause for leukemia, but what do you *really* think caused it?'' uncovers areas of guilt, blame, and punishment. Once the imagined cause is revealed, the person can be helped to deal with the possible irrationalities of that thinking.

Care Planning

Nurse-Physician Team. To meet the complex needs of a "dying family," a team approach is essential. Most important, the treating doctor and the consistent nurse or nurse team must work and communicate together. Nurses frequently relate their frustration of "being caught in the middle," when the family and physician refuse to share information with the ill person but the ill person requests such information from the nurse. Such situations could be avoided if all team members expressed their viewpoints openly and honestly.

The author has found a deeper understanding of physicians' cold, aloof, uninvolved attitude. Without such insulating protection from emotional bombardment, many of them would not be able to survive the responsibilities of their job. They are taught to treat and cure, not to counsel the dying. However, when both partners of the team realize the reason for the other's behavior, they are both better able to benefit the ill person and his family.

Nurse Team. The nursing team approach with the terminally ill child may include inservice and outpatient staff nurses, clinical specialist, private nurse counselor, public health nurse, oncology office nurse, and school nurse. Because of their diverse roles and separate locations, it is feasible for lines of communication and nursing care goals and services to become confused, fragmented, and duplicated. Unless one person takes the leadership role, the family will be dissected and treated by each nurse alone. Designating one nurse as the central primary agent for the family prevents such pitfalls and provides the family with a constant source of information and support.

For example, in one situation where the nurse counselor had no knowledge of the medical center staff and was unable to visit the child, she planned "long distance" care with the parents by exploring the reasons for the problems and suggesting possible interventions. She worked continuously with the parents over the telephone to evaluate the various alternatives and to support them through the long ordeal. The "long-distance care plan" was so effective that it resulted in a markedly improved parent-child relationship, which was noticed by the staff nurses. With some of the immediate hospital difficulties solved, the parents were able to concentrate their efforts on planning for the child's home care and their own preparation for his impending death.

Primary Care. Primary care seems to be particularly beneficial for children with long-term illnesses. The consistent, one-to-one nurse-patient relationship provides for a deeper understanding of the possible family problems and continuity in the assessment, implementation, and evaluation of care. The primary nurse is in a most advantageous position to offer emotional support, provided she is helped to deal with the family's reactions, as well as her own.

Implementation

Listening. The very act of listening may be the best intervention. Sometimes nurses forget this and, instead, avoid asking questions for fear of not knowing what to say. If they have begun to explore some of the areas previously outlined under assessment, intervention through the act of encouraging verbalization and listening to the responses may be the most beneficial therapy.

Telephone Contact. One method of implementation which is rarely used to its fullest is telephone communication. Even with the best possible physical and psychological care during hospitalization, parents need answers and help when at home.

For example, one mother called the nurse counselor and the physician seven times over a holiday weekend to inquire about her child's ear infection. Although she was given all the medical information possible, it was apparent that she had other worries, which she was not verbalizing directly. At one point, the nurse focused on the mother's urgent need for answers and opened the topic further by asking her what she thought was "really" happening. The mother finally admitted that she was skeptical about the doctor's cursory examination of the ear and feared that the symptoms of pain, irritability, sleeplessness, and loss of balance were due to a brain tumor. After discussing this as a possibility, the mother stated that she was very relieved to hear that the doctor was considering this possibility, but had not mentioned it for fear of unduly worrying her. The mother's concern was less over the brain tumor than the possibility of the physician missing such a diagnosis.

When intervening by telephone, nurses must assess the real reason for the call. Before answering a direct question the nurse must: 1) inquire about the events which led to this concern, 2) explore solutions that the parents have tried, and 3) ask them what they think is happening. In those situations when parents (or children) call but are unable to clearly identify their concern, the nurse asks them, "How can I help?" or "What is it you are asking for?" Most of the time, the question is answered by the other person because the nurse has facilitated the exploration of alternatives.

Evaluation

Identification of positive, adaptive behaviors, such as approach behaviors, may signal the need for less intervention, temporary cessation of intervention, or permanent termination of the therapeutic relationship. Identification of negative or avoidance behaviors or signs of morbid grief reactions may represent the need for more intensive, specialized psychological intervention.

With children, drawing and play are excellent evaluators. Through progressive play or art sessions, children can demonstrate their intellectual understanding, emotional growth, and self-confidence.

Record Keeping. Record keeping is essential for subjective and potential objective measurements. Record keeping may involve nurse's notes, detailed process recordings (written logs of interview session), or tape recordings. The latter is most unaffected by the record keeper's subjective opinion and interpretations.

Supervision. To ensure some measure of objectivity, nurses need supervision and support from others, such as colleagues, family members, and sometimes other professionals. The emotional drain of working with the dying is a significant psychological toll. One cannot always give unless one also receives. The danger of failing to realize one's own emotional limitations is overinvestment in the dying person to the point of losing perspective of whose needs are being met in the relationship. Part of the function of ongoing evaluation is prevention of such overinvestment and social attachment and the refocusing of priorities, goals, and responsibilities.

Follow-up. Another potential tool for evaluation is follow-up contact with the family after the death of the child. This may be a telephone call, home visit, or invitation to the family to visit in the hospital or professional's office. It is a time to talk about "how things are going with everyone." It should be goal-directed, using a casual, informal approach. It also presents an excellent opportunity for final termination with the survivors. Such a session conveys a special message to the family because it is initiated by the nurse and does not deal with a problem or difficulty. Instead, it focuses on the emotional health, recovery, and adjustment of the family members in a manner that reinforces the empathy, care, and sharing which was part of the nurse-patient relationship.

SUMMARY

The ill child is only one victim in the catastrophe of terminal illness. His parents, siblings, and other significant people in his life, including those health professionals who care for him, are deeply affected. Although the challenges of nursing the dying child frequently seem insurmountable and the correct answers vague and elusive, the rewards are equally great. The strength, love, and support each family member seems capable of demonstrating, even under the most adverse circumstances, helps those working with the family to endure the psychological and emotional burdens of their responsibilities. Nurses need only the courage to risk involvement in order to experience the innumerable personal satisfactions of helping families cope with the crisis of expected or unexpected grief.

The need for individualized, holistic, and sensitive care is always necessary, but in the case of a dying child, it is paramount because there may be no second chance for revision or improvement. Nurses' willingness to face the issues surrounding life and death, to explore their own feelings toward nonexistence, to understand and accept the reactions of children and parents to expected death, and to learn methods of intervening therapeutically for all family members prepares them for helping the child live as well as die.

REFERENCES

1. Babson, S. G. et al. *Management of High-Risk Pregnancy and Intensive Care of the Neonate.* St. Louis: C. V. Mosby Co., 1975, 1.
2. Kübler-Ross, E. *On Death and Dying.* New York: Macmillan Co., 1969, 38–137.
3. Lindemann, E. "Symptomatology and Management of Acute Grief." In Parad, N. J. (ed.). *Crisis Intervention: Selected Readings.* New York: Family Service Association of America, 1965, 7–21.
4. Sutow, W. W., T. J. Vietti, and D. J. Fernbach. *Clinical Pediatric Oncology.* St. Louis: C. V. Mosby Co., 1977, 4.

ADDITIONAL READINGS

1. Epstein, C. *Nursing the Dying Patient.* Virginia: Reston Publishing Co., 1975.
2. Fochtman, D. "Leukemia in Children." *Pediatric Nursing,* 2, 1976, 8–13.
3. Furman, E. *A Child's Parent Dies.* New Haven: Yale University Press, 1974.
4. Greene, P. "The Child with Leukemia in the Classroom." *American Journal of Nursing,* 75, 1975, 86–87.
5. Grollman, E. (ed.). *Explaining Death to Children.* Boston: Beacon Press, 1967.
6. Karon, M. and J. Vernick. "An Approach to the Emotional Support of Fatally Ill Children." *Clinical Pediatrics,* 7, 1968, 274–280.
7. Kavannaugh, R. E. "Children's Special Needs?" In Chaney, P. S. (ed.). *Dealing with Death and Dying.* Philadelphia: Intermed Communications Inc., 1976, 33–46.
8. Lowenberg, J. "The Coping Behaviors of Fatally Ill Adolescents and Their Parents." *Nursing Forum,* 9, 1970, 270–272.
9. Martinson, I. "Parents Help Each Other." *American Journal of Nursing,* 76, 1976, 1120–1122.
10. Morrissey, J. "Children's Adaptation to Fatal Illness." *Social Work,* 8, 1963, 81–88.
11. Nagy, M. "The Child's View of Death." *Journal of Genetic Psychology,* 73, 1948, 3–27.
12. Natterson, J. and A. Knudsen. "Observations Concerning Fear of Death in Fatally Ill Children and Their Mothers." *Psychosomatic Medicine,* 22, 1969, 456–465.
13. Northrup, F. C. "The Dying Child." *American Journal of Nursing,* 74, 1974, 1066–1068.
14. Potheir, P. *Mental Health Counseling with Children.* Boston: Little, Brown, 1976.
15. Schowalter, J. E. "Children's Reactions to Terminal Illness." *Pediatric Annals,* 3, November 1974, 93–100.
16. Waechter, E. "Children's Awareness of Fatal Illness," *American Journal of Nursing,* 71, June 1971, 1168–1172.
17. Wolf, A. *Helping Your Child to Understand Death.* New York: Child Study Press, 1973.

PERTINENT ORGANIZATIONS

NATIONAL
- *American Cancer Society, Inc.*
  National Headquarters
  777 Third Avenue
  New York, New York 10017
  Provides information and studies for prevention and treatment of cancer.
- *Leukemia Society of America, Inc.*
  National Headquarters
  211 East 43rd Street
  New York, New York 10017
  Provides information and studies on leukemia.
- *National Foundation for Sudden Infant Death, Inc.*
  1501 Broadway
  New York, New York, 19936
  Provides information on sudden infant death problems and local parent groups.

LOCAL
- Local hospital, community, or church groups aimed to counseling the family with a terminally ill child.

The Family at Risk Due to a High-Risk Parent

PART THREE

Just as any child at risk affects the whole family, any parent at risk also creates a family at risk. The parent's essential role in the family is emphasized when it is altered by a parental risk situation such as drug abuse or terminal illness among many others.

The following chapters will describe the family difficulties resulting from many specific parent risk situations and suggest nursing approaches. These specific parent risk situations are representative of the problems but are not meant to exclude other possible risk situations.

The Adolescent Parent

Charlotte Cram-Elsberry, R.N., C.N.M., M.S.N., and
Anne Malley-Corrinet, R.N., C.N.M., M.S.

CHAPTER ELEVEN

NINE MONTHS IS NOT ENOUGH

Adolescent pregnancy, which involves a great deal more than just the reproduction of a human being, has many implications for the mother, child, and family. Physically, the body of a young adolescent, still completing growth, is asked to sustain the growth of another. Although pregnancy is not an illness, it requires medical attention which is often a new concept and need for the adolescent. Psychologically, pregnancy often signals and demands entry into womanhood. This entrance is exhibited in the adolescent by: the accentuation of her struggle between independence and dependence; her obvious sexuality; the interruption of her normal maturational development process; and the demand to function as a parent while she is often still being reared by her own family. Socially, the pregnancy touches and affects the father of the baby, her parent(s), siblings, peers, significant others, herself, the future child, and the community.

The nurse working with pregnant adolescents is provided with the opportunity to administer nursing care in the broadest and most demanding sense. She must utilize her nursing skills to meet the interwoven physical, psychological, and social needs of the pregnant adolescent. Sound theoretical knowledge plus skills in communication techniques and clinical strategies must be implemented. The nurse's role is a challenging one, one that needs reevaluation and redefinition on a continuing basis, since the needs of the pregnant teenager are in constant flux.

While the general birth rate has dropped, the birth rate among teenagers has not fallen as sharply as among older age groups. The rate of births to women 15 to 19 years of age dropped from 97.3 to 58.7 per 1,000 births from 1957 to 1974, or from 10 to 5 percent. However, largely because of the increased number of teenagers in the community, the actual number of births to teenagers remained about the same from 1960 to 1974. Although there is a higher percentage of pregnancies among nonwhite women, in general the rate of teenage pregnancies for nonwhites is dropping while the rate for whites is increasing.[1] Teenage pregnancy, however, is a significant problem for both white and nonwhite populations.

The changes in the birth rate vary greatly among different age groups. While the birth rate is increasing for the younger teens, it is decreasing for the older teens. Table 11-1 shows the birth rate changes for different age groups. The birth rate increase

Table 11-1. Adolescent Birth Rate Change From 1970–1974

Age	Increase (%)	Decrease (%)
14	9	—
15	3	—
16	—	3
17	—	11
18	—	18
19	—	24

among the younger, 14 and 15 year olds, has added a new dimension to the problems of adolescent pregnancy. These girls are younger, more physically and emotionally immature, and are inclined to have high-risk pregnancies. They tend to be more dependent on outside help, both during and after the pregnancy.

Statistics on illegitimacy are rough estimates since definitions vary from state to state. Current statistics indicate that the total number of illegitimate births among teenagers is on the increase. The rate of illegitimate births is higher for nonwhites than whites; the trend in each group is not to select marriage during the pregnancy.

Teenage pregnancy, whether of a 15-year-old or 19-year-old, a white or nonwhite, or a married or unmarried woman is a significant problem for the teenager, the family, and society. The adolescent mother's needs continue and change from the time of conception through the pregnancy, delivery, and childrearing periods. The concomitant nursing approaches are planned and implemented during these periods. *Nine months is not enough* for the teenager's development into motherhood.

DEVELOPMENTAL CONCEPTS OF ADOLESCENCE RELATED TO TEENAGE PREGNANCY

Adolescence is universally described as an uncertain and fluctuating period between childhood and adulthood. The fluctuations occur because psychological, physiological, and sexual develop-

ment do not happen simultaneously or with equal intensity and completeness.

Adolescents vary greatly depending on their cultural background, individual lifestyles, educational background, parental and societal guidance, and personal needs. These influences provide many variables which can be both enriching and detrimental.

An important concept frequently not considered is that adolescence is just one aspect of the whole, which is life's continuum. When not viewed within this framework, expectations are unrealistic and result in unattainable goals.

Physiological Development

The various phases of physiological development can be very traumatic or can progress in a nontraumatic sequence. How the pregnant adolescent views these developments will depend upon her psychological and sexual readiness as well as prior attitudes and preparation for the changes.

Physical growth is not achieved harmoniously for all parts of the body. Initially, growth is centered in the arms, legs, face, and neck. This is why adolescents are frequently lanky with uncoordinated movements. The nurse will observe the effects of this growth imbalance in the teenager's reluctance to participate in general physical conditioning, specifically in performing preparation for childbirth exercises.

Other physical changes which occur are related to sexual development. These include establishing of menses, enlarging breasts, darkening of the areola, development of subcutaneous fat, and increased axillary and pubic hair.

Because the occurrence and pattern of the changes vary with the individual teenager, the nurse must gear her interaction to the individual's needs. The nurse's role may revolve around education, synthesis of knowledge and attitudes, counseling, and serving as a role model. Education may range from providing and clarifying initial information to correcting misconceptions. Teenagers frequently have misconceptions about when their safe and fertile periods occur in relation to menstruation. Synthesis of knowledge and attitudes is complex, as is reflected in a teenager's use of the common phrases, "my friend" or "the curse" to refer to her menstrual cycle. This particular example indicates the girl's previous preparation and current thinking relating to a physical change. Counseling requires the nurse to identify the goals to be achieved. Nurses, in acting as a role model, remember that being helpful or friendly to the adolescent does not mean being a buddy. It is healthy and normal for a teenager to emulate someone. A teenager may ask the nurse personal questions as a way of assessing ranges of attitudes and values which she may later choose to emulate.

Physiological changes associated with pregnancy tend to focus initially on the teenager's sexual organs. The noted changes include breast and nipple tenderness, amenorrhea, and breast enlargement. Another physiological change which occurs is leukorrhea. Because this is a newly experienced phenomenon for the teenager, its impact may be exaggerated. Nonsexual changes specific to pregnancy include weight gain, pigment changes, changes in metabolic rates, and increased peripheral vascularity. Most of these changes are newly experienced and create varying degrees of discomfort.

The pregnant teenager is likely to express physical complaints to the nurse. The nurse can provide comfort measures for the common complaints of pregnancy as well as assure that they are normal phenomena. The nurse can anticipate that the teenager will also use her peers for comparison and feedback. She may view herself as normal or abnormal according to what she sees as standard for the group. An expression of this which the nurse may hear is: "How come her stomach is bigger than mine and we are both six months pregnant?" Throughout the pregnancy, the nurse will need to deal with the girl's need to normalize herself in relation to peer standards.

Psychological Development

Physiological maturity does not correspond with psychological maturity. This is an important concept to maintain when working with pregnant adolescents. A physically mature girl may be psychologically immature and vice versa.

Because adolescence is a transitional period, it is normal for adolescents to exhibit conflict and inconsistencies in behavior and thought. Examples of issues which illustrate this period of adolescent psychological development are: emotional volatility, need for immediate gratification, impaired reality testing, lack of self-criticism, indifference to the world at large. These characteristics can trigger wide and rapid mood fluctuations in the adolescent. One of the dominant moods expressed by the teenager is anger. The health professional must not allow this anger to inhibit necessary interaction. Emotional volatility on the part of the adolescent frequently results in frustrated interpersonal relations. When this frustration occurs, the health care provider should not be discouraged from continuing to administer the care required at that time. The care provider needs to deal openly and honestly with the interaction conflict. This requires time and exemplifies why providing high quality care to adolescents requires more personnel and a smaller case load.

During pregnancy, the teenager will have the same adolescent behavioral and psychological needs, however, they tend to be accentuated by the added stress of making life decisions. Although they may not verbalize their dilemmas, many teenagers feel inadequate and insecure in making decisions on their own and the baby's future. Pregnancy also radically interferes with the establishment of a sense of balance between independence and dependence. All adolescents face the struggle between dependence and independence in which many issues of conflict revolve. Pregnancy automatically reduces the teenager to economic and emotional dependence upon others. Conversely, she may need to become more independent or isolated due to peer group rejection. All of these changes and stresses require energy. The accomplishment of psychological tasks may be retarded by the divested energies associated with pregnancy.

Sexual changes in adolescents are both physiological and psychological, and the level of sophistication in one area may not correspond with the other. In general, feelings may be summed up by two concepts: curiosity and ambivalence. Curiosity may lead to sexual encounters which may be explorative and exploitive. Many adolescents, especially the younger ones, have no in-depth knowledge of sexual functioning, and many learn through experimentation. This results in psychological and physical repercussions of their actions and ambivalence. The role of the nurse in sexual counseling usually revolves around a psychological issue: helping the adolescent achieve consistency between her attitudes and actions.

FAMILY DIFFICULTIES

Family difficulties due to an adolescent pregnancy include crises any time during and after pregnancy and special difficulties during the prenatal, intrapartum and postpartum periods. See Figure 11-1 for a concise list of difficulties.

Intermittent Crises of Teenage Pregnancy

Providing health care to the pregnant adolescent is challenging, time-consuming, frustrating, and easily leads to discouragement. This is because of the number of stresses inherent in this situation. These stresses are not singular but tend to be interwoven and compound one another. It is the number of stresses, timing, resources available, and past physio-psycho-social history that define the degree of risk at which the mother and her child are placed.

The pregnancy will have a rippling effect. It usually affects the girl herself, her family, including siblings and extended members, immediate friends, father of the baby, and perhaps his family. Indirect effects are also felt by society at large, since the girl will need to utilize special community resources. The multiple stresses may, but need not, continue throughout each phase of the maternity cycle.

The Recognition of Pregnancy. The first crisis usually occurs with the recognition of pregnancy. Often the recognition of pregnancy is delayed be-

Figure 11-1. Family Difficulties for the Adolescent Parent

Intermittent Crises of Teenage Pregnancy
The recognition of pregnancy
The adolescent crisis
The family crisis
Prenatal Difficulties
Termination or continuation of pregnancy
Special high-risk difficulties
Economic and medication needs
Nutrition and medication needs
Body image and exercise
Interpersonal relationships
Intrapartum Difficulties
Labor and delivery difficulties
Environmental control and depersonalization problems
Postpartum Difficulties
Adoption possibility
Body image changes
Breast feeding difficulties
Cesarean section problems
Environmental restrictions
Bonding difficulties
Birth control difficulties
Parenting difficulties

cause the signs and symptoms of pregnancy parallel those of a physically maturing adolescent. Recognition may also be delayed by denial or misconceptions of sexual facts leading to pregnancy. A false sense of security may be established when the initial acts of intercourse without contraception are not rapidly followed by pregnancy.

The Adolescent Crisis. There is a gap between suspicion and confirmation of pregnancy. This period may be particularly stressful because the pregnant adolescent will need to wait for obviously recognizable signs which occur at the fourth or fifth month of pregnancy or go to a health care facility for confirmation. This may or may not require financial payment. Neither of these solutions seems natural to the adolescent who focuses on the immediate handling of the situation. Seeking and initiating her own health care is often a foreign concept to her.

The pregnant adolescent may delay confirmation of the pregnancy because of fear, guilt, or confusion, which may continue after pregnancy is confirmed. Delay in confirming the pregnancy may also affect the possible resolutions. To the pregnant adolescent, pregnancy may mean a disruption in education and special activities, or changing relationships with peers, family, or boyfriend. The recognition of pregnancy may not always be a delayed occurrence. Alternate factors which motivated her to become pregnant may also motivate her to disclose her pregnancy early in gestation.

The Family Crisis. The initial strain pregnancy places on the interaction between the pregnant adolescent girl and her family frequently depends upon the situation and her motivations for pregnancy. Anger, guilt, tension, hostility, or acceptance may be found in any combination or degree and can occur at varying intervals throughout the pregnancy.

The girl's siblings frequently take cues from their parent(s) on how to interact with the girl and how to view the pregnancy. The siblings may see pregnancy as a way of achieving favoritism and change in responsibility. An example is when heavy, undesirable chores are relegated to them rather than to the pregnant sister. Jealousy is a natural response in this situation. The jealousy may impede healthy interaction between the pregnant girl and her siblings. If it is anticipated that the girl will bring the baby home to raise, changes in living arrangements may occur, placing additional stress on the family.

Pregnancy requires extra money expenditures for any family unit. The family may have to assume all or part of the added expense for prenatal and hospital care, clothing, preparation for the baby, increased dietary needs, and possible special education or living arrangements. These extra expenses may necessitate the pregnant adolescent's mother to return to work, the father to moonlight, or siblings to contribute money. If the family is unable to meet any of the added financial needs, the girl may be forced to apply for state funds. If she receives state funds, she may still be financially dependent on the family or her boyfriend for social needs.

When the family is unable to accept the girl's pregnancy, she may have to live elsewhere. At this point, she has several options. One is to live with the family of the baby's father. This arrangement may allow the boyfriend's family to allay their feelings of guilt over their son's actions. She may also elect to live with an aunt, uncle, grandparent, or other relative. Another possibility is for the pregnant teenager to live alone, in which case, she is faced with a set of very different problems. Being alone, she frequently experiences loneliness and lacks the social stimulation that promotes healthy psychological adaptation. She will also lack the physical help and support of others at a time when these needs are paramount. Living alone at this age is not a natural setting. It goes against the strong adolescent need and desire to be in the company of a group. A final option is to live in a home for unwed mothers. All the conditions present in living alone are present and further accentuated by transference to a foreign environment. Frequently, the maternity home is a considerable distance from the girl's home, thus limiting visits and opportunities for interaction among family and friends. All members of the family may not be in equal agreement over what is the best solution.

The nurse's role is to help the adolescent make a decision on where to live. A few of the following questions should be investigated in establishing a data base: Do other family members know about the pregnancy, and does the girl want this? Who is she presently living with and if the situation is not a positive one, with whom would she feel more comfortable living? If she is living alone, the nurse needs to refer her for social work assistance in transportation, obtaining Woman-Infant Care vouchers for food, and possibly arranging for a homemaker postdelivery. If the nurse learns about very strained family relationships, she may need to refer them for family counseling.

Some of the goals and expectations the parents had for their daughter may now be completely shattered or at least delayed. The family may be concerned that the pregnancy may result in her dropping out of school. They may feel it may interfere with their upward social and economic mobility. The nurse can recognize and anticipate these as normal feelings.

Prenatal Difficulties

During the antepartum course, the pregnant adolescent will encounter many new experiences and difficulties. This nine-month period sets the stage for resolution of problems and can influence her development in a positive or negative manner. How these difficulties are handled may have lasting influences and repercussions for her and the child long after the pregnancy has ended.

The care provided during this period will rely heavily on sound maternity nursing practice. Added knowledge and clinical expertise will be required in dealing with the additional risk factors that the nurse encounters when providing care to the pregnant adolescent and her family.

Termination or Continuation of the Pregnancy. Once the pregnancy has been recognized and confirmed, the girl needs to decide whether to terminate or keep the pregnancy. If she keeps the pregnancy, the next issue will be who will care for and raise the child. Options include abortion, foster care placement, her own family members, the father's family, or herself. Her choice will be influenced by the circumstances and motivation for pregnancy and parental viewpoints and values.

Once the choice for abortion is made, medical cooperation should be sought. Medical evaluation will determine the method of abortion if it is still a medically available option. If her abortion is performed in the first trimester, it can be accomplished easily without hospitalization or extended absence from school and home. An early second trimester abortion carries more medical hazards, the fear of hospitalization, and exposure to the family's awareness of the decision. Absence from school and home may not be easily covered over. If the girl decides on abortion as her resolution, she will need nursing and social work intervention and counseling. To achieve feelings of comfort with the resolution may take many weeks and help from health professionals both before and after the abortion.

Another option is carrying the pregnancy to term and placing the child for adoption. This is not an easy decision and the girl will have time during her pregnancy and perhaps after the delivery to make this decision. If she is unsure of adoption, the child may be placed in a foster home until such a final decision is reached. During pregnancy, the nurse helps the girl focus on making this decision rather than allow her to avoid the decision. The nurse must help the girl who is placing her child for adoption take pride in creating a healthy offspring rather than allow her to view the baby as something that can be misused, ignored, and not cared for.

As with adoption, the decision to keep the baby can be made slowly with the girl changing her mind as the reality of parenthood becomes more concrete. As a girl is considering the option of keeping the child, the nurse must help the girl focus on this reality and its demands. Part of the reality of parenthood is making long-term plans about who will raise or care for the child, where, for how long, under what circumstances, and who will provide housing and financial support for both the mother and her child.

It is difficult for the adolescent to take an active role in making the decision about how to resolve the pregnancy. She may express denial, passivity, or dependency. The nurse is responsible for helping the girl to identify and understand the implications of her decision. One way to accomplish this is by asking the client to write down how she perceives her future life following through on each possible alternative. Once she has decided which alternative to take, the nurse should gear all efforts to supporting her and helping her follow through with her decision.

The pregnant adolescent's initial decision about the resolution of the pregnancy may conflict with her family's desires. One of the confusing and difficult aspects of working with the family of a pregnant adolescent is that the situation may bring to surface many conflicting parental viewpoints regarding a resolution. Past unresolved issues may be reawakened. Efforts to learn and understand where their feelings come from is paramount in promoting communication between the girl and her family. Emphasis is on hearing and listening rather than judging the feelings as good or bad. In order for maximum growth to occur, the pregnant adolescent must be able to respect others' viewpoints, yet feel comfortable and secure with the final decision. For an ideal outcome, the family members should be in agreement on the resolution.

Special High-Risk Difficulties. When one becomes pregnant and assumes the parenting role, the need to be accountable and responsible is mandatory. Unfortunately, many teenagers have not matured enough to either achieve this or perform consistently. Specific examples of the teenager's lack of responsibility are late medical registration, noncompliance in taking medications, failure to keep clinic appointments for herself or her newborn baby.

Initially, it was felt that these girls were physically immature. However, it is now felt that this population is more at risk psychosocially than physically. Specific physical risks include: incomplete bone epiphyses if conception has taken place less than one year after menarche, resulting in small pelves; anemia; pre-eclampsia; increased incidence of vaginitis and cervicitis. Anemia and pre-eclampsia are associated with nutritional deficiencies.

The basic concern is that late registration for medical care has been highly correlated with increased fetal and maternal complications. Late registration precludes anticipatory guidance and prenatal counseling, which frequently reduce the risk factors. It may also make medical management more complicated, necessitating more complicated and expensive diagnostic testing.

The problem the nurse faces in dealing with a patient who is a late registrant is that she has so much to accomplish within a short time span. She may never have the opportunity to elicit or work on the patient's individual needs, refer her to other health team members for help or counseling, or allay fears of labor and delivery through teaching or participation of the girl in prenatal classes. She may find herself faced with a patient who has many unmet needs and feel frustrated and impotent because of the limited time she has to work in. The nurse may improve the situation by seeing the patient weekly until time of delivery and allowing more time for each visit. However, the girl's compliance in keeping weekly appointments is questionable because of her initial inaccessibility.

Economic and Education Problems. Although able to work during pregnancy, obtaining full or part-time work is all but impossible. This forces economic dependence on the family or state. When economically dependent, it is easy for the pregnant girl to become comfortable with the status quo. This fosters her passivity and interferes with a positive, capable self-image. Goals then become short-term rather than long-term.

In order to prevent cyclic economic dependency, the nurse gives intensive guidance and counseling so that the girl will be able to complete her self-maturation and realize long-term goals. Encouragement and follow-up on suggestions are consistently required. The nurse is not discouraged by behavior fluctuating between dependency and independency since this is common among all adolescents.

Attitudes toward adolescent pregnancy have changed in our society. One demonstration of this is the trend to keep the pregnant adolescent in school. Although her education is no longer interrupted by removing her from school, her extracurricular functions are interrupted. She may be prevented from achieving desired adolescent goals such as being a cheerleader, prom queen, athletic star, or class officer. Her dating may be restricted, and denial of male companions and lack of friendship may add to her feelings of rejection. Parental attitudes expressed through female and male classmates may be harsh and judgmental. In addition, pregnancy will require rest periods, frequent bathroom breaks, nutritional snacks, and timing of meals which are often incongruous with the school schedule. It may be difficult to avoid crowded corridors and stairs and to find uncrowded rest rooms. Although the pregnant adolescent continues to need structured physical exercise, appropriate substitutes for her frequently are not made. The physical design of chairs and equipment may not be conducive to the needs of a pregnant adolescent.

The teachers in the school may exhibit negative feelings either verbally or nonverbally.

A special educational program for pregnant adolescents placed in a separate institution answers many of these problems. The advantages include scheduling and structure compatible with the needs of pregnancy. Snacks and rest breaks are a part of the daily schedule. The teachers tend to be more aware of the girl's educational, physiological, and psychological needs. More intimate relationships allow the teacher to discover areas of special interest and can help to promote them. The major curriculum disadvantage is that it is difficult for the girl to enter her academic subjects at the same point she left off at her previous school. She may be removed from her peer group and forced to enter a new group with whom she may not have anything in common besides pregnancy. This may or may not be to her liking.

Continuing her education through homebound instruction involves the same curriculum problems as the special program. In addition, the girl may have to deal with increased social isolation and less academic stimulation. Homebound instruction requires the girl to study more on her own since the tutor usually is present only one to two hours daily or less. This may lead to educational failure if the girl does not have sufficient motivation or stimulation from family members.

The subject of continuing education may expose different expectations of parents and the adolescent. The parent(s) may have to change their expectations for their child and accept the reality that further schooling may be temporarily interrupted or discontinued. Conflict may center on the feeling that "You can make it through school if you really try."

The girl may not be able to deal successfully with the dual demands of education and pregnancy. The whole process of education may be affected because it is no longer the primary focus of the pregnant adolescent's life and energies. Her lack of concentration on academic subjects easily leads to a feeling of defeat. There may be a difference between her desire to perform academically and the actual outcome.

The nurse participates with others in encouraging the adolescent to continue and complete her formal education. The nurse can provide an important link between the medical care facility and school counselors and school health providers. Two facts to be remembered are that withdrawal from school leads to difficulty in reentry into education and an incomplete education usually leads to a state of economic dependency and subsequent deprivation for the girl and her child.

Nutrition and Medication Needs. The adolescent's dietary habits may place her and her child at risk. Adolescents are notoriously poor in obtaining consistent, well-balanced meals. There are many reasons for this. Their lifestyle contributes to picking up hurried meals from fast food restaurants to substitute for the many well-balanced family meals missed. Their limited income may lead to consumption of high carbohydrate, high calorie snack foods.

It is now believed that inadequate protein intake can result in inadequate fetal brain growth and intrauterine growth retardation. The effect may be irreversible. Inadequate protein intake also may predispose the pregnant adolescent to preeclampsia. When discussing nutrition, it is important to remember that additional quantities of iron, calcium, and protein are needed.

The nurse and nutritionist must stress the importance of meals being regular as well as nutritionally well-balanced. Long periods of starvation may predispose the mother and fetus to periods of ketosis and the resulting possible damage to fetal brain development. Also related to diet are drug use, smoking, alcohol, and pica. Any of these may be used as a substitute for proper nutritional intake.

Two perplexing questions the nurse deals with continually are how to make good nutrition fun and how to assess what the adolescent needs for optimum fetal and self-growth. A common mistake is to offer suggestions without obtaining an initial diet history. The patient is asked to bring in a three-day diet history. The history also includes a list of foods she likes and those she does not like, combined with type of preparation. The nurse or nutritionist can then use this as a guideline in offering nutritional guidance. Guidance centers on suggestions that complement or supplement her already existing patterns rather than restrict or eliminate foods. An example of this would be the addition of a slice of cheese to a hamburger and a milk shake in place of a coke. The addition of a tomato and lettuce would also help to balance the meal for optimal nutritional intake. Positive reinforcement of weight gain and fundal growth can serve as a motivating factor for the pregnant adolescent as long as she does not view a large abdomen as a detriment. Recommendations are consistent and fit into cultural styles.

The nurse works with and teaches the person in the home environment who is responsible for the cooking and the shopping. Both the nurse and this person often benefit from direct interaction either in personal meetings or over the phone. Inquiry is made as to whether the girl is enrolled in the Women-Infant-Care program which allocates food vouchers for milk, cheese, eggs, orange juice, and fortified cereals. Even though additional foods are made available through the WIC program, they may be dispersed to all family members, thus depleting the amount of protein the pregnant adolescent receives.

The amount of weight a teenager should gain during pregnancy is a difficult clinical question. It must be remembered that additional weight gain is probably necessary since the girl's own body is growing along with the fetus. It is for this reason that a nutritionist must be consulted before telling the girl that she is gaining too much weight.

During the antepartal period, the pregnant adolescent may experience a new responsibility for self-medication. Medicine previously taken was probably for a short period of time and controlled by someone else, usually the mother. Since all pregnant women are encouraged to take iron and vitamin pills, the practitioner may have to teach the adolescent how to take pills and constantly reiterate the value or purpose each one serves. The idea of pills for prevention rather than immediate remedy may be a foreign concept to her.

Body Image and Exercise. The most obvious and perhaps most difficult body change to accept is the increased weight gain and the protrusion of abdomen. Most adolescents desire a slim body and spend hours discussing it with their peers. Fears and ambivalent feelings about body image may be expressed through comments such as:

> Why am I bigger than she is?
> I must be due sooner because I'm bigger than her.
> This kid sticks out too much.
> This kid hurts me when it moves.
> When will my breasts stop growing?

The nurse may be quick to identify these feelings when the adolescent gives conflicting thoughts. She may exhibit enthusiasm over the pregnancy yet refuse to listen to fetal heart tones when given the opportunity. The nurse must not force the issue but emphasize the positive aspects of her body changes, including promotion of maternal-fetal bonding.

The common aches and pains associated with pregnancy can negatively influence the adolescent's body image. Backache, shortness of breath, ligamental discomforts, frequent urination, striae and pigment changes all contribute to a changing body and require adjustment time. Many of these conditions have no medicinal remedies. The caregiver explains the physiological basis for their occurrence and teaches palliative measures to decrease body discomfort and indirectly promote a better self-image.

The value of exercise during pregnancy is often unrecognized by the adolescent. Although pregnant, the adolescent still needs to experience the control, discipline, and mastery achieved in physical exercise. A new component to the exercise regimen is the learning and mastery of relaxation. This again is a foreign concept to the adolescent. Relaxation can be utilized during pregnancy to enhance sleep, relieve tension, and reduce some of the discomforts she experiences. Labor necessitates endurance of strenuous muscular exertion which requires good physical conditioning. Just as an athlete would not enter competition without previous conditioning, neither should a pregnant woman enter labor without conditioning. Although the direct responsibility of the caregiver may be to teach breathing and relaxation techniques, she also encourages the young woman to obtain maximum exercise. When no planned program of physical exercise is available, the adolescent needs to develop an individual program. This may include daily brisk walking and swimming.

Interpersonal Relationships. A primary task of adolescence is learning how to relate to others. During pregnancy, the adolescent will have to broaden this circle to many more individuals and analyze and articulate personal feelings and attitudes. The most important and influential group for the adolescent is her peer group. It is from this group that she seeks positive feedback about her attitudes, appearance, values, and behavior. When pregnancy occurs, it may place her in a group she previously had not been able to join or it may exclude her from her present group. The nurse investigates the social integration with peers and the extent to which this occurs. Frequently, a pregnant teenager who has not joined any group becomes increasingly withdrawn and isolated, which may indicate future psychological problems and require more intensive nursing input.

Today, although some relationships disintegrate with the realization of pregnancy, many adolescent girls continue their relationships with the baby's father. The fathers are more likely to take an active part in the pregnancy and continue with the relationship when the child is born. Once pregnancy is realized, conflict in the relationship may arise from decisions over pregnancy, resolution, and marriage. The father's social and economic dependency may prevent them from achieving mutual wishes. A typical reaction is that they would like to have a baby together sometime but cannot afford it now. Conflicts over sexual issues may be exaggerated because of the adolescent parents' lack of knowledge. This may lead to increasing frustration and misunderstandings. The father may interpret the girl's varying degrees of responsiveness as rejection or manipulation. The clinician evaluates the degree of involvement with the baby's father and his ability to be supportive. His support may be

psychological as well as economic. The girl with a continuing relationship may or may not expect economic support but does expect psychological support. It is more difficult for a boy to provide support when his peer group jeers him about being a "tied down old man" or when either family forbids the couple to interact.

The nurse evaluates the degree of support the father of the baby is able to give in a number of ways. Direct questioning of the girl or boy should be used. This is usually most successful if a general question is used initially, followed by more specific question(s); for example, the nurse might ask, "Who will be with you in labor and delivery? Have you thought about having the baby's father with you?" During conversation, the nurse may pick up direct or indirect references to the father which need to be explored. The nurse may foster psychological support by including him and encouraging his attendance at the prenatal appointments. If he cannot be present, an indirect way of including him may be to have the girl bring in his questions or ask her what his concerns are regarding the pregnancy.

The nurse working in the prenatal clinic may be able to lay the groundwork for future parenting by including the baby's father as much as possible. To encourage fetal bonding, the father listens to the fetal heart tones and feels fetal movements and growth. A father who is also aware of nutritional importance and special requirements of pregnancy is better able to acknowledge and take responsibility in helping the mother maintain a normal pregnancy and produce a "blue-ribbon baby."

Some programs have group sessions especially for the male partners or combined groups in which both partners participate. The need and demand for "father groups" is greater than ever since the number of couples electing marriage as a result of pregnancy is decreasing. Optimally, there should be a group during and after pregnancy. The group should allow individuals to express feelings about the situation and new demands placed upon them. The format also includes anticipatory guidance concerning presenting issues and counseling relating to role changes. The nurse does not assume or encourage the concept that responsibility for parenting occurs only in marriage.

The father of the baby who decides not to continue his relationship with the pregnant adolescent also has special needs. He too may need to have a therapeutic environment in which he can express and further articulate his feelings and attitudes.

If the adolescent is married, there may be an inherent stress on the marriage because of the baby. Usually, this relationship is not firmly established prior to the baby's arrival. Children can dissipate energy in a marriage as well as enrich it. If a large degree of energy is expended on the marital relationship, the child receives less. To find and maintain a proper equilibrium is difficult for a mature couple to handle effectively. The added difficulty for a teenage couple is obvious. The clinician needs to be aware of these stresses and assess the degree to which they are present during the postpartum check-up and interconceptional visits.

Since adolescents generally have difficulty in dealing and relating with authority figures and issues, the pregnant adolescent may have difficulty in relating to the caregiver, whom she may view as an authority figure. Indeed, the caregiver is in an authoritative position, but does not have to be authoritarian. The caregiver maintains a delicate balance between being consistent and directive in providing care and allowing flexibility for feedback and discussion about pertinent plans and feelings.

Intrapartum Difficulties

During the intrapartum period, the pregnant adolescent is exposed to a new set of difficulties as well as some that carry over from the antepartal period. Each difficulty has three common problems associated with it. The first is that she will have no direct control over the length of the intrapartum period. For example, there is no way of knowing exactly how long the time will be from the onset of labor to the birth of the baby. The second problem is that a small or large part of the intrapartal period will occur away from the girl's home and familiar surroundings, with varying degrees of contact from family and friends. The third problem is the issue of independence versus dependence. The pregnant adolescent may be frustrated by and resent the dependence on medical personnel during labor and delivery.

Labor and Delivery Difficulties. One of the questions frequently asked is whether or not the pregnant adolescent is at higher risk than the mature woman of complications during labor and delivery. If pregnancy does occur less than one year after menarche, pelvic bone maturity is not completed and the woman is more likely to experience cephalopelvic disproportion in labor. This can be absolute or relative, depending on the factors involved. As a result of these factors, the teenager is exposed to a longer and more arduous labor, utilization of more technological interference, an increased incidence of operative delivery, and the possibility of sustaining more lacerations.

Another medical difficulty commonly encountered by pregnant adolescents is pre-eclampsia. If the onset of pre-eclampsia is during the prenatal period, intrauterine growth retardation may result. Pre-eclampsia also predisposes the girl to a stressful, often precipitous, labor and increased chance for abruptio placenta. Fetal distress secondary to diminished oxygen transport found in pre-eclampsia and intrauterine growth retardation may result. The incidence of premature rupture of membranes may increase when either vaginal infections, herpes, venereal disease, or possibly cervical beta strep infection occur. Premature rupture of membranes can predispose the fetus to respiratory distress from a premature delivery as well as increased risk of systemic infection from amnionitis. Prematurity and infection may necessitate the infant being placed in a newborn intensive care unit, which requires increased medical and nursing attention and financial cost, as well as separation of mother and newborn during the critical phases of bonding.

These risk situations necessitate more continuous nursing care and demand knowledge and skill of medical nursing as well as obstetrical nursing. The nurse assesses the psychological needs of the new young mother, especially if her baby is in the intensive care unit. The nurse may follow the progress of the infant as well as take the mother to visit the baby frequently. She also explains situations to family members and significant others to allay their anxieties and concerns.

It is generally agreed that it is beneficial to a woman in labor to have a significant other with her to provide support and to serve as her advocate. For a pregnant adolescent, finding or choosing who should be with her may be difficult. Her choices usually involve the father of the baby, a boyfriend, a family member, or a peer. It is normal for her to want everyone who is significant to her present. It may be hard for her to select one. Particular conflict may occur if both the father of the baby and the girl's mother demand to be there. The nurse can help in making this decision by having the girl explore her own feelings about whether she would be more comfortable with a male or a female; whether she wants someone who can function in a supportive role and who is capable of doing this; and whether she thinks it would be helpful to have someone with her who previously has given birth. The nurse respects her choice.

During labor, the nurse will be faced with deciding how to effectively use this support person. Often this person has not had classes for labor and delivery preparation. If preparation is based solely on their own childbearing experience, their supportive care may reflect their own care during the experience. To be an effective supporter, many people feel that the person needs to be assertive and touch oriented. Is this a projection of cultural value? It has been observed that some patients receive support from a significant other who plays a passive role. Her developed pattern of functioning may be based on passive rather than active support. Some people find interruption and noise intrusive. Other individuals have learned to dampen multisensory stimulation. These examples illustrate the need for more individualized care.

During labor and delivery, many pregnant adolescents have difficulty with sexual exposure and intimacy. She must quickly become accustomed to body exposure, an intimidating posture, and intrusion of the organs. The intimacy which often develops between the adolescent patient and her female nurses may cause latent fears of homosexuality. In the delivery room, the teenager may view her genitalia for the first time. This may have a particular impact if she focuses on her distorted genitalia instead of the birth of the baby. Poor pushing may be a manifestation of this phenomenon.

Loss of control in labor is an important issue. The pregnant adolescent may view this as childlike rather than adult behavior. In the past, she could control unpleasant situations by removing herself from them. However, the process of labor prevents her from doing this. Once contractions begin, there is no recourse to stop them. The adolescent must work with these contractions from ten to 20 hours, a personal feat she suspects is impossible. In addition, medication does not totally eliminate the discomfort. The adolescent may make constant demands for pain relief, which may result in overmedication and increased loss of control manifested through irritability and increased activity levels. Some adolescents view the pain of labor and delivery as a form of punishment. This is especially evident in the patient who has received no prenatal preparation or the girl who has not resolved guilt feelings over the pregnancy. Although medication is available for pain alleviation, frequently it is administered by a needle. Many adolescents have exaggerated anxiety over needles. It may be difficult for the adolescent to separate pain from outcome. The result is a lack of immediate enthusiasm for the impending arrival of the baby.

She may further sense loss of body control if a precipitous bout of vomiting occurs. Also, during the pushing stage, bladder and bowel control are frequently lost. A final loss of body control may come when the girl's arms and legs are strapped down on the delivery table. Fortunately, personnel are becoming more aware that control can be maintained better with the use of fewer physical restraints. The adolescent responds to lack of control in an adolescent manner. She may go to the extremes of being physically and verbally hostile and demanding or becoming withdrawn and unwilling to do anything. This behavior, in turn, frequently evokes responses from medical personnel the opposite of what the girl wishes and needs. Instead of obtaining more attention and help, the girl is labeled difficult and overdemanding or unresponsive and uncooperative.

The nurse can do much to help the laboring adolescent maintain or regain psychological control. Whether in or out of control, the girl will respond best to a voice that combines kindness, confidence, and control with consistent and concise directives. Better control also may be obtained by having minimal change in personnel and by reducing the number of interruptions. The nurse remembers that the laboring adolescent is particularly afraid of being left alone and is prone to lose control when no one is with her. This is why the nurse encourages a significant other to stay with the girl according to her wishes. Significant others also can help the nurse with the girl who has lost control and refuses to cooperate. During this situation, the nurse should give specific directives to the significant other, who can communicate them to the girl. For example, the nurse may teach the significant other how to position the girl and have her push. The significant other should then actively coach the girl while the nurse aids and supports them.

Comments, or the lack of comments, from the nurse can do much to alleviate the girl's personal embarrassment over the loss of body control. If she inadvertently loses urine during pushing, the nurse may say nothing or she can comment on the normality of fluids escaping from the body during this process. Her responses may be determined by the patient's awareness and verbal or nonverbal embarrassment. Anticipatory explanations need to be timed appropriately with the mother's stage of labor.

Environmental Control and Depersonalization Problems. Regardless of what is done, hospitals will always impose more environmental controls and depersonalization than home. The most obvious examples include the drapelike nightgown; personnel in scrub instead of civilian clothing; hard beds with rubber mattress covers and sometimes paper bed linen; no or limited bathroom and kitchen privileges; and health care providers previously not known. A few personal belongings brought from home can help to personalize the environment. Allowing the pregnant adolescent to ambulate, to position herself to her liking and comfort, and to specify her preference for mode of pushing during delivery, when appropriate to the obstetric condition, also can reduce unnecessary controls and depersonalization.

The manner in which hospital personnel interact with the pregnant adolescent also may communicate depersonalization. The same courtesies all laboring women need should be extended to the pregnant adolescent regardless of how busy the unit is: She will need to know the names of those caring for her; how to call for help; and what, why, and how a procedure is done and what its outcome is.

The nurse keeps in mind that the pregnant adolescent is asked to adjust to new people, to a foreign environment, and to hospital controls and routines at a time when she may be experiencing varying degrees of discomfort and of support and presence from her family. These factors and the hurried, routine manner of personnel can contribute to the pregnant adolescent's inability to give accurate, complete, and specific history and respond optimally to her labor.

Postpartum Difficulties

Much of what dictates the care of the adolescent in the postpartum period is reflected in her prenatal preparation and her labor and delivery experience. The quick adjustments an adolescent has had to make through the childbirth experience is frightening as well as overwhelming if proper education and prenatal preparation did not precede it. It is during this time that the new mother may or may not focus on the reality of her new situation. Yet how realistic are these "realities" in such a foreign environment?

Adoption Possibility. If adoption is chosen, it is now generally agreed that it is psychologically healthier for the girl to see and care for the baby and to be reassured of its existence and its normality. It is better to accept the realities of being pregnant than to suppress them and have to deal with them later as a mother under different circumstances. The nurse discusses directly with the girl how she would like to separate from the baby. Each instance should be individualized to the girl's desires. Some may wish to part the night before leaving the hospital, and others may wish to care for the infant until the moment of discharge. Significant others also may need help in separating from the baby and in supporting the mother.

During the postpartum period the nurse should note the progress the girl is making in the grieving process associated with adoption separation. A healthy resolution is dependent upon successful progression through the grieving steps. A girl who has made little or no progress in grieving should be carefully assessed and followed after discharge from the hospital. If the girl shows a change of mind, the nurse must help her to make her decision rationally rather than relying too heavily on emotions which may be transitory.

The nurse actively discusses discharge plans and anticipated behavior the girl may display with the family or significant others. It is not therapeutic to have the girl reenter the family and act as though nothing had happened. Likewise, they should not dwell on the pregnancy. A Visiting Nurse Association (VNA) visit or more frequent postpartum visits are necessary. There should be a way to contact an appropriate health care giver if a problem arises.

Body Image Changes. As discussed previously, a major concern for the adolescent is her body and how it has changed or been changed through the prenatal and intrapartum course. The adolescent often has difficulty with the perineal changes resulting from labor and delivery. Her concern is expressed postpartally by such questions as: "Do you have to take the stitches out?"; "When do they fall out?"; "I feel little bumps when I wipe myself."; "Will my boyfriend know I have had stitches?"; "How do I know when I'm healed?" The caregiver can provide reassuring comments which make the girl aware that the stitches do not hurt as much today as they did previously. Also, she can point out that the patient is moving, talking, and sitting easier each day.

Breast Feeding Difficulties. For the breast feeding as well as nonbreast feeding mother, breast engorgement may be a painful experience. This has particular impact on the adolescent who often may not be comfortable with her breasts and their functioning as body organs. The nurse reassures the patient that this will usually last 24 hours. The discomfort may be lessened by analgesics, a supportive bra, no breast stimulation, and application of hot or cold packs to the breasts. Reinforcement of this phenomenon as a temporary change, with reassurance that normality will return, is extremely important to the adolescent. For the adolescent who elects to breast feed, the breasts change in focus from sexual to nurturing body organs. The new mother will need strong nursing support and input. Education about breast feeding, the special care of breasts and nipples, and fears coupled with embarrassment need to be addressed by the nurse. Breast feeding also requires a nutritious diet, which may not be adherred to if the young mother is concerned with getting back into shape immediately and severely restricting her dietary intake.

Because of the postpartum lochial flow, the nurse needs to emphasize the importance of body hygiene and consistent perineal care. The adolescent often is not interested in the self-administration of perineal care. She is not strongly motivated to initiate regimen and follow-through. The nurse needs to focus directions on explaining why healing and proper hygiene are interwoven. The nurse may have to be directive in the way of instruction. She may have to initially do the peri-care to illustrate and then check frequently to make sure it has been done by the patient.

Cesarean Section Problems. Many times a cesarean section is not anticipated prior to entering the hospital. Because the adolescent is struggling with the psychological inconsistencies of dependency versus independency, this event forces her into a more severely dependent role. Often it is the first surgery ever experienced and the side effects are always baffling for the adolescent. Initially, it is difficult for her to imagine herself as ever feeling better, and she has the added burden of feeling physically unable to care for her child. Consistent and supportive nursing care is mandatory for the adolescent at this time with provision for the many questions which invariably will come to the front.

Environmental Restrictions. Compared to labor and delivery, postpartum does allow more freedom, but the adolescent is still more restricted than in her home environment. One of the major values teenagers have is social interaction, but this may be one of the most restrictive factors. The girl can not choose her roommates. She may not know who else is on the floor with her, and visiting hours and the number of people allowed at one time are restricted. The family and peer visits are important aspects of postpartum care, but they should be interspersed to allow time between visits for rest and privacy which the new mother requires. It is hard for her to understand why she and her friends cannot all get together. She is also forced to spend time alone. She may cope with this by demanding a television set and spending many hours on the telephone with family and friends, neglecting caregivers' attempts at interaction. Conflict may occur when the rights of roommates to the telephone and sleep are jeopardized.

Sleep is a frequently manipulated variable in the adolescent's life. She delights in staying up late and getting up at her convenience without an alarm.

The choice of food for selection may not be compatible with the cultural, religious, or personal desires. This may prove to be frustrating to the patient as well as nutritionally unsound. The adolescent often has aberrant eating patterns and may request her family or friends to bring in her special favorites, thus helping her to bridge the gap between hospital and home.

Because of the restrictions placed upon her, unfamiliarity with the unit, and homesickness, the adolescent may react in a more overt, demanding fashion. This behavior exhibits itself when she turns on call lights frequently for insignificant requests. A whole circle of interaction may be established. These irritating and apparently selfish requests harass the staff members who soon stop responding to the calls.

The nurse exercises patience and understanding with a young mother. She makes herself available and checks in with the mother frequently, thus possibly avoiding the call light demands. The nurse may also have to set and consistently apply specific limits to the adolescent on telephone and television usage if these are disturbing to others. The period of adolescence, as previously described, is a time when limit-setting is important but may be reacted against strongly.

Bonding Difficulties. How the teenage mother bonds with her child and at what speed depends on many factors. Some variations are the result of the girl's cultural orientation, reasons for the pregnancy, difficulty with labor and delivery, fatigue, the hospital environment, and the attitudes and policies of medical personnel. Although difficult at times, the clinician must do everything possible to promote bonding because of its therapeutic effect of positive long-term maternal-infant interaction and relationship. Identifying the infant as an individual includes close, prolonged contact in task-oriented as well as nontask-oriented situations. The resolution of differences between what the mother perceived about the baby and what the real baby is like may impede or reinforce her bonding abilities.

When the nurse recognizes delayed bonding, the cause needs to be explored. It may be just a manifestation of physical discomfort. It may also indicate the patient is trying to cope with the reality that her mother or another family member will be assuming major responsibility for the care of the infant. It also can indicate poor adjustment or rejection. Regardless of the cause, the nurse needs to ascertain and validate with the mother the reason(s) for its occurrence. Special plans including VNA visits, family meeting(s) with a social worker, more individual time spent by the nurse with the mother and baby, and special bonding interventions discussed in earlier chapters may be needed.

Birth Control Difficulties. One of the main problems caregivers must deal with is how they can give successful help and information on birth control to an adolescent postpartally.

One cannot assume, when discussing contraception with the adolescent postpartally, that she perceives an obvious need for contraception because she has had a baby. Pregnancy itself does not automatically remove the inconsistent perception that she is not a sexually active woman. It is the rare and extremely motivated adolescent who does not become sexually active within the first year post-delivery, and she cannot predict what her sexual activity will be once she leaves the hospital. However, daily contraception may not be possible for the girl who still does not view herself as sexually active, and she will therefore be more vulnerable to unprotected coitus. She may also be increasingly exposed to sexual advances by males who know that she has been pregnant.

Counseling and repetition regarding birth control are usually part of the postpartum care. Although the adolescent may be initially motivated, while a captive audience in the hospital, her lifestyle and values are not addressed. Initial compliance with contraceptive methods later may be seen as intrusive and incompatible with her normal daily functions.

The nurse helps the adolescent focus on her needs and individual desires. Giving information on types of contraceptives alone is not enough. The nurse could elicit how the patient views herself, including her sexuality, her difficulty in obtaining birth control measures, her embarrassment in using foam and condoms or a diaphragm, her feelings about an IUD, the recognition that oral contraceptives must be taken every day to be effective, daily usage difficulties depending on lifestyle, and the degree of outside interference by boyfriend, mother, or peer attitudes.

Parenting Difficulties. The postpartum period marks the beginning of parenting responsibilities, as previously mentioned. Parenting requires consistent giving and caring, planning for safety and prevention of child injuries and illness, stimulation for physical and mental development, as well as physical care of the child. However, the demands of adolescence and of childrearing and parenting are often incompatible. Motherhood requires increasing comfort in initiating independent actions, but an adolescent may be in a dependent role because of her age and limited experiences. Even though she may have had babysitting or sibling care responsibilities, she may not automatically transfer these experiences to her mothering role.

Because abstract concepts such as attitude formation and values may be foreign to the adolescent, it is easier for her to respond to the physical needs of the infant than to the psychological or educational needs. Teenagers usually do well in caring for the child during the first year. Once the child reaches two and is becoming autonomous, she finds it difficult to teach social, psychological, and educational values and attitudes. The child may then make demands she cannot deal with, and she translates her feelings of rejection and frustration into physical abuse. It is more common for these children to be subjected to child abuse and negligent accidents. Once the loving relationship is interfered with, the teenager often becomes pregnant again to fulfill that lost need.

In the parenting process, peer pressure can be a significant influence. Even if the mother has a natural desire to be a "good parent," peer pressure may supersede this instinct and lead to a negative outcome. If this occurs, both mother and child suffer. Conversely, peer pressure can have a positive effect if it is strengthening and supportive of motherhood ideals.

Because of these potential parenting difficulties, long-term and long-range nursing care with frequent follow-up is required. The nurse utilizes the basic concept that adolescent teaching should be geared to the present, not the future. Although previous teaching may have familiarized the teenager with the subject and concepts of parenting, actual on-the-job training is required for learning and implementing the parenting process.

NURSING APPROACHES

The previous discussion has presented the special needs of the pregnant adolescent during the conceptional phase. In dealing with these special needs, the nursing care and approaches should be based on the following four concepts:

1. A pregnant adolescent is at psychosocial risk which may influence physical risks;
2. Pregnancy is an interruptional factor which necessitates intervention and guidance;
3. Consistent input, counseling, and follow-up are necessary;
4. Nine months are not enough for redirection of the adolescent and prevention of future unwanted pregnancies.

When dealing with the potential psychosocial-physical risks to which the pregnant adolescent may be exposed, the nurse must have background knowledge and understanding of the composition and interaction among the risk factors. She will need to assess them directly and indirectly with each individual client. In order to obtain this information, the nurse must interact with the patient in a firm, consistent, and caring manner. She should not fear direct confrontation with sharing of feelings. The nurse should not have or communicate the expectation that all information needed to identify risks will be obtained within the initial visits. This may be a reason why return appointments are made sooner and more frequently. The needed trust may be developed by honest sharing of concerns and problems between the caregiver and the adolescent. Once the risk situations have been identified, the nurse must direct the pregnant adolescent to the various appropriate resources available. The nurse may have the responsibility of coordinating the many facets of care rendered by the various resources. Appropriate feedback should be given to those involved in her primary care. When a specific regimen needs to be implemented outside of the health care facility, the problem and expected prescribed regimen should be communicated to those directly involved in its implementation. This may include the school nurse, boyfriend, or parent. In order to adequately deal with the risks of teenage pregnancy, more time and energy needs to be allotted with coordination and follow-through among the staff.

Frequently pregnancy temporarily interrupts and sidetracks the adolescent from progressing through the stages of adolescent development. This temporary interruption can become permanent if she is not guided in completing each maturational task before entering the next one. The individual goals devised by the adolescent and the nurse should be based on adolescent theory, since it is unrealistic to focus on adult goals and expectations. Acknowledgment of this fact will have direct and indirect implications for the decisions that will affect the adolescent's future. Since change is expected, long-term goals should reflect this fact and leave room for flexibility and mobility. A concrete example is the adolescent's expectation of immediate need gratification. If pregnancy represents the desire and need to have a love object of her own, this need is fulfilled with the birth of her baby. However, in planning for the care of the child, she will be exposed to the multiple problems inherent in parenting. She will be faced with the necessity to make plans for education, financial support, and daily child care at a time when she may want freedom to do what she wants, when she wants. Only by reflecting upon what stage of development the individual is in can realistic goals be set.

At a time of stress and insecurity in her life, the pregnant adolescent benefits most from consistent input, counseling, and follow-up. Consistency in frequency, availability, and accessibility of care or persons involved in care must be maintained. This will further enhance the sense of trust which promotes honest and productive interaction. The degree of success may depend on this factor.

Health care will play a major role in the care of the pregnant adolescent. The health care includes the preventive, immediate, and subsequent aspects. Education again should be based on adolescent theory. For example, adolescents want to learn but many are afraid to expose their ignorance of a situation. Easy accessibility to reading material and audiovisual aids should be provided in a nonobvious or casual manner. Pregnant adolescents will profit from both group and individual instruction. The group will provide a means of comparison and a sense of peer belonging. Individual teaching will allow questions of sensitive nature to be discussed prior to exposure in a group situation. The topics for prenatal education are basically the same as for any adult group of expectant mothers but with added emphasis on parenting. This educational process may need to be more repetitive. Help in individual clarification and application may be needed as a special nursing approach.

Since the pregnant adolescent lives in a community milieu, referrals are necessary. Common referrals include the Visiting Nurse Association, adoption agencies, social workers, nutritionists, physicians, psychologists, and nurse specialists. Darting can be a very effective method of referring and indicating a risk situation. Computer banks are now being used to coordinate and prevent duplication of referrals.

As previously stated, the amount of individual growth and responsibility required by a pregnant adolescent is great. Generally, the younger she is, the more intense the care and redirection needed. Attaining the responsibilities of adulthood and parenthood within the nine months of pregnancy is impossible. Any successful program must provide for long-term individual follow-up.

Because the pregnant adolescent or the adolescent mother and child are at risk, more frequent medical, nursing, or social visits are necessary. Frequent visits and follow-up should extend well beyond the six-week postpartum exam. Visits can be done in a number of ways: visits to the home, visits to the health care facility, visits to the school. Telephone calls are a vastly underutilized resource for maintaining contact and relating messages of positive concern.

Another reason for continuous follow-up and education is that the patient lacks experiences in dealing with life's issues. In order to obtain the full value of her conceptional experience, she will have to reach a level in maturational development where personal insight and the ability to work toward long-range goals is possible. This includes working toward economic independence.

A final reason for frequent long-term follow-up is that a teenager's state of equilibrium at the end of pregnancy is not necessarily the same in six months or a year. The difficulties discussed under

postpartum indicate that the difficulties do not end at delivery. Some chronic problems persist and some new ones occur. Parenting difficulties and concerns are of the utmost importance.

The follow-up care of the adolescent is geared toward the three aspects of health care previously mentioned. The nurse, who has worked consistently with the adolescent during pregnancy, may coordinate follow-up services. As new problems arise or old ones recur, she is often the first person the adolescent contacts.

SUMMARY

The crisis of adolescent pregnancy can be readily seen. The basis of sound care is founded on good maternity nursing practice. Additional awareness of the problems of the adolescent in general and the pregnant adolescent specifically is utilized by the nurse as she provides care.

An adolescent pregnancy truly necessitates a family-centered approach. Family should be interpreted in a broad sense to include the father of the baby, prospective grandparents, aunts and uncles, or significant others that may serve as family.

The cornerstone to successful parenting will be initiated by successful bonding. The nurse can do much to influence the environment to allow for this occurrence.

Idealistically, the pregnant adolescent should be cared for in a facility geared toward providing health care for all adolescents. Pregnancy is only one health issue which an adolescent faces. When viewed on a continuum, follow-up is more realistic, can be more easily obtained and geared toward more individual physio-psycho-social needs.

Nine months is often not long enough for the adolescent mother to complete the adolescent and mothering developmental talks. The nurse's role is to assist her in developing both as an adolescent and as a mother.

REFERENCES

1. Baldwin, W. H. *Population Bulletin.* "Adolescent Pregnancy and Childbearing—Growing

Concerns for Americans." Population Reference Bureau, Inc., Vol. 31, No. 2, September 1976.

ADDITIONAL READINGS

1. Adams, J. F., ed. *Understanding Adolescence —Current Developments in Adolescent Psychology.* Boston: Allyn & Bacon, 1968.
2. Brewer, T. H. *Metabolic Toxemia of Late Pregnancy: A Disease of Malnutrition.* Springfield, Ill.: Charles C Thomas, 1966.
3. Esman, A. H., M.D., ed. *The Psychology of Adolescence.* New York: International Universities Press, 1975.
4. Fischman, S. H. "Delivery or Abortion in Inner-city Adolescents." *American Journal of Orthopsychiatry,* 47 #1, January 1977, 127–133.
5. Gallagher, J. R., F. P. Heald and D. C. Garell. *Medical Care of the Adolescent.* New York: Appleton-Century-Crofts, 1976.
6. Kalafatich, A. J. *Approaches to the Care of the Adolescents.* New York: Appleton-Century-Crofts, 1975.
7. Osofsky, H. *The Pregnant Teenager—A Medical, Educational and Social Analysis.* E. C. Thomas, 1968.
8. Sorenson, R. *(The Sorenson Report) Adolescent Sexuality in Contemporary America.* New York: World Publishing Company, 1973.
9. "Special Issue: Teenagers U.S.A." *Family Planning Perspectives,* 8 #4, July/August 1976.
10. Stone, L. J. and J. Church. *Childhood and Adolescence,* 3rd ed. New York: Random House, 1975.
11. Waters, J. L., Jr., M.D. "Pregnancy in Young Adolescents: A Syndrome of Failure." *Southern Medical Journal,* June 1969, 655–658.
12. Young, A. T., B. Berkman, and H. Rehr. "Parental Influence on Pregnant Adolescents." *Social Work,* 20 #5, September 1975, 387–391.

PERTINENT ORGANIZATIONS

NATIONAL
- *International Childbirth Education Association, Inc.*
  Publication Distribution Center
  P.O. Box 9316 Midtown Plaza
  Rochester, New York 14604
  Provides educational material on childbirth and parenting applicable to adolescent pregnancy.
- *Nurses Association of the American College of Obstetricians and Gynecologists*
  One East Wacker Drive
  Chicago, Illinois 60601
  A nursing association focused on obstetrical and gynecologic nursing providing a journal, *JOGN Nursing.*

LOCAL
- Information on local services for the pregnant adolescent can be obtained from some city health departments, churches, medical clinics, or educational groups.

The Single Parent

Edith A. Tankson, R.N., M.P.H.

CHAPTER TWELVE

The single-parent family is rapidly becoming more visible in our society. In addition to rising divorce rates and fatal illnesses such as heart disease and cancer which frequently strike middle-aged parents, more unmarried mothers are electing to keep their children, more couples are deciding to live apart to pursue educational and career goals, and more single persons are adopting children than in the past.

Though not all single-parent families should be classified as high-risk families, single parenthood can create many problems that may place both the parent and children at risk. The fact that one parent must assume all of the responsibilities that are usually shared by two can create many problems for the family. In addition, other difficulties may be directly related to the cause of single parenthood, such as divorce, unwed pregnancy, or the death of a spouse.

As the number of single-parent families increases, it becomes evident that they are unique units with special needs and that nurses, and especially community health nurses, are often in an ideal position to play a vital role in helping to prevent or reduce the effects of some family difficulties.

BASIC CONCEPTS OF THE SINGLE-PARENT FAMILY

Female-Headed Single-Parent Families. The majority of single-parent families today are headed by women. Older studies have attempted to prove that children in female-headed families are at a much greater risk than are children of two-parent families for developing behavioral problems (juvenile delinquency), poor academic performance, and inappropriate sex role behavior (supposedly, boys behave in a feminine manner and girls are less able to develop and maintain healthy relationships with males later in life).

Current thinking does not support these "findings." There is no concrete evidence that a direct cause and effect relationship exists between absence of a father per se and poor school performance in children. Behavioral problems, such as juvenile delinquency, seem to be more strongly influenced by how the family functions, its climate, and the quality of supervision a child receives than by the number of parents in the home. In fact, some studies found that the presence of some fathers was more detrimental to children's well-being than their absence when they created stress and conflict in the home.[4] Finally, there is an obvious lack of evidence to support the belief that the absence of a resident father interferes with a boy's masculine identity and denies a girl the opportunity to interact with a good male model. To believe this would be to presume that nonresident fathers do not spend any time with their children and that there are no other males interacting with the family.[4]

Even though the above risk factors do not automatically apply to single-parent families headed by women, there are other more realistic risks that may affect them. The mother's psychological and behavioral reactions to her situation as a single parent are critical to the stability and functioning of the family unit. How does she cope with stress and conflict? Is she able to effectively fulfill her roles as homemaker and breadwinner? Is she able to exercise adequate supervision over the children? Is she in good health and does she have adequate psychological and physical energy to handle the increased responsibilities of single parenthood? For many single mothers, single parenthood "includes reduction in income, social status, and social activities, posing a struggle against resentment, isolation, and self-doubt." The single mother must deal with the tendency to be overpossessive, pushing the children to maturity, and feeling guilty for the cause or results of single parenthood.[4]

Although the importance of exposure to healthy male models in the development of children should not be minimized and certainly can be included with thoughtful planning on the part of the single mother, successful family functioning is greatly influenced by the mother's reaction to her situation. Therefore, practical assistance and support to facilitate the mother's adaptation is an appropriate goal for a nurse who is involved with the family.

Male-Headed Single-Parent Families. In recent years, the number of single-parent families headed by males has risen. This trend may be due to the women's movement, relaxation of sex stereotypes, and changing custody laws.

Since the coming of the women's movement, some women are able for the first time to admit that motherhood is not totally fulfilling and in increasing numbers are pursuing educational and career goals that compete directly with being full-time wives and mothers. Some are resisting social pressures to adhere to more traditional women's roles and are choosing not to take custody of their children following separation or divorce.

The relaxation of role assignment by sex, also influenced by the women's movement, reflects changes in society's attitudes regarding appropriate male or female behaviors. Men are becoming more assertive in areas concerning their rights as parents. Some are refusing to relinquish important decision making that affects their children's futures. Men are increasingly acceptng roles that were once considered feminine, such as child care and homemaking tasks. A degree of competence in these activities and the increased availability of child day care centers provide an alternative to speedy or premature remarriage for help with child-rearing for fathers of young children.

Another very important factor contributing to an increased number of single-parent families headed by males is the changing custody laws in some states, which make it easier for fathers to get custody of their children. In the past, fathers have not been considered qualified to assume the responsibility for child-rearing. The only chance a father had of getting his children was to prove that their mother was unfit due to nymphomania or sexual promiscuity, alcoholism, child abuse or neglect, mental incompetence, or lesbianism. Even if a father could prove that his ex-wife was unfit, the children were still often placed in a foster home rather than allowed to live with their natural father.[1] Custody laws, such as the Family Law Act of California, have eliminated the need to prove a mother unfit, creating a no-fault dissolution of marriage and making it less cumbersome for fathers to obtain custody.[6]

FAMILY DIFFICULTIES RELATED TO SINGLE PARENTHOOD

There are a number of potential difficulties shared by single-parent families, regardless of the

Figure 12-1. Family Difficulties Related
to Single Parenthood

Family Crisis
Redefinition of Roles and Responsibilities
   Role strain
   Leader strain
Child-rearing
Financial Insecurity
Stereotype Difficulties
Social Isolation and Loneliness

cause of single parenthood or the sex of the parent. Figure 12-1 concisely lists the common problems associated with single parenthood.

Family Crisis

Whatever the cause of single parenthood, an initial family crisis develops, and though it can be experienced in degrees varying from minor to overwhelming, it temporarily affects the family unit. This crisis is directly related to the sometimes dramatic and sudden changes within the family structure and its manner of functioning. The family often lacks preparation or experience for dealing with these changes and the resulting problems. For the family that is unable to make an immediate, harmonious adaptation to its new situation or to effectively resolve its problems, a crisis develops.

To illustrate this, we can consider the case of a family in which one parent, for whatever reason, leaves the home. The remaining parent must take on the unfamiliar tasks and responsibilities of the absent parent in addition to his usual ones. For example, the single father will have to concern himself with child care arrangements, household duties, meal planning, and other tasks that were previously handled by his wife. The family may initially eat many meals out or the father may have to miss days from work until he can find reliable child care. The single mother, who in the past has allowed her husband to handle most of the financial matters, may find herself in debt or overdrawn at the bank until she learns how to budget money appropriately. Relatives or friends may step in initially to fill the gaps, but eventually the family must redefine its members' roles and responsibilities and

realistically determine what ongoing assistance is available from grandparents, other extended family members, friends, or community resources.

Redefinition of Roles and Responsibilities

Redefining roles and responsibilities is a major concern and requirement for all single-parent families. The single parent is responsible for providing for the physical, emotional, and social needs of the family members. This task is usually shared by two adults and is more than a full-time job for a single parent. His attempts to meet the family's needs can lead to increased stress and decreased coping energy. "When a single parent must assume the responsibilities usually shared between two adults, he or she may experience 'role strain,' and almost always, 'leader strain.'"[2]

Role Strain. Role strain occurs when the parent has to do those things that he thinks he should not or cannot do. The parent may have low expectations of himself and tend to belittle himself while trying to perform those tasks. This condition occurs mainly in families where previously tasks were distributed along rigid sexual lines. For example, the single mother may still view financial matters as a task more suitably handled by a man. Therefore, she may assume this responsibility unwillingly, not expecting to do it efficiently. If in fact she does it poorly, this may further reinforce her belief that financial matters are the responsibility of men and make her even less motivated to master this task.

Several complications can develop when a parent is unable or unwilling to master certain tasks. They may be turned over to the child, who ends up assuming more responsibility than he should. For example, a single father may assign such tasks as meal planning and preparation, housekeeping, care and discipline of younger children and other "women's" tasks to a female child who is too young to handle them. This can, in turn, be very upsetting to the child who has had to sacrifice playtime and activities with friends because she is too busy satisfying family needs. As family members become more discontent, they become more critical of each others' roles which leads to less family cohesiveness.[2]

Leader Strain. The term leader strain describes what happens when a parent attempts to perform dissimilar tasks for which he does not have the time and energy. The parent, in this case, probably exchanged tasks with his ex-spouse according to each parent's availability rather than along sexual lines. Therefore, his family is less likely to develop the complications associated with role strain.

In many cases, leader strain is inevitable, due to the great number of tasks and the parents' limited energy, time, and preparation to do them. Leader strain may be manifested by parental fatigue, disorganization, and lack of personal time. It is unrealistic to believe that a single parent can or should continue to perform all the tasks usually shared by two parents over a long period of time. Those parents, who, because of guilt, feel they must be superparents to the children to compensate for the absence of one parent will eventually suffer both leader and role strain. They need help in deciding how tasks can be reduced, eliminated, or shared and if they can be done with less adequacy.[2]

Child-rearing

Child-rearing is a major concern for the single parent. The working parent may be torn between the roles of breadwinner and child-rearer. This can create significant problems for the single parent. First of all, the parent may feel extremely guilty about being away from the child for so many hours of the day. This guilt can cause the parent much anxiety that, in turn, will affect his concentration and performance at work. For example, the parent may be unmotivated to work harder or longer hours, be unwilling to assume added responsibility, talk excessively about his child, make frequent calls to check on the child on work time, and pass up opportunities to socialize with co-workers outside of work. This can have serious implications, since such behavior can adversely affect the parent's relationship with his employer and decrease his chances of advancement. Ultimately, this can affect earnings and the family's standard of living.

The parent's guilt can also have a direct and detrimental effect on the parent-child relationship. The parent, in an effort to compensate for the injustice he feels he has subjected the child to, may be too permissive, overindulgent, overprotective, or too controlling. He may try to spend every available moment with the child, sacrificing adult relationships and effectively interfering with the child's normal socialization. These conditions can lead to rebellion or excessive dependence on the part of the child and self-denial, loneliness, and eventual resentment on the part of the adult.

Another problem faced by the working single parent is finding a reliable caretaker during the parent's absence from the home. Depending on the child's age, this may need to be an all-day arrangement or just a few hours after school until the parent returns home. All parents want to know that their children are receiving the best possible care, but for the parent who already feels guilty about being away from the child, this may be the only consoling factor. Many parents do not know how to locate and evaluate child care services and, therefore, are at risk of their children receiving inferior or even unsafe care.

A child develops his ideas about the adult world through observations and evaluation of significant adults in his life. In most cases, the adults are his parents, whose beliefs and experiences greatly influence how the child will think about and respond to his world. For example, a child whose parents do not like a certain food or group of people will most likely have the same dislikes. A child who grows up in a household where watching television is a major source of entertainment for the adults is very likely to use television in the same way.

In our society, sex still dictates to some degree what experiences an individual may have. The child in a one-parent family is not provided with the role model of both sexes and, therefore, lacks the varied experiences that a child in a two-parent family has to draw from as he develops his ideas about the world.

The parent is the only authority figure in the one-parent family. Unlike in two-parent families, the single parent necessarily makes day-to-day decisions without the benefit of consulting another person. This can cause the parent anxiety and worry when he questions the correctness of a decision. Of course, two parents can also make a wrong decision, but if there is open communication between them, being able to discuss and consult with one another should decrease the chance of error and increase confidence about making subsequent decisions. There may also be some consolation in knowing that one was not alone in making a wrong decision, and it would be helpful to have another's input when it is necessary to reevaluate and change a decision. In order to avoid error, the single parent may attempt to be very consistent at the risk of becoming quite inflexible, controlling, and authoritarian. The child is at a disadvantage, because he has no choice of parent to go to for a decision. In contrast, the child in a two-parent family can approach the parent he thinks will be more sympathetic in a particular matter. If the single parent tends to be too controlling or authoritarian, the child, over a period of time, may show little initiative and increasing dependence on the parent or he may become rebellious.

Financial Insecurity

Temporary or chronic financial insecurity is a problem shared by many single parents. Either loss of income or having to spend more on services such as child care can create a serious deficiency. The single father may have an advantage over the single mother because he is more likely to have a better paying job. A single mother may be dependent on monthly child support checks or public assistance programs that are often insufficient. Inadequate education or skills may make it very difficult for men or women to find interesting, well-paying jobs with flexible hours.

Single parents may be the victims of discrimination in several important ways. Jobs may be withheld from single mothers because employers fear that their commitment to home and children will interfere with regular attendance and reliabil-ity. Single men, to a lesser degree, may be eliminated as job candidates because wives are important in jobs in which entertaining is stressed. In addition, single parents may experience discrimination when purchasing insurance and attempting to establish credit.

Social Isolation and Loneliness

The single parent often feels lonely and socially isolated. He no longer fits in with married parents and may feel uncomfortable with childless single people at first. Married friends may hesitate to invite single parents to social gatherings because they may be denying or avoiding discussions about problems within their own marriages that could possibly lead to divorce or separation. The widowed person may be excluded because others do not want to face the possibility of their partners dying. And, of course, in a mixed group, the single parent may be seen as competition by those of the same sex.

Because the single parent does not socialize much, companionship and sexual needs often go unmet. Some, particularly the widowed, feel guilty about needing companionship, while others find it difficult to find persons who accept their single-parent roles and get along well with their children.

FAMILY DIFFICULTIES AND NURSING APPROACHES RELATED TO CAUSES OF SINGLE PARENTHOOD

Single-parent families have potential difficulties that are related specifically to the causes of single parenthood. For example, a family in which the single parent is divorced may have different concerns from a family in which the single parent is widowed or was never married. See Figure 12-2 for a concise list of the difficulties related to the single unwed, separated or divorced, widowed, or adoptive parent.

Difficulties Particular to Unwed Parents

The annual decrease in the total number of live births, the relatively stable out-of-wedlock de-

Figure 12-2. Family Difficulties Related to the Causes of Single Parenthood

Unwed Difficulties
  Adolescent conflicts
  Social stigma
    social isolation
    discrimination in employment and housing
    punitive attitudes and practices of welfare agency personnel
    lack of sympathy and support from society and significant others

Separation and Divorce Difficulties
  Rejection
  Grief
  Children's guilt
  Children's separation anxiety
  Discipline
  Custody and visitation

Widowhood Difficulties
  Grief
  Intrapersonal problems
    developing independence
  Interpersonal problems
    establishing relationships
  Material problems

Adoption Difficulties
  Competition with two-parent family
  Discriminatory adoption practices
  Care of special-need child
  Explanation to child about adoption
  Social stigma

livery rate, and a diminishing in-wedlock delivery rate have combined to make out-of-wedlock births an increasing proportion of total live births.[10] In 1965, out-of-wedlock births numbered 291,200, accounting for 8 percent of all live births compared to 447,900 or 14 percent in 1975. Births to adolescents have become an increasing proportion of the total out-of-wedlock births. In 1965, births to adolescents came to 129,200 or 44 percent of all out-of-wedlock births compared to 233,500 or 52 percent in 1975.[9] Today many more adult women and teenagers are choosing to remain single and to keep their babies.

The Unwed Adolescent Parent. A fairly significant number of pregnant teenagers still marry, but only temporarily avoid single parenthood due to a high incidence of marital dissolution within this group. One study of pregnant teenage girls found that 33 percent were married by the time of delivery, another 27 percent by one year after delivery, and a final 15 percent within two years after delivery, bringing the total number of those married to

75 percent. "Ironically, most of the young mothers who managed to avoid single parenthood by marrying either before or shortly after delivery ended up as single parents several years later. And many of these women no doubt will never remarry. Therefore, it might be said that once an unplanned pregnancy occurs in adolescence, it hardly matters whether the young mother marries. In time, she may be almost as likely as the unwed mother to bear the major, if not the sole, responsibility for supporting her child."[3]

The difficulties of the unwed adolescent parent and related nursing approaches were discussed in the preceding chapter.

The Unwed Adult Parent. The increased availability of contraception and legalized abortion has not significantly influenced the incidence of unwed births to adult women. Not all unwed pregnancies are "accidents"; many adult women actually plan to become pregnant. Even though this is more common today, there still exists a degree of social stigma associated with unwed parenthood which may be manifested through social isolation of unwed parents, discrimination against them in employment and housing, and punitive attitudes or practices directed toward them by social service or welfare agency personnel. In addition to financial insecurity, stereotyping, and some of the other problems that were discussed in the section on problems related to single parenthood, the unwed mother, perhaps more than other single parents, may have to cope with relationship problems with parents, friends, and even the father of her baby. These significant others may strongly disapprove of the woman having sexual relations or conceiving outside of marriage, carrying the pregnancy to term, or keeping the child. Society, in general, is much less likely to sympathize with the unwed mother who is having difficulties and therefore tends to offer her less support than, for example, a mother whose spouse has died. The following case is one illustration.

Shirley was a 29-year-old single woman who had worked for seven years as a maid in a hotel. Soon after Shirley became pregnant, the hotel came under new management. Due to Shirley's past medical history, she was classified as being high risk for developing complications during her pregnancy and had to be seen by a doctor more frequently than most pregnant women. The new manager was very disturbed about this and asked Shirley to quit. She refused to quit and he had no legitimate reason to fire her because her work was thorough and she always notified him in advance when she had clinic appointments and brought a medical excuse when returning to work the following day. There had been an unofficial policy at the hotel to assign lighter duty to pregnant employees. The manager refused to do this in Shirley's case and began to give her more weekend and night assignments. She was convinced that it was because she was unmarried and pregnant. When encouraged by the clinic nurse to contact the legal aid office, Shirley backed down for fear of losing her job. She finally accepted a referral to the welfare department from which she received supplemental payments and assistance with her medical expenses. She was able to work part-time, which allowed her to keep clinic appointments. Shortly after delivery, she returned to work full-time.

In this case, the nurse was helpful by referring the patient to an appropriate community resource. Nurses working in a variety of settings can effectively act as advocate for the single mother and should support and encourage patients to be more assertive in obtaining what is rightfully theirs, be it employment, housing, medical care, or financial assistance. The nurse may also be able to help the unwed mother resolve some of the relationship problems mentioned earlier, through nurse-family counseling or referral to a mental health resource for this type of service. The nurse's involvement, of course, depends upon the problems presented. Individual assessment of the problems and needs for each single parent is essential.

Difficulties Related to Separation and Divorce

Almost any day, one can pick up a newspaper or magazine and read about couples who have decided to live apart so that one or both partners can

pursue individual educational or career goals in different geographical locations. Even though each partner in this arrangement benefits from the social status, financial resources, and shared decision making that accompanies being married, the major responsibility for child care on a day-to-day basis is usually assumed by one partner who, in a practical sense, can be classified as a "single" parent. This type of separation is voluntary and usually does not result from marital discord. There are ongoing communication, regular reunions, and mutual affection. The separation is usually temporary, with some target date for permanent reunion in mind.

Separation due to unreconcilable marital problems is much more common. It can be a permanent arrangement, but most often is a transitional stage leading to divorce after varying lengths of time. The ever-increasing divorce rate in this country is the single most important contributor to the increasing number of single-parent families. In 1973, three out of every five marriages ended in divorce, and in some parts of California the ratio was one to one.[11] One very interesting point is that even marriages of relatively long standing are dissolving. It is estimated that over 25 percent of all divorces involve marriages of over 15 years duration.[7] In most separation or divorce cases, the children go with one parent; less commonly, the children are divided so that each parent has custody of one or more children.

Single-parent families that result from parental separation or divorce present a different set of difficulties from those of the unwed parent. If the absent parent initiated the separation or divorce, the single parent often experiences feelings of rejection and grief similar to that associated with the death of a spouse. The grief process may begin prior to the actual separation or divorce, when it becomes obvious that the marriage is not working. Therefore, at the time of divorce, the individual may be in the final stage of grief rather than the first.

Marcia's case illustrates a single parent's progression through these stages of grief. Marcia and Jack had been married seven years and had two children who were ages three and five at the time they separated. They had been having serious marital problems for several years stemming from the fact that Jack was a heavy drinker and, consequently, frequently unemployed. Marcia worked full-time as a registered nurse, but they were deeply in debt. Marcia encouraged Jack to seek counseling for his drinking problem, which Jack refused to do. When he quit his job, after quarreling with his supervisor about his poor attendance, Marcia asked him to move out. She had done this several times in the past, but each time allowed him to come back "hoping" that things would change (denial). She was very angry at Jack because she had been forced to support the family alone and she was even angrier with herself for having tolerated his irresponsible behavior for so long (anger). Marcia continued to "date" Jack for several months after the separation to see if they could resolve their difficulties. She thought that, if she did not live in the same house with Jack for a while, maybe she could be less emotional and more understanding about his alcoholism. She even offered to enter counseling with him (bargaining). When Jack refused, Marcia filed for divorce. The divorce was not final for six months, and within that time Marcia sold the house and moved back home with her parents who were able to help her care for the children. Marcia became very depressed and was encouraged by her parents to seek professional counseling (depression). She began to attend a divorced women's group at a mental health center and, through this group, gained a much better understanding of her feelings and capabilities. She attended this group for nearly a year and, with the support and encouragement she received from its members, she was eventually able to move out of her parents' home and assume the major responsibility of caring for her children (acceptance).

The stages of grief do not usually occur in the order in which they are presented here for clarity. Two or more stages, for example, may coincide. Neither is there a set time in which individuals work through all of the stages of grief. Some never complete the process; they may never accept their divorce status or may remain extremely angry or dependent on others to care for them and their children.

The nurse's response or approach depends on what stage of grief the single parent is in. For example, during the denial stage the nurse must listen sympathetically but, whenever possible, help the single parent focus on the reality of the situation. If the parent is in the anger stage, the nurse must allow or encourage the parent to openly express himself, even though the nurse may at times be the target of misdirected parental anger. The nurse can promote the parent's final acceptance of his situation through honest discussion about his needs, limitations, capabilities, and new responsibilities. She may be able to offer practical advice about financial matters, housing problems, child care concerns, companionship needs, and other aspects of single parenthood that arise.

In addition to the grief process that the parent must work through, the children may also experience some fairly common problems. One important concern is the child's guilt about the separation or divorce. This is especially strong if, in anger, he has in the past wished the absent parent were out of the home. In his confusion and fantasy about the changes within the family, the young child may blame himself for what has happened. Because he feels responsible, he may make attempts to reunite the parents.

The anxiety experienced by young children on separation from the absent parent can result in somatic complaints, disturbances in activity, regression, behavioral problems, and withdrawal from reality. The child may feel rejected or helpless. Fearing that he will be sent away like the absent parent, he may become overly anxious to please the remaining parent to prevent this from happening.[12] His anxiety may be further increased by moving to a new home or apartment, a new school or caretaker, and any other changes created by the separation of the parents.

The nurse who is involved with the family before, during, or shortly after separation or divorce should encourage the parents, together if possible, to tell each child separately that there will be a divorce, why, and what arrangements have been made for him. The parents must use language that is easily understood by the child and be as truthful as possible without placing blame on either parent. The child must be reassured that he is loved by both parents, not only verbally, but by the parents' actions. The nurse should strongly emphasize the child's need for regularity in his life immediately following separation or divorce.[12] This is very important to stress, since the parents may still be too embroiled in fighting one another to focus on the child's need for order and consistency at this critical time.

If a child develops any of the manifestations of separation anxiety mentioned earlier, the nurse should reassure the parent that these things are not uncommon and will usually be resolved in time. The parent should be encouraged to be patient, understanding, and loving toward the child during this period of adjustment. If professional counseling is needed, the nurse can intervene by helping the family to locate the appropriate resources, making referrals and following up to see that problems are being addressed.

Discipline and limit setting can be a problem in the single-parent family that results from separation or divorce. Sometimes the parent feels guilty about the child not having a two-parent home and having had to suffer through perhaps years of the parents' fighting. The parent attempts to make up for whatever damage may have been done to the child; he overcompensates by being too permissive or relinquishing his personal identity. The parent develops an "over intense, possessive relationship with the child, building (his) whole life around him."[1] One example of this is the young divorced mother who spends almost every moment of the day with her child. She feels guilty about leaving the child with anyone else and, therefore, never goes anywhere without him. She sacrifices peer relationships of all types and may avoid dating for fear that this may in some way psychologically damage the child.

The nurse may need to help the parent look at discipline and setting limits. It might help to talk through the parent's feelings of guilt and how this can affect his relationship with the child. Together, the nurse and parent may identify specific problem areas in the parent-child relationship and develop a plan of action to resolve these. For example, in the case of the overintense, possessive relationship between a parent and child, the nurse and parent may set up a timetable of events that range from leaving the child for short periods of time with close friends or relatives to all-day attendance at a day care center. As steps are taken, the nurse and parent can evaluate their effectiveness and build on them as indicated. This is not an easy task for a parent, and he may become discouraged if there are no immediate results or if he slips back into old patterns from time to time. The nurse should be supportive and help the parent to look at progress realistically.

Custody and visitation are two other problems faced by the family. The type of relationship that exists between the parents will determine how custody and visitation will be handled. When much hostility and anger prevails, custody and visitation can be used by either or both parents as one more weapon in their war against one another. This obviously can be very disturbing to a child.

Alice and Bob separated when their sons were four and five. Bob was angrily opposed to the separation and divorce that soon followed, but willingly agreed that the children should live with Alice. At the time of the divorce, Alice insisted that Bob spend a day with the children each week; she felt that the boys needed regular contact with their father in order to develop healthy masculine identities. Bob agreed to every Sunday, but frequently failed to show up. This concerned and angered Alice, which is what it was intended to do. At the same time, however, it totally confused the children who took their father's behavior as a sign of rejection of them.

The custody and visitation questions may be handled through the courts. The parent should be encouraged to seek legal assistance and, again, the nurse may initiate referral. The nurse can help both parents to give adequate attention to the needs of the child during the custody-visitation dispute so that the child does not get lost in the vengeful game playing that can continue between parents over a long period of time.

Difficulties Related to Widowhood

The single parent who has lost his spouse through death must deal with the major problem of grief. The grief process as it relates to death is discussed in detail in the chapter on the "Terminally Ill Parent." Basically, grief is a progression of time-consuming stages through which a person learns to accept his loss and reorder his life.

Other problems for the widowed parent may be loneliness, guilt about the need for tenderness and love, financial insecurity, planning for the needs of children, lack of self-confidence and independence, making new friends, finding a job, and planning for the future.[8]

The widowed parent may find self-help or "grief" groups to be a source of support and useful advice. The nurse may be instrumental in organizing self-help groups either in parents' homes or at a community site such as a church or neighborhood service center. In the majority of cases, the nurse will be involved with the widowed parent in a one-to-one relationship. The nurse should be prepared to be involved with the family over an extended period of time; too often nurses end their nursing care immediately after the death of a spouse. As mentioned earlier, the grief process is time-consuming and nursing assessment and preventive intervention are needed as the family attempts to cope with difficulties that arise during the stages of grief. The nurse's intervention may include listening understandingly, focusing on the reality of the situation, encouraging parental independence and socializing, suggesting activities or new experiences in which the parent can realize his strengths and capabilities, and making appropriate referrals with follow-up.

Difficulties Related to Adoption

Adoption of children by single persons, though not commonplace, has become somewhat more common in recent years. Competition with two-parent families for adoptable children and the refusal of some private social service agencies to provide adoption services to single persons still create barriers.

The first problem that the single person faces when trying to adopt is competition with two parent families. "Most agencies, given comparable standards of health, stability, and other characteristics considered necessary in an adoptive home, would give a child to two parents rather than one."[5] Due to this discriminatory practice, the single parent is more likely to adopt what are called special need children. These children, who are passed over by couples interested in "normal" infants, may be older, mentally or physically handicapped, interracial or transracial. The single parent, therefore, has the added burden of coping with problems associated with the child's special needs. For example, an older child may have lived in a number of unpleasant foster homes or institutions before the adoption. This is a traumatic experience for the child and, because of his fear of being rejected again, he may not fully trust or express any affection for the parent. He may also be depressed or have other psychological disturbances requiring professional intervention. The child's unresponsiveness may cause the parent to feel angry, overwhelmed, or deeply discouraged.

The nurse, in this case, will have to be very supportive of the parent, who may be doubting his ability to parent. The nurse can help the parent understand the dynamics behind the child's present behavior and assure him that the child's response is a defense mechanism, unrelated to the parent's treatment of the child. This type of assurance helps the parent to be patient with the child until he feels more secure. Some adoption agencies offer ongoing counseling for adoptive parents and their children. The nurse should encourage use of this service if problems are very serious or persistent.

Another problem single persons must contend with is the stereotypes and myths associated with single persons, especially men, who want to adopt. A man may automatically be suspected of being homosexual and during the investigatory period prior to adoption, he may have to provide proof of his heterosexuality by revealing information about his intimate personal relationships. Single men and women both have to go through exhaustive interviews in which the motivation for adoption is the single most important issue.

The single parent may have difficulty deciding when and what to tell the child about adoption. If the community is predominantly two-parent families, the child may feel that he was discriminated against when he was given to a single parent. The single parent may be forced to explain adoption much earlier than two parents because the child is aware very early of the difference between his family make-up and other children's.[5] So the single parent finds himself in the position of trying to explain a very important issue to a child who may be confused by the explanation if it is not handled properly.

The nurse should encourage the parent to anticipate the child's questions and to begin early to think about how he will respond. This kind of preparation will prevent the parent from being surprised by the child's questions and giving a confusing or superficial explanation. The nurse may also explore with the parent what words would be easily understood by the child at his stage of growth and development. The nurse should stress that, as with most things, the young child will ask the same questions many times. The parent should patiently repeat the answers and try to be consistent.

The single parent may experience some problems in his interpersonal relationships as a result of the adoption. Friends may disappear as the single parent takes on new responsibilities of parenthood and has fewer things in common with them. Friends or relatives may not understand or accept the adoption, especially if the child has special needs. For example, interracial adoption can be a divisive factor if the single parent's friends and relatives have racial prejudices. Some older adopting women have reported losing friends who envied them for their courage to adopt. Other single women have had to deal with accusations of having illegitimate babies and lying about the adoptions.[5]

The nurse should listen understandingly as the parent expresses his feelings of hurt, anger, and loss about changes in his interpersonal relationships. The parent will need encouragement to establish new relationships. The nurse may refer the parent to local organizations of single parents such as Parents Without Partners, in which he can meet people with similar needs and interests. The adoptive parent, however, should also be encouraged not to limit his friendships to parents and their families.

NURSING APPROACHES

Reducing Crisis. The nurse can help the family through the crisis using crisis intervention strategies mentioned in a following chapter. These help the family members identify the crisis event and use problem-solving methods to find new ways of meeting their needs.

Redefining Roles and Responsibilities. Nurses come into contact with single-parent families in a variety of settings: health care facilities, community service agencies, and in their homes. The community health nurse may be in a better position to make a thorough assessment of the family's situation and recognize verbal or behavioral cues that indicate a parent is experiencing either role or leader strain.

Once a relationship has been established between the nurse and the family, the nurse can help family members to identify existing or potential role or leader strain difficulties and develop approaches to reduce or prevent strain. For example, if a single parent frequently complains of being too tired to go out with friends in the evening, the nurse may want to discuss what things he does during the day to cause such fatigue. The nurse should also explore the possibility that the reason the parent does not go out is that he feels guilty about leaving the children with a sitter and not just because of fatigue. This parent may need a lot of support and the nurse should verbally acknowledge that no one expects him to be a superparent. The nurse should encourage the parent to arrange his daily tasks according to priorities, perhaps even in writing. Some things can be spread over a period of days, while others can be appropriately assigned to other family members; older children can alternate washing dishes, vacuuming, or taking out the trash with the parent or other siblings. Establishing priorities and allocating time and resources will be the content of much of the counseling the nurse provides to a single parent experiencing leader strain.

The nurse may have to teach the single parent who is experiencing role strain, how to perform essential unfamiliar tasks. For example, a single father who lacks confidence in meal planning and preparation can be taught how to do this. This may be an excellent opportunity for the nurse to provide much needed nutrition counseling. Since meals have never been a concern to him, the father may have no idea what the four basic food groups are or what amounts of these are needed by children and adults for growth and energy. This kind of information can be the guidelines he needs to begin this new task. The nurse can help the parent plan a week's menu, suggest nutritious snacks, provide easy-to-prepare inexpensive recipes, or actually supervise the parent as he prepares a meal. If the parent requires more detailed or long-term instruction, the nurse can refer him to another resource. In the city of St. Paul, for example, there are nutrition aides, available through a university extention program, who can work with parents in their homes. These persons are knowledgeable in basic nutrition and can provide practical assistance with budgeting, shopping, meal planning, and meal preparation. For the more motivated parent, cooking classes at the local YWCA or through other community programs can be educational, entertaining, and may provide an opportunity for the parent to develop new relationships.

Admittedly, there will be some tasks that the single parent will never fully accept, even though the women's movement has brought about less task distribution based on sex. If the family is interested, the nurse can help the family decide what outside services would be most useful and how they can be paid for. For example, a working parent may need to hire someone to care for a young child during the day, clean house, or do laundry once or twice a week.

As mentioned before, the nurse can assist the family to identify those tasks that can appropriately be assigned to children. The nurse can perhaps suggest ways to implement a gradual transference of responsibility between family members so that children are not overburdened or given tasks that are more appropriately handled by the parent. Some families have become closer as they have worked together to meet family needs.

Child-rearing. When involved with a parent who feels guilty about leaving his child with others while he works, the nurse should encourage the parent to verbalize his guilt and whatever fears he may have about how his absence affects his child's development or the parent-child relationship. In addition to listening understandingly, when appropriate, the nurse should provide objective data about families with working parents. For example, the nurse might encourage the parent to think about single-working-parent families he is aware of that are functioning successfully. There may even be prominent people in the community who were either reared in single-working-parent families or are single working parents themselves; this is evidence that the children in such families are not necessarily deprived or doomed to maladjustment. Occasionally, newspaper or magazine articles report results of studies or surveys of single parents and their children; these may offer more encouragement for the single working parent.

The nurse can also point out some of the positive aspects of the child's separation from the parent, such as relief for the parent with an opportunity to pursue outside interests, promoting independence in the child, and the opportunity for the child to interact with others and develop a variety of new skills. The nurse should stress the fact that the quality of the time spent with the child can be much more important than the number of hours spent with him. The nurse should encourage activities that promote maximum interaction and sharing between parent and child and that are inexpensive, stimulating, and relaxing for both of them.

The nurse can assist the parent who is looking for a reliable caretaker in his absence. Many parents do not know what to look for or how to evaluate the care given. In addition to providing a listing of sitters or centers, the nurse will be aware of licensure requirements and may have firsthand knowledge about specific resources: whether they provide good physical and emotional care, age appropriate activities, adequate ratio of staff to children, and so on. A good understanding of normal behavior, growth and development, and the need for stimulation should be the basis for choosing a specific child care facility. Therefore, this can be an opportune time for the nurse to teach the parent about his child in relation to these factors.

As mentioned earlier, role models of opposite sex behaviors can and do provide children with a wider range of experiences. Some single parents have found parent substitutes of the opposite sex, either through personal friends, extended family members, or "friend" programs such as those sponsored by local welfare departments, YWCA, Big Brothers, or Big Sisters. Other parents may need the nurse's help to identify and encourage the use of resources that are available. At times this may require simply referring a parent to a community resource, but at other times it may mean helping the parent to list his friends and relatives who may have extra time and be interested in spending it with the child. It may be appropriate, once the parent has approached friends and relatives, for the nurse to meet with the parent and these persons to discuss the child's needs, suggest age appropriate activities, and so on.

Even though the nurse can not make decisions for the parent, she can be a sounding board, offer insights when appropriate, and facilitate better decision making by encouraging the parent to take advantage of resources designed to aid with this extremely important parental responsibility. Perhaps the best resources for the parent are other parents who have experienced or are experiencing many of the same things. Attending parent discussion groups at the YWCA, community mental health centers, child guidance centers, welfare departments, community-based activity centers, or single-parent organizations can provide an opportunity to share frustrations and to offer and receive practical suggestions about decision making in specific situations. If a parent for some reason is not motivated to go into a center, the nurse working in the community may be able to organize a small group of parents in her caseload who are having difficulties making decisions on a day-to-day basis. A group such as this could meet regularly in an agreed upon location, and if the nurse does not feel confident leading it, she could arrange to co-lead with or have the group led by a qualified resource person from an appropriate agency. This approach may be much less threatening for some parents and may motivate them to later make use of agencies that offer services to single parents and their children.

School and church personnel must not be overlooked as a valuable resource to single parents. Besides being supportive of the parents' efforts, school counselors, teachers, ministers, and other church members often have a wealth of insight and practical suggestions to share with parents. When the nurse makes a referral to a community resource, she assumes the role of coordinator and follows up to be sure the parent is receiving the help he needs.

Financial Insecurity. The single-parent family living on a fixed or limited income may be best helped by assistance with general budgeting and locating necessary items such as food and clothing at lower prices. If the single parent depends on public assistance, the nurse can act as an informed advocate to ensure that the parent is receiving the maximum benefits he is legally entitled to. Education about the welfare system can make it much less confusing for the parent and facilitate responsible use of its services. The nurse should encourage low-income parents, including those who are working, to investigate and apply for food stamps, federal food supplements, and medical assistance when appropriate.

If inadequate education or lack of job skills is

the obstacle to a better paying job, the nurse should encourage school attendance or refer the parent for job training, perhaps through a federal job training program that offers some financial incentive. The parent may need the nurse's assistance with more practical matters, such as obtaining and filling out applications, finding financial aid for educational programs, or arranging for child care or transportation.

Discrimination against single parents by employers, creditors, and others may be handled through the courts. The nurse should refer to and encourage the use of free or inexpensive legal aid programs if the parent thinks he has been victimized.

Social Isolation and Loneliness. Friendships can be established with co-workers, residents in the parents' apartment building or neighborhood, and members of church groups, adult classes, parent groups, local organizations for single parents, or other groups. The opportunities for friendship do exist, but some parents will need much support and encouragement from the nurse to reach out to others.

SUMMARY

Single-parent families have specific needs and problems related to single parenthood and its causes. Nurses can help these families to prevent, cope with, and resolve many of their difficulties through the use of nursing strategies (assessment, counseling, teaching, crisis intervention, referral, and follow-up) which are discussed in more detail in another section of this book.

The nursing approaches that have been suggested throughout this chapter may be helpful for all nurses, but are probably more likely to be used by the community health nurse who usually has a longer involvement with families than the hospital-based nurse and who, because she is a generalist, is able to intervene competently in a wider variety of family difficulties. It is important, however, that the nurse knows when and how to refer parents for more specialized or intensive treatment

of more serious problems. A major deficiency in human services is that, although there are a wealth of services available, too often they are attempting to function independently of one another. Lack of coordination results in duplication, gaps in services, fragmentation, and confusion on the part of the client. The role of the nurse working with single parents is often that of coordinator. Referring a family for service is not enough; she must follow up to be sure that there is a mechanism of communication between all agencies or professionals involved with a particular family, thus ensuring sharing of information and planning for the best possible service to that family.

REFERENCES

1. Biller, H. and D. Meredith. *Father Power*. New York: David McKay Co., 1974, 273–299, 590.
2. Blechman, E. and M. Manning. "A Reward—Cost Analysis of the Single-Parent Family." In *Behavior Modification and Families*. Eric Mask et al. (ed.). New York: Brunner/Mazel, 1976, 63, 70–75.
3. Furstenberg, F. F., Jr. "The Social Consequences of Teenage Parenthood." *Family Planning Perspectives*, 8, July/August 1976, 157.
4. Herzog, E. and C. Sudia. "Families Without Fathers." *Childhood Education*, 48, January 1972, 175–181.
5. Klein, C. *The Single Parent Experience*. New York: Walker and Company, 1973, 94, 104, 105.
6. Kübler-Ross, E. *On Death and Dying*. London: Macmillan Co., 1969.
7. McFadden, M. *Bachelor Fatherhood*. New York: Walker and Company, 1974, 20, 35.
8. Miles, H. and D. R. Hays, "Widowhood." *American Journal of Nursing*, February 1975, 280–282.
9. Minnesota State Health Department, Section of Vital Statistics, Minneapolis, Minnesota.
10. Osofsky, H. "Adolescent Out-of-Wedlock Pregnancy: An Overview." *Clinical Obstetrics and Gynecology*, 14, June 1971, 448.
11. Singer, L. J. "Divorce and the Single Life: Divorce as Development." *Journal of Sex and Marital Therapy*, 1, spring 1975, 255.
12. Sugar, M. "Children of Divorce." *Pediatrics*, 46, October 1970, 589.

ADDITIONAL READINGS

1.   Bemis, J. et al. "The Teenage Single Mother." *Child Welfare*, LV, May 1976, 310.
2.   Cutright, P. "AFDC, Family Allowances and Illegitimacy." *Family Planning Perspectives*, 2, October 1970, 4–9.
3.   Fischman, S. H. "The Pregnancy—Resolution Decisions of Unwed Adolescents." *Nursing Clinics of North America*, 10, June 1975, 217–227.
4.   Herman, S. J. "Divorce: A Grief Process." *Perspectives in Psychiatric Care*, 12, 1974, 108–112.
5.   Hope, K. and N. Young. *Momma: The Sourcebook for Single Mothers.* New York: New American Library, 1976.
6.   Kaseman, C. M. "The Single-Parent Family." *Perspectives in Psychiatric Care*, 12, July/September 1974, 113–118.
7.   McRae, M. "An Approach to the Single Parent Dilemma." *Maternal Child Nursing*, May–June 1977, 164–167.

PERTINENT ORGANIZATIONS

NATIONAL
- *Parents Without Partners*
  7910 Woodmont Avenue #1000
  Washington, D.C. 20014
  Provides information and groups for widowed, separated, divorced, or never married parents.

LOCAL
- Local groups such as religious organizations, community center groups, and phone "hot lines" help to serve the single parent.

The Abusive Parent

Carole K. Kauffman, R.N., M.P.H., and
Mary Kathleen Neill, R.N., M.A.

CHAPTER THIRTEEN

Throughout history children have been the recipients of physical and emotional abuse. Ancient and contemporary literature and history, religious teachings, and widely accepted educational and child-rearing practices have all condoned and even encouraged the maltreatment of children under the rubric of discipline, education, and salvation. Child labor was commonly accepted until the early nineteenth century when the first child labor laws were enacted. However, not until 1961 was this long-standing abuse of children, both in the family and society in general, specifically identified as a clinical problem, "the battered child syndrome."

The nurse working in pediatric, community, or school settings is in a key position to assess and intervene in the problems that children and parents present. The nurse's unique position of a close-working relationship with the family in many clinical settings places her in an essential position for prevention and early identification of child abuse.

The Child Abuse Prevention and Treatment Act of 1973 has defined abuse as "the physical treatment or maltreatment of a child under the age of eighteen by a person responsible for this child's welfare under circumstances which indicated that the child's health or welfare is harmed or threatened thereby."[11]

Abuse is generally associated with acts of commission that result in demonstrable external or internal physical injuries. The injuries are inflicted during extreme punishment, discipline, or physical assault on the child. They occur throughout childhood and adolescence, but the infant and young child are most vulnerable to irreversible damage.

Neglect, on the other hand, is usually associated with acts of omission, such as depriving the child of necessary food and emotional nurturing. These children are often underweight, have developmental lags, and frequently are apathetic. Neglect is most common among infants and the young child, but may also be seen in school-aged children.

Sexual abuse includes intercourse, rape, incest, exposure, and fondling. It is estimated that 75 percent of the offenders, most of whom are males, are known to the child or the child's family. Approximately 90 percent of the victims are girls ranging from infants through adolescence, with the greatest incidence occurring during prepubescence and adolescence.[11]

The above definitions are broad in scope and serve as guidelines. One can argue that they do not delineate where discipline ends and abuse begins. In determining abuse, the professional must consider the norms of child-rearing within different cultures and make judgments based on a multitude of factors, including the future physical and emotional safety of the child. At present this distinction is ultimately determined by the courts.

Incidence and Mortality

The incidence, mortality, and morbidity of child abuse and neglect are pervasive and of such a magnitude that this syndrome is one of the most challenging and critical health problems of our times. Unfortunately, accurate incidence and mortality rates are difficult to obtain. Approximately one half million cases of suspected abuse and neglect were reported in the United States in 1975. For that same year the Department of Health, Education and Welfare estimated the number to be 1 million. Others estimate the figures to range much higher, from 2 to 4 million a year.[5] It is suspected that approximately 10 percent of the injuries to children under 5 years of age seen in emergency rooms are the result of inflicted trauma.[9]

The wide discrepancy in such statistics is due to the iceberg theory that there are more actual cases than known cases. Reasons contributing to the existence of many more suspected than known cases of child abuse and neglect include failure of professionals to report suspected cases, misdiagnosis of inflicted injuries as accidental injuries, and the absence of child abuse as a listing in the International Classification of Disease (I.C.D.). Mortality ranges from 5 to 25 percent of the total abused cases.[6] Morbidity figures show that 25 to 50 percent of the children who have been abused have significant damage, in varying degrees, to the central nervous system.[7]

Child abuse and neglect affects all populations, socioeconomic levels, cultures, and religions, and occurs in rural, suburban, and urban communities. There is reason to believe that poor families may be more vulnerable because of environmental stresses, such as overcrowding and lack of financial re-

sources. More studies are needed to identify whether there are particular groups who indeed are more likely to harm their children than others.

Reporting

All 50 states have enacted legislation mandating reporting of child abuse. By 1970, 40 of the states included professional nurses in their statutes as reportees. Because of differences among the state laws regarding child abuse and neglect, it is incumbent upon the nurse and other health and social professionals to become knowledgeable about their state's child abuse statutes. Some of the differences include the legal definition of abuse, age of the child covered by the law, professional immunity for reporting, penalties for not reporting, agencies designated to receive reports, and criminal, family, or juvenile court proceedings.

Although many nurses are unaccustomed to the use of reporting as a prevention and treatment approach, reporting is essential to ensure the safety of the child and to initiate the delivery of services to the family. Legal involvement is recognized as an integral component of the multidisciplinary and community approach to child abuse. Judge Delaney writes: "Inherent in family law is the delicate balance between what is exclusively a matter within the family and what is of concern to society . . . . In the area of family, the court's true role is to define and protect the rights and enforce the responsibilities of the parent, of the child, and of the community."[5]* The child is placed in grave risk when one does not, after careful evaluation, report suspicion of child abuse and neglect. Children have died as a result of professionals' avoidance of or delay in reporting.

BASIC MULTIDISCIPLINARY CONCEPTS

Child abuse can best be understood when viewed as a symptom of family dysfunction caused by a variety of factors, frequently involving multi-

---

*Reprinted with permission from Child Abuse and Neglect: The Family and the Community, Copyright 1976, Ballinger Publishing Company, pp. 335–338.

ple determinants. The term itself refers to a range of behaviors from mild to lethal, including physical or emotional abuse and neglect. Many disciplines have made important contributions to an understanding of this complex and multifaceted problem.

The medical profession has played a critical role in the diagnosis and treatment of child abuse. In 1946 John Caffey associated subdural hematomas with fractures of long bones, a frequent radiological finding in child abuse. Silverman, a few years later, confirmed Caffey's findings, but it was not until 1955 that P. V. Wooley and W. A. Evans first attributed the findings of Caffey to intentional trauma. In 1962 Kempe coined the phrase "the battered child syndrome" and helped draw national attention to the problem. Doctors Helfer and Kempe stressed the importance of a multidisciplinary approach and initiated treatment programs for the entire family.[5]

Researchers in psychiatry and psychology have not been able to clearly define a specific child abusing personality nor to concur on the extent of psychopathology in abusing parents. However, there is general consensus that abusive parents may frequently present some or all of the following characteristics:[2,4]

1. A history of abuse in the parents' own childhood;
2. Unrealistic inappropriate performance expectations of their child;
3. Social isolation;
4. Immaturity;
5. Poor self-image;
6. Poor control of aggressive and other impulses;
7. A limited capacity to express their own needs.

Often the parents' own personalities have been molded by the lessons learned in early childhood. They believe that children are easily spoiled, that absolute obedience is the goal of child-rearing, and that physical punishment is the best way to achieve this goal. It seems natural for many of these parents to expect their children to meet their needs regardless of the fact that as children they were never able to satisfy their own parents. Their strong sense of right and wrong evolves from the con-

science they developed from the rigid expectations set years earlier by their own parents.[4]

Such experiences in childhood may result in a basically unhappy, unsatisfied parent who looks to his child for the emotional relationship he should have had with his own parents (sometimes referred to as role reversal). The child's inability to gratify these needs may serve to increase the parent's frustration and sense of rejection, resulting in impulsive physical abuse or self-righteous punishment.[4] These acts of abuse are often triggered by a minor event that is interpreted by the parent as a crisis, such as a glass of milk spilled on a clean floor.

Although the role of the nonabusing parent has not been adequately studied, it is clear that in many instances there is either frank compliance or passive participation in the abuse. Effective treatment of the abusive parent must include work with the "nonabusing" partner.

Anthropologists and sociologists have extensively studied the determinants of violent and aggressive behavior. Of particular interest is a study of child abuse and neglect conducted by David Gil. The results of this study led Gil to conclude that the single most important contributing factor to child abuse was the acceptance of any form of physical force as a means of training and disciplining children.[3]

In summary, a combination of theories has led authorities in the field to conclude that the following characteristics are most commonly found in abuse situations:[6]

1. The parent has the potential to abuse.
2. The child is viewed as different from other children.
3. There is a perceived crisis that triggers the act of aggression.

The at-risk child and parent may be identified, but the crisis situation that leads to abuse is more difficult to anticipate and thus to prevent.

FAMILY CHARACTERISTICS

Although individual characteristics within the family in which child abuse has occurred are as unique and different as those within "normal" families, some generalizations on the child's and parent's characteristics and the effect of situational crises are helpful.

Children's Characteristics

High-risk children, as discussed in preceding chapters, include the premature infant and children with physical, intellectual, or emotional handicaps. Although these children are considered at risk, certainly not every at-risk child is abused. It has not been possible to identify anything special or unique about many abused children that placed them at risk of abuse. The following examples demonstrate child characteristics that may precipitate child abuse.

High-risk Infant Factor. An infant hospitalized for one month because of prematurity and necrotizing enterocolitis was readmitted two weeks later with a skull fracture. The mother had visited only two times during the first hospitalization, had received different advice from many people on how to feed the baby, and was frustrated with her attempts with feeding at home. The family had recently moved into a paternal aunt's overcrowded home, the father did not have steady employment, and the family did not have a pediatrician or clinic to take the child to for follow-up.

Any of the above factors could place the infant at risk. The most important factor, however, is the separation of the infant from its parent at the time of birth. This is the most critical time for bonding to occur. A child who was ill and a fussy eater plus the overcrowding, unemployment, and lack of a primary physician compounded an already dangerous situation of disruption of maternal-infant bonding.

Special Child. A two-year-old child, product of a rape, was hospitalized for abuse and placed in a foster home. Three years later the grandmother pressured the mother to regain custody because the grandmother felt the mother should love that child. The mother had four other children who have never been abused. Seeing this child stirs up hatred for him because of the pain and humiliation she suffered during the rape and because she had wanted an abortion but never carried it through.

Although this is an extreme example, it illus-

trates that one child in a family can be the sole recipient of abuse. The child may remind the caretaker of someone from the past whom she dislikes, possibly her own self-image. Once the child is removed from the home, another child in that family may be abused. In some instances, as in the above example, only one child is injured.

Parental Characteristics

Alcohol or drug addiction, adolescent parenthood, intense emotional disturbance, and physical illness are among the factors that may place parents at risk for abusing their children. These factors are discussed in detail in other chapters. However, the most critical parental risk factors are a childhood history of abuse and the unrealistic expectation that the child meet the parent's emotional needs.

Childhood History of an Abuse. A 19-year-old mother threatened to throw her two young children out the window. The children had not been abused. The mother was a heroin addict at 14 years, attempted suicide at 17, and was hospitalized for depression following the birth of her second child. As a child she felt unwanted, having been shuffled back and forth between her parents, and had been beaten by her father.

With a history of having been abused as a child plus the very serious problems of addiction and self-destructive behavior, her threat to harm her children must be taken seriously. This mother was referred to a child abuse team for preventive intervention. Any threat of a parent to harm his child should be carefully evaluated. A "you wouldn't do such a thing" attitude is extremely dangerous, especially when the parent has a past history of abuse as a child.

Unrealistic Expectations of the Child. A five-week-old infant was admitted because of human bites and bruises. The mother said the baby only laid in bed and cried a lot and did not love the mother.

Parents who abuse their children are often unaware that children develop slowly over time and thus may have unrealistic expectations of the child's abilities. This mother was unaware that a new infant cries frequently and is incapable of a social smile let alone "loving" its mother. The abusive parent punishes the child for not meeting the parental expectations and needs.

Isolation and Longing to Be Nurtured. A young mother with a five-week-old baby and a two-year-old girl had recently moved to a new city. Without close friends or relatives, living alone in one room of a boarding house, she felt completely isolated. A temper tantrum by the two-year-old provoked a beating in which the girl was struck in the face with a paddle. When the mother began to cry in the E R because the authorities had been notified, the two-year-old wiped away her mother's tears and tried to comfort her with pats on the back.

Several factors are demonstrated by this example. One of the effects of her isolation and unsatisfied need to be cared for was to lower her threshold of tolerance for her two-year-old's behavior. Even very young children in such an environment frequently learn to adopt a comforting, nurturing role with their parents (role reversal). Another factor is that, frequently, the abusive parent is unable to reach out to friends and relatives during times of stress or, when in a new environment, to develop the kinds of friendships that can be supportive during stress.

Choice of Abusive Partner. During an argument the boyfriend of a young woman began hitting her while she held their infant. The baby was admitted to the hospital with a fractured femur. The woman subsequently terminated her relationship with the man and the baby was returned from a foster home to her. Two years later the same child was readmitted to the hospital with second and third degree burns of the lower extremities. The woman's new partner had submerged the child in a tub of hot water when the woman left the apartment following a fight with him.

Although this mother was not "abusing" her children, her selection of partners had twice resulted in serious injury to the children. Terminating her relationship with these men is not sufficient to ensure the children's safety. Unless she as the "nonabusing" parent receives treatment, her pattern of selecting abusive partners will continue to endanger her children.

Situational Crisis

Many situations from minor to major problems can precipitate a crisis. In some instances it is a series of events; in others, it is an isolated event that leads to abuse. Overcrowding, major illness, the loss of a job, or an event that is considered the "last straw" in a series of unfortunate occurrences are some examples.

Major Illness. An eight-year-old boy was hospitalized because of repeated whippings, referred by the school nurse. While he was hospitalized his mother was also hospitalized and died of terminal cancer that had not been diagnosed or treated. In pain, she had repeatedly struck the boy for not helping her enough.

This mother had no emotional or physical reserves to draw upon. In fact, she had a real need to be taken care of. Physical illness can be a precipitant to abuse. Without assistance from another adult—a "life line"—during a time of emotional or physical discomfort, the parent may be unable to cope with a child's behavior or needs.

The "Last Straw." A grandmother severely beat her seven- and 11-year-old grandsons with a strap and extension cord because she had asked them to clean their rooms and they had replied, "You can't tell us what to do because you are not our mother." The mother rarely cared for the children, leaving the child-rearing to the grandmother. The grandmother was devoted to the children and was distressed about her daughter's attitude toward them. It was a single incident of abuse, disturbing to the grandmother who subsequently sought and received counseling.

Statistics on the number of children who are injured seriously only one time are unavailable. Empirically this does happen, but in such instances the caretaker is in need of counseling to prevent a recurrence and to resolve the guilt.

FAMILY DIFFICULTIES

The very fact that a child has been abused suggests that there are significant problems within that family. The underlying pathologies in them-

Figure 13-1. Family Difficulties Resulting from Child Abuse

Impact on the Child
  Death
  Physical injury
  Neurological impairment
  Developmental deficits
  Emotional handicaps
  Perpetuation of the cycle of abuse

Impact on the Parent
  Termination of parental rights
  Relating to large numbers of people
  Angry hostile feelings from professionals
  Court proceedings and court-ordered treatment
  Reactions on family members and neighbors
  Financial obligations

selves are difficult to treat. However, the situation is further complicated by the effects of the abuse on both the child and parents. The family difficulties are summarized in Figure 13-1.

Impact on the Child

The effects of child abuse are far-ranging and influenced by a number of factors. Infants are more vulnerable to death and permanent disability than older, stronger children. Head injuries and burns that lead to permanent brain damage or body disfigurement are of more consequence and indicative of greater pathology than a single incident of bruising. The duration of trauma over an extended period of time has a greater consequence to the child's developing personality than a single incidence of abuse. The rate of recovery is influenced by the child's general state of health, nutritional status, and the overall quality of the relationship with the parent. Some of the effects of the abuse on the child are described in the following sections.

Death. Precise statistics are not available. Unidentified and untreated, 25 to 50 percent will be admitted dead on arrival.[6]

Physical Injury. The pain inherent in these injuries is obvious, as is the pain that frequently accompanies necessary medical treatment. The long-term physical effects may include scarring and obvious handicaps that seriously impair the child's functioning and further development.

Neurological Impairment. Significant neurological impairment has been documented in many abused children, including children who have no history of head trauma. Of particular concern is the interplay between neurological and psychological factors. Given the intimate and complementary relationship between neurological and emotional development, it is difficult to define clearly the exact roots of the neurological deficits that are observed in many abused children.[7]

Developmental Deficits. Developmental delays in speech, gross motor, and learning abilities are common. Maturation of these functions requires not only neurological capability, but also an environment in which there is sufficient stimulation and interaction to allow the child to direct energies toward learning and mastery. In the abusive environment the parents' needs often take preeminence over the needs of the child, thus the child's needs will be met at best inconsistently.

Emotional Handicaps. Normal behaviors such as crying, wiggling during diaper changes, or reaching for interesting objects may be perceived by the parent as rejection, willfulness, or stubborness. The child's inability to meet and satisfy the parent's unrealistic expectations results in the child repeatedly experiencing failure, criticism, and rage. Lack of positive experiences with his parent prevents the child from feeling that he is lovable and a source of delight to his family, that he has some influence on his world, and that he is successful in exploring and learning from mistakes that are accepted, and from developing a positive relationship with the adults in his world. One adaptation the abused child may make is to become a compliant, submissive child with the pain and fear masked by "good behavior." Such an adaptation may result in the child going unnoticed, viewed by teachers and others as "model children."

Perpetuation of the Cycle of Abuse in the Next Generation. The existing rates of child abuse and neglect attest to this critical outcome of unreported, untreated child abuse. As parents, many abused children are likely to repeat the cycle of child abuse they had experienced and thus imprint on their own children this continuing destructive pattern of parenting.

Impact on the Parent

The identification of abuse leads to a series of crises for parents ill-prepared to deal with stress and unable to seek and use help. Particularly stressful experiences include the following.

Termination of Parental Rights. In many communities the police, court, social and medical systems place the highest priority on protecting the child from further abuse. Often this protection is achieved by the abrupt temporary or permanent removal of the child from the parents' care. Frequently, parents do not want their child removed from their care. Although the child may be thus protected from physical harm, the suddenness of the separation creates significant additional stress for the parents, particularly when therapeutic support is unavailable or inadequate.

Relating to Large Numbers of People. Although successful intervention in child abuse requires involving many disciplines and community resources, the orientation and goals of these many disciplines may not always be consistent with therapeutic management of the child and family. In having to relate to so many individuals and institutions, the parents frequently receive confusing messages, promises that cannot be kept, and even threats. For parents who have a limited capacity to trust others, the complexity of the system is often inherently untherapeutic.

Angry Hostile Feelings from Professionals. Parents are often alienated from potential sources of help by the intense negative feelings child abuse stimulates in caregivers. Failure to greet parents during visits with their child, avoiding the parent, being overheard discussing the case, and making open critical remarks are among the ways staff communicate their negative feelings toward the parent.

Court Proceedings and Court-Ordered Treatment. Although procedures may vary in different communities, many parents who have abused their child must at some point face the trauma of a court proceeding, either civil or criminal. Often the parents do not understand the issues in the proceeding or the meaning of its outcome. When court proceedings are perceived as punitive, court-ordered treatment is likewise viewed as punishment rather than assistance and thus difficult for the parents to understand or accept.

Reactions of Family Members and Neighbors. Reactions of the parent's parents, brothers and sisters, neighbors, and others may vary widely and include positive helpful support, open rejection, and even denial of the incident of abuse or its significance. Efforts by the parents to accept responsibility and seek help may stimulate criticism about "needing a psychiatrist." A decision by the parents to relinquish a child is often rejected by the extended family, thus the parents may feel compelled to regain custody even when they do not want to raise that particular child. In other situations, some parents engage in elaborate efforts to keep their families and friends from knowing about the abuse, thus further isolating themselves from significant others.

Financial Obligations. In addition to the preceding stresses, parents who have abused their child may incur significant financial obligations from medical and legal expenses. Incidental expenses may include time lost from work, transportation costs, and babysitting costs for children left at home while parents are at court or visiting in the hospital.

NURSING APPROACHES

Prevention

Is prevention of abuse and neglect possible? Although controlled research evidence is unavailable, empirically one can say yes. Countless nurses and doctors with patience and understanding of the difficulties of child care and with their ability to offer supportive counseling and referral for parents experiencing these difficulties have helped prevent serious physical and emotional abuse of many children.

The nurse in pediatric, obstetric, and community settings has the opportunity to identify difficulties in parenting through observation of the parent-child interaction, history-taking (with an emphasis on how the parents were raised and critical events in their lives and those of their children), physical examination, and administration of developmental screening tests. She also has many opportunities to provide instructions on child care and, most important, the developmental needs of children.

Assessment. There are many signs that a family is in need of preventive intervention. It is important to note in the assessment of the family that one cue does not mean the parent will abuse or neglect his child; often a combination of factors must be present. Schneider and others are working on a predictive questionnaire whereby specific cues and their scores indicate a high-risk situation.[5] Gray, Cutler, Dean, and Kempe from the University of Colorado Medical Center have detailed important signals of risk in the perinatal period.[5] Information drawn from these works and others are included in the Preventive Assessment Guidelines in Figure 13-2. Assessment of the family for potential factors in child abuse includes observation of prenatal, labor and delivery, infancy, and childhood periods. Lack of maternal or paternal attachment as discussed in earlier chapters is also an important sign of potential child abuse.

Preventive Interventions. Assisting parents to accept help in decreasing stresses in child-rearing is a delicate process. For some parents role modeling helps; others need tangible assistance with food, clothing, or shelter before they are able to accept more esoteric help regarding human behavior; and others respond to a firm approach of setting limits and establishing contracts of agreement. Continuity of care is crucial to a helping relationship and determining which approach might be the most successful.

The nurse must have a repertoire of possible interventions to plan nursing actions. Community nursing, social service, medical, and psychiatric referrals and the community resources listed in the latter part of this chapter are sources of help. Counseling, crisis intervention, and other helpful strategies are discussed in later chapters. The nurse is cautioned when working with high-risk parents to focus on the parents' needs first in a nonjudgmental manner before attempting to focus on how they can meet the infant's or child's needs. Specific preventive approaches are listed in Figure 13-3.

A valuable general approach for prevention of child abuse and neglect are classes on growth and development and parenting skills. Nurses in a variety of settings provide this type of service. Included in these classes are means of identifying and enjoying an infant's developmental gains; how to provide sensory, motor, and auditory stimulation; how to make toys inexpensively; and group sessions designed to help one understand and express one's needs as a parent and an individual. Although the classes on child-rearing and child development are common for pregnant women or teenage parents, the range of possibilities for teaching development are limitless and include classes for fathers, adolescents, and senior citizens. It is through the nurse's imagination and motivation that very rewarding programs develop and prevention is achieved.

For example, the adolescent population is the next generation of parents. Focusing on their needs and familiarizing them with the responsibilities of parenthood may be one of the most important approaches in the prevention of child abuse and neglect.

At Children's Hospital National Medical Center, Washington, D.C., there is a specially designed program for teenagers which is known as "Rap." In this coeducational program, teenagers meet weekly over a period of time to discuss such topics as birth control, dating, premarital sex, reproduction, and life problems. The important emphasis is on understanding one's own value system and appreciating one's own individuality. The sessions are not aimed at the prevention of child abuse per se; rather they must be viewed as a method for teaching and exploring normal growth and development.

Identification

Except for the very blatant symptoms of child abuse that even a layman easily recognizes, the diagnosis of abuse is often difficult for profession-

Figure 13-2. Preventive Assessment Guidelines—High-Risk Cues of Potential Child Abuse

Prenatal Period
  An unplanned or unwanted pregnancy
  Unrealistic expectations of the newborn baby: e.g., hoping the presence of an infant will solve personal or marital problems
  Denial of pregnancy
  Over-concern about physical changes
  A history of having been abused or neglected or having multiple foster home placements as a child
  Nesting behavior absent in last trimester: e.g., no crib, baby clothes, no plans for feeding
  Psychosocial instability: e.g., addiction, alcoholism, unemployment, marital conflict, psychosis, depression
  History of having previous difficulties in raising children
  Difficulties with pregnancy: e.g., frequent calls for seemingly minor discomfort, persistent exhaustion, nausea, sleep disturbance
  Lack of personal support from spouse, friends, or relatives

Labor and Delivery Period
  Difficult and prolonged labor
  Supports unavailable or nonapparent
  Verbal or nonverbal expressions of disappointment in infant's sex or condition
  Avoidance of eye contact with baby—no "en face" positioning
  Avoidance or discomfort in touching, examining, or holding the infant
  Disparaging remarks about the baby or between parents
  Obvious rejection of baby
  Lack of joy in the birth
  Separation of baby and parent, placing strains on the bonding process
  Not naming the baby
  Postpartum psychological problems: e.g., depression, anxiety, memory loss, extreme mood swings
  Perceiving the baby's cry as rejection or feeling helpless or immobilized

Infancy Period
  No response or responses highly inconsistent to the infant's cry
  Feeding and digestive problems: e.g., slow feeder, finicky feeder, diarrhea, frequent changes in diet
  Minimal physical care: e.g., persistent unresolved cradle cap, diaper rash, dirty or underfed child
  Irritable baby: e.g., cries frequently or has excessive motor activity
  Persistent disappointment in baby's sex or activity level
  Disinterest in mothering activities: e.g., feeding, comforting, bathing or clothing the child
  Lack of eye contact, visual responses, cooing, rocking or cuddling
  Frequent calls to doctor, nurse, emergency room over minor problems
  Rigid time schedules
  Uncertainty, awkwardness, rigidity, or obvious continued discomfort in holding baby
  Misunderstanding and reacting inappropriately to child's developmental ability

Childhood and Adolescent Period
  Difficulties of management of a particular developmental state: e.g., toilet training, crawling, negativism of toddler or adolescent, sexuality of the adolescent
  Delays in developmental milestones with no underlying pathology
  Sudden changes in behavior: e.g., regression to bedwetting or thumb sucking, mood changes
  Language and speech delays
  School problems: e.g., learning difficulties, frequent absenteeism, falling asleep in the classroom, lingering about school before or after school hours
  Adolescents who run away, have extreme parental conflicts
  Problems with discipline and reward: e.g., harsh punishment, inconsistent rewards

als. There are various explanations for this difficulty in diagnosis such as the professional's lack of knowledge about symptoms and denial that caretakers can harm their children. Shared ethnic and socioeconomic background of parent and professional may increase the professional's denial, particularly when the parent is personally known to the professional.

Nurses who work in pediatric settings, especially in emergency rooms, schools, offices, and homes, are in an excellent position to identify possible abuse and neglect symptoms. After initial assessment of possible abuse, they should consult with other members of the health care team and make appropriate referrals for more definitive evaluation. As with any symptom, those that are associ-

Figure 13-3. Preventive Intervention Guidelines—Nursing Approaches

General
　Providing a relationship with the parents that allows freedom for them to discuss difficulties, fears, and fantasies
　Building upon parental strengths rather than focusing on their weaknesses
　Assisting parents to recognize the need for support systems and how to develop them
　Referring families for expert help for assessment and management of difficult problems
　Encouraging parents to meet their own needs as individuals

Prenatal
　Good prenatal care that includes individualized teaching on physical and emotional changes of pregnancy
　Encouraging significant others to be present during labor and delivery: e.g., partner, friend, or parent
　Providing counseling or referring parents who wish to interrupt the pregnancy or relinquish the child
　Assisting prospective parents identify support needed in the home during the postnatal period
　Exploring with parents expectations of parenthood and the unborn child

Labor and Delivery
　Allowing significant others to be present during labor and delivery
　Setting a tone of acceptance for any behavior by offering emotional support and avoiding confrontations
　Setting a tone and developing an environment conducive to parental attachment at the time of delivery: i.e., see, touch, and hold the newborn

Neonate and Infancy Period
　Nonthreatening explanations of baby's normal physiology, anatomy, reflexes, and individuation
　Providing opportunities for attachment, especially if there is interruption in bonding due to prolonged hospitalization
　Explaining that most babies need to and cry more the first month of life—they need consistent warm responses to their cry
　Alerting parents that shaking babies can lead to subdural hematomas
　Providing outreach to all parents experiencing difficulties: phone call within two days from unit staff following discharge from nursery, return appointment with primary caretaker within two weeks, availability of 24-hour phone consultation, community nursing referral

Childhood and Adolescence
　Ensuring well-child care
　Providing anticipatory guidance relative to growth and development (physical, emotional, and psychosocial)
　Assisting the parent to recognize and respond to the child or infant's unfolding personality and abilities
　Discussing with parents how they discipline their children and exploring with them alternative methods (other than physical)
　Providing anticipatory guidance relative to selection of babysitters and accident prevention
　Providing adolescents opportunities, individually or in groups, to discuss sexuality, parenting and role models

ated with abuse and neglect must be "worked up." One would not tell a parent that their child has leukemia based on an elevated white count. Similarly, one would not tell a parent that their child is abused because of peculiar bruising without consultation. Since serious emotional harm can occur by labeling a parent an abuser, identification of abuse must be carefully substantiated. Findings in the following areas may identify abuse and neglect.

History. The history may alert professionals of the need for an in-depth assessment. The following is a list of important signs.[6] A history by the caretaker that:

　• does not explain or is inappropriate for the extent or location of the injury on the child
　• conflicts with the developmental ability of the child

　• indicates inappropriate delay in seeking medical attention
　• reveals frequent injuries and/or frequent changes in hospital or clinic for treatment
　• accuses a third party of causing the injury
　• changes significantly with further questioning
　• reveals family discord

A history by the child that:

　• names the person who inflicted the injury
　• conflicts significantly with the caretaker's history
　• is unbelievable

For example, a six-month-old infant was brought to the emergency room with first and second degree burns of the face and buttocks. The caretaker said the child had pulled a pan of boiling water from the stove onto himself two days prior to their coming to the hospital. The six-month-old was unable to pull himself to a standing position; the burns were located in such an area of the body that they could not have occurred from a single accident: the burns were from two separate occurrences and the caretaker delayed in seeking medical assistance. On further questioning, the parent said the burns occurred when their pet cat jumped on the stove and overturned a pot of water.

Observation. Although parents and children react in different ways to stressful situations, there are some important observations the nurse can make. The following list illustrates some important behaviors.[6] When the parent:

- does not touch, look at, or make attempts to comfort the child
- reacts inappropriately to the severity of the injury
- shows loss of control or is overly controlled
- is detached or cannot be located
- overtly rejects the child

When the child:

- is apparently poorly cared for—dirty and/or inappropriately dressed
- is fearful of adults
- becomes frightened when another child cries
- comforts and gives care to the parent (role reversal)
- remains stoic during painful procedures
- is self-absorbed and does not seek comfort
- demonstrates indiscriminate affection to strangers

Physical Findings. Physical findings are often present from falls and other accidents and may be difficult to differentiate from nonaccidental injury. However, there are some physical findings that are frequently associated with abuse and neglect.[4] The following is a list of important physical findings:

- multiple injuries in various stages of healing (old and new injuries)
- injuries that are present which were not mentioned in the history
- strange appearing skin injuries such as strap and/or buckle marks, rope or cord markings,

cigarette burns
- circumoral bruising
- contusions of all descriptions
- ruptured abdominal organs
- an injury that is inadequately treated
- dehydration and/or malnutrition without obvious cause
- multiple fractures in various stages of healing
- fractures in a child less than one year of age
- gonorrhea
- bruises on or near the genitalia, vaginal bruises and tears
- subdural hematoma
- retinal hemorrhages, bruising around the eye

For example, late in the summer a public health nurse was performing follow-up vision screening tests on children who had been absent from a Head Start Program when other children had been tested. While testing a small, shy five-year-old girl, a bruise on the child's arm made the nurse pause. It was not particularly different from bruises seen on children of this age. Something, perhaps the location, created a "gut feeling." She unbuttoned the back of the girl's sundress and found the child's back covered with old scars, including a buckle mark and the imprint of an iron, there were no other new injuries. A protective service worker was notified (the person responsible for receiving reports in that state), the nurse in the school in which the child would be attending kindergarten was alerted by letter to make home visits for all absenteeism, but the nurse failed to refer the child to a medical center. The outcome of the referral to protective service is not known.

The following are physical signs frequently found in neglect:[10] surrender positioning, floppy legs, lack of visual affect, no snuggling when held, lack of social initiative and responses, uncharacteristic vocalizations, reluctance to reach for objects, rumination, rocking behavior, lack of purposefulness and specificity in behavior, and a lack of anticipatory excitement when someone reaches for the baby.

Differential Testing and Examination. Differential tests and examinations should be performed on suspected cases of child abuse and neglect in order to confirm the diagnosis. X-ray studies, such as a skeletal survey, can be diagnostic and uncover additional fractures. Bleeding and clotting times can rule out blood dyscrasias. Developmental testing such as the Bayley determines the extent of delay. Consultation with members of other disciplines such as social workers and psychologists helps to understand the factors that led to abuse or neglect.

Treatment

Once abuse or neglect has been confirmed, approaches must be carefully planned that are most beneficial for the child, the parents, and the family as a whole.

Special Considerations for the Nurse. The nurse may have difficulty in establishing a therapeutic relationship with the family due, in part, to the previously described personality of the parent but, even more significantly, to the feelings these parents stimulate in the professional.

Working with abusive and at-risk families is stressful, demanding work. Parental inability to trust, impulsivity, isolation, and other characteristics require that those offering help do so with a commitment to be available, flexible, and willing to provide continuity of care. Although the parents may break appointments, be chronically late, or not return calls, the nurse must be consistent in following through on commitments and promises made to the family. Follow-up and continual evidence of concern and involvement are critical. Gestures such as a phone call or hand-written note may be novel experiences for these parents and could be vital in underscoring the sincerity of one's commitment.

The anger and outrage one experiences in reaction to child abuse are real and natural. Regardless of how long one works with abusing parents, anger is almost inevitably part of the initial reaction and must be resolved before the professional will be able to help the family. Looking beyond the actual abusive incident to the abused child within the parent often makes it possible to extend compassion to both the child and the parent.

The difficulty of this work requires that the nurse have available supportive colleagues who can help in problem solving and evaluating one's practice. Simultaneously, the availability of other more immediately rewarding work, such as teaching, research, or other less difficult patients, may help reduce the stress experienced by the nurse.

Hospitalization. The hospital emergency room is the location where most abuse is first identified. Some of these children clearly require hospitalization either because of their injuries or for further diagnostic work. A significant number of abused children are admitted to the hospital to remove them from a potentially volatile home situation rather than because of medical concerns. In these situations the hospital is functioning as a protective environment providing time to mobilize other community resources such as foster care.

Valid questions can be raised regarding the appropriateness of these essentially "social" hospitalizations. The precipitous separation of the child from his family forces him to deal with not only the stress of the abuse and the abusive environment but also the separation from the parents and the highly stressful experience of the pediatric hospital unit.

Regardless of the reason for the hospitalization, whether medical or social, the needs of the hospitalized abused child present the nurse with some unique problems as well as opportunities for therapeutic intervention.

Crisis Related to Hospitalization. Hospitalization of the abused child is a crisis for both the child and parents. The precipitating crisis at home, the injury of the child, identification of the child as abused, hospitalization, and police involvement are among the factors creating an overwhelming crisis for the family.

A primary principle of crisis theory is that interventions at a time of crisis may have the greatest potential for having a meaningful impact. Thus it is clear that the nurse in the emergency room or the pediatric unit can play a critical role in helping both the child and parent. Maximizing nursing effectiveness requires that the nurse deal with feelings about child abuse and understand the dynamics involved.

In working with these families one must be

aware of the parent's extreme sensitivity to rejection and criticism. As much as possible one must be aware not only of verbal communication but equally of tone, facial expression, looks, and other body language. Unresolved feelings will often be expressed in these ways and can prove devastating to a beginning trusting relationship.

Nursing Goals for the Hospitalized Child. The goals of nursing interventions for the hospitalized abused child and parents include:

1. "Setting a tone of treatment rather than one of punishment.
2. Promoting a sense of parental adequacy.
3. Supporting strengths of the parent-child relationship.
4. Decreasing the trauma of hospitalization for child and parents.
5. Identifying needs of parents and child and sharing these with the team.
6. Promoting the child's return to wellness.
7. Implementing principles of crisis intervention.
8. Modeling for parents and the child alternate ways of handling behaviors, feelings, and interactions with others."[8]*

Nursing Interventions for the Hospitalized Child. The following nursing interventions facilitate achieving these goals. These approaches are essential in the nursing care plan.[8]

Nursing history: In taking a nursing history the nurse can begin to establish a positive relationship with the parents. In collecting the data, she can assess their knowledge of child development, support strengths identified, and communicate an appreciation and recognition of them as the child's parents. Through asking questions relative to the child's needs such as sleep rituals and food preferences the nurse illustrates that children have individual needs that should be recognized and met. Obtaining this data must be done with sensitivity to the stresses the parents are experiencing and recorded with accuracy.

---

*Copyright © 1976, the American Journal of Nursing Company. Reproduced with permission of MCN, The American Journal of Maternal-Child Nursing, March/April, Vol 1, #2 p. 119.

Orientation to the unit: The uncertainty that pervades the hospitalization of a child requires that the nurse take an active role in helping parents feel comfortable visiting their child and in participating in his care when possible.

Continued nursing observations: Nursing observations of parent-child and parent-professional interactions can provide valuable data for both diagnostic and planning purposes.

Consistent nursing care: Both the child and parents may have problems in relating to and trusting others that can only be dealt with when provided an opportunity to work with selected personnel. Specific primary nursing strategies discussed in Chapter 23 are valuable for the abusive family.

Preparation for procedures: Consistent with maintaining the principles of good pediatric nursing care, both children and their parents must be informed of and involved in preparation for procedures.

Management of child's and parent's behavior: Abused children and parents may present unit staff with a wide range of perplexing and troublesome behaviors. The nurse, in collaboration with the child abuse team and other resources, must be prepared to formulate appropriate ways of dealing with these behaviors that ensure consistent and therapeutic management. Adaptations of behavioral modification may prove useful in dealing with some of these issues.

Protection of privacy and confidentiality: Child abuse is a topic easily sensationalized. Visits by police and others to the nursing unit only tend to attract unnecessary attention and undermine sensitive care. Discussion of the child or family should be related to nursing care, based on fact, and addressed to appropriate sources.

Preparation for discharge or placement: Whether discharged to home, a foster home, or institutional placement, both the child and parents need support and help in making the transition and preparing for the next phase of intervention and treatment. Collaboration with the community-based nurse is particularly critical at this point.

Participation and multidisciplinary team: The nurse's observations and recommendations are necessary for team planning and the development of consistent interventions by the entire team.

Community Resources

The nurse uses the resources in the community which will help troubled families and acts as a catalyst for the development of new resources.

General Resources. There are many general services which, although not specifically designed for the abusive family, may prove helpful. As parents' needs change and their willingness to accept additional services grows, different combinations of resources will be required. These may include individual psychotherapy, group therapy, marital counseling, social case work, pastoral counseling, child psychotherapy, parenting classes, and services designed for the physically or emotionally handicapped child. Others may require services for their medical or psychological problems, such as drug rehabilitation centers, Alcoholics Anonymous, or psychiatric hospitalization.

Although the parent may be fearful of these sources of help, the nurse may gain the family's confidence to the point of accepting suggestions regarding these resources. Approaches that are helpful in obtaining parental acceptance of needed services vary.

For example, one nurse accompanied an intellectually impaired parent to agencies to help her fill out forms, the parent was then able to accept a teaching homemaker and a therapeutic nursery. In another case, a nurse visited a mother (with a history of neglecting her children) while the mother was hospitalized. During that visit the mother was able to accept the need for and followed through with psychiatric intervention.

Among the most readily available and beneficial general resources in the community are day care centers and preschools. Not only do they remove the child from a harmful environment several hours a day, but they also temporarily relieve the parent from the stress of child-rearing. Preschools in addition can be viewed as the child's group therapy—learning new skills and relating to peers and adults in healthy ways.

Specific Resources. In some communities pro-

grams have been developed specifically to meet the needs of the abused child and the family. Although these services are not readily available in all cities and rural areas, the passage of P.L. 93-247 (the Child Abuse Prevention and Treatment Act of 1973) has encouraged the development of child abuse programs in communities in need of specific services. Nurses play an important role in identifying the need for, planning, and referring families to these resources.

1. **Crisis nurseries** are designed to provide a safe environment during times of family crisis. Their primary goal is to prevent child abuse. A necessary component is that the nursery is available to receive children 24 hours a day, seven days a week. Personnel skilled in crisis management and child development and knowledgeable about child abuse are suggested prerequisites for staff.

2. **Parents Anonymous,** similar in concept to Alcoholics Anonymous, has been highly acceptable to parents who will not accept other forms of therapeutic intervention. Parents sharing similar problems help each other by outreach and discussion without dominance by professionals.

3. **Lay therapy** is a type of service generally linked to a treatment center. These paraprofessionals work directly with parents, generally in their homes and over an extended period of time. Their intervention involves an enormous amount of outreach, including assisting these parents in acquiring necessary services, providing transportation, and accompanying parents to appointments. The fundamental service is to provide a trustworthy relationship that provides nurturing to the parent. The lay therapists are usually selected according to the criteria of having raised children successfully and having experienced healthy and nurturing parenting as children.

4. **Residential Treatment Centers** are designed to provide residential treatment for the entire family. Some provide intensive psychotherapy, others focus on problems of child-rearing, and others on daily concerns such as budgeting and financing; some combine components of each. These centers are not widely available.

5. **Hot lines** are designed to prevent child

abuse by making 24-hour phone service available with a sympathetic, nonjudgmental listener who can refer callers to appropriate resources.

6. **Special preschool programs** (therapeutic nurseries) have been designed for the child who has been abused. Staff are generally highly skilled in child development and have available the entire range of medical, social, and psychiatric resources.

Evaluation of Interventions

The two primary evaluation factors, described by Martin and Beezley, for evaluating the effectiveness of treatment and the safety of the home are improvement in the parents' psychological status and improvement in behavior and attitude toward children.

Signs that the parents' psychological state has improved include decreased isolation, increased pleasure in life, increased self-esteem, ability to reach out to others for help, improved handling of stress and crisis, more realistic self-expectations, alternative ways of dealing with anger, fewer pathological interpersonal relationships, utilization of therapy and treatment.[7]

Improvement in the parents' psychological status is not sufficient to ensure that the child's needs will be met; there must be indications that the parent-child relationship has also improved. Signs of improvement in the parent-child relationship include the parents' ability to see the child as an individual, to enjoy the child, to have age-appropriate expectations, to tolerate the child's negative behavior, to accept other people's concern and affection for the child, to accept therapy for the child, and to demonstrate physical and emotional affection to the child without expecting the child to return affection.[7]

Nursing Research

With identification of abuse as a national problem, the federal monies now allocated for research in the field will result in new insights and improved therapies in the future. Of particular interest is the research that is being conducted by nurses. Dishrow, Dour, and Caulfield, nurses at the University of Washington, are developing criteria for the assessment of parents' potential for child abuse and neglect.[1]

The role of nursing in the prevention of child abuse and neglect is apparent. Research is needed to identify and document the success of nursing preventive and treatment interventions.

SUMMARY

Within the past decade there has been increasing awareness and commitment by communities to deal with the complex problem of child abuse and neglect. This new emphasis on child abuse has created a heightened awareness among professionals and laity that has resulted in increased referrals to hospitals and other community agencies to evaluate and treat these troubled families.

Nurses in hospital, office, school, and community services play a vital role in all areas of child abuse, including prevention, assessment, treatment, research, and participation in the multidisciplinary team. Nurses must clearly recognize the impact of their contributions on the abused child and his family.

REFERENCES

1. Dishrow, M. A. et. al. "Measuring the Components of Parents' Potential for Child Abuse and Neglect." *International Congress on Child Abuse and Neglect Abstracts*, September 1976, 97–98.
2. Galdston, R. "Observations on Children Who Have Been Physically Abused and Their Parents." *The American Journal of Psychiatry*, 122 #4, October 1966, 439–443.
3. Gil, D. *Violence Against Children: Physical Child Abuse in the United States.* Cambridge, Mass.: Harvard University Press, 1970, 135–141.
4. Helfer, R. and C. H. Kempe, eds. *The Battered Child.* Chicago: University of Chicago Press, 1974, 41–42, 61–86, 95, 107–108.
5. ———, eds. *Child Abuse and Neglect: The Family and the Community.* Cambridge, Mass.: Ballinger Publishing Co., 1976, xvii–xviii, 3–23, 335–338, 377–407.
6. Kempe, C. H. and R. Helfer, eds. *Helping the Battered Child and His Family.* Philadelphia: J. B. Lippincott Co., 1972, 65, 73, 103.

7. Martin, H., ed. *The Abused Child: A Multidisciplinary Approach to Developmental Issues and Treatment.* Cambridge, Mass.: Ballinger Publishing Co., 1976, 76, 143, 251–263.
8. Neill, K. and C. Kauffman. "Care of the Hospitalized Abused Child and His Family: Nursing Implications." *Maternal-Child Nursing,* 1, March/April 1976, 119.
9. Schmitt, B. and C. H. Kempe. "The Pediatrician's Role in Child Abuse and Neglect." *Current Problems in Pediatrics,* 5, March 1975, 7.
10. Robinson, M. "The Deprived Child in the Hospital." paper presented at the Clinical Nursing Supervision Short Course, Walter Reed Army Medical Center, October 1970.
11. ———. *Child Abuse and Neglect: The Problem and Its Management.* Vol. 1, Department of Health, Education and Welfare Publication OHD 75-30073, 3–7.

ADDITIONAL READINGS

1. Debuyst, C. "Etiology of Violence." *Violence in Society.* Council of Europe, Strasbourg, Vol. XI, 1974, 230–250.
2. Hopkins, J. and C. H. Kempe. "The Public Health Nurse's Role in the Prevention of Child Abuse and Neglect." *Public Health Currents,* 15, March 1975, 1–4.
3. Josten, L. "The Treatment of an Abused Family." *Maternal-Child Nursing Journal,* 4, September 1975, 23–34.

PERTINENT ORGANIZATIONS

NATIONAL
*   *Department of Health, Education and Welfare National Center on Child Abuse and Neglect*

U.S. Children's Bureau
Office of Child Development
P.O. Box 1182
Washington, D.C. 20013
Provides information on programs in individual states, publications and training materials.

*   *National Center for the Prevention and Treatment of Child Abuse and Neglect*
Department of Pediatrics
University of Colorado Medical Center
1205 Oneida Street
Denver, Colorado 80220
Provides a current and informative newsletter on child abuse prevention and treatment, *National Child Protection Newsletter.*

*   *National Committee for Prevention of Child Abuse*
Suite 510
111 East Wacker Drive
Chicago, Illinois 60601
Provides a current newsletter on the prevention of child abuse, called *Caring.*

*   *Parents Anonymous*
2810 Artesia Boulevard
Redondo Beach, California 90278
Provides information on the services and how to establish Parents Anonymous groups in the community.

LOCAL
*   Community hot lines, day care centers, and religious organizations.

The Drug Abuse Parent

Carol Edgerton Mitchell, R.N., M.N.

CHAPTER FOURTEEN

The thought of drug abuse invokes images that are ominous and loosely defined: a house burglarized to support someone's heroin habit, a high school sophomore popping barbiturates, a skid row derelict unconscious in the gutter, or, perhaps, an emergency room staff rescuing another amphetamine overdose. Seldom do the images focus on families, or even on the victims as family members. Seldom, too, do they incorporate the reality of drug abuse: the housewife unable to function without alcohol, the husband who alternates between amphetamines and tanquilizers, their son or daughter trapped in still other patterns of "peer group drug experimentation."

Finely tuned to the communication of each of its members, a family system is remarkably sensitive to the implications of drug abuse. Substance misuse, especially when it is of the psychoactive drugs (methamphetamines, alcohol, barbiturates, narcotics, and hallucinogens) translates into an abundance of physical, emotional, and social problems. Each problem becomes an insidious and insistent stressor to the family system, amplifying other problem areas both for the family as a unit and for each of its members.

With a professional goal of health promotion, nurses are committed to detection, assessment, intervention, and evaluation of the various family health problem areas, including drug abuse. Working with individuals and families, in general hospital units, emergency rooms, outpatient clinics, school and industrial health offices, mental health clinics, and community agencies, nurses are involved in almost every phase of prevention and treatment.

BASIC CONCEPTS OF DRUG ABUSE AND ITS EFFECTS ON THE FAMILY

Perhaps there is no substance without present or historical evidence of being distorted into abuse. Sometimes through ignorance or disregard of the danger, or, perhaps, as either a challenge or mockery of its evident hazard, use becomes misuse and the user becomes the used.

The intensity of the repercussions from abuse on both the abuser and the whole interacting family system will vary some-what according to the particular drug involved. The degree to which its usage is socially sanctioned—or stigmatized—will greatly influence perceptions of its abuse. The ensuing messages given to, and by, both abuser and family reflect these social judg-ments. All of the prescription drugs, considered medically and morally acceptable for therapeutic usage, are viewed with consternation when illicitly obtained for individual purposes. Also, if depend-ency on a tranquilizer is established and main-tained through legitimate prescription, its abuse may be considered unfortunate but certainly not immoral. It is primarily the illegal status of mari-juana that is reflected in our society's disparaging view of its usage while alcohol use, encouraged for socialization, is met with disgust, stigmatization, and legal consequences only when it physically or emotionally threatens others.

Our society's perception of the incidence of drug abuse will also modify its reaction to individ-ual cases. As epidemiology detects various patterns of abuse, the apparent threat inherent in each pat-tern will be translated into the society's response to the abuser. While alcohol, with an estimated 9 mil-lion abusers or "alcoholics," is both our favorite and our most devastating drug, its very commonal-ity dulls its threat.[4] We recognize its sanctioned position in our culture and hesitate to acknowledge its danger. Except, that is, for our children. A socie-ty's young represent its hope for continuity; a threat to their well-being provokes retaliation. Alcohol abuse is increasing among the young along with public concern with this segment of abusers.[2] A drug of even more limited usage, heroin is esti-mated to have between 250,000 and 350,000 addicts in this country, largely clustered in urban centers.[1] The drug is relatively expensive and largely sup-ported by illegal activities. Within this context, the related social message of fear and dismay are un-mistakable.

Understanding of the physical danger of the particular abused drug will also influence its per-ception by both the family and the abuser. Mari-juana, illegal but especially favored by groups of young adults, was described just a few years ago as highly addictive and physiologically explosive. Its use was socially interpreted as dangerous abuse and the accompanying stigma was woven into family tension. Both legal and social reactions have been modified as more favorable reports have been pub-licized. On the other hand, LSD was initially ac-cepted as "safe" and creative by the same age group but, as laboratory and personal reports warned of psychoactive problems, its usage has declined. This concern with physical effect can be compelling, though often it remains secondary to social threat. Alcohol, theoretically and experientially estab-lished as a serious threat to every organ system, is culturally considered far less dangerous than her-oin, which, like the other opiates, is both toxic and addictive but apparently is not organically damag-ing through long-term use.[1] Both amphetamines and cocaine can also be dangerously toxic, but the former, sanctioned for medical use, is culturally far more acceptable than the latter.

Terminology also makes a difference. Health professionals, accustomed to subtle levels of differ-entiation, recognize that "tolerance" refers to an organism's metabolic adjustment to a substance, an adjustment that will necessitate larger and larger quantities of the drug to create the same effect. Physical dependence or addiction means that the organism has come to require the substance for "normal" function and forewarns of withdrawal problems in the drug's absence. Further, even as the substance has been experienced as a buffer from psychic pain, so will the need for its special "as-sistance" with problem solving grow into emo-tional dependency. It is this emotional dependency, interwoven with physical addiction, that results in "dependency." Drug tolerance, addiction, and de-pendency—the nomenclature may communicate to the professionals, but it obscures the message for the public. "Drugs" suggest overdose and addic-tion; "medicine" is linked with "therapy"; and "drinking" means that someone is having a good time.

Partly because of this confusion and stereo-typed reaction to the very word "addiction," and partly because the physiological dependence, basic to its proper use, is often obscure, the term "addiction" has generally given way to "abuse." Cutting through professional language with a clear message, abuse more vividly suggests the harmful physical and emotional consequences of drug misuse. It also bypasses the controversial area of etiology and better acknowledges the circular cause-effect-cause relationship of drug abuse that represents our working problem, for the etiology of a dependency on barbiturates, or any other drug, is less important than the complex of interacting physical, emotional, and cultural conditions that encourage its continuation. It is this painful continuous complex, a dynamic spiral rather than a specific instance, that is central to the challenge of drug abuse.

PHYSICAL DIFFICULTIES FOR THE SYMPTOMATIC MEMBER OF THE FAMILY

Difficulties associated with drug abuse of the individual family member will quickly become generalized into family system difficulties such as those listed in Figure 14-1. Of the myriad of particular problem areas, the physical difficulty is most accessible to health interventions. Perhaps, too, the area of legal difficulties may initially seem most clear-cut while psychosocial difficulties appear most painful. In reality, all areas defy neat categorization. The same dynamic spiral that blends cause into effect is evident here; difficulties with motor coordination, as an effect of drug use, may lead to second degree burns of the hand, further decreasing physical dexterity, and may eventually result in an automobile accident or household fire. Acknowledging this tendency toward spread, four fairly well-defined areas of physical difficulty do emerge: drug specific physical difficulties, difficulties with nutrition, difficulties arising from alterations in coordination, difficulties with pregnancy.

Drug Specific Physical Difficulties

Associated with and aggravated by a tendency toward generally poor hygiene, victims of

Figure 14-1. Difficulties of Drug Abuse

For the Symptomatic Family Member
  Physical difficulties
    drug specific
    nutritional
    alterations in coordination
    pregnancy—fetal alcohol syndrome
  Psychosocial difficulties
    mood swings
    distorted reality
    secrecy

For Family Members
  Physical difficulties
    abuse and neglect
  Psychosocial difficulties
    perception of reality
    emotional confusion

For the Entire Family
  Legal status difficulties
  Financial problem difficulties
  Social isolation difficulties

drug abuse suffer various physical difficulties in response to their drug use. The pharmacologic properties of the various drugs will determine certain physical indicators of their abuse, while the route of administration will influence others. Local and systemic infections mark heroin's hypodermic routing, and irritation of the nasal mucosa is associated with cocaine. Amphetamines, chosen for their excitatory action, stimulate the central nervous system, increasing wakefulness while decreasing appetite. Physical fatigue and paranoia may follow heavy or continued usage; tolerance is rapid and toxicity leads to convulsions. Restlessness, excitability, insomnia, all the "flying high" symptoms associated with the drug, may present as difficulties. Central nervous system (CNS) depressants, such as tranquilizers, alcohol, and barbiturates, may further complicate amphetamine abuse. These "downers" may be used to moderate the excitation of the stimulants. For both, tolerance may be swift, dependency strong, and withdrawal symptoms hazardous. Abuse of both alcohol and the barbiturates will reduce motor coordination and mental clarity. In addition, alcohol is especially dangerous to the body's various organ systems: from brain to peripheral circulation, alcohol follows body fluids to every organ, and clients may complain of the drug's action on heart, stomach, liver, or skin. Opiates, including heroin, are CNS depressants with analgesic properties. Tolerance is rapid, dependency is persistent, and toxicity is severe; generally, the intensity of withdrawal corresponds to the heaviness of usage.

The various physical problems are not only the most conspicuous, but are also generally considered the most approachable area of difficulty. Concern for obvious physical health may be the practitioner's strongest ally in a complex family situation of discouragement and fear. Knowledge of normal function and awareness of patterns of malfunction enable the nurse to capitalize on this advantage and detect problem areas, assess them in detail, and intervene with appropriate referrals. Interventions include discussion of dependency potential of barbiturates, or the significance of liver disease as well as alcohol treatment programs. Perhaps there will be a request for consultation related to apparent tranquilizer dependency or any one of a full repertoire of other personalized intervention strategies. The crisis of an acute health situation may provide the strongest motivation for corrective action.

Difficulties with Nutrition

Alteration of consciousness, common to most drugs of abuse, is an underlying factor in malnutrition of the drug victims. Abuse, whether of alcohol, heroin, or barbiturates, generally is antithetical to both activities and interest associated with the "real world," and, as such, the preparation and enjoyment of balanced meals is quick to be abandoned. But, over and beyond this far-ranging disinterest, various substances interfere with nutrition in specific ways. Opiates, through their smooth muscle action, interfere with peristalsis, while stimulants, such as amphetamines, depress the appetite either as a sought for primary action or as a gratuitous side effect. Whichever, the drug abusing family member's disinterest in eating coincides with a stimulated metabolic rate that demands an augmented nutritional intake. The incongruency may result in complaints of fatigue, irritability, digestive upsets, and poor resistance to minor infections.

Alcohol disrupts nutritional balance through a variety of actions. An irritant to the digestive mucosa, it may trigger anorexia, nausea and vomiting, gastritis, and diarrhea. Its concentrated load of "empty" carbohydrate calories can initiate a weight gain accompanied by general malnutrition. This can be further aggravated both by the drug's pharmacologic ability to neutralize vitamins and its alteration of consciousness. Again, the abuser's complaints may include fatigue, malaise, digestive disorders, "ulcer" pain, fluctuations in weight, and susceptibility to infections.

Detection is the first nursing intervention for all of the drug-related nutritional difficulties. Based upon knowledge of norms and deviations from them, this detection requires a sharply focused assessment of nutritional status of all the family members. Inquiries that elicit detailed information rather than vague generalities make the difference. Amount, frequency, and circumstances of drug use are discovered and form the basis for nutritional teaching of both client and family. Motivation for change is inherent in the distress of the client's present symptoms.

Difficulties Arising from Alterations in Coordination

Coordination is influenced by all the drugs of abuse, especially the CNS depressants and alcohol in particular. Even while judgment deteriorates, reaction time slows, and the visual field narrows, motor coordination is measurably impaired by one to three alcohol-based drinks. While the alcohol syndrome has long been the butt of tired old jokes, it is this interplay of cognitive, motor, and perceptive distortion that lies behind the annual cost of alcohol abuse, which includes half of all our highway deaths, half of our homicides, one-third of suicides, almost half of all arrests, untold fires, drownings, divorces, assaults, cases of child neglect and abuse. All together, the economic cost of alcohol abuse totals $25 billion and the social cost defies enumeration.[4]

The symptomatic family member comes to the emergency room, physician's office, or neighborhood clinic complaining of scalds from spilled coffee, burns from unattended cigarettes, contusions, lacerations, and fractures from falls and automobile accidents. When detected, these complaints demand further analysis. It may be unknowing or deliberate cross-drug use (such as concurrent, and potentiating, use of barbiturates and alcohol), single drug abuse or, perhaps, a problem that requires referral for neurologic or visual evaluation. Whatever the underlying cause, the present health predicament can become a springboard for effective preventive health teaching.

Difficulty with Pregnancy—Fetal Alcohol Syndrome

If the drug abusing woman is pregnant, an additional difficulty is posed. Focus of current research, the fetal alcohol syndrome (FAS) is of considerable international concern. Initially detected in France in 1968, babies with this condition suffer irreversible growth and mental deficiencies as well as craniofacial, structural, and general musculoskeletal anomalies. Probably 1,500 American babies, one in every 2,000 births, are born with this syndrome each year.[3] While many details are yet to be discovered, it seems that a fairly high blood alcohol level, during a fairly short fetal developmental period, is causative. Safe drinking levels during pregnancy have not yet been established, but apparently six alcoholic drinks a day, especially during the period between three and four and a half months of pregnancy, establishes risk. Even one to three ounces of alcohol a day may be hazardous.

During prenatal care, the nurse incorporates detailed information regarding FAS into physical assessments and health teaching. The returns may be immeasurable. Mothers raising their FAS-crippled children have bitterly commented on how differently they would have managed their pregnancy, if only they had known, if only someone had told them of the risk.

PSYCHOSOCIAL DIFFICULTIES FOR THE SYMPTOMATIC FAMILY MEMBER

While many of the physical difficulties of abuse are specific to a particular substance, the psychosocial difficulties tend to be both more inclusive and more unique. Careful dissection may separate and identify them as individual difficulties, yet the various emotional and cultural disturbances of one particular drug of abuse may duplicate those of another. Conversely, the syndrome of difficulty occurring for one symptomatic client may never be duplicated, regardless of how many other clients are seen as victims of the identical drug.

Difficulties with Swings of Mood

Discontent with one's prevailing interaction style has long initiated drug use. Alcohol dilutes shyness and constraint, morphine disassociates pain, the barbiturates induce tranquility, and amphetamines "promise" elation. As individuals experience their mood of choice through their drug of choice, both their drug dependency and the certainty of their drug-induced emotional reactions increase. Clear-cut "have" and "have-not" emotional states are apt to emerge. Shy or bold, tranquil or distressed—these dichotomized affects then reinforce the individual's perception of consistent need. This reliability of the drug response seems comforting. Far less interpersonal energy need be expended, since greater certainty of effect is "guaranteed" than would be possible through natural, normal efforts. As the drug becomes its victim's preferred strategy for coping with stress, other more active coping strategies fall into disuse and the drug's abuse is perpetuated.

The mood swings between the drugged and nondrugged states can be uncomfortable for both the symptomatic member and the family. Love to hate, depression to euphoria; confusion and uncertainty will influence all family members. Family members will not know if their actions will produce praise or blame. Children severely punished for an action when a parent is angry may be ignored for the same action when a parent is euphoric on a drug.

Difficulties in this area, long suffered in private, may surface through complaints of the symptomatic member or of his associates, such as the following: "can't work with him . . . emotionally all over the place," expressed at the industrial clinic;

"can't live with her . . . emotionally unstable," stated to the marriage counselor; "can't teach him . . ." at the school health office. The complaints mirror individual difficulties. Nursing interventions to identify family difficulties center on clear communication. When the nurse picks up oblique references to a problem of this kind, it is important to openly restate what has been heard, say a little about open and adaptive communication, and then encourage client or family members to identify their related concerns. Mention of community services available and, perhaps, provision of leaflets or phone numbers "that might be useful" can also facilitate a problem-solving approach to a troublesome family concern.

Difficulties with Distorted Reality

As mood alterations are sought through use of drugs, "reshaping" of any aspect of reality can be pursued in the same fashion. Even when not actively desired, it is a common corollary of the drugs' psychoactive function. Cannabis distorts perception of time and space, somewhat as do the hallucinogens, and the opiates decrease visual acuity. Through its action on brain centers, alcohol rapidly distorts reality and is often the drug of choice for this purpose. While "choice" implies active decision making, many of the issues and difficulties surrounding reality distortion represent old decisions, decisions by default, and habits currently overgrown and obscured by their patterned consequences. The aspect of deliberate choice may have long vanished. In its place, the symptomatic family member is apt to sense an alienation from self-responsibility and will frequently express this lack of responsibility as helplessness. The abuser may then use his unreal "reality" of helplessness as an excuse for innumerable irresponsibilities, encouraging self and family members to permanently assign to him the nondemand role of "incompetent." The role is assumed with a degree of ambivalence—relief, but guilt and hostility as well; additional drug use may seem the way to cope with this, too.

The difficulties associated with this problem

include all of the pragmatics that can ordinarily glue a family system together: bills paid on time, steadiness in employment, appointments and responsibilities met as scheduled, support services such as laundry, meal preparation, and child care provided as expected. When discharge of these responsibilities becomes a "maybe" thing, the family becomes "unglued." The system's confusion and disorganization may almost seem designed to encourage the symptomatic member's further withdrawal. Interventions emphasize both reality and responsibility. Nonjudgmentally, the nurse facilitates a delineation of reality and the sympomatic member's recognition of self-responsibility. "But who breathes for you? And who directs your feet and hands?" As simple cause-effect relationships and the distress that accompanies them are identified, energy may become available for adaptive change. Again, individually appropriate referrals may be the best nursing intervention, both to assure consistent follow-through and to encourage the initial change to be permanent.

Difficulties with Secrecy

Whether the drug is licit or illicit, secrecy will probably shroud its abuse. Unless the abuser is truly ignorant of the assorted dangers of the situation, he will attempt to mask its use. A possible exception might be abuse intended as either challenge or aggression, in which case secrecy would defeat the purpose. But generally abuse is embedded in secrecy, guilt, and suspicion. Classic examples include marijuana growing in the pansies and a whiskey bottle hidden in the chandelier. In actuality, little humor and much bitterness are associated with such subterfuge. As the abuser invests more and more energy in the mystique of his addiction, its protection and maintenance become all-encompassing. Intricate strategies will be designed to cover the time, place, and quantity of drug use. Since the strategies are defensive, they are also exclusionary, dividing the family into abuser versus others. A certain paranoia colors the abuser's perception—a daughter's frantic search for her missing school book takes on the significance of a narcotics raid. Suspicion breeds further secrecy, another downward spiral for the stressed family system.

Complaints of this difficulty are similar to those of mood swings; either the abuser or his associates angrily list examples of deception, defensiveness, and suspicion. Nursing interventions follow the same sequence as for the other psychosocial difficulties: sensitive listening, open communication, establishment of both reality and responsibility, and probable referral for evaluative follow-up.

PHYSICAL DIFFICULTIES FOR THE FAMILY MEMBERS

Difficulties with Abuse and Neglect

Abuse and neglect seem to be the major physical difficulties suffered by the family. Both result in human misery. Domestic tension, exacerbated by at least one family member's drug abuse, easily erupts as domestic violence. Trigger events may be innocent in themselves, but be perceived as symbolic of either challenge or insult to the aggressor. Other events may be deliberately selected by the victim to tease or torment the abuser. Their payoff is always harmful and sometimes deadly; placation may bring bruises or fractures, sarcasm may lead to homicide. The strategies and complementary roles of both victim and victimizer seem to be readily learned; children play them almost as smoothly as do their adult models. Perhaps because of their hopelessness and powerlessness, the roles tend to repeat throughout an individual's life span and into the following generation.

Physical abuse includes sexual assault. Perhaps there is no more devastating blow to a family system than such assault, for rape and incest stigmatize the victim as much as the aggressor. They are doubly distressing, through both their emotional trauma and the guilt and secrecy their stigmatization enforces. The victim may experience fear, helplessness, worthlessness, and ambivalent rage, while despair, confusion, hostility, and guilt may be the overriding emotion for the aggressor, unless drug-related reality distortion interferes.

Physical neglect, though lacking the explosiveness of abuse, may be equally corrosive. Usually vulnerable through the extremes of age or the helplessness of poor health, the victims include toddlers who have fallen from windows or down stairs, failure to thrive infants, and invalids unable to care for themselves because of chronic afflictions or to elicit necessary care from the drug abusing family member. A model neglect case is that of untended youngsters of an alcoholic mother, consistently left to fend for themselves. Even when physical harm does not accompany such neglect, emotional distress is usually present. A sense of personal worthlessness tends to accompany the experience of neglect, and to be further complicated by hostility and its close associate, guilt.

Nursing interventions for both abuse and neglect emphasize speedy detection. Physical and emotional safety of the victims is the primary concern. "Accidents" demand careful assessment, as do malnutrition and furtive half-complaints that hint at interpersonal fear or danger. The assessment, done with meticulous detail and personal warmth, can suggest the presence of viable support services in the community. Description of particular services available through the community's social services and specialized private agencies for abuse is helpful. Its intense emotional charge may be lessened by an explanation or discussion of the commonality and seriousness of the problem, as well as its potential for modification. Since the self-perpetuating pattern of physical abuse and neglect has its best chance for reversal if intervention is available during the period of turmoil, the accessibility of help needs to be well publicized; response to pleas for help must be swift.

PSYCHOSOCIAL DIFFICULTIES FOR FAMILY MEMBERS

Although interventions for certain categories of difficulties may be fairly discreet, this is frequently not the case. Psychosocial difficulties, although interrelated, can be identified.

Difficulties with Perception of Reality

Rooted in experiences of physical abuse and neglect, of the abuser's twisted reality and fluctuating moods, difficulties are inherent for the family members' perception and recognition of an objective and fairly stable reality. As the drug abusing member experiences, and translates into action, distortions of reality, the family system will struggle with its efforts to reorder their actual reality into a framework that can somehow accommodate the deviant member's deviance. Efforts may include denial, or "unawareness," of the problem area as well as rationalization, or elaborate "explaining away" of the situation. Such efforts, since they are further distortions of reality, may seem to be effective for short-term family consolation, but they tend to further complicate the situation for all the family members.

As children observe one parent incongruently reacting to the behavior of the other, they must question their own perception of what is real and what is distortion. As each family member observes the behavioral and emotional fluctuations of the drug abuser, the same perplexing incongruency is evident. Which behavior is real? "Is father loving and kind? Or is he a roaring monster?" "Mother was thoughtful, warm when we left for school—but now she staggers through the apartment talking dirty and crying." "John was himself when he left for work, and now, at return, . . ." Role models and behavioral patterns of congruency and rationality are lacking; in their place are role models and increasingly rigid habits of maladaptive interaction styles, of distorted coping strategies that seek chemical action for problem solving. As the patterns repeat, they encourage their own repetition; as the irrational replaces the rational, it becomes the New Reality. The ensuing self-doubt can be devastating. Unable to validate one's sense of the real through consensus with trusted others, the individual easily loses faith in his own perception. Members of such high-risk families may eventually abandon their efforts to sort out the real from the false, electing to trust themselves to the unthinking habit patterns that have been so vividly demonstrated within their homes.

Difficulties with Emotional Confusion

Emotional confusion interweaves with physical abuse and distorted reality to become an intricate problem for family members of the drug abuser. Our culture holds love and affection to be the normative emotions for family members; love is generally the root emotion between marital partners and between parent and child. As the cohesion of such positive emotions becomes distorted through angry encounters, guilty withdrawals, and transparent deceptions, schisms split the family system. The self-protective tendency is to isolate, to identify the abuser with the drug of abuse, and to wall them both out of the family system. If the drug of abuse is one that is enjoyed or tolerated by other family members, the moral judgment facilitating such isolation is especially difficult. If the drug is disfavored by the family though sanctioned by the community, or, easier yet, stigmatized by both community *and* family, the moral pronouncement against the drug is eased, but is still difficult relative to privileged family status. "Should I not still support/love/honor my husband/wife/parent/child? Is this not my responsibility, in spite of her/his bizarre behavior, which may be but a temporary thing? Indeed, am I not the one to cure this poor wretch?" Then may come the thought, "Is it really intolerable?" and, finally, "Or is it just the way I'm reacting? Is there something strange about the way *I* see it?" Conflicting responsibilities to partner, children, and self interact with conflicting drug and nondrug realities, become aggravated by the abuser's mood swings, and almost guarantee emotional confusion throughout the family.

The love-hate confusion of these parental and parent-child relationships is evidenced in many ways. Children's achievement in school may fall while all the "acting-out behaviors" of delinquency—as well as such self-defeating behaviors as compulsive over- or undereating and hypochondriasis—become common. The abuser's partner may experience mood swings almost as severe as those that accompany the drug itself. Such fluctuations as between aggressive hostility and passive guilt may translate into tiresome nagging for behavior change, quickly followed by another half-hearted rescue effort. The failure of this effort then allows further nagging. The spiral is the same: action and reaction, cause-effect-cause; the result is encouragement of intricate entanglement.

Interventions for Psychosocial Difficulties

Nursing interventions for the family members' various psychosocial difficulties are similar to those designed for the symptomatic member. The goal is self-responsibility; the process is reinforcement of the various members' confidence in their own perceptions. As objective reality is reintroduced through the practitioner's matter of fact description of what she hears and observes, the family members are encouraged to thoughtfully assess their own perceptions, trust their judgments, and take responsibility for their own evaluative problem-solving process. Health education's emphasis is on this self-responsibility as much as on facts and figures of health problems. As the family is introduced to objective data of drug abuse in this context, and considers its physiological and emotional ramifications, both the heavy moral tone and the sense of powerlessness evaporate. As the family members recognize the misery and the naturalness of their cause-effect spiral, their energy tends to become freed for more rational problem solving. The nurse may be able to initiate and follow through this process of change when she first detects the difficulties, or she may need persistent and consistent contact and demonstrated concern to even establish a foundational entry. Whichever the beginning, individualized referrals to local support services are often the appropriate follow-up. Not only must current difficulties be recognized and altered, but space also needs to be built into the family system to allow the deviant member to become reincorporated without permanent loss of status. If "ghosts of errors past" are forever to haunt him, this reincorporation is doubtful. The vexing problem of restitution and reinvestment needs to be honestly addressed.

DIFFICULTIES FOR THE ENTIRE FAMILY SYSTEM

Difficulties with Legal Status

Almost all drug abuse poses legal hazards for the abuser and, through system interactions, for the abuser's family. Illicit drugs, such as heroin, with their intrinsic risk of arrest and imprisonment for use, immediately come to mind. Other drug abuse, such as that of alcohol, is legal in use and illegal in certain instances of abuse. Public drunkenness, drunken driving, and alcohol precipitated assaults are illegal and subject to fines, imprisonment, or both. Such legal action not only threatens the abuser with incarceration, but also the family with all the various disruptions of separation and demoralization associated with imprisonment of a family member.

Fear of legal difficulties may restrict abuse in some instances and encourage it in others. While some individuals are concerned with the implications of these practicalities, others see the legal threat as a personal challenge and will either test the system with flagrant abuse or circumnavigate it through intricate deception. Others, suicidally committed to disaster, will use their abuse to ensure their own, and sometimes other's, destruction. Drug overdosage, drunken driving, and cross-drug usage may all exemplify this intent. Nursing interventions are reality oriented. Emphasis of legal practicalities and facilitation of appropriate support systems are central, and closely accompanied by legal efforts to protect the safety of others.

Difficulties with Financial Problems of Abuse

Another aspect of total family system concern is financial. From cheap wine through "under the counter" amphetamines to cocaine, drugs, in themselves, form a spectrum of budgetary drain. As the habit intensifies, the cost for "effectiveness" rises. Dependency dictates a central budgetary concern for the drug; shelter or food for self or family become secondary. Indeed, unless the abuser's wants are small and income generous, family support becomes problematic. In the case of heroin abuse, a 1970 study indicated that an average addict's $30 per day habit was typically financed: 45 percent through drug pushing, 30.8 percent through prostitution, 22.6 percent through shoplifting, 19 percent by burglary, 7.5 percent by larceny, 5.4 percent by pickpocketing and 3.3 percent by robbery.[1] With so high a degree of energy expended on maintaining a drug supply, not much is left for other activities.

A further financial constraint is posed by the various drugs' interference with motivation and performance. With motor coordination, cognition, and reality distorted, energy levels altered, and labile emotions, the abuser's demonstrated performance is apt to shatter cultural norms. Indeed, employment instability is sometimes the key to detection of drug abuse. Difficulties in the work world are such that alcohol abuse, alone, costs approximately $10 billion a year in lost worktime.[4]

As drug effect compounds the financial strain of drug expense, difficulties become evident throughout the family system: underemployment, another job loss, rent in arrears, a shabby personal appearance that embarrasses the children at school and the family within its neighborhood, carbohydrates replacing protein in the diet, health care inconsistent, dental care impossible. Nursing interventions, as before, are reality based. Threatened employment loss is sometimes the strongest motivation for reduced drug use; when realistically explored, this may be the factor that initiates adaptive change. Regardless, support systems will be necessary for dependent family members and alternative sources of income may be available for others.

Difficulties with Social Isolation

As all of the earlier areas of difficulty have suggested, family systems stressed by drug abuse tend to withdraw from the very support systems that might be of help. Both symptomatic and other family members perceive themselves as "different" and strangely inferior. It may be a moral note of character weakness, the financial reality of spiraling poverty, the fear of discovery, or the stigma of legally defined deviance, but whatever the apparent roots, social isolation is the general outcome. While this tendency toward withdrawal is accentuated in communities with a low tolerance for social deviation, it is present, to some degree, in all. How is isolation manifest? Perhaps through the family's brusque defensiveness, designed to counter expected rejection, or perhaps through passivity or uncommitted withdrawal. Children may distance themselves from peers or absent themselves from classes; adults may physically withdraw from community contact, drop out of their social groups, or, through curt messages of anger and distrust, emotionally separate themselves from former supports: friends, church, relatives, work, and neighborhood associates.

Intervention is difficult. Through isolation, these families have pretty much closed the door to their accessibility and seem to be, in spite of their apparent need, unable to invest any trust in a helping relationship. Accessibility may come through one or more of the other difficulties. As any of them force a break from the painful status quo, the practitioner can use this fleeting opportunity to encourage hope for adaptive change and to demonstrate the effectiveness of even initial interventions.

NURSING APPROACHES

Again and again, nursing approaches to the difficulties of drug abuse have emphasized careful general assessment based on a nonjudgmental analysis of the behavior patterns that facilitate or comprise such abuse. Health counseling replaces moralistic scolding and emphasis is on client responsibility for decisions and actions. Hope bolstered by the secure knowledge that this is another treatable health problem replaces both client helplessness and professional denial.

Through nursing's concern with holistic—

body-mind-environment—health, its practitioners have a great potential ability in the area of assessment. Yet, since assertiveness initiates and facilitates this whole process of analysis, this is an area where traditionally the advantage has been unrealized. As able health practitioners, nurses have an exceptional foundation of integrated physical and social sciences to support their holistic approach to clients. Professional assertiveness acknowledges and encourages the richness of this approach. Generally, various state nursing practice regulations also recognize and encourage this ability. Through the specifications of health counseling, nurses have a mandate and professional responsibility to follow-up their clinical hunches with appropriate assessment and counsel. Assessment and strategy guidelines from other chapters help the nurse.

Under the umbrella of assertiveness, a sequential approach to intervention is possible. With concern for the specific client situation as a given, mutuality of approach between client and nurse must be the next concern. Little more than resistance follows a unilateral, or "professional as all-knowing director," intervention. Such an approach parallels the unfortunate "rescue" efforts that typically mark the ambivalent abuser-significant other interactions and tends to decrease the client's independence and responsibility. As client participation is encouraged—and expected!—the likelihood of energetic follow-up increases, for no outsider can grasp the reality, or the potential, of the situation as well as its actual participants. While their perception may be temporarily skewed by anxiety and hopelessness, with appropriate facilitation clients will resume effective leadership in their own lives. This is the challenge and opportunity of mutuality.

Through mutuality, the nurse may establish an effective working team relationship with the client, but consultation and various referrals are usually necessary to fully implement intervention strategies. Knowledge of the community's available services (and the philosophies behind them as well as their various degrees of assessability) enables the nurse to nicely tailor referrals to client need. If she is a school nurse, she may consult with her young client's teachers, with the school psychologist, with family members, the family physician, religious advisor, and others. Client referrals, carefully considered and discussed with the client, may be to Alateen, to the school's vocational testing facilities, or to a reading diagnosis center. To maintain continuity and demonstrate interest, the nurse maintains personal contact throughout the referral period, checking with the client to ascertain effectiveness of the various connecting links. This team effort broadens areas of expertise and better assures the client of a proper fit.

Evaluation needs to be built into each phase of the intervention. Professionally indispensable, it can be implemented through a simple "How does that seem to you?" or through thoughtfully detailed checkouts following various intervention strategies. Such evaluations help keep the intervener on track. As other evaluations accumulate as final summaries, they indicate general directions that tend to be effective in the various categories of situations. Objectively detailed evaluation, a form of clinical research, enables the nurse to better generalize the successes and to more smoothly avoid the failures. Surely there is no area of health with a greater need to generalize and publicize its success than the area of drug abuse!

SUMMARY

The problems of drug abuse are intricate and pervasive. While most surely they will occur in mutations and complex interactions, rather than in clearly differentiated categories, they are approachable; they do offer an opportunity for success. Interventions can be systematic and effective. Nurses have a unique capability and professional obligation to intervene in the various health problems of drug abuse. Each success touches the lives of many, offering hope to others and freeing energy for adaptive change.

REFERENCES

1. *Dealing with Drug Abuse, a Report to the Ford Foundation.* Drug Abuse Survey Project. New

York and Washington: Praeger Publication, 1972.

2. *N.I.A.A.A. Information and Feature Service.* 18, November 26, 1975, 4.

3. *N.I.A.A.A. Information and Feature Service.* 39, September 8, 1977, 1.

4. U.S. National Institute on Alcohol Abuse and Alcoholism. *Facts about Alcohol and Alcoholism.* L. C. Hall (ed.). Department of Health, Education and Welfare Publication No. ADM 74–31. Washington, D.C.: U.S. Government Printing Office, 1974.

ADDITIONAL READINGS

1. *Alcohol Interactions.* Philadelphia: Smith Kline and French Laboratories, 1974.

2. Mitchell, C. E. "Assessment of Alcohol Abuse." *Nursing Outlook,* 24 #8, August 1976, 511–515.

3. Morgan, A. J. and J. W. Moreno. *The Practice of Mental Health Nursing: A Community Approach.* Philadelphia: J. B. Lippincott Co., 1973.

4. Parachini, A. *Reporter's Guide: Drugs, Drug Abuse Issues, Resources.* Washington, D.C.: Drug Abuse Council, Inc., 1975.

5. Presnall, L. F. *What about Drugs and Employees?* Long Grove, Ill.: Kemper Insurance Companies, 1975.

PERTINENT ORGANIZATIONS

NATIONAL

- *National Clearinghouse for Drug Abuse Information*
  5454 Wisconsin Avenue
  Chevy Chase, Maryland 20015
  Resource material and referral service for local and statewide programs.

- *National Clearinghouse for Alcohol Information*
  Box 2345
  Rockville, Maryland
  Resource material and referral service for local and statewide programs.

- *Alcoholics Anonymous*
  P. O. Box 459, Grand Central Station
  New York, New York 10017
  Resource material and referral service.

LOCAL

- *Community Mental Health Services*
  Information and referral of local resources for drug abuse.

- *Alcoholics Anonymous*
  Local groups with information and assistance for the individual problem drinker.

- *Al-Anon, Family Group*
  Local groups with information and assistance for the problem drinker's family members.

- *Alateen*
  Local groups for assistance to teenagers.

The Emotionally Disturbed Parent

Carolyn Hill Krone, R.N., M.S.

CHAPTER FIFTEEN

A parent's emotional disturbance has a significant impact on the family. Families often respond in many different ways to an emotionally disturbed parent, and any family can show more than one type of response. Family difficulties are not static; they constantly change and evolve as the family copes with their situation. The disturbed parent does not exist in a vacuum, but in a dynamic relationship with those around him.

The emotionally disturbed parent may not come to a psychiatric facility initially, but may be identified in other sectors of the health care system and referred for psychiatric assessment and intervention or for supportive services through community resources. Obstetrical and pediatric nurses work closely with families and can often identify couples whose behavior raises questions about their emotional ability to care for their children. Public health nurses are often involved with families in which a parent is emotionally disturbed. Nurses in any parent or child setting have an important role in identifying emotionally disturbed parents and assisting them in obtaining treatment. In addition, nurses can provide supportive measures to help parents utilize their strengths and cope with their problems.

The incidence of emotional disturbance in adults is difficult to determine, partly because it is such a vaguely defined term. There is no systematic method of determining who is emotionally disturbed, what kind of disturbance they have, and how extensive the disturbance is. It becomes even more confusing when you realize that not all disturbed people are in psychiatric treatment and not all of those in psychotherapy are emotionally disturbed. As an estimate, perhaps up to one-third of the total population of the United States may need mental health services at some point in their lives. Therefore it is reasonable to estimate that the emotionally disturbed parent is fairly common and that nurses may encounter family members with emotional difficulties on a regular basis.

In order to develop an accurate nursing assessment of a family with an emotionally disturbed parent, it is necessary to be acquainted with the basic concepts of emotional disturbance and the effects of an emotionally disturbed parent on the family unit.

BASIC CONCEPTS OF EMOTIONAL DISTURBANCE

Emotional disturbances are thought or behavior difficulties that interfere with a person's ability to function within the usual standards of society. Specific disturbances are characterized by different behaviors, degrees of severity, and duration of the disturbance. An understanding of these variations is essential to planning nursing interventions. It is also valuable to have some knowledge of the critical periods which may trigger a disturbance. If the nurse is aware that a family is more vulnerable to emotional disturbance than usual, she may be able to respond more quickly and effectively to the family's needs and perhaps prevent a severe disturbance.

Behaviors Characteristic of Emotional Disturbance

The emotionally disturbed parent is a person who varies from the acceptable normal range of behaviors by having changes of mood or disorders of thought. Changes in mood may range from a mild depression or unhappiness to suicidal depression or hyperactivity. Disorders of thought are irrational or illogical ideas and may include delusions and hallucinations. A person with a thought disorder may be viewed by family and friends as having strange ideas or being out of touch with reality.

Behaviors showing emotional disturbance range from severe to very slight abnormalities. Behavioral extremes include constant activity with little or no sleep and withdrawal marked by minimal communication and slow physical and verbal responses. Many aspects of daily living may be affected, since the organization required to complete tasks may be disrupted. In extreme conditions the person may not be able to meet his own needs for food and safety or he may be aggressive toward others. The disturbed person may have illogical or irrational thoughts or perceptions in which he believes he is someone else, has unique powers, or sees things which are not real. People with religious backgrounds may feel extreme guilt for an actual or imagined sin. They may be especially fearful or

suspicious and believe they are the target of some malevolent activity.

Less severe disturbance may be shown by heightened anxiety, feelings of depression or hopelessness, sleep disturbance, mild confusion, or inability to concentrate. It is often difficult to determine if a mild behavior change is a sign of a short-term crisis reaction or a longer term emotional disturbance.

Relationships between parents are adversely affected when one person's behavior is different from what is expected. Abrupt anger, crying, or other behavior which can be considered inappropriate to the situation may prevent relationships from developing and frighten the partner. Emotional disturbance may affect the person's ability to give and receive affection, which can have a strong impact on parenting relationships. An example of this would be a mother who feels extreme guilt for the illness of her child, which makes her feel like a terrible person who is unlovable. Any support and attention from her husband would be negated if not rejected because of her belief that she is unworthy of love.

Parenting behavior can be affected to the point that the parent is not able to provide for the physical care and safety of the children. Disturbed parents can overload children with input, or they may understimulate the children, depending upon the pattern of their disturbance. A major concern with infants and small children is that the parent, due to his own emotional difficulties, will misinterpret the child's cues for care and interaction. The development of effective parenting is based in part on the parents' ability to establish their role depending on the child's needs. The disturbed parent may force-feed the child when he is not hungry or keep him awake to play when he is ready to sleep. The parent may attribute grossly unrealistic feelings and motivations to the child, and respond according to that interpretation. In response to a young infant's persistent crying, for example, the parent may believe that "He's just doing that to harass me, because he hates me. He knows he has nothing to cry about."

Young children rely on their parents to interpret their environment for them, and parents who have delusional ideas or are extremely suspicious may communicate to their child an inaccurate account of what is happening (or might happen) in their world. The mother who keeps her curtains closed against imagined spies communicates to her child a sense of vulnerability in a hostile world and models the behaviors of isolation rather than social interaction. It may take the child many years to realize that not all people behave as this mother and that mother has a special problem in trusting others.

In less severe disturbances, the child is still subject to the moods and behavior of the parent. If father is experiencing pressures which keep him from sleeping, the family may experience him as being crabby, complaining about the children's behavior when he usually would not, uninterested in playing with them, and generally difficult to be with. Each member of the family then responds to the father in his own way: perhaps being supportive, helping him to relax at night, or perhaps being resentful, complaining about his complaints. Even when the parent's problems are mild rather than dramatic, the other members of the family are affected, and their responses in turn influence the behavior of the disturbed parent.

Severity and Duration of Emotional Disturbance

Although any emotional disturbances may potentially be serious, the duration of the disruption is often as important as the degree of the disruption. Individual and family interactions may be quickly reorganized or take several months to several years. Duration and severity tend to go together, so that the sooner intervention supports reorganization the more likely the potential for serious consequences will be diminished. Emotional disturbance can be grouped into three levels of duration-severity: 1) situational crisis, 2) acute emotional disturbance, and 3) chronic emotional disturbance.

Situational Crisis. An unexpected change for a family, a situational crisis, may lead to an emotional disturbance. This is generally of short duration but may occur frequently for the parents and

families presented in this book. A situational crisis for the high-risk family is usually precipitated by an external event, for which they are unprepared, such as the death of a child, illness of a family member, or a change in status or role of any member. The manifestation of a crisis disturbance may be physical, such as sleep problems, palpitations, headaches, or anorexia, or there may be interpersonal problems, such as marital discord, inability to perform the parental role, or disruptions in other relationships. Severe thought or mood disorders are not common in situational crises, but the crisis disturbance can lead to a more severe disturbance when the parent has coping behaviors which are inadequate to handle the situation. At times the parent will handle the situation with denial, such as the mother of a premature infant who does not call, visit, or make preparations at home for the infant. When a parent has had previous emotional disturbance, perhaps to the point of hospitalization, a situational crisis may precipitate another serious disturbance. For example, one mother who had had one previous psychiatric hospitalization responded to her three-year-old daughter's death in a home fire by becoming severely disorganized, and required another hospitalization.

Crises caused by external events of death, illness, life passage states, and role changes can be resolved with the family returning to their previous level of functioning. A family or individual can grow stronger and closer by successfully resolving a crisis, but there is the potential that if the crisis is not resolved, the impaired functioning can become a chronic situation. If the family whose infant has died suddenly continues to blame the mother because she did not take the child to the doctor for an upper respiratory problem, they may never reach a point where they can fully acknowledge their own grief, accept and believe that the situation was outside their control. Many months of resentment and anger do not strengthen a marriage or the parents' sense of competency in their role.

In a situational crisis the family can benefit from support provided by relatives, friends, and neighbors. Church affiliations and special support groups are often an excellent source of compassion, concern, and assistance to the family for resolution of a situational crisis.

When the family is separated during a crisis it is more difficult for them to cope as a unit and support one another. Hospitalization of a family member or temporarily sending the children to live with relatives requires the family to respond more as individuals than as a unit, even though this separation may provide necessary help to an individual. The more the family is physically apart, the more difficult it is for them to pull together, support each other, and learn new ways of coping with problems.

Typical family interaction patterns can be intensified by stress. A person who tends to resolve problems in his own head, without consulting with his spouse, may do this more during a crisis to the point where he seems to withdraw. A family who tends to scapegoat by blaming one member for their problems may do this more when they are trying to cope with stress. If a coping behavior works to make a person feel better, he will continue to use that behavior when stress threatens his sense of equilibrium.

Acute Emotional Disturbance. A parent with an acute emotional disturbance may have incapacitating mood changes, bizarre behavior, or peculiar ideas. The parent may be immobilized by depression—that is, he may spend long periods in bed or just sitting, be unable to work in any respect, be unresponsive to the physical needs of the children. In a different form of emotional disturbance the parent's ability to determine reality may be impaired. An example of this is the parent who fears he has a terminal disease when he is known to be healthy, or the parent who hears voices instructing him to behave a certain way. Impaired reality testing is generally referred to as psychosis. These behaviors are viewed as unexpected and inappropriate and usually reflect sudden, pronounced changes in personality. The parent may be taken to a psychiatric facility either as an outpatient or inpatient. With treatment, medication, psychotherapy, and a supportive family, the acute episode usually resolves in several weeks to several months with full recovery in one year. Some parents have recurring acute episodes throughout their adult lives, but are able to function adequately between the episodes. An acute disturbance is more severe than a crisis disturbance although it may also be triggered by external crises. High-risk parenting situations can be the triggering event. The previous example of the mother who required psychiatric hospitalization after her child died in a home fire illustrates this situation.

It can be especially frightening for the family to witness the sudden emergence of an unusual behavior in a parent, such as the loss of contact with reality or the expression of suicidal thoughts. The methods and language used by the psychiatrist, to whom the family turns in this moment of confusion and fear, may be quite unfamiliar and frightening in themselves. Many people make a virtually complete recovery following a single episode of acute disturbance, but the family may be so overwhelmed that they find this hard to believe. Since it is difficult to predict how long recovery will take, many people are alarmed when recovery does not occur quickly. They may begin to doubt that the parent will ever recover or become critical of the disturbed parent, implying that he could get well if he wanted.

If the parent is hospitalized or unable to perform his role functions at home these functions will need to be performed by other people. The nurse can assist the family in determining what needs immediate replacement, who can do it, and how to initiate the plan. When a spouse feels guilty for "causing the problem" he may try to be both parents or otherwise make up for his perceived contribution by doing double duty. The nurse can encourage the spouse that this is neither wise nor healthy in its extreme, and she can provide support for the parent and urge him to accept help from others until the home returns to normal.

The same resources of relatives, friends, neighbors, and church are important to the family with an acutely disturbed parent. However, many people are afraid of an emotionally disturbed person and may be unwilling to help the family as they would if the problem was a physical illness. Encouragement from the nurse that an emotionally disturbed person is not dangerous or contagious may help them become more comfortable dealing with the emotionally disturbed parent. Especially helpful is suggesting what specific aids the family needs, such as babysitting, help with meal preparation, or transportation to therapy. Community agencies may be necessary to augment family and friends. Public health nurses are especially good at devising ways of supporting families. The local community mental health center may have a variety of support services and people skilled in working with acutely disturbed parents. The nurse can make a significant contribution by maintaining a consistent and continuous relationship with the family.

Chronic Emotional Disturbance. An emotional disturbance can be considered chronic if the person has psychotic or depressive episodes which result in his continued inability to function in an acceptable role in the community. This parent requires multiple psychiatric hospitalizations or continuous outpatient treatment. Although the illness may be attenuated by medication and psychotherapy, the person may never gain full functioning. One type of chronic emotional disturbance is labeled by psychiatrists as schizophrenia. Usually an acute disturbance is differentiated from a chronic disturbance only through retrospective analysis.

A parent with a chronic disturbance has a persistent impairment in functioning, although not all areas of functioning are affected. It is possible for a person to maintain work performance even though he may have bizarre ideas. Usually he has learned to restrict expression of this part of his thoughts. With this continuing condition, the family often accepts it as the norm and just a part of the family member's personality. In many families a chronic emotional disturbance is regarded as a chronic medical illness such as diabetes. It may be a source of concern, but the family responds to the ups and downs, supporting and taking care of the parent when necessary. If the parent has long-term or frequent hospitalizations the family may learn to organize as if the parent did not exist and place the parent in a marginal family role.

Other aspects of a chronic emotional disturbance which can affect the family may include aggressive and destructive actions, restrictions of family activity due to morbid fear, and anxiety which prevents participation in normal family activities. For example, the parent who intermittently beats and injures the wife and children creates fearful watchfulness and perhaps avoidance by the family member victims.

Subsequent disturbance in the children is most likely when a long-term disturbance exists in the parent. The effect on the children depends on the extent to which they are involved in the parent's symptoms and the affectional relationship between them and the parent.

Causes of Emotional Disturbance in Adults

While there are a variety of causes of emotional disturbance, such as genetic predisposition and biochemical imbalances, the two most common and important for nurses to consider are psychological vulnerability and stress accumulation.

A psychologically vulnerable person has a weakness or an "Achilles heel" in their personality and, when subjected to certain stresses, may become emotionally disturbed. This vulnerability results from childhood experiences, relationships, and expectation which in the adult can become acute or chronic problems. Some situations are fairly obvious, such as when a person goes against parental expectations. An example might be the son who becomes a carpenter rather than a doctor as his parents had wished and encouraged. A person's failure to meet his own (possibly unrealistic) expectations can also lead to an emotional disturbance. Many sources of emotional disturbance resulting from psychological vulnerability are more subtle. Childhood environments often reinforce concepts of inadequacy or craziness. "You'll never be able to handle childbirth, you're too weak." "You're crazy just like your father."

Stress accumulation is a fairly common situation leading to emotional disturbance and the cause most likely to be seen by nurses. Most people have the ability to cope with stress up to a certain point, since their physical and emotional energy plus coping mechanisms, internal resources, and external supports carry them successfully through many problems. But each person has his breaking point, and nurses often hear a parent say, "I don't know how much more I can handle." Emotional disturbance may result from multiple losses of relatives, friends, possessions, or roles. People who are always taking care of others, nursing them in illness, solving their problems, listening to their worries, being the pillar of the family, are vulnerable to emotional disturbance if their own support needs are not met along the way. High-risk families are often victims of accumulated stress, especially if the family has been subjected to more than one stress in a short period of time. It is not uncommon for a nurse to see a family in which the father is unemployed, mother is pregnant, and one child has a chronic illness.

The stress accumulation theory of emotional disturbance emphasizes that not just one event but a series of challenges can lead to disturbance. Families or individuals may be assessed to be coping adequately with single events, but there remains the potential for breakdown if they are stressed over time by multiple events. The multiple crisis events of middle age, such as child-rearing and physical aging, put pressures on the middle-aged parent.

Ms. E was a woman in her mid-fifties, who was married and had four daughters. The oldest two were married but lived nearby. The youngest daughter was a high-school senior.

Ms. E had always taken care of the family. The oldest daughter had polio as a young child and Ms. E took care of her at home, treating her with hot packs as they would have in the hospital. Later, the second daughter broke both arms and required a great deal of care from her mother. The third daughter was mentally retarded and at age 21 was functioning at about a six- or seven-year-old level. About the time that daughter was four, Ms. E was pregnant with the last child, and because of placenta previa she spent most of the pregnancy in

bed. In recent years she had taken on the responsibility for the care of both sets of grandparents in their own homes.

Rather abruptly, with no apparent increase in external stress, Ms. E started accusing the neighbors of malicious deeds and generally became very disorganized and unable to manage her usual activities. She was hospitalized in a psychiatric facility for several months, followed by a slow recovery period lasting another four months. The family was jolted by her illness and very confused since she had been regarded as the pillar of the family.

This woman seemed to give until she had depleted her supply, and neither she nor her family had been concerned about her ability to handle stress. Her family not only were perplexed by her illness but had difficulty mobilizing alternate leadership to reduce the chaos. Her husband had never assumed that role in the family, so he was not able to step into the void. The older daughters were able to spend some time away from their families to help out and the youngest daughter did pick up some more home chores. The mentally retarded daughter needed the constant supervision that the mother had provided, and the family had difficulty filling in that gap.

Ms. E worried about things which were not getting done in her absence. The older daughters were the most understanding and supportive. The mentally retarded daughter tried hard but was often overlooked as a source of support. The youngest daughter gave considerable time and effort to stabilize the family, but she was obviously embarrassed by her mother's problems and did not discuss them outside the family. Mr. E was the most bewildered, as he had never given much thought to his wife's needs though he cared a great deal about her. He was at a loss as to how to handle her agitation and depression. The family members were very uncomfortable with her dependency and need for supervision. Mr. E began to wonder if she would ever recover and was greatly encouraged when she showed progress.

Because of her illness they began to discuss having someone else participate in the care of their parents and began to make arrangements for the mentally retarded daughter to live in a home-halfway house for mentally retarded adults. When they began to discuss these issues, Ms. E made steady progress.

Critical Periods of Emotional Disturbance

From the viewpoint of both psychological vulnerability and stress accumulation, the family may be particularly susceptible to the onset of parental disturbance at certain critical points in its development. For example, one of the most critical times for parents is the period of pregnancy and postpartum. Pregnancy, birth, and postpartum are a complex series of physiological, psychological, and social changes leaving both parents vulnerable to loss of psychic equilibrium.

Many people are psychologically vulnerable during this critical stage because of internal conflicts about childbearing, that is, what it means to them to be a parent, their expectations of themselves as parents, and what impact they expect the child to have on their lives. People may be psychologically vulnerable when the pregnancy was unintended or when the child will pose financial or social difficulties.

A pregnancy in addition to other stresses can push the parents near or beyond their ability to cope. A family who has experienced repeated stresses, such as illness, death, a recent move, a handicapped child, or loss of income, may find that pregnancy and a new child are simply too much to handle.

Women can experience the full range of emotional disturbances, both depression and loss of reality base. The disturbance may be a mild postpartum depression or severe disorganization requiring psychiatric hospitalization. Severe maternal emotional disturbance (incapacitating depression or loss of reality base) will have significant impact on mother-infant attachment as well as throw the family into a state of confusion and disorganization until they are able to arrange for care of the infant and mother.

Although there is not yet much literature or research on emotional disturbance in fathers during the puerperium, fathers do seem vulnerable to emotional disturbances during this period because of changes in role expectations. A prospective father may have difficulty when the mother needs more emotional support during her pregnancy than he is willing or able to give. Other fathers are unable to adapt to the inclusion of a dependent child in the family and refuse to perform fathering behaviors.

Primiparas are at greatest risk for emotional disturbance, although 20 percent of women having difficulty with the first pregnancy will have emotional disturbances with a later pregnancy. A large portion of severe postpartum disturbances will occur in the first two weeks, but many more will develop as late as six weeks postpartum. Since obstetrical hospitalizations are usually only three days, this means that many problems will develop after discharge.

Most pregnant women have contact with a health care system during their pregnancies and for well-child care after delivery. The nurse coming in contact with these women and their families needs to be alert to any cues that a disturbance exists or that there is potential for problems. In addition to being tuned into the problems of the family, the nurse needs to know where and how to refer parents for therapeutic intervention in their own communities.

Because of the critical nature of pregnancy and birth for the well-being of the family, and because nurses are frequently in contact with families during this time, most of the case examples found later in the chapter will be drawn from this population.

FAMILY DIFFICULTIES

Families can respond to the emotional disturbance of a parent in a variety of ways. Actually, of course, each family responds in several ways, but for the moment we will discuss several types of response as though each one could occur by itself. Figure 15-1 concisely lists the family difficulties. After considering some nursing approaches to the problems experienced by the family with a disturbed parent, we will turn to some case examples

Figure 15-1. Family Difficulties

The Family Ignores the Problem of an Emotionally Disturbed
Parent
The Family Makes the Parent the Patient
The Family Has Unmet Parenting Needs
The Family Seeks Help Without Direction
The Family Seeks Preventive Intervention

in which a variety of parental problems and family responses occur simultaneously.

The Family Ignores the Problem of an Emotionally Disturbed Parent

Ignoring or denying that a person is emotionally distressed can be a protective coping behavior. However, it is not a productive behavior. By pretending not to see the problem or saying that it does not exist, the family may find comfort, but the disturbed parent is then left with the responsibility for solving his own problem. When the disturbed parent is in this position, he may seek outside help on his own or be forced to escalate his behavior perhaps to the point of attempting suicide in order to elicit the attention of the family. When asked about the behavior of the emotionally disturbed parent, the family who is denying a problem may say: "Oh, she's been like that before, she'll snap out of it" or "That's just the way he is." Also, the family may emphatically tell an outside person to mind his own business and leave them alone.

Nursing approaches in the situation of a family denying the problem usually work toward the goal of the family allowing the emotionally disturbed parent to be recognized, assisted, or treated. While the family may never come around to seeing the situation as the nurse does, there are many intermediate steps which are still helpful. The nurse may have difficulty getting into the home or into conversations with the family, so her first task is to build some trust with the family. Building trust may be a long, slow process and the nurse must be patient. Once the nurse has established some degree of comfort with the family, she may begin teaching them about emotions and problems with emotions. When speaking about and to the emotionally disturbed parent, references to "normal" and "abnor-mal" are avoided. It is generally more productive, and certainly less judgmental, to phrase comments about the need for change in terms of being happier, more relaxed, more energetic, or enjoying life more.

Denial serves a purpose, and the nurse may not be able to eliminate it. When this is the case, she can often work around it. Alternatives for working around the denial might be to enlist the help of trusted friends and neighbors, their minister or priest, someone who has access to the family but is not regarded as a threat. If the disturbed parent is a threat to the children, and the family denies the problem, then the nurse may need to contact the local protective services agency for official intervention.

The following example shows the problem of gaining access to a family and establishing trust with them. Families with a chronically disturbed parent are often "closed" families who are suspicious of others and do not reveal themselves easily. The ill parent may be kept isolated from the outside world. The family may have developed a tolerance or acceptance of eccentric behavior. In some families it has been observed that a particular family member's bizarre behavior is subtly encouraged and more normal behavior is not rewarded. Family relationships may be distorted and the children may have problems moving between family and community.

Ms. D was ready to go home after delivering her second child, a girl, when her sister talked with the nursing staff, expressing concern that Mr. D would abuse the baby as he had his wife and six-year-old son. When asked, Ms. D indicated that he had been abusive but felt it was not significant. Ms. D was passive and dependent, slow to respond, but able to form attachments to her children and other adults. The father dominated the family. He had some rigid religious beliefs, which, combined with extreme suspiciousness and an explosive temper, had a very effective lock on their interactions with others in their community. This man had limited ability to form relationships. He consistently discounted his wife's and son's competency and convinced them of their inadequacy. His beliefs also interfered with his fathering behavior with the infant daughter; he did not believe she had any skills or ability to interact with others and therefore he consistently misinterpreted her cues, did not perceive them, and had minimal interaction with her. The father had many bizarre ideas and fears about women, especially concerning their physical characteristics. As might be expected, the six-year-old son picked up many of his father's ideas and fears, especially his distrust of people, which jeopardized the child's school functioning.

Mr. D's family felt powerless to help or intervene because they feared his temper. A nurse identified the difficulties in parental attachment and the father's explosive behavior and called on a mental health therapist knowledgeable in parental difficulties to help the family. Slowly the therapist gained access to the home and very slowly Mr. D allowed some trust to develop. Ms. D virtually bloomed when the therapist praised and encouraged her mothering behaviors. As the therapist consistently pointed out how the infant interacted and modeled appropriate interaction with the infant and older child, Mr. D gradually demonstrated positive fathering behaviors.

This family will always be handicapped by the mother's passivity and the father's extreme suspiciousness and temper, but the potential for abuse can be lessened with continuous support.

The Family Makes the Parent the Patient

Frequently, the nurse encounters a family which not only does not deny that one parent is disturbed, but actually seems to dwell excessively on the identified patient's abnormalities. The family who scapegoats an emotionally disturbed parent does so to avoid any responsibility for the parent's problems or to prevent awareness of other problems in the family. The family may insist that the parent seek psychiatric help for the express purpose of changing the parent to meet their expectations. Frequently, the designated emotionally disturbed parent is a passive person who tries hard to please others, and the family capitalizes on this personal-

ity. From an outsider's viewpoint, the person whom the family identifies as the patient may actually seem less disturbed than other members of the family. The rest of the family seems to have tacitly conspired to say, "He's the crazy one, there's nothing the matter with us!" In spite of their complaints and their initial insistence on psychiatric help for the identified patient, this type of family may abruptly decide that therapy is doing no good and refuse to let the parent continue. Such a withdrawal from treatment is likely to occur at the moment when the patient is actually starting to improve.

The nurse trying to assist this family may find that she feels very confused about what is happening. Because of the games that the family plays with each other, it is best to treat the family as a whole rather than focus on individuals. However, due to probable resistance from the family and the scarcity of family-centered treatment centers, the nurse may be the one to attempt alternative intervention. The nurse may have little choice but to work primarily with the parent who is the designated patient. In conversation with the parents the nurse would find out what their concerns are, what they want, and whether they feel "abnormal." In essence, the nurse switches the focus from "What does my family want of me?" to "What do I want?" Then the nurse encourages and praises nonpatient behavior, attitudes, and activities. Often the nurse finds that perfectly normal aspects of the parent's personality have been labeled as "sick," and her acceptance and support can help the parent to redefine himself. The parent remains a scapegoat only as long as he agrees to accept that role.

The Family Has Unmet Parenting Needs

The emotionally disturbed parent may leave a void in parenting if he is inadequate in meeting physical or emotional needs even though he is present in the home. If there is severe emotional illness and the parent is hospitalized, there will be a void in parenting. The family will feel this lack of parenting, and in some situations the family may become quite disorganized both physically—in meal, laundry, housekeeping routines—and emotionally, with feelings of shock or being deserted. The family may be able on their own to regroup, redistribute the parenting, or seek external supports.

When the nurse encounters the family who has unmet parenting needs, her initial assessment should include the family strengths as well as the unmet needs. In some instances the family can reorder parenting priorities, especially if there are older children who can temporarily do more than usual. The nurse might instruct and encourage older children in meal preparation or housekeeping chores.

When the nurse helps the family to help themselves they can develop a sense of competency in a situation that could leave them feeling very vulnerable. Therefore any assistance which minimizes the family's sense of vulnerability should be sought by the nurse working with a family with unmet parenting needs. This is a situation where the nurse must be creative and sometimes bold to find resources for the family. First on the list are free and nearby supports such as extended family, friends, and perhaps the family's church. Secondary resources might be agencies which have low-cost supportive services, such as public health nurse, day care centers, homemaker services. When the nurse is seeking out supportive services, she should be as specific as possible about what the family needs and for how long; for example, "The family needs a person who can fix the evening meal and do their laundry for the next two weeks while the mother is hospitalized." Volunteers will know better what they are agreeing to do, and agencies can make efficient assignment of personnel when the needs are specific and time defined.

Unmet parenting needs are illustrated in this example. When a psychiatric illness is associated with the birth of a former child, the family may feel especially vulnerable when the next child is expected. Preventing a recurrence is possible but may require advance planning and options for managing problems.

Ms. C had a psychiatric hospitalization after her first pregnancy at age 21, and during her second pregnancy two years later she was concerned about the possibility of it happening again. With her first pregnancy she had had no preparation and delivered in a small rural hospital with general anesthesia. She remembers some unusual thoughts about who she was and what she was doing, which occurred immediately after delivery and increased over the next three days, along with other symptoms such as not sleeping. Her husband remembered that he could not keep her in touch with reality and he became progressively alarmed when she would not respond to his questions and had a very distant, glazed look to her eyes. She had contact with her infant the first day but remembered little of that. She also remembered a severe, persistent headache and nightmares. Her family, upset and very concerned about her behavior, elected to hospitalize her at a private facility while an aunt took care of her infant. She recalls nothing of the first week of the three-week hospitalization. She was treated with antipsychotic medication and psychotherapy. She was fully recovered in six months but had a very tenuous relationship with the child because of their separation, first with her hospitalization and then his for medical problems unrelated to her psychosis. Her husband was spending his energy trying to work at a new job, see his wife, get acquainted with his son, and keep his home together. Other family members did help take care of the home and visit Ms. C in the hospital.

Midway through her second pregnancy she requested help to prevent another psychiatric illness. With the help of a mental health nurse, she and her husband reviewed their previous experience and its effects on them and their family. They identified key symptoms and when they had occurred, such as when she first started to have peculiar thoughts. They reviewed the psychiatric intervention and then set up plans for how to handle any recurrence of symptoms or feelings that things were not going quite right. They also reviewed their current life situation, their strengths and concerns. They participated in Lamaze training through which the combination of education, understanding, and practice made them feel much more in control and able to actively participate in labor. They requested that the mental health nurse attend the delivery. She was to monitor the emotional aspects and assume responsibility to manage any psychiatric symptoms. This permitted the couple to focus their energies for the labor and delivery and to acquaint themselves with their newborn.

This was an effective method of managing a potential problem. The couple were very pleased with themselves. As the woman passed each critical point, compared to her first experience, she gained confidence and felt more competent in handling her infant.

The Family Seeks Help Without Direction

A family may seek help for an emotionally disturbed parent, but they may not do this in a straightforward manner. They may not know how to describe the problem. They may not know about emotional disturbances or they may be frightened of them. When a family does not know that the problem is an emotional disturbance, they may seek inappropriate resources which compound their confusion. In addition, the family may not know where or how to seek help. Often the family will emphasize physical symptoms such as headaches or tiredness. When the family reports physical symptoms they may expect a medical cure with medication or hospitalization for rest. Many people assume that when one has a problem one goes to the doctor, he prescribes some pills and in a couple of days everything is all better. Unfortunately, many physicians do have a tendency to prescribe tranquilizers or antidepressants as the only intervention. Even if the family does recognize an emotional problem, they may not know possible resources or how to ask for help. When the family recognizes that a parent needs to talk with someone, they might first think of their minister or priest. If their problem is not of a religious nature, they might not follow through on that resource.

The nurse has a series of tasks to accomplish with the family who know they have a problem with an emotionally disturbed parent but cannot specify the problem and do not know where to go for help. First the nurse helps the family identify and describe the problem beyond "She's so tired." A later description might be, "She's been worried about her elderly parents, our last child is finishing high school, and she hasn't been sleeping past four o'clock in the morning." If the parent needs counseling but the family does not know where they can go, the nurse might begin by asking if they know of agencies or people from whom friends or relatives have obtained counseling. If there are no options with that idea, perhaps they could ask their minister or priest for a referral. If these ideas are not productive, then the nurse goes on her own knowledge, even if that consists only of opening the phone book. The local phone book will list the community mental health center, child guidance agencies, child and family service agencies, Catholic social services, marriage counselors, and psychotherapists. The nurse can devise with the family a method of approaching unknown agencies to find out if they are appropriate to help the family with a specific problem. Over the phone the family can request information about services, qualifications, and kinds of counselors, hours, and fees. Without revealing their name, which may be important to some people, especially in a small town, the family can decide if they wish to make an appointment. They can be encouraged to contact several agencies and the nurse can review the information and agency response with the family before they make a final decision.

The Family Seeks Preventive Intervention

The family who has experienced an emotionally disturbed parent or who fears that a parent may become emotionally disturbed may seek reassurance that it will not happen or look for ways of warding off the problem. The pain and disorganization which are remembered can be powerful motivators for seeking insurance against repetition. The family may have the feeling they did not know what happened or why but they recognize their vulnerability. When a family is overly anxious about the potential for emotional disturbance their perception may be distorted to make many insignificant behaviors seem to be leading to an emotional disturbance. The family may lose their awareness of the normality of fluctuations in mood, behavior, and physical sensations.

Nursing approaches would first focus on the past problem: what happened, in what sequence, what were the key symptoms, and what were possible causative factors? Most families have arrived at an explanation which makes sense to them, and the nurse uses that explanation as well as additional ideas from her own understanding of the situation to develop a framework of the problem. The nurse helps the family compare "then" to "now," and assess what things about the family have changed and what have not. The current and potential stresses are identified as well as how those can be managed by the family on an ongoing basis. The family needs to be encouraged to take care of themselves, perhaps to reorder priorities for investment of energy. The assurance and reassurance that the family is looking for might be in the form of an arrangement for regular or periodic monitoring which could be accomplished by a public health nurse. An additional source of insurance might be a written account of key symptoms with the notation stapled inside the family phone book of who and where to call if they need help.

NURSING APPROACHES

The nurse is in a position, regardless of the setting, to pick up on cues from families that they have an emotionally disturbed parent. If the nurse is acquainted with the family over a period of time, she can identify problems in their early stages or anticipate potential stress situations and help the family mobilize coping behaviors. The nurse identifying a situation might intervene directly with the family or assist them to find appropriate resources.

Assessment. When making an initial assessment the nurse should take note of all family members because the most obvious problem is often not the only problem. Do not be overly concerned with labels or psychiatric diagnosis, since the most helpful assessment will be one that describes behavior. A behavioral assessment more quickly shows what intervention is needed, when, toward what goal, and its potential effectiveness.

The nurse observes for disturbances in the person's daily activities, interactions between family members, and interactions with the environment. When one parent has been designated as emotionally disturbed, the nurse observes how the family responds to that parent and what impact the parent has on the day-to-day functioning of the family.

In addition to assessing the family, the nurse can examine her own responses to the family for useful information. Does she feel angry at them, helpless, protective of certain members, or afraid of the disturbed parent? This self-assessment will help the nurse to be aware of her own reactions and to identify the behaviors causing these responses. The behaviors that create negative feelings in the nurse may also cause difficulties in family members.

While the nurse may spend much of the assessment identifying problems, she must remember that every family has strengths and resources. Taking note of what goes well in the family, what they take pride in, and what they do cope with adequately will allow the nurse to encourage those aspects of the family to help them contend with the current problems.

Teaching. The nurse can teach families about emotional stress and disturbance to help them understand their own particular situation and to avoid future crises. The nurse often discusses how stress accumulates for families with multiple crises, the course of a chronic illness, normal grief reactions for the grieving family, family disorganization for families with an emotionally disturbed parent, and the effect of emotions on physiology for families with physical symptoms. In her teaching the nurse points out that emotional disturbance is not being lazy or weak-willed and applies the information to the family's individual difficulties and strengths.

Prevention. Prevention is a difficult task to

accomplish, but the nurse can make a significant contribution by preparing families for stressful events such as surgery, helping them to understand the course of an illness, listening to the family describe their concerns and experiences, and being alert to and responding quickly to a family's need for support. The nurse should be available to help the family solve problems, to give them encouragement, and to tell them how they are doing. Waiting for a family to ask for help may not always be appropriate as the nurse may assess a potential problem more rapidly, or the family may not be the kind who ask for assistance even if they are aware of a problem.

In general, prevention means taking mental health services to the people in the community. Counseling and crisis intervention need to be accessible and acceptable and can be made an integral part of obstetrical services, intensive care areas, pediatric services, and public health agencies. Mental health services can be effective by supporting people with low level stress and uncomplicated crises. Prevention is helping people build up and upon their health.

Crisis Intervention. The nurse uses crisis intervention techniques to reduce emotional disturbance related to crisis events. After an initial assessment the nurse arrives at short-term goals and appropriate intervention which not only can prevent further decompensation but also can communicate to the family that something is being done to help them. The nurse can begin crisis intervention before knowing if the emotional disturbance is a crisis disturbance, an acute disturbance, or a chronic emotional disturbance.

Primary Nursing. Vulnerable families, especially those with an emotionally disturbed parent, respond well to a consistent person. Depending on the major health care need of the family, a public health nurse, pediatric nurse practitioner, or psych-mental health nurse can function as a primary nurse to the family over an extended period of time. Some nursing services are formally organized to provide primary care even if it is simply that one nurse calls the family on a regular basis.

Counseling. The essence of counseling is not which theory or philosophy is used but a warm, concerned, sincere relationship. The nurse counselor usually depends on a verbal relationship and offers lots of support. Support includes encouragement, problem solving, and feedback on behavior. Counseling assists the client to maintain or achieve a perspective on his life circumstances. With the emotionally disturbed parent, a variety of counseling strategies such as those described in a later chapter may be helpful.

Referral. The emotionally disturbed parent may need specialized psych-mental health assessment and intervention, but it is imperative that all professionals involved with a family work cooperatively. The nurse works closely with the social worker, psychologist, psychiatrist, and other mental health counselors. With the permission of the family, information can be shared and comprehensive care plans developed. If an individual nurse is making referrals, it would be wise to check with the agency in advance to assure that the referral is appropriate and well timed. Depending on the situation, the nurse may make the referral or the family can make the initial approach. The nurse should not do for the family what they can do for themselves. Often the referral can be planned with the client so that it is a growth experience for them, taking advantage of an opportunity to focus their efforts and identify their needs. Also many agencies respond better to the consumer who asks for assistance than the professional making the referral on behalf of the client. Families who make their own calls are often more motivated to follow through with an appointment.

SUMMARY

The emotionally disturbed parent is a significant challenge to the family, the community, and the health professional. High-risk situations frequently precipitate emotional disturbance, while, in turn, emotional disturbances of parents place the family at even greater risk. Because the emotionally disturbed parent often has temporary or permanent changes in functioning, all family members and the family unit are influenced. The nurse can reduce the incidence of emotional disturbances for high-risk families by intervening during crisis events and can reduce the effects of the emotional disturbances on the family through early identification and treatment of the family difficulties.

ADDITIONAL READING

1.   Aguilera, D. and J. Messick. *Crisis Intervention*. St. Louis: C. V. Mosby Co., 1974.
2.   Anthony, E. and T. Benedek. *Parenthood, Its Psychology and Psychopathology*. Boston: Little, Brown, 1970.
3.   Herzog, A. and T. Detre. "Psychotic Reactions Associated with Childbirth." *Diseases of the Nervous System*, April 1976, 220–235.
4.   MacDonald, J. "The Emotional Cripple—A Family Problem." *Nursing Times*, February 1974, 236.
5.   Rodnick, E. and M. Goldstein. "Premorbid Adjustment and the Recovery of Mothering Functioning in Acute Schizophrenic Women." *Journal of Abnormal Psychology*, 83 #6, 1974, 623–628.
6.   Rutter, M. *Children of Sick Parents: An Environmental and Psychiatric Study*. London: Oxford University Press, 1966.
7.   Silbermann, R., F. Reenen, and H. deJong. "Clinical Treatment of Postpartum Delirium with Perfenazine and Lithium Carbonate." *Psychiatria Clinica*, 8, 1975, 314–326.

PERTINENT ORGANIZATIONS

NATIONAL
*   *National Institutes of Mental Health*
    Bethesda, Maryland 20014
    Provides research and information for the prevention and treatment of mental illness and growth of mental health.

LOCAL
*   Check with the local Community Mental Health Board for supportive organizations within any geographic area.

The Terminally Ill Parent

Jane C. Williams, R.N., M.S.W.

CHAPTER SIXTEEN

Today's nuclear family lacks the support once provided by the extended family. Society often does not provide an opportunity for parents and children to familiarize themselves with death before the crisis, and most people now die in hospitals where the family is fractured. As a result, families have more difficulty coping with the death of a parent than ever before.

The death of a parent radically alters the lifestyle of the family and the future of each individual. Although the family who loses a parent experiences grief similar to the family who loses a child, the former has special difficulties. When a parent dies the remaining parent has all the responsibilities and parenting roles without the support of a spouse. The children must understand the meaning of the death of a parent and cope with the shift in parenting roles onto one parent.

The nurse is often in an excellent position to help the family adjust to the death of a parent. Nurses in emergency rooms, medical-surgical units, and many community settings frequently come in contact with the family adjusting to the death of a parent. Nurses in maternal-child settings may also identify the single parent who is having difficulty from the recent death of the spouse. In addition, because of the nurse-family contact during the terminal illness of the parent, many families already accept the nurse as a person who is concerned for their welfare and may be willing to communicate with her about their family health and stresses. Therefore the nurse is often the ideal member of the health team to coordinate the services of many health professionals and follow the family throughout the grieving period.

The nurse's goal is to help the family members cope with the terminal illness and death of a parent by working through the grief and reestablishing effective family roles which meet the individual and family needs. If the family can move along together in the stages of grieving, supporting, and sharing feelings, they may meet the death situation in a deeply meaningful and growing way.

BASIC CONCEPTS

Heart disease, cancer, and accidents cause most of the deaths to adults in the middle or parenting years and place many families in the position of coping with the potential or actual loss of a parent. The actual death of a parent is only the beginning of the stressful experiences for the family. Although heart disease and accidents are frequently the cause of a sudden death, they, along with cancer, can also cause a preceding illness and anticipated death. Although sudden death is caused by an unexpected event and anticipated death is preceded by a prolonged illness, families experiencing both types of death often have common problems.

Shock and denial are usually present, since preparing for the death of a loved one is difficult regardless of the length or severity of the illness. Deep inside, people feel that death will come "to thee and to thee, but not to me," as stated by the Psalmist. The thought of death is usually frightening and is easier to avoid thinking and talking about than it is to confront.

Regret and guilt are common feelings for any family following the death of a parent. Family members frequently remember with sadness the days that were filled with disagreements or emptiness and experience guilt over their past actions. The words of kindness not spoken and the actions left undone become painfully haunting when a family member dies. Often the remaining spouse tries to reduce his guilt and make up for his previous actions through funeral planning. One family in which the father died from a sudden heart attack experienced shock after the death and guilt over things that might have been but never were said or done. Although the guilt has been reduced, it recurs at times even years later.

Along with guilt, some family members may blame themselves for the actual death of the parent. The survivors will often frantically search for the cause of the tragedy. Some wives blame their cooking habits if their husband dies of a disease they associate with nutrition such as a heart attack. The family member may blame himself for one possible cause rather than recognizing the many factors frequently leading to the event.

Sudden Death. The sudden death of a parent often caused by heart disease or an accident, fre-

quently creates some special problems for the family. Sudden death may be easiest for the one who dies and most difficult for those left behind. The dead person does not have to grieve; the remaining family is left alone with their grief.

Following a sudden death the family members are frequently confused, stunned, and panicked. They often need help with immediate decisions and needs such as selecting a coffin, making funeral arrangements, and eating nutritious meals.

Often, sudden death leaves members of the family outside the emergency room, in strange surroundings, with nowhere to grieve openly. Acknowledging the shock, allowing privacy or company for grieving, and allowing grieving near the body are important nursing actions.

In the turmoil of sudden death, the surviving spouse must tell the children about the death with no time for rehearsals on how to approach the subject. Honesty and gentleness are important from the first encounter with the child. Children should be included as much as possible in the grieving and funeral preparations, although the child should never be forced into doing something he or she does not want to do, such as kissing the body or going to the cemetery. Since the spouse knows the child's age, temperament, and how he has talked with the child in the past, the nurse can support him in finding the right approach for his child. The parent who talks openly to the child about his shock and grief allows the child also to grieve openly.

Prolonged Illness. Prolonged illness provides more opportunities and also more pitfalls for the family than sudden illness. When the illness is prolonged, although there is often enough time for family members to express love and complete much unfinished business, there is too much time for grief and pain. For some, the intermittent crises of prolonged illness are too much to deal with and the tension of drawn out suffering too long. Family members frequently find watching a parent in continuing pain more difficult than death and wish for an end to the illness. The pain of surviving family members is expressed in the many court proceedings where survivors question the continuation of life-saving procedures for their loved ones, preferring a peaceful death.

FAMILY DIFFICULTIES

The death of a parent may place the family in a state of turmoil. As one role in the family is left vacant by the death, each member must compensate for that loss. In addition, each member's journey through the grieving process may result in loneliness, confusion, and often frightening feelings. These problems may be increased when, within a month after the funeral, the family finds itself abandoned by friends and relatives who believe they have had enough time and support by now to adjust. When the phone calls stop, and friends do not visit as frequently, the loss and emptiness may become even more of a reality. Health care workers, who make a point of visiting a bereaved family a month after the death, often find many opportunities for intervention and prevention.

Like physical injury, grief usually comes quickly and unexpectedly. However, grief's wound takes far longer to heal. Although the grief reactions and process are normal and healthy, delays or other problems may occur to produce added difficulties. One young mother had developed a stress ulcer four and a half weeks after her husband's death.

The family situation is more complicated because each individual personality is dealing with grief in a unique way. There is no medication to reach the bereaved—no pill to fill up the emptiness, calm the loneliness, or quiet the fear. Human caring is the most vital source of support and healing that the nurse can give.

When death strikes a parent, many severe family difficulties arise. Some of these troubles occur early in the illness and time following the death. Others are delayed. Often the delayed difficulties are more critical as the family members become discouraged. Physical illness, insomnia, nightmares, suicidal ideations, and withdrawal are only a few of the problems. Children's, spouse's,

Figure 16-1. Family Difficulties of a Family with a Terminally Ill Parent

Children's Difficulties
  Perception of death
  Withdrawal or aggression
  Confusion about death
  Fear of loss of other parent
  Relating to peers
  Relating to parent
  Nightmares
  Physical symptoms
Spouse's Difficulties
  Grieving: anger and depression
  Saying goodbye
  Discussing death with children
  Funeral arrangements
  Loneliness
  Getting support
Family Interaction Difficulties
  Reordering of roles
  Effects of spouse's reaction on children
  Effects of child's reaction on parent

and family interaction difficulties are common as described in Figure 16-1.

Children's Difficulties

Children's difficulties are related to the age and temperament of the child and the environment in which the death of the parent occurred. The more cohesive the family unit was before the death, the more supportive the members will be to one another following the death.

Perception of Death. A child's age and level of growth and development are means of determining his possible reactions to the death of a parent. The reactions of children of different ages described below are guidelines for assessing an individual child's reaction. The idea of death grows with a child. A preschooler and a teenager, though both classified as children, look at death in radically different ways. Children need individualized explanations in accordance with their level of understanding. "What does it mean to be dead?" A reply to a teenager would contain more depth and intensity than an answer to a four-year-old. Both would be honest answers.

Unresolved grief, guilt, and anger can affect development for the rest of the child's life. Words that are spoken around the time of death often linger in the child's mind for years. The guilt, often present in adults, is magnified in the child's fantasy world and psychological framework. The complex relationship between parents and children often leaves the child with the feeling that he is to blame for the misfortunes that occur. Children may see death as a punishment or a result of their naughty behavior.

Birth to three: Up to the age of three, children usually have little concept of death itself. The very young child does, however, experience loss such as when the mother leaves, a favorite blanket is lost, or a parent dies.

Preschool: The preschool child is very preoccupied with bodily function. The child often associates death with mutilation, envisioning it as a temporary phenomenon. Television has reinforced this idea: the person who gets shot this week is on TV again next week. Most children experience death for the first time when a pet dies, a dead animal is found on the road, or insects are killed. Children at this age often want to dig up the goldfish they bury.

Because the preschooler often believes death is temporary, it is common for him to wish someone were dead. Adults are seen as all-powerful, making the child perform or behave in certain ways; the death wish may compensate for this. The death of a parent at this age is very critical because the child often takes the blame for the death upon himself. Even when a child has death explained, and is included in the funeral, the memory of the "I hate you" and "I wish you were dead" lingers. The child perceives the death as brought about by his own wishful thinking or bad behavior. A young child of seven was overheard praying that God would tell his Daddy he was sorry for being naughty. Then Daddy would not be angry anymore and would come home from heaven.

The ages of three to six also hold innumerable complex questions such as: "How will Daddy go to the bathroom when he's buried in the ground?" or "How will Mommy eat in the cemetery?" The child

will usually ask repeatedly when the deceased will return.

Early school age: The early school age child (approximately six through nine years) begins to personalize death as a skeleton or figure from a scary story commonly shared by friends. He is often intrigued by spooky books and television stories with ghosts and monsters. The child is usually concerned about details. What does the body look like after it is in the ground? Does the skin get real dry or does the body really turn into a skeleton? Do the fingernails and hair still grow?

Most children's experiences with death involve an older person. Death is viewed as very remote, something that only happens when you are very old. The child still believes death to be avoidable if one is careful.

By the age of nine, a child has usually developed his concept of death to the point of recognizing it as permanent, involving the cessation of all bodily activity. Now the focus is on social questions. "Who will take care of us now that Daddy is dead?" "Who will tuck me into bed now that Mommy is in heaven?"

Adolescent: Because of the emotional extremes experienced in this period of life, teenagers have a difficult time coping with death. They are usually concerned with deep questions exploring the meaning of life and death. Emotional states are very labile and crisis is not handled easily. When a peer is grieving, the adolescent is not usually very supportive and often avoids contact with the troubled friend. Following his father's death, a sixteen-year-old found his friends to be stunned and aloof. The friends were uncomfortable in his presence, abandoning him for several months following his loss.

Withdrawal or Aggression. Children tend to react in one of two ways: withdrawal or acting out in an aggressive manner. The withdrawn child, unable to express deep feelings troubling him, is usually in more difficulty than the aggressive one. In the midst of crisis, the quiet, good little child is forgotten or spoken of as adjusting so well. Often this withdrawn child goes months or even years without help. The longer the needs of the bereaved child are left unmet, the deeper and more enduring the problem becomes. A child who does not miss the dead is either too young or is having serious emotional difficulty.

A six-year-old child who had been included in his mother's funeral, and who was behaving very well, was observed placing an apple outside of his bedroom window each night. His grandmother noticed and questioned his action. "Mommy loves apples," he said. "I thought if I left one she wouldn't be mad at me anymore and come home."

The nurse and family members have to identify the child's questions and concepts regarding death. Once the problem area is identified, gentle discussion and repeated explanations can help the child release himself from blame. Setting aside definite times to talk about the dead parent, and being prepared to take time whenever it appears the child needs to talk, are important means of intervention. Reading children's stories on death is another helpful avenue for conveying correct information. Some of these books are listed in the bibliography at the end of this chapter.

The aggressive child's behavior is such that his trouble cannot be ignored. This child often acts out in school, beats up other children, or may perform severe acts such as starting fires. Unfortunately, the general parental response is often punishment. Since the punishment includes parental attention, it reinforces the aggression. A young boy became the terror of the neighborhood following his father's death. He beat up all the children he could catch. The public health nurse asked him why he beat up children. He said, "Maybe I'll get dead one of these times and I can be with Daddy."

The approach for the aggressive child is similar to the withdrawn child. Assessment of the child's idea about the meaning of the death, increased parent-child discussions and closeness, and realistic consistent limits for behavior are important.

Confusion about Death. Just because a child is told about the death and included in the funeral does not mean he totally understands and all his needs have been met. Death is a mystery to every-

one. It is extremely difficult to answer questions and no one's complete understanding should be assumed.

For example, a mother carefully explained to her six-year-old daughter her own belief that the part of Daddy they knew and loved was now with God. Only Daddy's worn-out body was in the coffin. Two months later the child was still wondering where Daddy went. After the distraught mother reminded the child that all of that had been explained before, she replied, "Mommy, I didn't understand any of those things you said."

Fear of Loss of Other Parent. After the death of one parent, children experience a deep sense of panic that the healthy parent will also die. For younger children, this often shows itself in clinging behavior. The healthy parent cannot get away even for a few minutes without the child reacting fearfully. If the healthy parent becomes sick or injured, no matter how slight, it is a very traumatic experience for the child.

This puts an added strain on the grieving parent. The nurse can prepare the parent for this behavior by explaining it and forewarning the parent before it occurs. Anticipated behavior can be met with understanding. Providing comfort to the child will bring about the return of trust. A child needs to believe that there is security for him. Fearfulness of being separated from the surviving parent can be lessened by arranging for a familiar person to stay with the child when the parent needs to be away. Telling the child the time when the parent will return is also important.

All difficulties have the potentiality of causing later problems. The sooner a difficulty is recognized, acknowledged, and dealt with appropriately, the less likely problems will develop later. Common sense is often the best guide. Each situation is unique and there are no easy answers.

Relating to Peers. Other children are not always very supportive of grieving children. Unknowingly, they often say and do harmful things. They may hurt the child of a deceased parent by making comments such as "Your Daddy was weak" or "You are an orphan."

Generally, teenagers avoid their troubled friend. The death of someone else's parent reminds them that they, too, could lose a parent. If there is time before the death to explain this to a teenager, and open the door for relating to other adults, it will make the grieving time less painful and lonely.

Relating to a Parent. During the illness, and following the death of a parent, children may have difficulties relating to the ill or surviving parent. This depends on the ages of the child, the parent, and their previous rapport. Behavior following a death is usually consistent with past behavior during frustration or crisis. Generally, younger children develop clinging behaviors, unable to let the surviving parent out of their sight. Older children tend to be more stoic and aloof, avoiding contact with the surviving parent.

The dying parent often requires family routines to center around him. The child may resent the dying parent, who has become the center of attention. On the other hand, children may become so solicitous and concerned that they have no time left to be children or maintain outside contacts.

It is difficult to discern whether the behavior is adaptive or maladaptive, and a real problem. The best measure is to determine if the behavior is moderate or extreme. Both the ill and the surviving parent should understand that these expressions of grief are normal. Together, the nurse and parents can anticipate grieving patterns by examining past behaviors.

Nightmares. The deep fear and anxiety that children experience at death is commonly expressed in nightmares. Their vividness makes it difficult for a parent to be reassuring. They may occur for a year or more, but usually become less frequent a few months after the death. Often the child must be slept with for many nights. Gradually, as the fear ceases, the child will go back to his or her own bed. Leaving a light on at night may help the child to orient to reality quicker than if he awakens in the dark. It must be reinforced that a nightmare is only a dream.

Physical Symptoms. The following is an example of how a child's grief may result in physical symptoms. A five-year-old girl woke up in the middle of the night, screaming and incoherently pointing to her vagina, indicating it itched. The sleepy mother tried to comfort her, but the child became more hysterical. Mom tried to wash the area, but the child stiffened and screamed louder, "I itch inside!" The mother said she would call the doctor, and the child's hysteria grew worse.

In desperation the mother said, "Be quiet, now, and listen to me. Mommy had the same thing happen to her." The child grew strangely silent. Mother continued, "I went to the doctor and he told me I was upset about something. You know how you get hives on your skin that itch? Well, that can happen in your vagina, too. Why don't we talk about what's bothering you?"

The child began to cry softly and said, "No one loves me. Daddy died. And you just holler at me all the time."

The mother was shocked at the radical reaction. She held the child, saying, "You are my beloved, my angel. I love you more than anyone in the world. Since Daddy's dead, you and Mommy have to try to help each other."

The child, listening intently, then asked, "Who else loves me?"

The mother named people who loved her, and what they did to show their love. The child quieted down completely by this time. Then they talked about how much they missed Daddy. Mother told her she was sorry for being irritable, but that it was very hard not having Daddy around. The child said she was sorry for being so naughty. After 45 minutes of talking, the child fell soundly asleep.

This is a rather dramatic example of a child's grief difficulties resulting in physical symptoms.

Spouse's Difficulties

The death of a spouse leaves one completely alone in a couple oriented society. Activities of financing, housekeeping, and childbearing, once shared, are now to be carried out alone. This involves the incredible task of being both mother and father and carrying out various other responsibilities of heading and guiding the family complex.

Additional difficulties related to single parenting are discussed in the chapter, "The Single Parent."

Grieving: Anger and Depression. Although men and women experience a similar grief process following the loss of a partner or child, there are unique difficulties. The remaining parent experiences the grief stages of denial, anger, bargaining, depression, and acceptance as described in the chapter, "The Terminally Ill Child."

Anger and depression are the two most difficult stages for the family to handle. Most of us react to anger by either getting angry in return or ignoring the anger totally. When a dying person's anger is met with anger, guilt usually results for both, especially the initiator. Ignoring anger allows no release and eventually blocks a person's move toward acceptance. Depression usually elicits attempts on the part of others to distract or cheer up the depressed person. Encouraging the depressed person to cry or express feelings is difficult but essential for assuring completed grief work.

The feelings of anger and depression are real and legitimate. Permission must be given to honestly express all feelings. If the focus is on helping one another and being accepting of one another's feelings, the difficulties can be mastered more readily. People who work through a crisis together usually find their relationship deepened by the experience. Strengths are discovered and focused upon, and support is given.

Often, the family members are not in the same stage in their grief work. This can cause family strife. When the terminal parent's anger at his or her pending death is directed at the family members, it is taken personally, leaving individuals deeply hurt. The same thing is true of a family member's anger at the impending loss of a parent.

Saying Goodbye. One of the heaviest pains is the spouse's feeling that there was not enough time spent alone with the dying partner. Many widows and widowers recount later how they were rushed out of the emergency or hospital room after a brief stay. A young widow told how important it was for her to stay and say goodbye to her dead husband: "I could not believe it, I just had to stay by his bed and hold his hand until I got enough strength to leave." Since each person has individual needs, the nurse assesses each spouse to determine his need for being near the dead person and for company or privacy.

Discussing Death with Children. The strain of being asked unanswerable questions by children is a dreaded experience for most single parents. Questions such as "Why did God take Mommy when we need her?" "Where is dead?" "Does it hurt to be dead?" are difficult to answer. The parent must extend himself at a time when there is hardly enough emotional energy for self-survival, making it difficult to resolve his own grief while aiding the child. Questions about the cause of death or the future may be similar to the parent's own questions. Simple, truthful explanations are the most effective.

At one particular funeral, two school-age children of the dead father asked their mother, "Daddy's hands are so cold, couldn't we get a blanket and cover him?" It was difficult for the grieving parent to support the children's concern for the deceased parent, while explaining why this was not possible.

A preschool child asked everyone who came to the funeral home where heaven was and to help her dial the phone so she could talk with Daddy. It was difficult for the parent to attend to her grief while also discussing the complicated question of heaven.

Death should not be described to a child in terms of the usual type of sleep. Children then become very frightened of sleeping at night and often become restless, sleepless, and experience nightmares. It is helpful to use a religious context if that is relevant for the family. Death is a mystery and very difficult to relate in tangibles.

Funeral Arrangements. Anticipatory funeral plans can be made among the entire family. Some parents have preferences for their own open or closed casket viewing, burial or cremation, and location for their remains. These preferences can be shared between spouses and noted in a will along with directions for care of the children if both parents die. During a potentially terminal illness, spouses may make even more plans when the spouse has preferences, such as for pallbearers or a specific resting place. Knowing the preferences of the dead spouse helps the survivor to make decisions with the comfort that they are best for the family. For example, one parent who loves the ocean told his family that he would like to be cremated and his ashes thrown in a favorite location at sea.

There are also the difficult questions of how to involve the children in the funeral, especially if they are young. Everyone has advice about what the children should know and how they should be involved. It seems best to invite the child to participate as much as possible, but never to force him against his will. Careful explanations are needed. Trying to anticipate questions and discuss them in advance saves much trauma at the scene. Explanations should include how the deceased parent will look and feel, people who will be there, what the funeral home looks like, and what they should do.

A poignant example is a fourth grade child attempting to climb into the coffin with his father while the rest of the family is taking a short break in the back room. Although the parent could ask friends or relatives to stay with the children, they probably need the closeness of the remaining parent to share their grief. This places a heavy burden on the parent. Thoughtful friends or relatives will try to provide extra support and relief periods for the parent.

Loneliness. Loneliness and a sense of longing for the dead person are predominant feelings for the spouse. Suddenly there is the need to adjust to being single again. The spouse may experience difficulty with decision making, discomfort in socializing, and the pressure of single parenting. Emptiness is a troublesome feeling. Sleepless nights follow long, frightening days.

Grieving people have various ways of compensating for the loneliness. They may become overactive in community affairs, take medications to numb feelings, or develop the same physical symptoms as the dead spouse. Others contemplate and may even attempt suicide. A young widow shot

her two children, her mother-in-law, and herself three days before Thanksgiving, so that the family could be together again.

It is an unexplained phenomenon that many widows and widowers die within the first year following the death of a spouse. The majority die from cardiac arrest without prior history of heart disease. Medical personnel often speak of these people as having died from a broken heart. There is no scientific evidence, only statistics, to prove the "old wives' tale."[1]

This emphasizes the need for continued follow-up and support for months after death occurs. The first year is critical, as it involves a series of "firsts" without the partner: the first Thanksgiving, the first Christmas, and so on.

Getting Support. The bereaved parent frequently has nowhere to turn for help. The person is usually emotionally paralyzed and unable to reach out to anyone, although the need for support is tremendous. The thoughtful friend or relative will gently make small decisions of daily living and be quietly present for the bereaved spouse. Major decisions must be delayed until a more stable environment has returned.

There are several community organizations available to the grieving person day and night. A sensitive clergyman may also provide great support and comfort. A thoughtful person would ask the bereaved if this support would be helpful.

Family Interaction Difficulties

Following a parent's death, family members struggle to find a new place and a new definition of how to live as a family. As family roles change, interaction difficulties occur until new patterns are formed.

Reordering of Roles. A woman finds herself the head of the family and responsible for the total financial and emotional support of herself and the children. If she has not been working, she will face the difficulty of finding a job and arranging for child care. If she has been working, the job now becomes a matter of necessity rather than choice.

Financial responsibilities are a new burden and hard for many women to adjust to.

A widower will find himself in an equally precarious position of having to run a household and care for the children. Men who have never operated a washing machine, fried an egg, or done other household work will have the most difficulty. The widower will now need to provide for the care of the children during his absence for work.

Widows and widowers become the sole child-rearer. The remaining parent will have to provide all the discipline, love, and other parenting needs. Parents frequently find it more difficult to be sole models for the opposite sexed children. Mothers just do not quite fit at father-son banquets, nor fathers at mother-daughter teas. Whether widow or widower, the changes are drastic and more than double the normal demands of family living.

Older children now find added responsibilities such as doing extra household chores. All of the children will be forced to grow up faster with more chores and responsibilities to help the family through each day.

Effects of Spouse's Reaction on Children. Children's behavior reflects their sensitivity to tensions and discomforts in their parents. When a parent responds with anger, children may withdraw to avoid irritating the parent. When a parent responds by withdrawing, children may act out, trying to regain attention that has been lost.

The more cohesive the family unit has been in the past, the less traumatic the transition. It will be therapeutic for all if a parent can feel comfortable in sharing his feelings with the children. An apology from a parent for a quick temper can have a deep meaning for a child. The child will begin to recognize that he is not the cause of the wrath, is still loved, and can possibly help the parent by responding in a different way.

A young widow spoke of being uncomfortable at mealtime. She wanted to cry, but felt she should be strong for the children. As she was encouraged to express her sadness by crying openly and talking about missing her husband, the children felt free to express their own feelings. The family could cry and talk together about how much they all missed Dad. Mutual support and the closeness related to grieving together should be encouraged by the health care worker.

Effects of Child's Reaction on Parent. Whatever pain the child experiences will be felt and added to that of the parent. The parent cannot grieve for the child, since each human being must do his own grieving. Like adults, children will continue to have many questions. The ability of the parent to be as open, honest, and supportive as possible will greatly help the child. Likewise, the parent will benefit as he watches the child resolve painful issues.

Young children may be found playing funeral with their friends. Again, this is a way for children to work out their feelings. The parent can help plan opportunities that allow freedom of expression, such as helping a child bury a pet that dies or reading stories involving the death of an animal.

Sometimes children, especially older ones, will seek out another person to share deep feelings. This often hurts the parent, who feels left out and a failure. The child should be made comfortable and given permission to share feelings with whomever he chooses. The nurse helps the parent understand that older children may need to talk with other peers or adults and that this is due to their need for independence not poor parenting.

NURSING APPROACHES

Before a nurse can examine any approaches, she must examine her own feelings on death. How can anyone with fears about a problem help someone else with that same problem? The results would be rather ineffective. It may be helpful to quietly contemplate one's own death and the feelings that arise.

The nurse needs to be aware that bereavement is a continuous process including three main stages: denial, recoil, and restitution. Denial, similar to initial shock described by Dr. Elisabeth Kübler-Ross, is a brief period usually lasting three to five days. Recoil, lasting from a few months to a couple of years, incorporates the many feelings involving depression, guilt, anger, pining, and remembering. Restitution is a better word than acceptance, as a person never fully accepts the death of a loved one. It is much more difficult to talk about bereavement than death. Dying ends, bereavement does not.

The nurse assesses each family member's reactions to the illness and death of the parent, recognizes his individual responses in the bereavement process, and plans specific interventions for the family. General nursing actions include crisis intervention, team approach, teaching, counseling, and follow-up. More detailed descriptions of nursing strategies are described in the last section of this book.

Crisis Intervention. The major approach in the situation involving death is crisis intervention. Crisis intervention is a continuous strategy since parental death brings a series of crises such as what to do at vacation time, how to handle finances, what to do on holidays and anniversaries. The crises frequently occur through the terminal illness, if there is one, and for six months to a year following death. The larger the family, the more complex and numerous are the problems as each individual reacts differently and individual reactions affect the adjustment of the family as a whole. The nurse must institute crisis intervention early to reduce the immediate problem and prevent other family complications causing additional stresses.

Team Approach. The team approach is essential for the family with a terminally ill parent. The main supporter should be someone who can comfort the grievers and feel comfortable himself. This person needs to be aware of his own limitations and have a knowledge of other resource persons with whom the family members can better relate. Social workers, clergy, physicians, nurses, dieticians, physical therapists, and occupational therapists all have a role with the patient and the family.

Teaching. Some hardships can be avoided, or at least made less painful, by preparing for them ahead of time. If the grieving process is explained to the parent and children, they will be better pre-

pared to support and understand the behavior of the dying person. Likewise, if the dying parent is aware of the normal anger and depression involved, he will not be so troubled with experiencing these feelings. Fear of the unknown is a terrible pain; human fantasy usually makes the situation worse than the reality. If appropriate, there is excellent literature, for all age levels, dealing with death. Parents appreciate books which explain death to children.

Counseling. The helping person must be comfortable with whatever intervention technique is used. Crying with a patient or family can provide a deep bond and sense of comfort, but only if it is genuine. If the helper is able to deal with people in an open, nonpushy way, it will permit the griever opportunity to ventilate and express what lies buried deep inside. Nonverbal communication is also important. Touching a hand, stroking a forehead, offering a Kleenex will often provide an opening for ventilation.

Grieving persons deeply appreciate an expression of concern and understanding. What is said is not nearly as important as the warmth and concern which lies behind it. Sharing one's own grief experience often helps to let the person know he is not alone in an experience or feeling. Sharing, however, should not reduce listening to the family's unique experiences with death.

Follow-up. The continued involvement of the health team is often overlooked. A follow-up system can prevent many problems and provide care for the family troubles that occur following death.

Within a month after a death, the phone calls and cards stop coming. Other people's lives are back to normal, but for the grieving family the reality of their loss is just beginning to sink in: the children may begin having trouble in school; the spouse may develop an ulcer; and emptiness may become overwhelming.

Very soon after the death, the family should be contacted regarding the scheduling of follow-up visits. If possible, follow-up care should be mentioned before the death. The family will know they have continued support in the difficulties ahead.

Regular meetings with the family usually enable quicker adjustments. The griever may feel more comfortable with home visits. On the other hand, some bereaved persons may welcome a chance to get out of the home and visit professionals in the office.

Acknowledging the difficult areas and reflecting willingness to discuss them are goals of interaction. There are many questions and statements of concern that may pave the way for discussion. "How have you been sleeping?" "You look tired." "Are you eating regularly?" "How are the children doing in school?" "It's hard being a single parent."

SUMMARY

The death of a parent is one of the most severe traumas for the family. While grieving the loss of the parent, the surviving family members must shift their roles to continue to meet all the family needs. The nurse assesses each family's reactions to the death and helps them to identify and solve their own difficulties. Family members who work together to master their feelings of loss and role change strengthen their family ties.

REFERENCES

1. Parkes, C. Bereavement. New York: International Universities Press, 1972.

ADDITIONAL READINGS

1. Chaney, P., ed. Dealing with Death and Dying. Jenkintown, Pa.: Intermed Communications, 1976.
2. Fassler, J. My Grandpa Died Today. New York: Behavioral Publications, 1971.
3. Grollman, C., ed. Explaining Death to Children. Boston: Beacon Press, 1967.
4. Harris, A. Why Did He Die? Minneapolis: Lerner Publications, 1965.
5. Hoffman, D. Yes Lord. St. Louis: Concordia, 1975.
6. Kastenbaum, R. "The Kingdom Where Nobody Dies." Saturday Review, December 23, 1972.
7. Lewis, C. S. A Grief Observed. New York: Seabury Press, 1961.
8. Miles, M. Annie and the Old One. Boston: Little, Brown, 1971.
9. Ross, E. K. Death: The Final Stage of Growth. Englewood Cliffs, N.J.: Prentice-Hall, 1975.
10. ———. On Death and Dying. New York: MacMillan Co., 1969.
11. ———. Questions and Answers on Death and Dying. New York: Collier Book, 1974.
12. Shepard, M. Someone You Love Is Dying. New York: Harmony Books, 1975.
13. Shoenberg, B., ed. Anticipatory Grief. New York: Columbia University Press, 1970.
14. ———, ed. Loss and Grief. New York: Columbia University Press, 1970.
15. ———, ed. Psychosocial Aspects of Terminal Care. New York: Columbia University Press, 1972.
16. Williams, J. C. "Understanding the Feelings of the Dying." Nursing, March 1976.
17. Zelligs, R. Children's Experience with Death. Springfield, Ill.: Charles C Thomas, 1974.

PERTINENT ORGANIZATIONS

LOCAL

*   *Naim.*
    Organized for widowed persons. Sponsored by Archdioceses throughout the country. Naim provides a social and therapeutic group atmosphere. Check with any Catholic church for location of meetings.

*   *Live One Day at a Time.*
    Orville Kelly Groups, providing social and emotional support, are set up for the entire family before death occurs. Check with a local social service agency or church for the nearest available groups.

*   *Widow to Widow.*
    Programs for support, located in some form in all major cities. Counseling, self-help, and social activities are dealt with. Check with local social service agency or church to locate nearest groups.

*   *Hospitals.*
    Some hospitals recognizing need for after-care, hold ecumenical memorial prayer services monthly.

*   *Churches.*
    Many churches sponsor groups for the dying and bereaved. The local pastor should be contacted.

Nursing Strategies for the High-Risk Family

PART FOUR

The nurse who is most successful in preventing and reducing the difficulties for the high-risk family has a repertoire of strategies from which she selects the combination of interventions for the particular family. A strategy is a tactic involving various specific interventions aimed at meeting a goal. There are many strategies which may be used alone or in combination to prevent or reduce the high-risk family's problems and to meet their goals.

Counseling strategies including crisis intervention, behavior modification, role theory, and transactional analysis strategies help the family identify their own difficulties from the risk situation and plan ways to prevent or reduce them. Teaching, primary nursing, cultural, and financial strategies respectively help reduce the added stresses of the unknown, multiple health professionals, noncultural health practices, and financial strains which create even more stress on the high-risk family. The following chapters describe these strategies and the ways the nurse combines them to help the family at risk.

Counseling Strategies

Margaret Shandor Miles, R.N., Ph.d.

CHAPTER SEVENTEEN

Nurses are becoming very skillful in all areas of assessment, but one of the major challenges confronting the practitioner is deciding how to intervene to help the family who has been identified as high risk. Counseling is a general term that is often used in describing the process of helping someone in need. Because it has been used rather loosely to include almost any human relationship in which people help each other solve problems or grow, the definition of counseling is difficult to determine.

Counseling is seen as a specific role of many different professionals such as physicians, ministers, social workers, lawyers, teachers, and psychologists. Nurses, working in a variety of settings including public health agencies, hospitals, and clinics, are also involved in counseling individuals and families who come to them with a wide variety of health, social, and personal problems.

Counseling is often seen by nurses as the process of advising or telling others what they must do; however, this author views counseling as a process helpful to the family's own problem solving. Counseling, for the purposes of this chapter, is defined as a step in the intervention phase of the nursing process whereby a professional nurse helps an individual or a family cope more effectively with their life situation. Counseling is also seen as a process, that is, a sequence of events which takes place over time.[6] The result of counseling not only results in a resolved problem, but can also help a family reach a higher level of maturity, greater self-esteem, and closer relationships.[17] The ultimate aim of counseling should be to help the individual and family attain self-sufficiency, self-help, and an increased sense of responsibility for meeting their own problems.

The purpose of this chapter is to present an overview of counseling strategies that can be used when working with high-risk individuals and families. Counseling strategies are the basis for most other strategies. Transactional analysis, behavior modification, and crisis intervention are specific types of counseling. Teaching is most effective when counseling is used to help the individual act on the new knowledge that is given. Counseling is also the vehicle for strategies such as financial assistance.

Counseling strategies are extremely valuable for helping the high-risk family, because of the complexity of their needs and problems. No one approach is completely effective with these families, and the helper needs to have a rich repertoire of intervention strategies to use when attempting to help the family deal with stress, handle problems, and grow.

BASIC CONCEPTS

There is a broad range of theoretical and philosophical beliefs that affect the nurse's approach to the counseling process. Since theory provides the rationale for the counseling process and helps guide the nurse in establishing goals and directions, it is vital that nurses be aware of their own philosophical and theoretical frame of reference when working with high-risk families.

The nurse determines her philosophical framework by examining the following beliefs:

1. Basic beliefs about man, including the development of personality, basic needs and
   goals, behavior, and the role of the family.
2. Basic beliefs about how individuals and families grow, change, and mature.
3. Basic beliefs about nursing, including process, roles, and expectations.

Beliefs on these issues are influenced by psychological, personality, counseling, and nursing theories. These theories are generally explored to some degree by nurses during their educational courses in liberal arts and nursing. Nurses working with high-risk families may need to do further reading as they examine and define their basic beliefs which affect nursing intervention with families.

Characteristics of a Good Helper

It is also vital that professionals working with high-risk families be knowledgeable about the characteristics of a good helper and aware of the

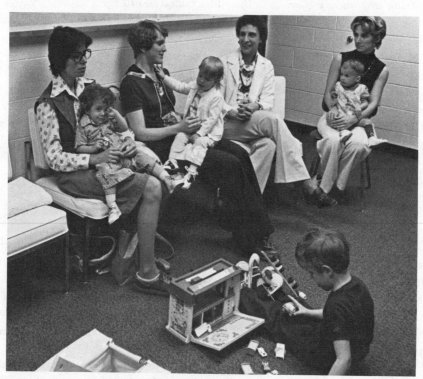

Figure 17-1. Group counseling of high-risk parents allows the parents to share experiences, concerns, and successes with each other. These parents are sharing family concerns about heart defects. Permission to reproduce photograph from Margaret Miles.

strengths that they bring into the situation. Specific personality traits of effective helpers have been identified from extensive research studies and from personal experiences of experienced counselors and psychologists. Characteristics of helpers can be divided into two categories: attitude traits and helping skills.[4]

Attitude Traits. The manner in which we use ourselves and our personalities as instruments in helping others is involved in attitude traits. Rogers emphasizes the importance of having a positive attitude toward other persons. This includes feelings such as warmth, caring, liking, interest, and respect.[16] Combs and his co-workers found that good helpers see other people as able, friendly, worthy, interesting, motivated, dependable, helpful, capable of solving their own problems, and able to manage their own lives.[5] Jourard also pointed out the importance of self-disclosure in helping people. Self-disclosure is the process of revealing oneself to another. Self-disclosure on the part of the professional helps the client feel more at ease and more self-disclosing himself.[12]

Helping Skills. The specific behaviors which can be used to help people are considered helping skills. These will be thoroughly discussed under the section entitled counseling strategies. The helping skills which are important in assisting the high-risk family cope with stress and grow toward maturity will vary depending upon the professional's frame of reference, his personality, and the family's needs and characteristics. The most basic skill for any intervention, however, is skill in interviewing. It is not the purpose of this chapter to discuss at any length specific interviewing skills. Several excellent texts have been developed for this purpose and are included in the References for this chapter.[2,3,4,8]

COUNSELING STRATEGIES

The following section of this paper describes some of the counseling strategies that might be considered when working with high-risk individuals and families. They fall into four basic categories:

Figure 17-2. Counseling Strategies

Relationship Strategies
  Use a family-centered approach
  Clarify expectations
  Establish a trust relationship
  Be a good role model
  Plan termination

Communication Strategies
  Be a good listener
  Help the family develop better communication skills
  Provide new information
  Use positive reinforcement

Problem-Solving Strategies
  Define the problem
  Help the family become problem solvers
  Use confrontation and feedback when appropriate
  Build on the family's strengths
  Manipulate the environment when necessary
  Make appropriate referrals

Personal Strategies
  Get supervision
  Be responsible, not "omnipotent"
  Become aware of "burn out"
  Learn how to cope with the stresses

1) relationship strategies, 2) communication strategies, 3) problem-solving strategies, and 4) personal strategies. See Figure 17-2 for a concise list of the strategies. These strategies are ones the author has implemented and found successful with high-risk families. Not every strategy, however, is appropriate to every family. The decision on which strategies to use must go hand in hand with the assessment of the family's problems, needs, and strengths described in the assessment chapters.

Relationship Strategies

One of the keystones to successful counseling is the ability to establish a meaningful relationship with the individual and family and to learn how to use that relationship to help them change and grow.

Use a Family Centered Approach Whenever Possible. Based on the family systems theories, the best approach to counseling high-risk individuals is an approach which in some way involves or considers all members of the family. Family systems theory views the family as an interacting, reacting system which is delicately balanced and struggles to maintain that balance. A change or problem in one member of the system, thus, affects the entire system.[13,17] The focus of counseling, is on the family system rather than on the individual.

A family might include grandparents, aunts, uncles, or cousins if they are closely involved with the family. The family can also include friends who live with the family or who are closely involved with them.

The skilled professional, working with the entire family, can help them to examine problems, strengths, and weaknesses and develop solutions to their problems. She can also help the family improve and develop their system of communication, sharing, and loving which ultimately will increase the maturity of individuals within the family and the family as a group.

Obviously, it is not always possible to work with the entire family group. Some members may be resistant to professional help. Other members may be separated from the family by long distances. However, the professional who has access to working with one or two members should always keep the entire family system in mind. Changes in one person can affect the entire family positively or negatively.

The author was recently working with a young couple whose first child was born with multiple congenital anomalies. Although she met with both parents on several occasions, the father was so hostile about the birth of a defective child that he resisted any type of help. Working with the mother, the nurse was able to help her cope with the stress of caring for this very sick infant and gain an understanding of what her husband was experiencing. As a result of her experience, the mother became more self-confident and was able to be patient and kind to her distraught husband. Although unable to meet with all the family members, the nurse focused on the impact of this sick infant on the entire family system.

Clarify Expectations. Whether working with an individual, couple, or family group, it is important for the nurse to establish some type of contract with the family to help clarify her role and their expectations. A contract is a working agreement between the nurse, patient, or family which is continuously negotiable. Contracts can be written or verbal but should serve to set some parameters and goals on the relationships.[18] Clients need to know who you are, what your qualifications are, what you want to help them with, the frequency of contact, and how long you will be available to work with them. The nurse, on the other hand, needs to know who the individual and family are, their needs and problems, the help they want, and the changes they desire to make.

Because the aim of counseling is self-sufficiency and an increased sense of responsibility, it is vital that the individual or family being helped be an integral part of the counseling process. Establishing a contract with a family includes them in the development of goals and directions. Counseling, then, becomes a process of doing something with people rather than for them.[4]

The nurse will need to be creative in establishing a contract. Contracts need to be made at the right time. During an acute phase of illness, long discussion of a contract is not appropriate. When a person appears to be resistant and threatened, a contract geared toward meeting the problem behavior may be too threatening, whereas, a contract to help the client in a less threatening area may be acceptable. For example, although the nurse assessed that one mother was overprotecting her four-year-old son and treating him like a baby, the mother was not concerned with his behavior. She was, however, concerned about his delayed speech. A contract was made to work on his speech problem, and gradually the nurse was able to focus on his other problems with the mother.

Contracts also need to be geared to the client's level of understanding. It is vital that the nurse attempt to learn what the client understands about the contract. For example, arrangements were made for one couple to have counseling to help them cope with the stresses of caring for a very sick infant. As the problems of the infant improved and they began to cope more adaptively with her care, the mother suspiciously asked the therapists what they thought of their marriage. Her question implied that her view of the counseling sessions was for the counselors to evaluate their marriage and then point out problems to them. During the next several sessions, expectations of both the parents and the counselors regarding the purpose of the counseling were clarified. The parents decided they were satisfied with their marriage and the focus of the counseling sessions remained on their adaptation to caring for their sick infant.

Sometimes contracts need to be modified or completely changed. The family crisis may be resolved quickly, leaving the family with less desire for help. A new crisis may arise which requires a change in focus or more intensive help. For example, the original reason for counseling with one couple was to help them find ways to cope with the demands of their chronically sick child. However, when their child was hospitalized in critical condition and not expected to live, the focus of counseling changed to help them cope with their grief.

Contracts can help prevent the nurse from experiencing "burn out" or "battle fatigue" which is created by developing unrealistic expectations for herself and the family.[14] Goals become more realistic and attainable and satisfaction can be obtained from seeing the family develop increased ability to define and solve their own problems. For many high-risk families, goals must be narrow, short-term, and few in number, despite the fact that the professional sees many problems and needs. Several attainable goals provide positive rewards and motivation, while unattainable ones result in feelings of failure for the family and the nurse.

Establish a Trust Relationship. Many high-risk families have had so many professionals working with them that they may be distrustful of the professional's commitment to them and suspicious of her motives. Making a contract or working agreement with them which gives them some responsibility and defines the time limits on the relationship can help to facilitate trust.

Trust is also facilitated when the family feels valued and accepted and when they feel the professional is truly interested. This can be shown by a caring attitude, by giving the family positive

strokes, and by remembering little things about their interests or activities that are important to them. Sincerity of purpose on the part of the professional is also an important behavior that promotes trust. Sincerity is shown by consistently following through on plans that are made with the family and not breaking the family's confidentiality by telling peers or other family members about problems or needs which are discussed.

With some high-risk families, trust may take a long time to develop. It has been estimated by professionals working with abusive families that it can take up to one year of continual contact, along with much testing by the families, for trust to develop. Once developed, however, much can be done to help the family.

One father of a very sick child was suspicious of the medical and nursing staff caring for his child. The nurse specialist accepted his rejecting behavior and anger and continued to make contact with him in a caring and sincere manner. For example, instead of focusing solely on the infant, she always asked how the father was doing and asked specific questions about his job. One day when he was angry about an incident, she helped him express his anger by sharing her perceptions of his emotional state with him. "You seem very upset and angry to me. What's bothering you today?" He immediately turned to her and said, "But I'm not angry with you. You're the only one around here that I can trust." It took a lot of time and effort, but the results were rewarding as the father started sharing some of his concerns with the nurse.

Be a Good Role Model. Modeling is vicarious learning occurring from observation of another person's behavior and its consequences.[1] This means that people can learn new behavior by imitating the behavior, values, and attitudes of others. Three conditions seem to be important for modeling to occur: the client must see a need for the behavior, the behavior must appear to be effective, and the model must be seen as a person of influence and prestige.[6] In addition, once the behavior has been imitated, the client must experience a positive reinforcement for it. A warm, understanding nurse who has developed a close relationship with a high-risk family can become a powerful model.

In using modeling as a counseling strategy, then, it is important for the helper to see himself as a model who is likely to be emulated by the client and then to behave in ways which he believes will be helpful to the effective functioning of the client. The nurse can be an effective model by modeling positive reinforcement by giving positive reinforcement whenever possible; modeling clear communication by always being precise, clear, and honest when communicating with the family; modeling relaxation by attempting to be relaxed during sessions with the family; and modeling warmth, empathy, understanding, and genuineness, characteristics which the counselor should exhibit in all his encounters with the family.

Modeling is a very good, indirect, nonthreatening method of teaching parenting skills to a high-risk family. A parent can be shown new and more positive parenting skills through the behavior of the nurse toward the children. The advantage of using modeling is that the parent does not need to be taught the skills in a didactic, superior manner but can learn through imitation.

Modeling has been effective in working with a teenage parent of an infant who was admitted for failure to thrive caused primarily by inadequate parental contact. While the mother was visiting the baby, the nurse sat in a rocking chair next to the mother and talked with her about her needs and concerns while holding her baby in a cuddling position and playing with him. After several such visits in which the nurse modeled mothering behaviors with the baby, the mother began picking him up and mimicking the nurse. The nurse immediately gave the mother praise for her actions and also helped her see how the baby responded to the mother's behaviors.

Modeling can be very effective in communicating new behaviors and attitudes which are important additions to the skills of high-risk families. As with other counseling strategies, modeling is usually used along with other approaches such as teaching and positive reinforcement. The important

element of modeling is the fact that the professional is deliberately demonstrating through his own behavior new skills which he wants the high-risk individual or family to emulate.

Plan Termination. Termination of a therapeutic relationship usually is accomplished in one of the following ways: premature termination by the counselor, premature termination by the client, or coagreement between the client and counselor because of successful outcomes.[6] Regardless of the manner in which termination is accomplished, both the counselor and the client usually have some important feelings related to the ending of the relationship.

High-risk parents who may already feel inadequate are especially vulnerable to emotional injury by termination by the counselor. If premature termination by the counselor is necessary, the client needs to know the reasons for the termination and to have help in expressing the emotions that such a closure can create and in transferring his trust to a new counselor if that is planned. One way this can be done is by bringing the new counselor into the last session with the client and introducing him at that time to the client. Once the first counselor has terminated from the case, she should not interfere with the new relationship that is developing with the new counselor. For example, if the client calls for help, he should be referred to his new helper.

Although contracts are less recognized on a hospital ward, the nurse has an informal contract with the patient when she cares for her over a period of time. If the nurse's assignment changes, she needs to consider all of the previously mentioned facets of premature closure to help her patient cope with the change.

One mother had been a patient on the high-risk maternity unit for two weeks because of bleeding secondary to abruptio placenta. A graduate student nurse, who had been her primary nurse during that two-week period, had developed a trust relationship with the mother while helping her to share some of her concerns and anxieties. Although the nurse was scheduled to take a trip out of town with her family and would be gone when the mother was going to have her cesarean section, she was careful to gently remind the mother several times about her planned departure and helped her to express her feelings of loss and her concerns about delivery. The nurse also found another nurse who began to relate to the mother and stayed with her during and after the cesarean section.

Premature termination by the client can occur at any time during the counseling relationship. Sometimes individuals will just neglect to return for the next session, or they may cancel meetings for several weeks in a row. In public health nursing, the nurse may find that no one answers the door after an appointment has been made. Some clients will discuss their desire to terminate before leaving. In any case of premature closure by the client, the counselor usually needs support and guidance in sorting through the possible reasons for the client's termination and her feelings of rejection and anger. The individual or family may have been fearful of the impact the counseling might have on them, they may not have been ready to face and deal with their problems, or they might have had a difficult time establishing a trust relationship with the helper. Not all individuals or families can be expected to establish a trust relationship with a given helper. Sometimes personalities just do not fit well together. If a client has terminated without an opportunity for discussion, it may be important to attempt to contact him to let him know that you are still interested and to find out the reasons for the termination. If he still does not want the help offered, the helper should leave the door open in case he might wish to return later.

When a high-risk family has been seen for counseling for a long period of time, it is often the family who reaches the decision for termination before the counselor. The counselor may see the family as one that still has a multitude of problems to work on. However, the family may have reached a plateau; that is, they have made some real gains but need a rest, an opportunity to solidify these gains. Some families, on the other hand, just are not willing to face and work on all of their problems. Once the crisis has passed, they are ready to termi-

nate and go on with their lives as before. In either case, the counselor should leave the door open by telling them to come back at any time should they decide to return later for help.

When termination by mutual agreement has been reached, both the helper and family should have reached a point of mutual satisfaction with the experience. The main emotion to be handled is the feeling of loss experienced by all parties. The helper should also help the family review and summarize accomplishments and let the family know the impact the counseling experience has had on him. The family may feel some anxiety about whether they will continue to make progress once the counseling is terminated. If anxiety is intense, termination might be accomplished by gradually reducing the frequency of contacts until the client or clients feel more secure.

Communication Strategies

The ability to communicate openly and honestly and to interview appropriately and effectively is at the heart of all counseling. Being a good listener, helping the family to learn new and more adaptive ways of communicating with each other, providing new information at the right time, and using positive reinforcement whenever possible are all important communication strategies.

Be a Good Listener. Creative and skillful listening can be one of the most important strategies in working with high-risk individuals and families. Some clients may talk to many people about themselves, their needs, and their problems, but it is surprising how few persons (professional as well as laymen) truly listen to what is being said. One father began telling the nurse how frightened he was when he saw his newborn son in the neonatal intensive care unit hooked up to monitors and tubes. The nurse attempted to reassure him that his son was doing well and had a good chance of living. The father, however, was not as concerned about his son's survival as he was about the appearance of his son and how he felt about the equipment.

Listening is an attempt to perceive the verbal

and nonverbal communication of another person and to convey to him some level of understanding about that communication.

Implied in the process of listening is seeing behind what a person is saying or doing to the meaning or perceptions producing his behavior. Thus, in true listening, the helper implies to the client that he is interested in *his* internal frame of reference.[2] Listening involves hearing what is said, the way it is said, and what is not said (feelings which lie behind what is expressed verbally and nonverbally).[7]

When the goal of listening is truly understanding the client, it is hard work and requires the full attention and energy of the helper.[2] A professional, working with a busy schedule and moving from one person or activity to another, may have a hard time in tuning out all of the other experiences in order to tune into the client. Because of the stress level and number of problems for many risk families, the nurse may be able to handle only a few high-risk families at one time. If we are preoccupied with something else, clients will quickly sense our emotional state and lose interest in revealing themselves. A busy professional, then, must learn to tune out other activities and tune into the client. This can be done more easily in a quiet setting or if the professional takes a few minutes between activities to relax. When making home visits, the nurse may want to pick a time of day when the children are napping, in order to be able to truly listen to the mother's concerns. In many homes, it may be important to ask the mother whether she would mind turning off the television to enhance communication.

Silence is an important listening technique for high-risk families since it helps the family member to pull his thoughts and feelings together or express himself more fully. Questions from the helper should be minimal, carefully phrased, and geared to help the client rather than to satisfy the helper. Open-ended questions can be useful in eliciting further verbalizations. "You said that you were confused yesterday about the operation. Can you tell me how you feel today?" A similar question about the same topic, phrased as a closed question, would elicit a narrower response from the client: "Are you still confused about the operation?" Questions can also be used to clarify what the helper thinks he has heard or to assist the client in clarifying the problems expressed.[2] "I'm not sure what you meant when you said that Suzy is the cause of your problems. Can you explain that to me?"

The nurse must listen to each individual family's problems related to the risk situation. The family difficulties presented in early chapters are potential problems which help the nurse make a more detailed assessment, but the nurse should never assume the presence of a difficulty without listening to the family's description of their problems.

Help the Family Develop Better Communication Skills. It has been suggested by family systems theorists that many high-risk families have dysfunctional communications systems.[10,13,17] Perhaps one of the most important strategies to use when working with these families is that of helping them improve their internal and external communication patterns. In a healthy family, communication is usually direct, clear, specific, and honest, whereas, in a troubled family such as high-risk families, it tends to be rigid, vague, dishonest, and unclear.[17]

Helping families change to more open and honest communication is a long-term process. The professional should begin with small steps, perhaps by pointing out simple areas where communications could be improved and the consequences of the problem communication. "I noticed that John just asked you a question but I really didn't understand your answer. Could you give him your answer again more clearly?" This kind of remark lets the parent know that his communications were not clear and allows him to attempt to correct the communication. Sometimes the helper will need to be even more specific. "I hear Connie saying that she needs to know whether or not you care about her. Could you tell her how you feel about her?"

In the stress of high-risk situations, parents frequently misinterpret each other's messages. The helper may also need to help the family members learn how to check out the meanings of statements which were made. "I heard you say that you were worried about George, but I'm not sure George understood what you meant by that. Did you understand what she meant?" Some families need help to become aware of the incongruence of messages which are given. "You have just told us that you aren't worried about the financial situation, but your face tells me something else. Can you share with us your gut level concerns?"

Provide New Information. Providing new information in the form of verbal discussion, verbal instruction, or written articles and books can be an important approach to helping high-risk individuals and families. Such information is best absorbed and used when it comes at the right time for the client. The right time is when the client begins asking questions about that problem and wants new ideas to formulate a solution.

New information should not be given in the form of advice or an order. Advice giving is more a teaching strategy and may interfere with the attainment of counseling goals by impeding the goal of helping the high-risk individual or family become more self-sufficient and responsible.

Offering new information in the form of suggestions and options is more a counseling strategy, provided that the family is encouraged to consider the alternatives and consequences and make the decisions for themselves. Some of the approaches to achieving this goal include verbal instructions such as telling a person how to do something, mutual discussion of a new concept such as informing a parent about the newer theories on infant feeding, provision of reading material followed by discussion, and interpretation of new information which has already been obtained by the parent.

In high-risk situations the new information may need to be given in very small units over several sessions. One mother was overwhelmed with the medical problems and daily needs of her infant with severe congenital heart disease. Although it was obvious that Kim was also showing signs of developmental delay, the mother could not cope with this problem at first. Gradually, the nurse introduced the idea of a developmental stimulation program for Kim. When Kim was eight months old,

the mother began to ask more specific questions about ways to help Kim learn to sit and crawl. The nurse, sensing her readiness at this time to learn, provided her with written instructions about ways to work with Kim, demonstrated these techniques, and gave the mother a pamphlet on infant stimulation.

Use Positive Reinforcement. One of the easiest and most common sense strategies that can be used with high-risk families is that of positive reinforcement or positive stroking. Positive reinforcement is based on the principle of human behavior that any positive stimulus which follows a behavior or response will strengthen that response.[6] Positive stroking or positive reinforcement means recognizing the need for all individuals to have signs of recognition, affection, appreciation, and love. Positive strokes not only help to reinforce behavior, but are also extremely important in increasing the self-esteem of the individual and family.[11] Since most high-risk individuals or families have a lowered self-esteem, any strategy aimed at raising self-esteem will be especially effective.

Positive reinforcers or strokes can be verbal or nonverbal responses made by the professional. The following are some examples of verbal reinforcements: complimenting a mother on the good care she has given her infant ("You have been so patient and careful with Janie during this recent illness."); noticing a positive change in appearance in a mother who usually looks very bedraggled ("You look so pretty today."); showing approval to a father for some behavior ("I'm so pleased that you were able to take Johnny on that overnight."); or telling a parent something that you like about them ("I like the way you ask questions when you aren't sure about something."). Nonverbal reinforcers include smiling at a mother as she tells you how she positively handled her child's misbehavior, nodding approval when a father tells you that he has found a better job, or hugging a mother who has just told you that she has accomplished her goal of telling her husband how much she needs his help.

The professional should also assist the high-risk individual or family in both giving and receiving positive strokes between each other. One couple were being seen for family counseling because of emotional instability of the wife and stresses in their relationship. Although the nurse working with the family frequently heard the husband compliment his wife in a kidding manner, the wife never seemed to hear the compliments. Gradually the nurse pointed out to the wife the many compliments coming from her husband. She began to hear and accept them.

Individuals in high-risk families must learn how to give themselves positive strokes and find activities in their daily lives that are reinforcing, because the stresses of the high-risk situation frequently cause guilt and loss of self-esteem as discussed in preceding chapters. One mother felt guilty about her past involvements with the church because she had been told that they kept her away from her emotionally disturbed child too much. The nurse and mother explored her reasons for the church activities. Before long, they had both discovered that these activities were very reinforcing to the mother and made her feel important. She was helped to arrange appropriate child care and was then encouraged to continue some of her church involvements in order to meet her own needs.

Problem-Solving Strategies

High-risk individuals and families may bring to the professional a multitude of problems and concerns. Helping these individuals or families through a problem-solving process is an important aspect of counseling. Problem-solving strategies include defining the problem, helping the family become problem solvers, building on the family strength's, using confrontation and feedback when appropriate, manipulating the environment when necessary, and making appropriate referrals.

Define the Problem. A professional who attempts to solve all the problems brought to him by many high-risk families is doomed to fail. It is imperative that the helper assist the individual and family to clearly define one or two solvable problems which they want to work on. "Now, you've just mentioned a number of problems that are both-

ering you, I wonder if we could decide on which of these problems is bothering you the most and that you would like to work on."

It is extremely important that the professional involve the high-risk family in the problem identification phase of problem solving. If the problem chosen by the helper to work on is not the problem identified by the client, the family's problem will continue without help. The insecure young mother of a two-year-old son came for help because she felt her son was hyperactive. Further assessment revealed that he was not hyperactive but was behaving normally for a two-year-old boy. The professional then attempted to focus on the mother's feelings about herself and her child, feeling that the problem lay in the mother's attitudes or expectations. She withdrew from counseling within two sessions because she was not ready to focus on herself. In retrospect, it would have been much more effective to focus on the two-year-old for a longer time until she was ready to discuss her problems or needs.

When working with a family group, the professional should help the entire family reach some sort of consensus about the problems and which problems they want to work on. What may be a problem to one member of the family may not be a problem to another.

The word "solvable" implies that a solution for the problem can be found within a reasonable amount of time if the family is truly committed to trying. Not all problems are solvable, and this needs to be recognized by both the professional and the client. One husband began discussing with the nurse the many problems which were causing him to become depressed and apathetic. The main problem which he wanted to solve was the fact that his wife had left him and filed for divorce. He wanted the nurse to help him get her back. His wife, however, refused to return to the counseling sessions and was quite firm about her decision to divorce him. The nurse had to help the husband refocus on the solvable problems of being a divorced man, including his feelings of loneliness, failure, and grief.

Help the Family Become Problem Solvers. In order for the effects of counseling to have long-term implications for family growth, it is important to help the individual and family learn how to use the process of problem solving rather than always have professionals solving problems for them. High-risk families frequently have multiple or intermittent problems to solve.

The process of problem solving involves the following steps:

1. Clearly defining the problem.
2. Determining goals related to the problem.
3. Describing existing conditions related to the problem.
4. Discussing all possible alternatives to solving the problem and the consequences of each.
5. Deciding on an approach to try.
6. Evaluating the outcome.
7. Making future plans.

The problem-solving process is illustrated in the case of a nurse who helped an abusive parent who was worried about hurting her three-year-old child. The problem was defined: "I'm afraid I will beat my child." The goals related to the problem were discussed: "I don't want to hurt my child. I don't want them to take her away from me." The mother was encouraged to discuss the existing conditions related to the problem: "I get lonely, depressed, and angry about my husband's leaving me and then I lose control with her." She was helped to discuss all the possible alternatives and the consequences of each: "When I get upset, I could put Jennifer in her crib and leave the room for a few minutes until I calm down. This might not be enough help and the feelings might return. I could call Parent's Anonymous and talk to another abusing parent who would understand and help. Then I would get immediate help in venting my feelings and being understood. I could also call you (the nurse). This would also help me discuss my feelings." The mother then decided on an approach: "The next time I get upset with Jennifer, I will put her in bed, call Parent's Anonymous, and if that doesn't work, I'll call you."

On the next visit, the nurse helped the mother evaluate the outcome: "I got upset with myself and almost hit Jennifer. Then I remembered our plan and I put her in bed with some toys and called Parent's Anonymous. It really helped." The nurse then helped the mother make future plans: "I think I'd like to start going to the parent's groups meetings so that I can learn more about myself. How do I do that?" By involving an individual or family in a problem-solving strategy like this, the nurse can help them eventually learn to evaluate their own problems, come up with their own solutions, and evaluate the outcomes themselves.

Not all clients can come up with their own solutions and may need suggestions from the helper. However, it is futile and detrimental to counseling to suggest an alternative, which the family has already tried and found unsuccessful. The suggested solution should have the least amount of negative consequences and be consistent with the basic values of the individual and family.

If the professional has used a problem-solving strategy during a session with a high-risk family, it is imperative that the outcome of the strategy be discussed thoroughly at the next meeting. A successful outcome may encourage the client to work on another problem. An unsuccessful outcome may indicate the need to come up with another alternative. In the situation where the planned intervention was not carried out, the client might need more encouragement, the problem might be too overwhelming, or the problem might not be as important to the client as it previously seemed. Continual reevaluation of the problems and alternatives is essential.

Use Confrontation and Feedback When Appropriate. There may come a time during the problem-solving process when confrontation or provision of feedback to the family is important. Confrontation means helping the client come face to face with some of his difficulties, problems, or behavior.[9] Confrontation may involve pointing out the differences the helper sees between what the client is saying and nonverbal behaviors such as tone of voice, bodily movement, and facial expressions. "You are telling me about some very sad experiences which you have had, and yet you are smiling. I sense that there are some tears behind that smile." Discrepancies between what the client is saying and what he is doing might be pointed out to him. "You keep telling me that you want to divorce your husband, but when he comes to the house you always let him come in. That confuses me." Confrontation can also clarify differences the helper has noted between what the client has said and what the helper has observed. "You have been telling me that both you and your husband are worried about Jim's behavior, yet John is never here when I come to discuss ways of modifying and improving Jim's behavior. I wonder if John is really concerned."

The purpose of confrontation is to provide feedback to the client in order to help him better understand his situation, behavior, and needs. It directs the client's attention to something he might not be aware of at the time.[8] Confrontations should not be phrased as a question, since the helper is not seeking an answer but rather is attempting to help the client see and discuss a problem. Open-ended phrases that emphasize what the helper has observed should be used. The client can then either discuss the issue or ignore it. The use of the word "I" linked with what the helper has observed is more appropriate than starting a statement directly with the term, "You"! "I've observed that you seem angry this week," rather than "You're angry about something."

It is extremely important that confrontation be used with sensitivity and tact, because confrontation should not be a hostile act. The helper should examine his motives before using confrontation. Is the helper feeling angry with the client? Has the situation stirred up some unresolved conflicts on the part of the helper?[9] If the helper is unsure of his own feelings about the situation, he should seek supervision before using confrontation techniques. Confrontation is not an excuse for anger, but a strategy based on individual assessment of the family's needs and reactions and continual evaluation.

It is important that confrontation as a strategy

not be overused because it could turn into nagging and lose its therapeutic potential. Confrontation also needs to be used with caution because it may cause the client to become defensive, to erupt in a panic state causing him to flee from the therapeutic relationship, or to become depressed.[9] Confrontation as a counseling strategy therefore needs to be used with careful consideration given to the purpose and the expected outcomes.

One family had been seeing the nurse for family counseling for several weeks. Although the problem of allowing their mildly retarded, teenage daughter more independence had been discussed several times and alternatives to the problem explored and decided upon, the parents never acted on the solutions between sessions. The nurse finally said to them, "I'm confused. We discussed last week Jane's need for more independence in going to school events with her friends, but you have not followed through on the solution discussed." For the first time, the father admitted that he did not agree that his daughter needed more independence and he certainly did not agree with the solution of allowing her to go out with her friends, even though he had been involved in the solution when it was outlined. Following the confrontation, the nurse was able to draw the father out and deal with his concerns about his daughter's needed independence. He disliked one of her friends and he was very fearful that she might get pregnant. Planned confrontation helped this family identify their difficulty, and counseling sessions could then focus on the problem of this father's fears.

Build on the Family's Strengths. High-risk families and the professionals working with them are much more aware of their problems and difficulties than of their capacities and potentials. The professional working with high-risk families needs to use every opportunity possible to help them discover and use their strengths for productive family functioning. The discovery and use of hidden strengths can result in a feeling of accomplishment and satisfaction for the family and may have a positive effect on family self-image, pride, and functioning.[15]

Otto suggests several methods that can be

used to identify family strengths. These include helping the family do a self-survey of strengths together, family discussions of ways to use and build on strengths, and strengths bombardment wherein one family member is helped to see and discover his strengths.

Manipulate the Environment When Necessary. Environmental manipulation includes any attempt to deal with the client's problem by removing or modifying disorganizing or problem elements in his environment. Although it is always desirable for the client himself to manipulate or change his environment, there are individuals and families, especially those in the initial crisis of a high-risk situation, who may need a helping start.[9] Contacting an agency to find a job, house, or financial assistance for an individual are examples of ways in which the nurse can assist the client in crisis. Appropriate use of social resources such as halfway houses, foster homes, and free clinics can also be effective in helping burdened clients. It is frequently a good idea to pave the way for the insecure or undecided client by getting in contact with the agency to learn about how they operate and to inform them of the client's needs.

A young, teenaged mother of a retarded and terminally ill infant was having increased difficulty in taking care of her baby who was extremely hard to feed. Because she had little support from her own family and her husband had recently left her, the mother reached the conclusion that she would need to place the baby in a residential crib home. She was not, however, able to make the initial steps needed to apply for this care because of her feelings of guilt and her depression. The nurse made several contacts with the agency to learn about the process of applying for such help and to alert an individual in the agency about the mother's needs and problems. The nurse was then able to give the mother more information about what to expect when she called the agency, including the name of someone there who would be aware of her as an individual.

When working with high-risk families in a hospital setting, the nurse may have to manipulate the hospital environment by getting permission for rules to be adapted or by assisting the health care team to plan together for the family's needs. The first infant of one couple died suddenly and unexpectedly of sudden infant death syndrome. When their second infant was three months old, she was found to have a congenital heart defect that required a hospitalization and cardiac catheterization. Knowing the past history of the family, the present anxiety, and the fact that the mother never left her baby with anyone, permission was obtained to have the mother care for the child in the nursery and go to the cardiac catheter laboratory.

Make Appropriate Referrals. Referrals are based on a thorough assessment. It has been the author's experience that many nurses and other professionals as well are too willing to refer the high-risk family to another agency or professional for help, once the many problems of the family have been identified. This may be a means of avoidance for the health worker. Referral must be based on an assessment of the family's needs and nurse's abilities. Some of the assessments a nurse should make before using a referral include:

1. The nurse's own strengths and weaknesses in helping this family.
2. The relationship that the family has already formed with the nurse and the ability of this family to make another trust relationship at this time.
3. The resources available to assist, guide, and support the nurse if she continues to work with the family.
4. Other professional resources available to help the family.
5. The family's desire for additional help and their motivation to follow through if a referral is made.

It has been the author's experience that troubled families often have a difficult time establishing a trust relationship; thus, referral to another professional or agency should not be taken lightly once a trust relationship has been established. In addition, many high-risk families are not as motivated to seek help as the referring nurse who views them as very needful. Another professional or agency may be viewed suspiciously or negatively by the family.

Referrals, therefore, should be made only after careful assessment, problem identification, and planning with the family.

Perhaps one of the most effective approaches to working with the high-risk family is a multidisciplinary approach involving one or more professionals working with the family to help them cope with their needs and learn how to grow. Close collaboration and a trust relationship between all professionals involved with the family is important.

Personal Strategies

Working with high-risk families is not easy for any professional. It is important for the nurse working in high-risk situations to think about the impact these families have on her personality and to think of the kinds of help which she needs to continue working effectively with them. Getting supervision, setting reasonable goals, becoming aware of "burnout," and learning how to cope with the stresses are all important personal strategies which make the nurse a more effective counselor to high-risk families.

Get Supervision. All professionals working with high-risk families need some kind of ongoing supervision or consultation from a peer, another professional, or a supervisor. Supervision, in this case, means discussing a family with another professional for the purpose of getting help with assessment of their problems, evaluation of intervention approaches which have been tried, planning of new intervention approaches, and evaluation of outcomes.

The best approach to supervision is using tape recorded interviews or process recordings to evaluate both the family and the professional's responses. This kind of supervision has traditionally been thought of as an exercise for students, but all professionals are students when working with high-risk individuals and families. Supervision is an opportunity for the professional to learn new approaches, receive reinforcement for the work she is doing, and objectively evaluate mistakes which have been made. Good supervision can be a growth experience for the professional as well as the supervisor.

Be Responsible, Not Omnipotent. It is important that the professionals working with high-risk families realize their own limitations and that of the families they are trying to help. As mentioned earlier, the setting of realistic contracts and goals for these families is essential. Many families have numerous problems and frequent crises, many of which are unsolvable and unpreventable. Sometimes professionals feel omnipotent in that they feel they can or should change a family overnight or solve all their problems quickly. It is easy for such professionals to feel a sense of failure when a family does not change quickly enough or adequately solve their problems.

Professionals may feel a sense of failure when a family who was beginning to show signs of integration suddenly falls apart during what seemed like a minor crisis. After numerous crises and problems, a young mother whose infant daughter had recently died of multiple congenital anomalies seemed to be coping with her loss adequately. She was calling the nurse less frequently because of depression or anxiety and had found a part-time job. One evening, however, she called and said that she was extremely upset and that she did not know why. The nurse listened to her and helped her to problem solve. An appointment was made for the next morning, but the nurse learned that the mother had taken a overdose of drugs and been admitted to a local hospital. At first the nurse felt as if she had failed the woman, but when she discussed the situation with her supervisor, she realized that the woman was responsible for her act and she had been given enough information to find additional help for her crisis if she had chosen to do this. Later, the nurse learned that the crisis had the positive outcome of prompting the woman's husband for the first time to agree to counseling, and together they saw the psychiatrist which helped them work out some of their unsolved marital problems.

Thus, setbacks and crises must be expected and should be viewed objectively by the professional. Supervision, contracts, and setting reasonable goals all help the professional be responsible to her families without becoming "super-reasonable" and thus creating unrealistic expectations.

Become Aware of "Burn Out." The professional who works intensively with individuals and families who have psychological, social, and physical problems may reach a point where she cannot cope with this continued stress and "burn out" can occur.[14] The beginning signs of burn out include vague anxieties about work related situations, depression, a dislike of going to work, a loss of objectivity and increase in subjectivity, and an inability to get organized or concentrate. The end result of burn out can include loss of concern and feeling for clients, increased focus on the negative, cynicism, treating people in detached or dehumanized ways, labeling people, becoming distant from clients, and using abstract, scientific jargon.[14]

Burn out can also affect the professional's personal life by leading to long depressions, increased use of drugs, alcohol or tobacco, and acting out behavior with family and friends. It can also affect one's physical well-being, causing various health problems.

It is imperative that professionals become aware of the impact their work has on them, realize when they are experiencing the beginning signs of burn out, and find ways to resolve and reduce the stress. Burn out is more likely to occur when a professional has a high case load, sets unrealistic expectations for herself and her clients, and gets little or no support from the system.

Learn How to Cope with the Stresses. In order to reduce or avoid burn out, professionals need to learn how to cope with the pressures and stresses of working with high-risk families. Each individual will find her own unique needs and methods for coping. The following are some suggestions:

Set a realistic case and work load and refuse to burden yourself with more clients or families than you can effectively help.

Develop opportunities to withdraw when needed. Be sure to take adequate time out with rest periods, lunch breaks, coffee breaks, days off and vacation time. Use these periods to get completely away from the work problems. Take a day or week off to attend a professional meeting or workshop which will help you to get some new ideas and strength. Change some aspect of your job to make it less stressful and more interesting.

Get support from your supervisor, peers, spouse, or friends. Professionals working with high-risk families have a strong need to talk about their experiences and have a right to do so. This can be done with a supervisor, consultant, or in group sessions with co-workers. Although confidentiality of clients must be preserved, certain aspects of job related stresses can also be shared with significant others who will understand your feelings and care about you.

Learn to separate work from personal life at least to some degree. Time away from work needs to include doing special things that are fun, relaxing, and rewarding to the professional. Family life, hobbies, professional activities, and church activities are all ways in which a professional can develop a satisfying life that can be a support to her job.

SUMMARY

Nurses are becoming very skillful in all areas of assessment, but one of the major challenges confronting the nurse is that of deciding how to intervene to help the family who has been identified as high risk. This chapter presents an overview of counseling strategies which can be used when working with high-risk individuals and families. Counseling is defined as one step in the intervention phase of the nursing process whereby a professional nurse helps an individual or family cope more effectively with their life situation. Counseling not only can result in a resolved problem, but also may help an individual or family reach higher levels of maturity, a greater sense of self-esteem and closer relationships.

The most valuable counseling strategies for the high-risk family are relationship strategies, communication strategies, problem-solving strategies, and personal strategies. Counseling strategies are extremely valuable for helping the high-risk family because of the complexity of their needs and problems. No one approach is effective with these families, and the professional needs to have a rich repertoire of intervention strategies to use when attempting to help the family deal with stress, handle problems, and grow.

REFERENCES

1. Bandura, A. *Principles of Behavior Modification.* New York: Holt, Rinehart, and Winston, 1969.
2. Benjamin, A. *The Helping Interview.* Boston: Houghton Mifflin Company, 1969.
3. Bernstein, L. *Interviewing: A Guide for Health Professionals.* New York: Appleton-Century-Crofts, 1974.
4. Brammer, L. M. *The Helping Relationships: Process and Skills.* Englewood Cliffs, N.J.: Prentice-Hall, 1973.
5. Combs, A. W., D. L. Avila, and W. W. Purkey. *Helping Relationships: Basic Concepts for the Helping Professions.* Boston: Allyn & Bacon, 1972.
6. Delaney, D. J. and S. Eisenberg. *The Counseling Process.* Chicago: Rand McNally, 1972.
7. Ekman, P. "Body Position, Facial Expression, and Verbal Behavior During Interviews." *Journal of Abnormal and Social Psychology,* 68, 1964, 295–301.
8. Enelow, A. J. and S. N. Swisher. *Interviewing and Patient Care.* New York: Oxford University Press, 1972.
9. Getz, W., A. E. Wiesen, S. Sue, and A. Ayera. *Fundamentals of Crisis Counseling.* Lexington, Mass.: Heath, 1974.
10. Haley, J. *Problem Solving Therapy: New Strategies for Effective Family Therapy.* San Francisco: Jossey-Bass, 1976.
11. James, M. and D. Joneward. *Born to Win: Transactional Analysis with Gestalt Experiments.* Reading, Mass.: Addison-Wesley, 1971.
12. Jourard, S. M. *The Transparent Self.* Toronto: D. Van Nostrand, 1964.
13. Lewis, M. et al. *No Single Thread: Psychological Health in Family Systems.* New York: Brunner/Mazel, 1976.
14. Maslach, C. "Burned-out," *Human Behavior,* 5, 1976, 17–21.
15. Otto, H. A. "Plan to Build Family Strength." *International Journal of Religious Education,* 43, 1967, 6–7, 40–41.
16. Rogers, C. R. "The Characteristics of a Helping Relationship." In D. L. Avila, A. W. Combs, and W. W. Purkey. (eds.). *Helping Relationships.* Boston: Allyn & Bacon, 1972.
17. Satir, V., J. Stachowiak, and H. A. Taschman. *Helping Families to Change.* New York: Jason Aronson, 1975.
18. Sloan, M. R. and B. T. Schommer. "The Process of Contracting in Community Health Nursing." In B. W. Spradley (ed.). *Contemporary Community Nursing.* Boston: Little, Brown, 1975.

PERTINENT ORGANIZATIONS
LOCAL
Local organizations who help the family or health professional with counseling strategies are Catholic charities, Jewish family services, Christian family services, welfare departments, community crisis centers, and mental health centers.

Crisis Intervention Strategies

Sally Felgenhauer Baird, R.N., M.S.N.

CHAPTER EIGHTEEN

Danger, yet opportunity, is the dual meaning given to the Chinese character "crisis." How aptly this describes our meaning of crisis, for it is a state of upset and disequilibrium, but also a time when an individual or family has the opportunity to grow, mature, and become better able to handle future life problems. Crisis intervention is a strategy designed to take advantage of this growth potentiality by timely intervention during the crisis period. As a method for dealing with high-risk families in crisis, its theory is basic, its scope is broad, and its application is appropriate for a wide range of professionals.

BASIC CONCEPTS OF CRISIS INTERVENTION

Crisis is defined as an upset in steady state. This definition is based on the postulate that man strives for homeostasis by constantly using his coping mechanisms to maintain equilibrium. When situations arise which threaten to upset this equilibrium, a person uses his usual problem-solving techniques to return to a state of mental balance. Occasionally, events arise which cannot be handled by the usual problem-solving techniques, thereby provoking a crisis. The individuals involved soon find themselves upset as they try various ineffective methods of coping, experience rising tension, and find the problem continuing without resolution. Finally, the tension acts as a powerful stimulus to mobilize internal and external resources, resulting in redefinition of the meaning of the event, utilization of new ways of coping, and possible resolution of the crisis. If the problem cannot be solved, avoided, or altered in a way that makes it tolerable, major disorganization of the individuals and family generally occurs. The outcome of the crisis is dependent on the person's coping behaviors and his interaction with others during the crisis period.

There are three variables that determine a crisis situation: the event itself, the meaning of the situation for the family, and the family's resources in dealing with the event.[1] Figure 18-1 shows this model of crisis intervention.

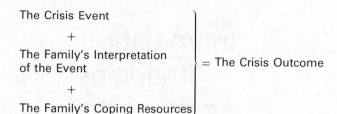

The Crisis Event

+

The Family's Interpretation
of the Event   = The Crisis Outcome

+

The Family's Coping Resources

Figure 18-1. Model of Crisis

The Event. The event which precipitates the crisis can be the type of threat, disaster, or life change which induces a crisis in nearly all individuals. Generally, these hazardous life events meet two criteria: they have great importance to the individuals involved and they are difficult to solve by familiar methods. Examples of these events may include the death of a family member, divorce, the birth of a defective infant, an incapacitating illness, important role changes such as entering school, acquiring a new job, addition of family members, moving, and a wide variety of other occurrences. Most high-risk situations include one or more crisis producing events. These problems demand solutions which are often novel in view of the individual's previous life experience. They also may revive old conflicts which can be symbolically linked with the present event.

The Family's Interpretation of the Event. No crisis precipitating event has quite the same meaning for every family. An event can appear very threatening on the surface, but may not be perceived as a crisis provoking event by the individuals involved. For example, a divorce may actually mean relief from anxiety and worry if both participants have agreed that separation from one another is in their best interest. On the other hand, a situation such as the confirmation of a pregnancy will not seem too anxiety provoking to most people, but the unwed teenage girl with few resources will be thrown into severe disequilibrium. Stressful events become crises if the individuals view them as such.

The Family's Resources. The resources the family has will also determine the crisis state. A stable marriage, a supportive extended family, friends, religious faith, and professional guidance may be viewed as stabilizing resources. The fami-

ly's previously successful coping mechanisms in other crisis situations will also prove to be a valuable asset. The more resources a family has, the less likely it is that there will be a severe crisis.

Crisis-prone individuals can be viewed as having low resources: specifically, poor family integration and poor family adaptability. Family integration is defined as a sense of unity, common purpose, and economic interdependence running through family life. Family adaptability involves the family's capacity to meet stressful events and solve problems as a family. Therefore, the family with marital discord, diverging views on goals, and little contact with outside people to help make adjustments is at high risk for crisis to develop.

Crisis Outcome. The outcome of the crisis is dependent on the three variables just discussed and is influenced by the help or hindrance of friends, neighbors, and professionals during the period of disequilibrium. An adaptive outcome is one in which the individuals in crisis resolved the situation in a healthy manner. A maladaptive outcome is resolution to a lower level of functioning, where the individuals can no longer cope with previously nonthreatening situations. An example may be the mother who no longer plays with her two-year-old child because of the birth of a premature sibling.

Crisis Intervention. Crisis intervention means entering the life situation of individuals or families in crisis in order to reduce the stress of the crisis event, mobilize resources to deal with the event, and use the present crisis situation to help those involved not only resolve their present problem but also be better able to adapt to and cope with future stressful experiences. The rationale for crisis intervention stems from the observation that a person in crisis is totally involved in a subjective experience and is psychologically open to outside assistance. This predictably more susceptible person in crisis may come through his experience in a healthy way depending on the quality of help he receives during the crisis. Intervention can then be a decisive factor in the outcome.

A crisis is characteristically self-limiting, lasting up to four to six weeks. Although some high-risk families appear to be in crisis longer, on closer assessment they are experiencing a series of crises from intermittent causes. Intervention is most effective during the four to six week time period for each crisis and ideally should be applied as close to the crisis as possible. The therapist using crisis intervention focuses actively on the current problem and its resolution, without attempting to engage in psychoanalysis or psychotherapy. The aim of crisis intervention is not that of restructuring the personality or removing psychotic symptoms. It deals with the present problem, relying on past history only as it pertains to this problem.

Minimum and maximum therapeutic goals can be set by the therapist and client. The minimum goal is psychological resolution of the immediate crisis and restoration to the same level of functioning existing prior to the crisis. The maximum goal is personal or family growth resulting in a better ability to cope with stresses in the future. A person not only resolves the immediate situation, but also learns from the experience to face future life problems with greater resources and problem solving mechanisms. For example, a couple thrown into crisis by the birth of their first baby should be able to deal with the birth of a second child more effectively.

The strategies used to achieve the goals of crisis intervention follow the problem-solving model. This approach is familiar to most nurses who have already become skilled in assessment, planning, intervention, and evaluation. The role of the person using these strategies can be that of direct, suppressive, and active participant. The techniques used vary but generally include helping the individual gain an intellectual understanding of his experience, assisting in recognition of feelings, exposing past and present coping methods, finding and using resources, and anticipatory planning to reduce the possibility of future crises.

Crisis intervention is partly a theory and partly a method. It makes its boundaries explicit by limiting the focus to the four to six week period and has internal consistency, since its concepts are interrelated. Crisis intervention theory predicts future events for persons involved in crisis by showing that a person who successfully copes with his present crisis will better handle subsequent crises. Theorists of crisis intervention have synthesized their theory into an equation, including the event, interpretation of event, and family resources. Figure 18-1 is a model of this equation.

Although there are still important questions that need to be answered by future use of the theory, such as, "How can we identify those individuals and families who will recover from a crisis on their own versus others who will not adapt without specific intervention?," the crisis intervention methods are valuable to a wide variety of people and settings.

SCOPE OF CRISIS INTERVENTION

The scope of crisis intervention is very broad. It can be used to predict crises that will occur with certain events to particular groups of people. This attribute allows health professionals to plan for high-risk family crises and be available at the appropriate time for intervention. Crisis intervention can be used by a variety of health professionals with much success. Its strategies can be used effectively with people from all walks of life, be they rich or poor, black, white, or yellow. And it can be used for a time-limited period, thereby discouraging a long-term commitment and client dependency.

Predicting Crises

The state of crisis and the opportunity for crisis intervention can arise at any point in an individual's life, regardless of his or her socioeconomic or sociocultural status. There are, however, specific situational and maturational events occurring to particular population groups which predictably result in crises for many people. Many potential crises producing events can occur during a high-risk situation.

Situational Events. A situation which threatens an individual or family's biological, psychological, or social integrity may produce a crisis. For the high-risk family, there are a number of situations which predictably disturb the family's integrity. The unwed teenage mother, the unwanted pregnancy, the premature baby, the baby born with birth defects, the stillborn, the baby who succumbs to sudden infant death syndrome, the hospitalized child, the abusing parent, the addicted parent, and other troubled parents are all examples of crisis-prone, situational events. Quite often, these high-risk situations produce expected family stresses and reactions which help in anticipating and planning strategies for the crisis. Many specific stresses and family difficulties are discussed in the earlier chapters on high-risk child or parent situations.

For example, a 15-year-old unwed girl has her pregnancy confirmed in a prenatal clinic. Her initial reaction is, "But I'm not that kind of girl, I didn't plan to have sexual relations." The nurse recognizes these are honest, predictable feelings, but in the final reality they can often be a means of avoiding the responsibility for one's actions. The girl leaves the clinic in a shocked, dazed state but promises to return for her next appointment. As the nurse plans her future care, she realizes that the girl will now not only be coping with the stresses of adolescence, but with the additional feelings of the loss of control over her future, erosion of an evolving moral system, the immediate need to assume the roles of woman and mother, and the acute body alterations imposed by pregnancy. Her biological, psychological, and social integrity are certainly threatened—a fact which causes the nurse to plan for crisis assessment and possible intervention as soon as possible.

Maturational Events. Normal growth and development introduces many changes, periods of disequilibrium, and potentials for crisis. Infancy, childhood, adolescence, and the various stages of adulthood are steps of increasing maturation which must be overcome before the next stage is tackled. When a person has excessive difficulty resolving a developmental step, a maturational crisis occurs. Examples of maturational crisis events include the infant who cannot trust his environment, the toddler who has limited initiative for exploration, the adolescent who cannot confirm his identity, and the young adult who avoids interpersonal contacts. When a situational event such as the birth of a congenital anomaly infant occurs during a maturational event such as adolescence, even greater family disorganization can result.

Pregnancy and parenthood are additional potential maturational crisis periods which are particularly relevant for the high-risk family. Pregnancy represents a period of increased susceptibility to and occurrence of intermittent critical events. The nine-month gestation is a period all its own, when hormonal balance changes, psychological preparation for a new role begins, and old conflicts arise. Likewise, new parenthood is now recognized as a crisis period when the romanticism of parenting is dissolved by the realities of life with a new baby. As with situational crisis events, these two potential crisis periods include recognizable stresses and reactions which aid the therapist. They also are periods where if the crises are overcome in a healthy manner, the positive outcome means real gains in parent-child relationships.

For example, a maternal-infant nurse receives a call from a concerned mother who is now one week postpartum. The woman says that ever since the baby arrived, she and her husband have been tired and argumentative. Several times during the call, the mother questions her ability to be a good mother and asks for any suggestions the nurse has to offer. The nurse realizes that the couple is experiencing the crises of parenthood and is very susceptible to outside assistance. As she plans her visit, she considers the usual factors which contribute to parental crises: the loss of sleep, the creation of new responsibilities, the loss of a second income, the decrease in social activity, and role change brought about by the new infant. This information will be invaluable as the nurse helps the family plan coping methods to handle the specific stresses caused by a new infant.

Use of Crisis Intervention by Professionals

As crisis intervention has become more widely recognized, its use by a variety of professionals has become popular. The skills needed to employ the intervention are possessed chiefly by nurses, physicians, psychologists, and social workers. In some settings, a team approach is used, while in others, individual counseling is done, with or without psychiatric back-up.

For the family in crisis, the professional closest to the client must begin the strategy, in either an inpatient or an outpatient setting. In many cases, this is the pediatric nurse, the public health nurse, the clinic nurse, or the social worker who sees the client initially and often over a four to six week period of time. These professionals can then often carry the intervention to completion without referral to a long-term agency. In a short-term setting, such as the postpartum ward, the strategy can still be used in a modified form. Most nurses have the advantage of being with the client for eight-hour shifts and can intervene several times a day. They also can recognize and assess the crisis behavior better than any other professional because of their proximity to the family.

Another advantage offered to the professional is the ease in which nonmental health professionals can use the strategies. If the therapist is familiar with the characteristic patterns of behavior occurring in most crises, she can form her plan of care around the phases of the particular crises, without having to focus on the psychodynamics of the individuals involved. This approach to crisis intervention has been found to be very effective in the resolution of most crises. For example, if a nurse is working with a couple who has just delivered a premature infant, she can expect four phases which the parents must work through before they can accept the child. They must realize that they may lose the baby, they must acknowledge failure in carrying a full-term infant, they must resume a relationship with this baby, and they must prepare for a caretaking role. With this knowledge, the nurse can support the various feelings of the couple and help them work through the phases necessary for parent-child bonding.

The setting used by the professional can be either individual or group, inpatient or outpatient. Although individual use of the strategy is the most common, very effective results have come from the application of crisis intervention to groups of parents of defective infants, parents of premature infants, and new parents of normal infants. These groups can run over a four to six week period or can be ongoing, with couples entering and leaving as they experience crisis and later resolution.

The type of professional carrying out crisis intervention strategies will depend on the setting and can include public health nurses, hospital nurses, clinic nurses, social workers, probation officers, teachers, pastoral counselors, and a host of others.

Advantages of Crisis Intervention to Client. Crisis intervention is focused only on the immediate crisis, is time limited, and costs relatively little since it can be applied by a variety of professionals. These factors make it a very desirable strategy for most people, particularly those who want relief from tension without long-term therapy commitments. Another advantage for many people is that the therapist makes no attempt to delve into a family's living pattern and make major characterological changes. The strategies focus on the here and now, reviewing only coping mechanisms of the past to help resolve the crisis.

Crisis intervention has been called "Band-Aid" therapy because it strives for immediate relief of symptoms. It is suggested that people will avoid needed psychotherapy if anxiety is lessened in crisis intervention. However, there is little evidence that this phenomenon occurs; more likely, there seems to be enhanced motivation from the present success in dealing with the crisis.

CRISIS INTERVENTION STRATEGIES FOR THE HIGH-RISK FAMILY

The goal of anyone applying crisis intervention to a high-risk family situation is always the same: to restore the individuals and family to their precrisis or higher level of functioning. All efforts are directed toward this goal.

The strategies in crisis intervention are interrelated and are used in a variable pattern, however, they do follow a typical sequence of phases including assessment, planned intervention, intervention, resolution, and anticipatory planning. The nurse is very flexible as she proceeds through the above phases since the coping methods used for resolution by each family may be very different. Figure 18-2 concisely lists crisis intervention strategies for the high-risk family.

Assessment

Assessment includes identifying the crisis reaction, event, onset, supportive people, coping behaviors, and risk. Since every person interprets

Figure 18-2. Crisis Intervention Strategies for the High-Risk Family

Assessment
    Determine if the client is actually in crisis
    Identify the precipitating event
    Ascertain crisis onset
    Identify client's perception of problem
    Determine situational supports
    Identify past coping mechanisms
    Assess suicidal or homicidal risk

Planned Intervention
    Determine degree of disruption on family
    Consider alternative coping methods

Intervention
    Relate the precipitating event and present crisis state
    Provide opportunities for expression of emotions
    Test alternative coping methods

Resolution and Anticipatory Planning
    Determine resolution of crisis
    Reinforce successful coping methods

and reacts to a crisis differently, this individual assessment is essential.

Determine If the Client Is Actually in a Crisis. The initial step in assessment is to determine if the family is actually in crisis. Although high-risk situations involve many potential crisis producing events, not all families will have a crisis. Symptoms of crisis are rising tension and disorganization related to the inability to cope with an event occurring four to six weeks or less in the past. Many individuals will appear disorganized by crying frequently, feeling exhausted, tense or depressed, and complaining of insomnia and altered appetite.

The therapist should observe the client's general appearance and behavior. Does she tell you she is very upset? Does she appear tense and nervous? Is she neat or grossly untidy? Is her speech pressured or relaxed? How does he describe his feelings? Is the family's behavior inappropriate? Some families may not demonstrate physical symptoms so much as they alter their usual living pattern. An example may be parents who have just received the diagnosis of leukemia in their oldest child completely ignoring the needs of their other children. It is important to realize that some families will experience a crisis when faced with a seemingly small problem, while others will have enough coping mechanisms to withstand most stressful events.

Identify the Precipitating Event. Once the crisis state has been determined, the therapist should identify the precipitating event. This is the occurrence which triggered the crisis in the family. In some instances, this will be very obvious, as in the cases of premature birth, stillbirth, death, or the delivery of a child with birth defects. In other situations, the precipitating event may be the "last straw" in a series of life problems. The individuals in these cases often may not recognize what precipitated their behavior, thereby making assessment more difficult. Questions to the client may include: Why did you come for help *today*? When did you begin to feel tense? What occurred at that period of time? Did you receive any unexpected news? Did you receive any visitors then? Is there a new baby in the home, a new job or loss of a job, or an illness or death in the family? The therapist may find such diverse precipitating events as that of a mother-in-law visiting an already upset home, the news of a job relocation, the recognition of alcoholism in the family, or the diagnosis of failure to thrive.

Ascertain Crisis Onset. The crisis onset is that period of time when the precipitating event caused the crisis. If the length of time since the onset or the beginning of the crisis is ascertained, the therapist has an idea of the amount of time there is to apply crisis intervention strategies. For example, if the birth of a defective baby occurred five weeks prior to the application of crisis intervention, the clients may no longer be susceptible to its strategies. On the other hand, if the person who initiates the intervention is present the day of the child's birth, initiation of crisis intervention is likely to be successful. This is not to say that no individuals will benefit from crisis techniques after the four to six week crisis period, but the strategy's usefulness will decline as the individuals involved become less susceptible to external help. For some high-risk families the crisis may be produced by a later event such as the time the parents first take their premature infant home. Continual assessment of crisis onset is needed.

Identify Client's Perception of the Problem. The next strategy is to determine the family's perception of the problem. This will give the therapist an idea of why the precipitating event provoked a crisis. An example is the diagnosis of pregnancy in a successful career woman who perceives a child as a threat to her self-image and career. For this woman, the diagnosis of pregnancy is coped with very differently from the healthy woman who wants children, the woman who is over 40 and finds herself pregnant, or the woman with a family history of birth defects. Answers to questions such as What does this event mean to you? How have things changed? How do you believe it will affect your future? will give the therapist an idea of the family's view of the event.

Determine Situational Supports. Assessment of the family's situational supports is the next strategy. Situational supports are those people in the family's environment who might give support and help during and after the crisis period. Many high-risk families call on neighbors or relatives to help with household chores during the crisis period. The individuals in crisis will know better than anyone else who could give them the most help, so this data should be elicited from them. Often the individuals will come up with names of people who were previously not recognized as supports. Typical questions include: Do you have anyone to help you care for the child? Who do you turn to when you have questions or problems? Whom do you trust? Who is your best friend? With whom do you live? Are they helpful? Do you have relatives who might be helpful? neighbors? Are any other professionals involved? The more people the therapist can involve in supporting the family, the better. These people can also be used for continued support after the crisis resolution.

Identify Past Coping Mechanisms. The family is then questioned about their past coping mechanisms. This history includes all methods the individuals involved have used previously to reduce tension or stress. Examples of these methods include taking a walk, playing the piano, going away for the weekend, getting a babysitter more frequently, talking with a friend, painting, biking, and gardening. Questions may include: Have you ever had an experience like this before? What did you do? How do you usually relieve tension and anxiety? Have you tried that method this time? If not, why not? What do you feel would reduce this stress? The couple may remember methods of coping that they have not used for years. They may also discuss methods that worked before but would not work in this situation. If these coping methods will not work, the therapist must ask herself why. What will work in this situation? Because adaptive skills are so individual, the therapist must work with the couple to determine what will decrease the stress for them.

Assess Suicidal or Homicidal Risk. A crucial part of the assessment is discovering possible suicidal or homicidal risk. People in crisis may exhibit behavior that they would normally be incapable of.

An abusing, alcoholic, addicted, or emotionally disturbed parent will need special attention. The therapist's previous assessment of the client's behavior since crisis onset will be most helpful. Does the client appear to be tearful, jolly, silly, or indifferent? Can he express his mood in terms like, "I feel as if . . ."? Does he appear not to care about anything? Does he express aggression? If the therapist suspects the client is potentially suicidal or homicidal, his questions should be direct: Are you planning to take your life? Have you ever thought of harming your children? Can you tell me your plans? How desperate have you felt? Some clients may begin to express relief that their desperation is recognized. If the client is thought to be too great a risk to himself or others, psychiatric referral is made immediately. If there is no suspected danger, planned intervention can proceed.

Planned Intervention

Planning the individual interventions for each family is based on a consideration of the family's present disruption and of possible effective alternative coping behaviors.

Determine Degree of Disruption in Family. The amount of disruption in the high-risk family will determine what intervention the therapist will plan. For example, a woman who is so stressed by the care of her physically disabled child that she no longer cares for herself, the house, the meals, or the child will require immediate intervention for substitute child care and home care. The therapist may ask Is the family continuing their daily functioning of work, school, house care, and child care? How are significant others in and near the family being affected? Are they also in crisis? Are the children receiving adequate mental and physical management? Are they upset? Answers to these questions will be vital to successful intervention.

Consider Alternative Coping Methods. Next, the therapist and the family examine the alternatives open to them for restoring equilibrium. Usually these are the methods that seem most feasible or that have worked well in the past. These alternatives are examined in the light of why the problem

is causing a crisis and what will restore balance. For example, the mother who feels like abusing her colicky baby proposes that she share the child's care with others until the colic passes. In another instance, parents who feel their premature baby may die choose to be told the exact status of their child and then help in his care to alleviate some of their anxiety.

Intervention

After options are explored, intervention is initiated. Intervention techniques are highly variable and depend on the skills and creativity of the professional as well as the individual needs of the family. The goals of the intervention phase are to help the individuals involved gain an intellectual understanding of why they are in crisis, bring into the open feelings which may have been suppressed, explore new ways of coping with this experience, and restore family functioning.

Relate the Precipitating Event and Present Crisis State. The therapist discusses the relationship between the present feelings of crisis and the defined precipitating event. This action clarifies the problem and causes the high-risk family to focus directly on their present situation. It is particularly helpful to the family who sees no relationship between a previous situation and their current stressful feelings. For example, a disturbed family may not recognize the mother-in-law's visit as the crisis precipitating event until it is pointed out to them. Since some high-risk families develop a crisis because of an event actually following the risk situation, the nurse helps the family to identify the initial or later cause. Parents who adapt to the birth of a premature infant may react to crisis later if the infant is transported to a regional center. The crisis state and intervention are then related to the separation of the infant from the family.

Provide Opportunities for Expression of Emotions. Another intervention strategy designed to reduce tension is that of providing opportunities for expression of feelings. Many individuals will suppress their emotions of hate, grief, or guilt over an event. This may be especially true for the parents who have a less than perfect baby. They characteristically feel shock, denial, shame, envy, bitterness, and rejection over their fate. Many of these feelings are not readily admissible in our society, but they are real and must be brought into the open if anxiety is to be lessened. Openers into this conversation may include: "It's often very hard for people to accept something like this when it happens to them. Many parents are very angry (or bitter, shocked, envious, and so on). Do you have any of these feelings?" The therapist should be prepared for the feelings that are expressed by supportive listening and understanding.

Test Alternative Coping Methods. The main intervention method involves trying and evaluating the alternative coping methods explored in the planning stage. Specific guidelines, either written or spoken, on what could be tried may have to be given. This provides the family in crisis with concrete steps to take toward their goal of reducing tension. After each alternative is carried out, it must be evaluated. If it was not successful, the family and therapist explore other options. For example, if the baby with failure to thrive does not respond well to a specific formula (thereby causing his mother great anxiety), another formula, nipple, or method of handling during feeding should be tried.

If a thorough assessment and adequate planned intervention were carried out, the coping methods tried during this phase quite often will be successful. This leads to a resolution of the crisis.

Resolution and Anticipatory Planning

Determining that the crisis has been resolved is very satisfying for both the family and the therapist. Immediately after resolution of the crisis, the family is often open to ideas which may anticipate or prevent future crisis.

Determine Resolution of Crisis. If the high-risk family in crisis realistically examine the problem, have adequate help from relatives, friends and health workers, and are able to develop new ways of coping, the crisis should be resolved four to six weeks after the event. The therapist can evaluate at that time whether the family returned to their usual or higher level of equilibrium because of the crisis. Some observations showing resolution of the crisis are a more positive mood and a decrease in such psychosomatic symptoms as depression, insomnia, altered appetite, crying, and headaches. The therapist looks for a return to the family's usual level of functioning in their home, child and self care. Signs which show additional growth are use of adaptive behaviors which allow the family to cope with additional stress and perform on a higher level than before. An example is improved communication patterns between the parents of a sick child. It is hoped that every crisis has some growth-promoting potential for all concerned.

Reinforce Successful Coping Methods. The therapist reinforces the family's newfound coping mechanisms by reviewing the experience and the action taken, allowing the family to feel satisfaction with the progress made. This provides the family with an additional experience of being rewarded for their resolution of the crisis and possible growth in coping with the stressful event.

The nurse discusses how the present experience may help in coping with future crisis. The family has now added more coping behaviors to their repertoire of life experiences. An exploration of the ways in which these new behaviors can be applied to future life stresses allows for additional growth from the current crisis. For example, the parents who resolved the crisis precipitated by their child's premature birth should be able to apply these same helpful coping mechanisms to another similar event. They should have learned and grown from this crisis.

CRISIS INTERVENTION STRATEGIES APPLIED IN A HIGH-RISK FAMILY EXAMPLE

Assessment

Determine If Client Is Actually in Crisis. A three-month-old male was admitted to the hospital with a broken arm and dislocated shoulder. Mrs. F, the child's mother, stated that the child rolled off the bed when she had turned her back. Child abuse could not be ruled out, so a referral was made to the public health nurse to evaluate the home condition.

During the home visit, the nurse found Mrs. F to be an attractive woman in her early 20s. Although she appeared calm when she greeted the nurse, she later began crying as she described her situation. She stated that ever since the birth of this baby, she had felt tired, irritable, and depressed. Her husband worked during the day and frequently socialized with the "boys" at night, leaving her alone with a 15-month-old and a three-month-old. Both the house and the oldest child appeared dirty and unkempt. Mrs. F stated that she considered herself a good mother and housekeeper, but could not cope with her present situation. Initial assessment by the nurse indicated that Mrs. F was indeed experiencing crisis.

Identify the Precipitating Event. The nurse initially thought of the birth of the baby as the crisis event, but since delivery occurred three months previously, she began to search for a more recent stressful period. Mrs. F stated that she had been tense and tired since she brought the baby home, but really began to be upset after her mother-in-law's visit. She felt that her care of her family had been unduly criticized by the mother-in-law. As the nurse continued her questioning, it was decided by both Mrs. F and the nurse that the mother-in-law's visit had tipped the scale toward crisis.

Ascertain Crisis Onset. In the case of Mrs. F, the mother-in-law's visit occurred one week prior to the child's injury and one and a half weeks before the nurse's visit. This provides a maximum period of two to four weeks for application of crisis intervention strategies.

Identify Client's Perception of Problem. The nurse recognized the mother-in-law's visit as the crisis event but needed to determine how Mrs. F viewed the situation. With questioning, Mrs. F stated that she had never gotten along well with her mother-in-law and had always considered her a critical, demanding person. Mrs. F realized that the mother-in-law's behavior reminded her too much of her own childhood, when she felt she could not live up to her parent's expectations. The nurse began to recognize the pattern of an insecure child with overly demanding parents, now being threatened by another critical adult. The nurse later asked Mrs. F what she expected of her own children. "I want them to love me, but all they do is drive me crazy," was Mrs. F's reply. Identification of Mrs. F's perception of the mother-in-law's visit provided invaluable clues to the nurse's recognition of and intervention for child abuse.

Determine Situational Supports. The nurse asked Mrs. F about friends or relatives who could help her with some of the infant's care. Mrs. F ruled out her parents and her mother-in-law, but mentioned that she did have a sister in a nearby town and had become acquainted with a neighbor across the street. The nurse also scheduled a meeting with Mr. F to determine his support of his wife. He was shocked to learn of the nurse's concern over his wife's feelings and admitted that indeed he had not assumed too much responsibility at home, but said he could try to help out with the children more. The sister, neighbor, and husband were all later used to decrease the crisis for Mrs. F.

Identify Past Coping Mechanisms. The nurse scheduled a later meeting with both Mr. and Mrs. F. Questions included: How did you handle your mother-in-law's visits before? Have you tried that method this time? What do you feel would lessen the feelings you now have? Mrs. F felt she could cope with her mother-in-law's criticism before, but now could not handle two babies and the mother-in-law. On previous visits, Mr. F had coped by leaving the house, while Mrs. F involved herself with intense housecleaning and cooking to relieve tension. As his wife continued talking, Mr. F began to see what a strain his wife was under during these visits and asked if his presence would lessen his mother's effects. Mrs. F said, "I've wanted you to help out at home for so long, but I have given up."

Her past coping mechanism did not seem appropriate now, but the offer of the husband to stay home more was identified as a possible adaptation to the stressful situation.

Assess Suicidal or Homicidal Risks. Since one

child was in the hospital, suspected of being abused, the nurse was very concerned about the safety of the oldest child. The nurse asked Mrs. F, "When you feel very tense and tired, do you ever feel like harming your children or yourself?" Mrs. F began to cry and said, "Sometimes the baby cries and cries and I just can't handle it. The oldest one never did this; why are the children so different? Right after my mother-in-law visited, he began crying and would not stop. I thought I would lose my mind without some help. I did hit him and now I feel so guilty I could die." The nurse stated her recognition of the strain Mrs. F was under. She asked her if she ever felt like harming her other child. Mrs. F said no, that he did not make her as irritable as the new baby.

The nurse assessed that Mrs. F's new baby was probably the only person at risk, although she did notify the physician and social worker of her findings. Frequent home intervention was planned while Mrs. F's new baby remained hospitalized.

Planned Intervention

Determine Degree of Disruption in Family. The disruption caused by the crisis was assessed. Mrs. F was unable to continue her usual level of house care and child care. Mr. F had continued his work as usual and did not appear as upset over the situation. This knowledge became valuable in planning for workable coping methods.

Consider Alternative Coping Methods. Now that the crisis event and resulting abuse on the baby were out in the open, the F family and the nurse began to explore alternative coping methods. The exploration of past coping behavior did not provide useful methods to relieve this stress. New coping methods suggested by both parents and the nurse included more frequent assistance in child care by Mr. F, asking the mother-in-law not to visit the family, providing babysitters on the days Mrs. F feels she cannot cope, giving the family the crisis line telephone number for the periods of extreme stress, and enrolling the couple in a parent discussion group at the local young family resource cen-

ter. All these alternatives were based on the identified problems of Mrs. F's inability to comfortably handle two small children alone, Mr. F's previous reluctance to assist in child care, and the added stress of a critical mother-in-law.

Intervention

Relate the Precipitating Event and Present Crisis State. Initially, neither Mr. or Mrs. F recognized the mother-in-law's visit as the crisis precipitating event which tipped the scale in an already disturbed home. Once this was pointed out, the couple began to discuss the difficulty of caring for two small children, especially when criticism rather than praise is received. Mr. F began to see the effect his mother had on his wife, as well as the consequences of his own lack of participation in the home. He said he did love his wife and children and would try some of the options considered.

Provide Opportunities for Expression of Emotions. Mrs. F's angry feelings toward her situation had been inappropriately released in an attack on her child. This behavior only added guilt to her list of negative emotions. The nurse asked both Mr. and Mrs. F how they felt about the present situation, stating that it would be very normal to feel anger, guilt, and bitterness over the past experience. Mrs. F again began to cry and stated it was a relief to tell someone just how she felt. Mr. F said he felt guilty over the outcome of his avoidance of the situation. The provision of a suitable outlet for emotions was essential for reducing the tension in this family.

Test Alternative Coping Methods. Mr. and Mrs. F were now ready to test the coping methods they had chosen. The baby had been returned to the family, so specific directions and close supervision by the nurse were essential. The nurse advised them to try two of the alternatives now and two later. Specifically, it was decided that Mr. F give his wife one night "off" a week when she could be free to visit friends, go shopping, or pursue any other interests without being responsible for the children. This alternative was chosen to temporarily relieve Mrs. F of the large responsibilities and stresses of two small children and was also seen as a way of involving Mr. F in child care. The other coping method chosen was to ask Mrs. F's mother-in-law not to visit them anymore. This option was selected because the mother-in-law was seen as an additional irritant in a tense family. The family was given two weeks to test the alternatives.

At the nurse's next visit, it was obvious that things had been going well. The couple was freely and happily exchanging comments throughout the visit. Mr. F had babysat two nights in the last two weeks and said he did not understand how his wife coped with the children by herself all the time. He related that they had been quite a handful and he had had to call the neighbor and the sister once to ask what to do to stop the baby from crying. Mrs. F stated that she had enjoyed her night "off" so much that she felt like a new person, ready to face the responsibilities of her home.

Asking the mother-in-law not to visit had not been as successful. The mother-in-law was very hurt by the request and accused Mrs. F of taking her grandchildren away. She said that now she had no one and was alone in the city. Mrs. F felt so bad about this that she allowed the mother-in-law to visit but only if she called first and came when her husband was home. This was agreed upon by all concerned. In this case, though the initial coping behaviors were not successful, a more acceptable method emerged from it.

The nurse complimented the family on their excellent progress and began to explore the possibilities of enrolling them in a parent discussion group for support and education.

Resolution and Anticipatory Planning

Determine Resolution of Crisis. Four weeks after the initial contact had been made, the nurse evaluated that the family had resolved their crisis. Mr. and Mrs. F were able to realistically view the problem of child care responsibilities and a critical mother-in-law, they received support from one another, the neighbor and parenting center, and a professional nurse, and they developed new ways

of coping with their situation. Mrs. F said she no longer felt tension, anger, and bitterness over her situation now that her husband supported her in her role, although the guilt over attacking her baby would probably never leave. Mrs. F was now able to care for the house and children as she once did. Additional growth for this family could be seen in many areas: the husband now helped in child care at least one night per week, they were enrolled in a parent discussion group, the mother-in-law's visits were realistically viewed and restricted, and supportive resources in the community were made available to the couple. Although a case of child abuse should be followed over a period of time, this couple showed many signs of new strength and adaptive behavior.

Reinforce Successful Coping Methods. The nurse reviewed the progress made by Mr. and Mrs. F over the past four weeks. Both Mr. and Mrs. F seemed pleased at their success. Mr. F said the nurse's support was especially helpful to him because there were some weeks when he really did not want to help his wife but now knew that it was a necessary part of his role as husband and father. Repeated reassurance and an examination of progress will be necessary as this family continues to adapt to their situation.

After the nurse had reviewed the new coping methods adopted by the F family, she asked the couple if they felt these behaviors would be useful when future problems arose. A prolonged visit by the mother-in-law, continued crying episodes by the infant, and the birth of a third baby were specifically suggested as potential crisis events which this family may experience. The F family stated that if any of these situations arose, they now knew they could rely on one another and on community resources for support. The nurse reinforced these feelings by stressing the importance of communicating with each other when problems arose and by giving the couple a list of parent services within the community, both preventive and crisis related. This information later proved to be invaluable as the couple coped with emerging independence in their toddler and frequent cases of otitis media in their infant. The support they gave one another and the guidance they received from community agencies averted any further child abuse situations.

SUMMARY

Since crises occur frequently for high-risk families, crisis intervention strategies are a valuable adjunct to any nurse involved in potential high-risk family situations. The intervention can be applied by the nurse in any setting, is time limited, focuses directly on the problem at hand, and offers the family not only relief from their anxiety but also the potential for growth and maturity with which to face later crises.

REFERENCE

1. Hill, R. "Generic Features of Families Under Stress." In *Crisis Intervention: Selected Readings*, H. Parad (ed.). New York: Family Service Association of America, 1965.

ADDITIONAL READINGS

1. Aguilera, D. and J. Messick. *Crisis Intervention, Theory and Methodology*. St. Louis: C. V. Mosby Co., 1974.
2. Baird, S. F. "Crisis Intervention Theory in Maternal-Infant Nursing." *JOGN Nursing*, 5 #1, January-February 1976, 30 +.
3. Brose, C. "Theories of Family Crisis." In *Family Health Care*, D. Hymovich and M. Barnard (eds.). New York: McGraw-Hill, 1973, 271–283.
4. Caplan, G. *Principles of Preventive Psychiatry*. New York: Basic Books, 1964.
5. Daniel, J. and J. Hyde. "Working with High Risk Families: Family Advocacy and the Parent Education Program." *Children Today*, November–December 1975, 23 +.
6. Hoffman, D. and M. Remmel. "Uncovering the Precipitant in Crisis Intervention." *Nursing Digest*, Summer 1976, 25–27.
7. Kale, J. and A. Kale. "Managing the Individual and Family in Crisis." *American Family Physician*, 12, November 1975, 109–115.
8. Kuenzi, S. and M. Fenton. "Crisis Intervention in Acute Care Areas." *American Journal of Nursing*, May 1975, 830–834.
9. Langsley, D. and R. Yarvis. "Evaluation of Crisis Intervention." *Current Psychiatric Therapies*, 15, 1975, 247–251.
10. Robischon, P. "The Challenge of Crisis Theory for Nursing." In *Family Centered Community Nursing—A Sociocultural Framework*. A. M. Reinhardt and M. Quinn (eds.). St. Louis: C. V. Mosby Co., 1973, 245–253.
11. Shields, L. "Crisis Intervention: Implications for the Nurse." *Journal of Psychiatric Nursing and Mental Health Services*, September–October 1975, 37–42.
12. Williams, W. V. et al. "Crisis Intervention: Effects of Crisis Intervention on Family Survivors of Sudden Death Situations." *Community Mental Health Journal*, 12 #2, 1976, 128–136.

Behavior
Modification Strategies

Suzanne Hall Johnson, R.N., M.N.

CHAPTER NINETEEN

The principles of behavior modification are naturally and frequently used by parents to reward desired behavior or punish undesired behavior in order to guide their children to socially accepted actions. In some high-risk parenting situations, maladaptive behaviors of the children or parent have not been controlled by the intuitive responses and may become a threat to the family. When this occurs, planned behavior modification may help to direct them to more socially accepted behavior.

Behavior modification is most useful for two types of behaviors in a high-risk family. First, behavior modification can help to reduce the actual risk behavior, such as the drinking of an alcoholic parent, aggression of an abusive parent, or overactivity of a hyperactive child. Second, it may help to reduce unacceptable coping behaviors that are caused by the risk situation, such as a parent leaving because of his drinking, a father avoiding interacting with his terminally ill son, or a sibling regressing because of attention being focused on his ill brother.

Since the nurse works with the high-risk family in many settings, including the home, school, clinic, and hospital, and frequently follows them over a period of time, she can help the family develop and implement a behavior modification plan. Her background and interest in focusing on behavior and including all family members in the health plan makes her an excellent person to identify the possible effectiveness of the behavior modification therapy for the family.

The nurse uses behavior modification along with other strategies for high-risk parents. Behavior modification involves both teaching and counseling strategies. Teaching strategies emphasize the need for an immediate reward for a learned behavior, and counseling strategies highlight individualizing the behavior therapy plan to the family. Crisis intervention, cultural, and financial strategies are also used along with behavior modification techniques to reduce other problems of the high-risk family.

The nurse's purpose in using behavior modification strategies is to help the family reduce the risk situation or cope with it. When parents are taught how to reduce problem behaviors and how to prevent future unacceptable behaviors, they are in more control of their own family interactions and better able to cope with the other high-risk problems. Unfortunately, behavior modification has too often been associated only with punishment and very formal techniques, but it can also be a very positive rewarding experience for the family. Using rewards for positive behavior fosters closeness and acceptable behavior between family members. The strategies in this chapter will emphasize the supportive aspects of behavior modification for use with high-risk families.

BASIC CONCEPTS

Behavior modification applies teaching theory to increase desired behavior or decrease undesired behavior. Since behavior is seen as a response to the environment and interactions with other people, any change in the environment or interactions will in turn change behavior. By controlling the environment and interactions, behavior can be modified as explained in the two basic theories of classical conditioning and operant conditioning.

Classical Conditioning. Classical conditioning emphasizes that whatever comes before a behavior influences that behavior. An antecedent event influences the responding behavior. This is illustrated in the following model.

Antecedent Event ⟶ Behavior
Figure 19-1

Operant Conditioning. Operant conditioning stresses that the behavior is also influenced by the response that follows it. A behavior that is followed by a negative response will be diminished, while a behavior followed by a positive consequence will be increased. The following model shows the operant conditioning concept.

Behavior ⟶ Consequence
Figure 19-2

Model of Behavior Response. Applying both models, behavior is seen as resulting from an antecedent event and also being influenced by the consequence. The following model incorporates both concepts.

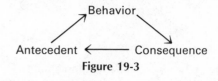
Figure 19-3

PLANNING MODIFICATION OF BEHAVIOR

Using the above model of how behavior may be modified, the nurse and parent can plan how to decrease undesired behaviors and increase desired ones.

Decreasing Undesired Behavior. Undesired behavior may be decreased by changing the antecedent event which causes the behavior, punishing the behavior after it occurs, or both. Punishment includes adding a negative event such as a spanking or removing a positive event such as a meal. Ignoring a behavior by omitting the positive smile or other acknowledgment of the person may also decrease the behavior without the use of physical punishment. The model for decreasing undesired behavior is illustrated below.

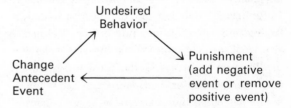
Figure 19-4. To Decrease Undesired Behavior

Increasing Desired Behavior. Desired behavior may be increased by changing the antecedent event to one which will elicit the desired response, by reinforcing the desired behavior after it occurs, or both. Reinforcement includes adding a positive event such as a hug or removing a negative event such as an early bedtime for previous bad behavior. The model for increasing desired behavior is illustrated in the following figure.

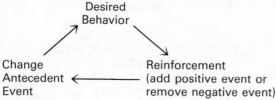

Figure 19-5. To Increase Desired Behavior

Changing Behavior. Too frequently, behavior modification is used to decrease undesired behavior by punishment without reinforcing the positive behavior. A combination of punishment and reward is a more supportive approach for the family members. In the early stages of an undesired action, ignoring the behavior while reinforcing desired behaviors is enough to change the behavior. Most parents find this system an effective and supportive method for parenting. Guiding their children to acceptable behavior through supporting rather than punishing leads to more self-respect for all members and a positive family relationship.

Due to the family crisis, feelings of inadequacy, and habit formation of the undesired behavior, many high-risk families are already using punishment as the major form of discipline in the family. This is frequently found in families with failure to thrive, hyperactive, abusive, or alcoholic family members. Unfortunately, punishment continues to reinforce feelings of inadequacy and guilt in a cycle of negative feedback. The nurse's role in using behavior modification is to assess the present system of antecedent, behavior, and consequences. When a family has fallen into a pattern of negative consequences and punishment, the nurse helps the family plan and use the more positive ways of changing behavior while fostering more positive self-respect and relationships for all family members.

For example, the parents of a hyperactive child may have reached physical and emotional exhaustion trying to control their child. With the loss of patience and intermittent crises, a behavior such as the child breaking a toy will result in the parent yelling at the child, telling him he is clumsy, or possibly violently abusing him. The nurse can help the family to change their pattern of antecedent behavior and consequences and thus influence the

child's behavior. By buying well-built wooden block toys rather than thin plastic ones, the environment and antecedent event will be changed and the toy breaking behavior will decrease. Helping the parents recognize their own stress and need for relaxation and planning for child day care will make the parents better able to tolerate the stress so they can ignore undesired behavior and reinforce positive ones.

BEHAVIOR MODIFICATION STRATEGIES FOR THE HIGH-RISK FAMILY

The nurse's function in using behavior modification with the high-risk family is to reduce the cause of the behavior problem whenever possible. Second, when this is not possible she helps the family change or cope with the behavior through behavior modification strategies. Third, she helps prevent future risk or coping behavior problems by helping the family apply the strategies before the problem behavior becomes a pattern. The nurse performs this role by using behavior modification strategies in her nursing process of assessing, planning, implementing, evaluating, and teaching. Basic behavior modification strategies are listed in Figure 19-6.

Assessing

The nurse assesses the family interactions to determine the target problem behavior or desired behavior and the antecedent and consequences of

Figure 19-6. Behavior Modification Strategies for the High-Risk Family

Assessing
  Pick specific observable behavior

Planning
  Select one or two target behaviors
  Communicate the plan to significant others

Implementing
  Change the antecedent event
  Provide reinforcement and avoid punishment
  Provide immediate feedback
  Reward progress

Evaluating
  Evaluate continually

Teaching

that behavior. She works closely with all family members to determine what behaviors they consider problems.

Pick Specific Observable Behavior. The nurse helps the family to select a target behavior that is specific and observable so the family will know if the treatment plan is helping to change the behavior. Both the negative behavior and the desired behavior are described so that reinforcement may be used more than punishment for the high-risk family member. The nurse helps the family record the frequency as well as the quality of the behavior, since both may change. This record is a base record that will be used in the behavior modification plan and evaluation to determine progress.

For example, a community health nurse working with a family with a congenital defect child helped the family develop a plan to reinforce the child's use of her weak legs. The parents described the undesired behavior as the child pulling herself along with her arms and the desired behavior as the child pulling herself up onto her feet or using her legs to reach a toy. The family recorded the frequency of both the desired and undesired behaviors and described how far the child was pulling up and putting weight on her legs. This baseline assessment was helpful in evaluating the effectiveness of the behavior modification plan they tried later.

Planning

After assessing the family situation, all family members are included in planning the change of antecedent event and different punishment or reinforcement consequences.

Select One or Two Target Behaviors. Frequently high-risk families identify many specific problem behaviors or desired behaviors for family members. When this occurs, the nurse helps the family to select one or, at the most, two behaviors which they consider to be of highest priority. Instituting a behavior modification program for many behaviors is confusing to the target family member and to the other members. Reinforcement is less likely to be immediate and consistent when several different behaviors are used. If there are several specific desired behaviors which are similar, such as the child previously mentioned using her legs in a variety of ways, then the plan may include a pair of desired behaviors to be rewarded in the same way. Frequently one undesired behavior may be replaced with several desired behaviors. The nurse helps the family select the one undesired behavior and plan the rewards for any of a set of related desired behaviors.

Communicate the Plan to Significant Others. The nurse helps the family to communicate the behavior modification plan to significant others such as the schoolteacher, babysitter, relatives, the hospital nurse, and others who will be responding to the target behavior. Since many high-risk behavior problems have been well established, consistent immediate feedback is needed to help change the behavior. By including significant others in the behavior modification plan, reactions to the desired and undesired behavior will be consistent in any setting. In some high-risk situations the significant others are actually included in developing the plan from the beginning of identifying the problem behaviors. For example, for the hyperactive child the schoolteacher or relative may be very helpful in identifying the problem and initiating a behavior modification plan with the family.

Implementing

Each one of the following actions is first planned and then carried out when the behavior modification plan is implemented.

Change the Antecedent Event. In some high-risk family situations, only the antecedent event causing the undesired behavior needs to be changed. This one change may elicit the desired behavior. For example, siblings of high-risk children often react to the decreased attention on themselves by either acting out or regressing to younger behavior. One child whose sister was hospitalized with a terminal illness would have a temper tantrum when he was left with a babysitter while the parents drove to the distant medical center. The parents recognized the antecedent event of being left at home and decided to take the child with them to the medical center. There they arranged day care where each parent could visit the well child several times during the day. The nurse encouraged the family to take the ill child outside in a wheelchair on a nice day for a family picnic with both children. The temper tantrums stopped.

Provide Reinforcement and Avoid Punishment. The nurse helps the family recognize the importance of reinforcement and the risks of punishment. Punishment involves applying an adverse event and results in a negative, blaming interaction between the family members. As already mentioned, because of the guilt, blame, and low self-esteem already present in most high-risk families, punishment should be used sparingly. Punishment is appropriate when the risk of not punishing would be greater, such as when a child is running into the street or hurting himself or others. Punishment that is used to stop a dangerous activity should be followed with a plan to reinforce acceptable behavior. The reinforcement and support of acceptable behavior will foster a closer relationship between family members.

Reinforcement is a very effective strategy for helping to change adult behavior as well as children's. A husband who is having difficulty because of his wife's drinking may identify a target behavior as his wife's failure to cook nutritious meals for the family. By using reinforcement for cooking and changing the antecedent event from blaming her to asking if he can help her, the husband may be able to reduce the wife's behavior that is a problem to him. Although behavior modification and other treatment plans may focus on the drinking behavior, the husband may decide to focus on the home behaviors while the drinking is still occurring.

Provide Immediate Feedback. Since many high-risk behavior problems have developed over time and may be a habit before the family seeks help, the most effective behavior modification plan will provide immediate and consistent feedback for the target behavior. When a new problem behavior is just being formed, intermittent feedback by reward or punishment is often satisfactory to change the behavior. Actually most families naturally reward or punish with some inconsistency due to environment or mood changes, yet this intermittent behavior plan is effective in guiding appropriate behavior. When it

is not effective, a specific behavior modification plan needs to be developed and implemented with immediate consistent feedback.

Reward Progress. Frequently rewards are initially used as positive feedback for a behavior approximating the desired behavior. Before the actual behavior has been displayed, rewards are given for behavior that will lead up to the final desired behavior. In this way the rewards are used to shape a desired behavior. Rewarding progress is important in high-risk situations, since the child or parent needs positive feedback for attempts and behaviors that will later grow into the desired behavior. Because behavior changes over a period of time, rewarding progress allows the behavior to continue to develop.

For example, rewarding progress is essential for the mentally disabled child. Rewarding a behavior of the child, such as playing with a button, may lead him progressively to grasping the button and later buttoning his own jacket. Recognizing the importance of initial behaviors provides more opportunities for reward. By slowly changing the desired behavior to more complicated behaviors, progress is achieved. As in any behavior modification plan, the reward must be one desired by the child or parent whose behavior is changing.

Rewarding progress is also helpful in establishing desired behavior which is realistic for the individual. An initial target behavior of walking is often unrealistic for the child with a congenital defect of her legs. By rewarding realistic behaviors such as pulling up on her legs and slowly rewarding more complex behaviors until walking is achieved, a feeling of success is maintained throughout the learning.

Evaluating

The nurse evaluates the progress of the behavior modification plan.

Evaluate Continually. Evaluation should be a continuous process. The evaluation includes a review of the effectiveness of the reward by determining immediate change in the behavior and a study of the changes in the behavior over time as it is shaped.

The family is encouraged to keep a chart of the frequency and quality of the desired and undesired behavior. This chart helps the family to see progress as the undesired behavior is reduced and replaced by more desired behavior.

The nurse recognizes the different stresses and crises for the family at risk and understands that progress in changes in behavior are therefore likely to be intermittent. She helps the family to recognize that one bad day is usual and progress is cyclic. The overall trend should be toward increased desired behaviors, however setbacks may occur for the high-risk family. Crises resulting from the risk situation, such as increased illness of the terminally ill child or increased drinking of the parent, will affect other family members and may cause a temporary increase in the undesired behavior. The family that recognizes these stressful periods will not worry about temporary setbacks such as the congenital defect child regressing to crawling instead of the newly learned walking for a few days. Parents in less stressful situations find that developing new behaviors involves this up and down progress, however, high-risk families tend to forget this as they are in need of continuous support and feelings of progress. Without the nurse's support, even temporary and expected setbacks may cause a crisis for the family.

Teaching the Family

The nurse teaches the family about the major strategies of behavior modification to allow its use in the present situation and to prevent behavior problems in the future. Teaching the family the importance of identifying target behaviors, using immediate consistent rewards, shaping a behavior, and evaluating progress encourages them to identify and solve their problems and receive the satisfaction of working together to enhance their family relationship.

SUMMARY

Behavior modification is a useful strategy to help the family members reduce problem behaviors caused by the risk situation or inappropriate coping. By including the family in the plan and stressing rewards instead of punishment to shape desired behaviors, the nurse helps the family to reduce disruptive behaviors, foster satisfaction, and prevent future difficulties.

ADDITIONAL READINGS

1. Berni, R. *Behavior Modification and the Nursing Process.* 2nd Ed., St Louis: C. V. Mosby Co., 1977.
2. Jaffa, E. B. "Behavior Modification in the Hospital: A Patient's Application." *Supervisor Nurse,* 7, April 1976, 40–41.
3. Katz, R. C. and S. Zlutnick. *Behavior Therapy and Health Care.* Elmsford, N. Y.: Pergamon Press, 1975, 14–29.
4. Kazdin, A. E. *Behavior Modification in Applied Settings.* Homewood, Ill.: Dorsey Press, 1975, 20–24.
5. Mash E. *Behavior Modification Approaches to Parenting.* New York: Brunner/Mazel, 1976, 19–24.
6. Murray, A. "Implementing a Behavior Modification Programme." *Nursing Times,* 73, February 3, 1977, 171–174.
7. Steckel, S. B. et al. "Contracting with Patients to Improve Compliance." *Hospitals,* 51, December 1, 1977, 81–82.
8. Tharp, R. G. *Behavior Modification in the Natural Environment.* New York: Academic Press, 1969.
9. Zangger, B. "Behavior Modification in School Nurse's Office." *Arizona Nurse,* 29, November 1976, 17–20.

Role Theory Strategies

Suzanne Hall Johnson, R.N., M.N.

CHAPTER TWENTY

Role theory stresses relationships, not static behaviors. A role is a sequence of acts performed by a person to complement other roles. For example, the mother role includes sequences of acts that are complementary to those in the father role. The most valuable perspective of role theory is not defining set role behaviors, since these change according to individual preferences, cultural background, and the risk situation, but recognizing the importance of parents' roles being reciprocal to each other and the child.

Role theory provides very valuable strategies for the nurse working with high-risk families. Since role theory focuses on the reciprocal nature of relationships between people, it identifies the effects of high-risk situations on all of the family members and helps to identify effective strategies for helping families to cope with high-risk problems.

While a high-risk situation involves a major role change for the symptomatic family member, it also includes a complementary role change for all family members. When the family members have difficulty coping with the high-risk situation, their roles often become independent of each other, resulting in confusion and crisis. For example, the family with a newborn physically disabled child must adapt to the inclusion of this new baby into their family structure. The parents must not only acquire the usual parenting behaviors, but they must also learn to care for a baby with additional physical disability and developmental needs. The birth of a physically disabled child therefore results in reciprocal changes for all the family members. How the family responds to this role change greatly affects the future of the family.

Role theory strategies are applicable to most high-risk situations because such situations are very likely to alter abruptly the roles of parents and children. The inclusion of a physically disabled, mentally disabled, or premature infant will often cause a major change in the roles of the parents. The failure to thrive infant and hyperactive child not only influence the roles of the mother and father, but may actually be symptoms of difficulties between the parents and the child. Since the death of a child often involves as much of a role change as the birth of the child, the terminally ill child causes major role changes in the family. The abusive, alcoholic or addicted, or emotionally disturbed parent displays behaviors that influence other family members' roles and behaviors. The adolescent and the single parent must make major changes in taking on the parenting role along with their other responsibilities. And, finally, the terminally ill parent influences the roles of the other family members, who must adapt to the possible loss of that member.

Role theory strategies fit very well with other strategies for the high-risk family. Counseling strategies, crisis intervention strategies, and transactional analysis strategies are useful before or with role theory strategies to help identify the parents' individual difficulties, reduce their stresses related to crisis, and analyze the family transactions. Teaching strategies and cultural strategies complement role theory strategies when the teaching involves role change and includes the individual cultural traits of the family. Finally, primary nursing strategies strengthen role theory strategies by including all family members in the role changes and providing one nurse to follow the family over a period of time.

For example, a combination of crisis intervention, counseling, teaching, and role theory intervention helped one family cope with the birth of a child with a clubfoot deformity. Crisis intervention techniques helped to reduce their initial fright and anxiety reactions, counseling and teaching strategies helped them identify the realistic risks and concerns and reduced their unfounded fears, and role theory strategies helped the parents develop a satisfying caring relationship with their child.

The nurse is in an optimal position to use role theory strategies. Since she already legitimately works with the family, often over an extended period of time and in different settings, the nurse is in a good position to see role changes and conflicts in the family and to intervene with role theory strategies. When the nurse and family have established a trust relationship during the medical treatment phase, the family is more likely to express their family stresses related to the illness. The family members often enjoy telling the nurse about their progress and enjoy her visiting in different settings such as the hospital, clinic, and home. Role theory

strategies can be applied very effectively by the nurse since she can include the family members affected, follow the family through their changes, and use the most effective settings for helping the family.

ROLE THEORY CONCEPTS FOR THE HIGH-RISK FAMILY

Role theory helps analyze interactions between family members, identifies possible role conflict problems, and suggests interventions for the family. Role theory helps organize observations of family interactions to determine who is having the difficulties and what the problem is. Although role theory itself is rather complex with new vocabulary and theoretical concepts, the basic concepts are actually quite clear and easy to apply to the high-risk situation. This section will focus on the basic concepts and some of the most essential vocabulary. Figure 20-1 is a summary of the basic vocabulary used in this chapter.

Multiple Roles and Intrapersonal Role Conflict

A role is a "goal directed pattern of acts, tailored by the cultural process for the transactions a person may carry out in a social group or situation."[5] In other words, a role is a set of behaviors or pattern of acts which is learned through past experiences and cultural upbringing. A role is a behavior performed among other people or in a social group, since it is not possible in isolation. Society places expectations for behaviors and responsibilities on roles. These expectations and responsibilities guide the person in when, where, and how to perform the role.

The basic concept underlying role theory is that behaviors are symbols which can be grouped together and described as different roles a person plays. This concept comes from symbolic interaction theory. For example, feeding a child, rocking him when he cries, and changing his diapers can all be grouped into roles called "mothering" or "fathering." Lying in bed during the day, drinking tea,

Figure 20-1. Basic Role Theory Vocabulary

Appropriate role—role in which the actions fulfill the requirements of the person, are efficiently and effectively satisfying to the person, and are acceptable to society.

Cue—input into the organism that comes from the "relevant other."

Misleading cue—a cue that is correlated low with the specific behavior but high with extraneous factors or behaviors.

Relevant other—a role's related partner role.

Role—"a goal directed pattern or sequence of acts tailored by the cultural process for the transactions a person may carry out in a social group or situation. It is conceived that no role exists in isolation but is always patterned to gear with the complementary or reciprocal role of a role partner."[5]

Role behaviors—actions expected and performed in a certain role.

Role conflict—when the expectations or behaviors of one role are incongruent with the expectations or behaviors of another role.

Role expectation—anticipation of certain actions and qualities within a role.

Role modification—changing of a role.

Role perception—locating the position of the "relevant other."

Role taking—adopting the perspective or attitude of the other.[4]

Valid cue—a cue that is correlated with the specific behavior and low to other extraneous factors.

and receiving cards and presents are all part of the role identified as the "sick role."

A person enacts more than one role. For example, a woman may be a mother, a wife, and a business woman while a man may be a husband, a father, and a businessman. These multiple roles blend well when behaviors fit into more than one role—for example, cooking fits into both the wife and the mother role—or when behaviors alternate, as in talking to the husband for a certain amount of time (wife role) and then playing with the children (mother role).

Overall conflict occurs when behaviors of two roles are not compatible as when the mother-worker has to leave work to attend to her very sick child. Here the woman's mothering role conflicts with her working role.

A high-risk situation frequently causes role conflict for the individual family member when his usually compatible set of roles becomes incompatible. For example, it may work very well for a father to be a traveling salesman when his child is healthy and playing with friends while he is gone and when he plans time with the child between trips. However, when the child becomes ill in any high-risk situation the father's working role which requires him to be out of town for long periods of time and his parenting role of caring for the ill child will be in conflict. Although the several roles that every person performs are usually compatible, a high-risk situation frequently causes intrapersonal role conflicts for the family members.

Reciprocal Roles and Interpersonal Role Conflict

A role does not exist in isolation, but is reciprocal to roles of other people. Every role has a role partner or "relevant other."[3] The mother role is complementary to the child's role. For a quiet child a mother can use more subtle means of discipline, while for a very active, noisy child the mother may need to use a loud reprimand or punishment as discipline. Another excellent example of complementary roles is the nurse and physician roles. Over several years the nurse's role and the physician's role have both been changing in a reciprocal fashion. For example, a pediatric nurse practitioner is doing more well baby examinations than she did previously and her physician partner does fewer, focusing more on illness problems. This is a reciprocal relationship between the two role partners that continues to change.

Interpersonal role conflict involves a difficulty between two people, whereas intrapersonal role conflict involves a conflict between two roles enacted by one person. The change in role of the high-risk member influences the roles of the other family members. If the family does not adapt by changing to complementary roles, interpersonal role conflict results. Although it is infrequently described, there is often an interpersonal role conflict for the children in a high-risk family. If a child is ill, the other sibling may need to take more responsibility for home measures while the parents are dealing with the ill child, and he may resent the loss of the attention and love from the parents. If a parent is ill, the child may actually change his role to do some of the caretaking for the ill parent at home. Since the ill person's role change affects all of the roles in the family, a risk illness frequently causes major role changes and role conflicts between family members.

Role Change

Learning a new role or changing a role can be very stressful. Developing a new role is stressful even in normal development, such as going to school for the first time, dating, taking a first job, marrying, or becoming a parent. These normally stressful periods are made even more stressful by high-risk situations. An adolescent struggling with her own independent and sexual development has a very stressful time if motherhood role changes are added to the normal adolescent changes. A couple who are developing parenting behaviors for the first time will find it more difficult to establish comfortable nurturing behaviors if the child is premature or physically disabled and is unable to respond normally to their nurturing.

Effective role changes are developed on a gradual basis and are directed to meet the person's own and other people's needs. A role change is not completed in one step and does not result in one static role behavior; it is a slow and continuous change of role based on changes in the person's and family member's needs. A good example is how the mothering and fathering role change as the child develops new abilities. Parents originally need to nurture their new infant, play with him by toddler age, and act as advisors by adolescence.

The flexibility and ability to continually change roles to meet the most important family needs determines the family's ability to cope with a high-risk situation. Family members who have already learned to be very flexible in assessing each others abilities are able to change their roles when one member becomes ill. This permits continuous family unity and reduces the stress on the family. Many people find role change very difficult and are inflexible to changes in their role, and when a family member becomes ill the roles among the family members are no longer coordinated. Some family members, although flexible in the past, have difficulty when a high-risk situation occurs because of the increased stress that interferes with their normal flexibility. These family members frequently recognize the conflict in the family but find it difficult in the crisis to determine what changes would reduce the stress. The nurse uses role theory strategies to help the family members identify role conflicts and decide what role changes would meet their needs and reduce their stress.

Any role change involves several steps. Although these steps are related and taken simultaneously, it is helpful to look at the parts of the role change process to determine where a family member is having difficulties and where intervention would be most successful. Every step must be completed successfully in order for the role change to be effective in meeting the needs of the person and his family members. These steps of a successful role change include identifying the role of the relevant other, identifying expectations for the new role, developing abilities for it, taking on the new role, and modifying it. Figure 20-2 is a model of the role change process.

Identify the Role of the Relevant Other. In this step the person recognizes the changes in the behavior of his "relevant other" or partner role. The person recognizes cues from his partner which show an unmet need and suggest a behavior change to adapt to the partner.[2] For example, a wife who recognizes that her husband is under unusual stress will recognize such cues as sighs and frowns. These alert the wife to a change in the role of her relevant other, the husband. Other cues that alert people to

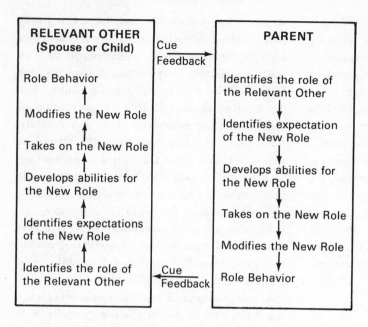

Figure 20-2. Model of the Role Change Process

the change of a role are a baby's cries which indicate to the mother a need of more nurturing, a baby's cooing that encourages the parents to continue playing and talking to the baby, and nervousness or drinking which alert the partner to the presence of increased stress. There are innumerable cues that a partner will give to another family member to indicate difficulties and need for a role change.

The partner that will be changing his role must be able to appropriately identify and interpret cues that direct the type of role change needed. When a person is under great stress, as in a high-risk situation, he frequently has difficulty perceiving cues from the other person. Sometimes the cues are not recognized at all, and sometimes they are misinterpreted. In either case, the family member who misinterprets cues will be unable to develop a role that coordinates with the other family member, and interpersonal role conflict will result. When cues are realistically identified they act as guidelines for the person for the desired role change. Identification of cues from the relevant other is an essential first step toward a successful role change.

For example, one mother had an emotional disorder following the birth of her first child. After several previous miscarriages, she was fearful this child would die. The mother had intermittent periods of fright and depression. Unable to handle either mood, the husband ignored his wife for many months by staying at work for longer periods of time and working more on the weekends. Unfortunately he was unable to identify his wife's cues which were asking for both support and quieting during the frightful period and loving and hope during the depressing periods. The mother's stress reactions were identified by an obstetrical nurse who referred them to the community mental health nurse. The community mental health nurse helped the husband to identify his wife's cues and support her by providing quieting or hope. Although the mother required additional psychiatric help, the husband's newly developed ability to identify her cues made it possible for her to stay home and not be institutionalized while she was receiving the psychiatric treatment.

Identify Expectations of the New Role. Before taking on a new role, a person must identify his own plus other people's expectations for that role.[3] Roles such as the mother role, father role, child role, nurse role, business role, and sick role involve expectations and responsibilities for the role behaviors. For example, from the fathering role people often expect financial support, emotional support, and child-rearing behaviors. A person's expectations of his new role come from his past experiences and cultural upbringing. As a child reaches adolescence and adulthood, his expectations of adult behavior have already been formed from his earlier experiences with his parents and other adults.

When a person's expectations and society's expectations of their new role are similar, the person has a fairly clear picture of the role behaviors that need to be performed. However, when there is a discrepancy between what the person expects and what society expects, it is much more difficult for the person to identify how he should act when he takes on the new role. One example of a conflict of expectations caused by a high-risk situation is when a mentally disabled child grows into adulthood. Society may expect him to take on all the normal decision-making behaviors of an adult but he may be unable to do this fully. When a person's and society's expectations are clear and consistent, role change is more successful and less stressful.

Develop Abilities for the New Role. Since a new role involves new behaviors, the person often needs to develop new abilities before enacting the new role. New abilities may include normal developmental abilities or other special abilities. For the adolescent to take on the adult role, he must have developed the ability to provide his own food and shelter, establish emotional supports, and communicate with other people in society. In high-risk situations the family members often have to develop special abilities to take on a role that adapts to the high-risk person. For example, the mother with a cleft lip child will not only have to learn the usual developmental abilities related to mothering, but will also often have to learn new skills such as special ways of feeding her child. A family member must develop the abilities needed to enact the new role in order to successfully change his role.

Take on the New Role. Taking on the new role includes performing the behaviors of the new role.[4] When a person takes on a new role he performs the

behaviors that he expects and which others have designated and he performs them with the appropriate abilities. When a person first tries a new role it may seem fairly awkward and cause some tension for him, although the role behaviors will be performed. Parents of high-risk infants frequently experience great stress in taking on full caretaking at home because they fear harming the child.

In order to successfully take on the role, not only do the behaviors have to be demonstrated but a certain quality or feeling is often expected to go along with the behaviors. For example, when the mother develops her new mothering role she is not only expected to feed the child but also to stroke and talk to the child and perform other caressing behaviors which demonstrate her love. She takes on the responsibility of caring for the child. Both the behaviors and the feelings related to a role must be taken on in order for the role to be successfully demonstrated.

Modify the New Role. The final step in a successful role change is the modification of the new role to meet the individual's and partner's needs. After a new role is taken on, some of the fine aspects of the behaviors must be individualized to fit with the individual's own personality and other roles. For example, a mother who is very conscious of nutritional needs for her whole family may take on the mothering role of feeding her child but modifying it to fit her own personality by making her own baby foods with no preservatives or food colorings rather than buying ready made baby foods. This mother could take on the normal mothering role including the normal feeding expectations, however, the modification of the role to fit her own style and family needs is the most successful role change for her.

The stress of high-risk situations frequently interferes with the parents' ability to modify their new roles. For example, the mother with a premature infant may take on the mothering role when the child returns home, but it often takes her many more months to become comfortable and adapt her mothering performances to her own lifestyle. Some parents, fearful of harming the child, continue caretaking procedures exactly as demonstrated in the hospital with no individual changes. Modification of the new role involves incorporating the new role into the person's and family's other roles and results in successfully meeting the individual and the family needs.

ROLE THEORY STRATEGIES FOR THE HIGH-RISK FAMILY

Role theory not only analyzes the relationship between family members, but also suggests specific nursing strategies that will help the family adjust to the high-risk situation. Role theory helps the nurse determine who is having difficulties, where the difficulties are, and what the nurse can do to help the family. In many clinical trials the author has found the following strategies the most helpful for families in high-risk situations. Figure 20-3 concisely lists these role theory strategies.

Assess Role Changes of All Family Members

Any high-risk situation involves a major change in the behavior of the "ill partner" as well as the other family members. The birth of a child results in a stressful family role change when the child is a high-risk premature infant or congenital anomaly child. This high-risk child often requires more medical attention and specialized nursing care and causes greater concern for the parents than the expected normal child. The alcoholic parent changes his behavior by increasing drinking and decreasing responsibility for his own health or the needs of the other family members.

The nurse must identify the impact of the high-risk situation on the symptomatic family member and the other family members. Her assessment includes questions such as: What did the symptomatic member do before the high-risk situation occurred? What behaviors have changed in the symptomatic member as a result of the high-risk situation? What have been the effects of these changes on the family since the high-risk situation occurred? The nurse also assesses the parents' abilities to adjust to the role changes in the family by asking questions such as: How have the family members changed since the high-risk situation? How did the family members cope during other role change periods such as change of jobs or first parenthood?

In one family with a hyperactive child, the nurse found that the child's hyperactivity, including fidgeting, kicking, and throwing foods, occurred most often during the day when the mother was caring for the child and least often in the evening when the father was caring for the child. In assessing the changes for all the family members the nurse found the child was increasingly hyperactive, the mother was finding it increasingly difficult to handle the child and was becoming more nervous, and the father did not identify the problem because the child was fairly well behaved when he played with him in the evening. In this case the change in the child mainly affected the mother and was very distressing to her. In assessing the parents' flexibility with previous role changes, the nurse found that the father was very flexible in changing roles when his wife was ill and the mother was normally fairly flexible in her role. Along with other medical and nutritional approaches to decrease the hyperactive behaviors, the nurse counseled the parents on role changes that might help the family handle the stress from the child's behavior. The father decided to take care of the child on weekend days because this was the most hyperactive time and the mother would have this time to relax. The mother decided to take the child outside

Figure 20-3. Role Theory Strategies for the High-Risk Family

Assess Role Changes of All Family Members
Identify Role Conflicts
Clarify the Cues of the Relevant Other
Clarify Expectations About the Needed Role
Strengthen the Family Members' Abilities to Enact the New Role
Assist the Family Member in Performing the New Role
Reward the New Role Taking
Help the Family Member to Modify the New Role
Reinforce the Feedback of the "Relevant Others"
Evaluate the Family Members' Roles

to a playground during the week days because she found that the hyperactivity of running and yelling did not bother her at the playground as it did at home. Although the child is still having difficulties with hyperactivity and aggressive behaviors, the parents have developed ways to support each other and to cope with the behavioral changes in the family. In this high-risk situation, as in others, it is important for the nurse to assess the type of changes in the symptomatic family member and their impact on the other family members.

Identify Role Conflicts

Based on the assessment of the family members' reactions to the high-risk situation, the nurse determines the presence of any role conflicts. Interpersonal role conflicts are more common than intrapersonal conflicts for the high-risk family, however both are potential problems.

For example, a failure to thrive child nine months of age was admitted to the hospital because of poor physical development and malnutrition. Initially the child would tense whenever he was stroked or held by any of the nurses, but after continued nurturing by a primary nurse the child began clinging to her and enjoying physical closeness. Apparently this child needed both his nutritional needs and nurturing needs met by a mother or mother substitute. The mother came infrequently to visit the child in the hospital and avoided touching him or being close to him when she did visit. She preferred letting the nurse care for the child and stayed for only a short time. A community health nurse visited the teenage mother at her home and found that the mother was very concerned about being popular among her friends. The mother would frequently take the child with her to eat at "quick food" places, giving the child some of her french fried potatoes. An interpersonal role conflict existed between the child's and mother's needs, however, an intrapersonal conflict also existed between the mother's own adolescent and mothering needs. The nurse used role theory strategies to help the family recognize and cope with the role conflict. The grandmother was included in the nurtur-

ing and caretaking of the child, and a schedule was planned between the child's mother and the grandmother to provide the child with adequate food and caressing and the teenage mother with time for both mothering and adolescent behaviors.

When the nurse identifies a role conflict in the family, she helps the family to identify the source of the conflict and to recognize that the conflict is a natural result of the high-risk situation and its effects on the family. Quite often during the nurse's assessment her questions and the family's answers increase their awareness of the problem. The most valuable nursing actions are for the nurse to state and to show acceptance of the problem. For example, for the single adolescent mother the nurse can state, "It must be very difficult to want to be with your friends and be accepted by them and at the same time to be with your child and be a loving mother to him." The statement includes both a description of the problem and of the difficulty it must involve for the person experiencing the problem. This type of statement helps the nurse communicate to the family that she understands not only the problem but how the family is actually experiencing their difficulties.

After determining the role conflict and identifying it along with the family, the nurse uses the following strategies to help the family members develop successful and satisfying roles.

Clarify the Cues of the Relevant Others

Since one of the main difficulties for the family members in a high-risk situation is increased stress and an inability to identify the cues of other family members, one of the nurse's main strategies is to help the family members identify the significant cues of the other members. The nurse may first need to use crisis intervention strategies to decrease the family's stress level so that they can be alert to each other's behaviors and the impact of these behaviors on others. Then the nurse can help clarify the cues of other family members by simply stating what other members are doing, asking other family members what needs they have, and increasing verbal cues between family members.

For example, one father of a child with leukemia refused to let the physicians or nurses tell the child about his illness or its possible fatal result. The father stated that he wanted to be kind to the child and spare him the fear of dying. Meanwhile the child was already demonstrating behaviors that showed worry and fear of pain and mutilation, if not of death. The child was crying, kicking, and getting more and more out of control during repeated blood drawing procedures. He kept asking the nurses if he would ever return to school and was overheard telling his friends that he might never return home. The father's own stress at the child's possibly terminal illness made it very difficult for him to recognize the cues from his son that the son was already very afraid of what was happening to him and wanted to discuss it with the nurse or other people.

The primary nurse requested all of the nurses to write down the cues from the child that showed his concern over mutilation and dying. The primary nurse discussed this list with the father and helped the father recognize several of his son's cues while he was present. The father realized his son wanted to talk about the seriousness of his illness and the reasons for all the tests. He immediately started talking to the son about his illness, and together they discussed what procedures had been done that day and what procedures would probably be scheduled for the next day. Although it was still a critical situation for the child and very distressing for both the child and his family, the clarification of cues between the parent and the child helped them to meet each other's needs more adequately.

Clarify Expectations About the Needed Role

The nurse helps the family members to identify their expectations about the new role or change in roles. The family members recognize their expectations for each other and discuss discrepancies. Also the family members identify conflicts between their expectations and society's expectations.

For example, one mother with a premature infant felt inadequate about her ability to care for the child. Although the mother had been included in caretaking of the child intermittently during his hospitalization, she felt that since the child had 24-hour nursing care, she would be unable to adequately care for him at home. Here the mother actually had extremely good mothering skills, as she demonstrated in caring for the child during hospitalization, but her expectations about what the child needed and her mothering ability were unrealistic. The child no longer needed the 24-hour nursing care and observation that he had needed in the beginning of the hospitalization. When the nurse clarified that the child only needed normal feeding, diapering, holding, and caring, the mother's anxieties decreased and her satisfaction and ability to take on the mothering role increased dramatically.

The father may also have difficulties with unrealistic expectations. For example, a child who had been admitted to the hospital with broken bones, bruises, or burns approximately five times in one year was found to be abused by his father. When the community health nurse along with the social workers and other professionals worked with this family, they found that the father had been brought up in a home where the parents were always right and the child was always expected to be perfect. The father expected the son to be a strong man, never to cry, and to be perfect. Whenever the child cried or showed any "weakness," the father became very upset and would punish him by striking or pushing him. The father's unrealistic expectations interfered with his ability to take on a successful fathering role. Psychiatric counselors were needed to help him work through his unrealistic expectations about his child's behavior.

Strengthen the Family Members' Abilities to Enact the New Role

The nurse determines what physical or developmental abilities or skills are needed for the family member to enact the desired new role and plans ways for the parent or child to develop these new abilities.

The role theory strategy of strengthening the family member's abilities and teaching strategies reinforce each other. In order to strengthen the family member's abilities, teaching strategies are used to help the person develop new skills or abilities. For example, the nurse teaches the mother of a premature infant how to stimulate his sucking by turning the nipple in his mouth, the adolescent mother about many of the mothering skills and the child's needs for stimulation and development, and the alcoholic parent about foods that will provide the most nutrients and reduce the physical symptoms of malnutrition. Through teaching new skills and knowledge, the nurse helps the family member prepare for a new role.

The members of a family with a terminally ill father, for example, actively learned new skills to take on a more satisfying role in his care. The father was expected to die fairly soon from a malignant tumor that was causing him extreme pain. His main wish was to return home to the family, since there was no more that the physicians could do for him. All of the family members discussed the feasibility of the father returning home and initially felt that the other family members could not care for him to provide the range of motion and turning every few hours, the nutritional intake, and other nursing skills required for a very weak patient. After several days the family members decided that they would like to try to care for the father while he was in the hospital to see if it would be possible for them to keep him comfortable. With the help of the nurse, family members each selected certain tasks that they would be responsible for. The wife was responsible for blending the foods so that they could be swallowed easily and choosing foods that were most nutritious. The sons and daughters developed a schedule in which each would be responsible for range of motion, turning, and hygiene needs for a certain length of time each day. With these learned abilities, the family returned the father to the home where he was comforted and loved during his last days. Strengthening the family members' skills provided the opportunity for them to take on this more nurturing role.

Assist the Family Member in Performing the New Role

The nurse should help the parent to take on the new or changed role. She can do this by helping the parent to plan a schedule of taking on behaviors one at a time, leading to the desired roles. For example, the mother who would like to take full care of her premature infant but who is anxious about it can learn the diapering, feeding, and bathing one at a time. The nurse can also help to support her in taking on the new role by being physically near to observe, help, and reward the mother as she performs the new role.

In one case, the mother of a young child left the husband and the child without notice. The father was left as the single parent for the young child. He needed assistance and support in learning and performing the new role performed before by the mother. He asked for help from a personal nurse friend who visited him on several occasions and talked to him about the cheapest place to buy food, the quickest way to prepare food, and other hints that would help him to take on the mothering role within his energy limitations. She helped him plan for mother substitute help from a reliable cleaning lady and a quality day care center. The nurse assisted the father to plan and perform the new role.

Reward the New Role Taking

The nurse rewards the family member's efforts and behaviors in taking on the new role that will more successfully meet the family members' needs. Although a generalization such as "You did that nicely" can be rewarding, the most rewarding feedback for a new role describes the actual positive outcome. For example, when a father learns how to feed his premature infant who has a weak suck by moving the nipple in his mouth to remind him to suck again, the nurse should reward him by saying that he is doing well and stating the outcome that the child is taking a large amount of the formula. Describing the desired outcome of a new behavior increases the satisfaction of the family member and strengthens the new role. Rewarding the parent for taking on a reciprocal role that meets the needs of the family is similar to the behavior modification strategy of rewarding the desired behavior.

Help the Family Member to Modify the New Role

The nurse helps the family member to modify the new role by helping him recognize how it fits in with his other roles and needs. The stress on the parents in high-risk situations frequently makes it difficult for the family member to modify the new role to his own individual style. It is quite common to find the mother of a premature infant demonstrating an effective feeding procedure or bathing procedure *exactly* as it was demonstrated to her, without any individualization or changes because she is afraid of hurting the child. The mother has difficulty becoming comfortable and satisfied with the role even though she seems to perform it successfully. Mothers with premature infants frequently return on clinic visits with feeding complaints and uncertainty about feeding procedures when actually the children have been very well nourished. The nurse helps the mother modify her role by discussing how the mother may like to do the bathing or other procedure at home. The mother can modify the timing or the location, by using the bathtub or the sink, or make other individual modifications if the nurse teaches her the essentials of the procedures along with the behaviors themselves. As the mother modifies the role, she expresses more satisfaction in parenting and is better able to take on new roles in the future.

The nurse should be alert to parents who return a demonstration of a procedure exactly as it was shown to them without any individual modifications. These parents will probably demonstrate increased stress and fear because they are afraid of the new behaviors and do not understand or incorporate them into their own behaviors.

Reinforce the Feedback of the "Relevant Others"

After a new role has been learned and reinforced by the nurse, it is important for the continual reinforcement to come from the actual family members. The nurse helps the family member to identify the outcome of his behavior. The outcomes are actually valid cues that reinforce his behavior. Parents in high-risk situations often see negative unrelated behaviors and think they are a result of their behavior. For example, when the parents of a premature infant first touch the child the infant frequently goes into a Moro's reflex where he cries and tenses his extremities due to his immature reflexes.[1] The parents, unaware that this is a natural response, frequently think that their touching the child has hurt him and therefore are fearful of touching him and do so less often. The nurse helps the high-risk family to realize that these negative behaviors are not related to their own behaviors but to part of the problems of the high-risk situation.

At the same time parents in a high-risk situation frequently ignore valid cues that show that their role behavior is excellent. In the previous example of the premature infant, the parents frequently complain about their difficulty feeding the child when actually the child is very comforted, sleeps well after feeding, and is growing normally. The nurse helps the parents by decreasing their focus on the negative cues which are unrelated to their new role and decrease satisfaction while increasing their awareness of valid cues that reinforce their parenting and lead to satisfaction.

Helping the parents to recognize the valid cues to reinforce their new roles is similar to the initial strategy of helping them recognize the child's cues to help them change their role. Helping the parents to recognize valid cues that are either positive, to reinforce their role, or negative, to show a need for a role change, encourages them to change unsuccessful behaviors to ones that meet the family needs. The nurse not only helps the parents develop a new role but also teaches the parents how to identify needed changes for future flexibility.

Evaluate the Family Members' Roles

The nurse's final role theory strategy is to evaluate the effectiveness of the strategies by determining if the family roles are reciprocal and if they meet the majority of their needs. This is similar to the initial assessment of the family members' roles and needs. If it appears that the needs of the children and parents are adequately met and the parents demonstrate their ability to identify the cues of the other family members and adjust their roles accordingly, the nurse will know that her role theory strategies have been successful. If the same role conflicts remain, then the nurse knows the approaches she used were ineffective. The nurse then develops other individual approaches for applying these strategies. Sometimes on evaluation the nurse finds that one role conflict has been resolved but another has occurred. When this happens the nurse should help the family members to go through the same steps in the role change, such as clarifying the cues of others, clarifying expectations, strengthening abilities, and performing the reciprocal role. Frequently the family members need less help in identifying and solving the problems than they did on the first role conflict.

Since many high-risk situations are long term, causing potential role conflicts over a long period, the nurse continues to assess the family for role conflicts. High-risk situations causing potential long-term role conflict problems include the premature infant who is transported to a regional center and hospitalized for a long period, the single adolescent mother who needs to develop the mothering role over time, the alcoholic parent who continues drinking or intermittently returns to the problem, or the terminally ill child or parent who may be ill intermittently over a period of time. Role theory strategies are useful on a short-term basis to help the family develop a new reciprocal role or on a long-term basis when many role changes are necessary.

SUMMARY

High-risk families frequently experience role conflicts because of the behavior changes in the symptomatic person and the effects of these changes on the other family members. The nurse uses role theory strategies to identify role conflicts and assist the family member in developing a new role that is reciprocal to the other roles and meets the needs of the family members. Helping the parents through the role change process during the stressful high-risk period helps them meet present needs, learn the process, and establish supportive relationships.

REFERENCES

1. Johnson, S. H. and J. Grubbs. "The Premature Infant's Reflex Behaviors: Effect on the Maternal-Child Relationship." *JOGN Nursing*, 4, May–June 1975, 15–20.
2. Roy, M. C. "Role Cues and Mothers of Hospitalized Children." *Nursing Research*, 16, Spring 1967, 179–182.
3. Sarbin, T. "Role Theory." *Handbook of Social Psychology*. G. Lindzey (ed.). Reading, Mass.: Addison-Wesley, 1954, 223–300.
4. ———. "The Concept of Role-Taking." *Sociometry*, 6, 1943, 273–285.
5. Spiegel, J. "The Resolution of Role Conflict within the Family." *Psychiatry*, 20, 1957, 1–16.

ADDITIONAL READINGS

1. Robischon, P. and D. Scott. "Role Theory and Its Application in Family Nursing." *Nursing Outlook*, July 1969, 52–57.

PERTINENT ORGANIZATIONS

NATIONAL
American Psychological Association
1200 17th St. N.W.
Washington, D.C. 20036
Association of psychologists and educators for the advancement of psychology as a science and profession.

Transactional
Analysis Strategies

Virgil Parsons, R.N., M.S.

CHAPTER TWENTY-ONE

Transactional Analysis (TA) was developed in the 1960s by Dr. Eric Berne as an approach to counseling and psychotherapy. This theory has become an important framework to help people handle problems as well as understand themselves. Like other conceptual frameworks, TA works to describe an individual's personality and way of problem-solving, and can be used by the nurse to assess family members as individuals, to observe the interactions of the members, and to assist in problem-solving during a high-risk situation.

Transactional Analysis includes many activities and exercises which can be utilized or adapted for a variety of nursing situations, and uses words that are simple, easily understood, and direct. Also, TA has been successful with adults, children, and families needing help and has techniques that are useful in high-risk parenting situations. Its focus on transactions between people makes TA a useful framework for intervening to assist parents in preventing or coping with interaction stresses from high-risk situations. It is especially helpful in working with a high-risk parent such as the abusing or battering parent and the alcoholic or addicted parent.

Since TA is based on the assumption that any person can learn to trust himself, think for himself, and make appropriate decisions, the nurse can use TA with the many other counseling and teaching strategies which share this problem-solving focus. In addition, concern for immediate intervention links TA and crisis intervention; the focus on family interactions connects TA and role theory strategies. Specific interventions related to these "partner" strategies are described in the chapters on the other strategies.

BASIC TA CONCEPTS

Transactional Analysis involves analysis of a person's interactions with others. The analysis includes assessing a person's *ego state transactions,* ways of giving and getting *strokes,* and ways in which *time is structured.* The nurse must also analyze her own interactions as well as those of the high-risk family members to determine the most effective interventions. Some of the basic concepts of TA will be presented in this section, and nursing strategies will follow.

Ego State Transactions

According to TA, everyone has three parts to his personality or self: a Parent, an Adult, and a Child. These parts are called ego states. When capitalized, the words Parent, Adult, and Child refer to ego states, not to actual parents, adults, or children. The ego states are similar to the Super-ego (Parent), Ego (Adult), and Id (Child) of Freud's psychoanalytic theory. One ego state dominates a transaction, an interaction occurring between the ego states of two or more people. However, a person can move from one ego state into another during interactions. For example, parents when relating to their children most often interact from the Parent, but may switch to the Adult or Child as needed for the circumstances.

Parent. This ego state contains the attitudes and behavior incorporated from external sources, primarily parents. It is expressed in prejudicial, critical, or nurturing behaviors—or all three. For example:

Prejudicial Parent—"All patients are sick and helpless."

Critical Parent—"They don't know how to take care of themselves."

Nurturing Parent—"I should help them by teaching them health practices."

Inside the person, the Parent ego state is experienced as old parental-type messages which influence present functioning, including "shoulds," "oughts," and "don't's." Phrases or words frequently used by the Parent include: "should," "never," "if I were you," "let me help you," "there there." Nonverbal behaviors are pointing an accusing finger, a pat on the back, a condescending tone of voice, a scowl, or an encouraging nod. An illustration of an overpowerful Parent ego state is the abusing-battering parent who might be caught up in the Critical Parent state, believing a child "should" receive corporal punishment. A mentally disabled child may demonstrate an inadequate Parent in not grasping behaviors he "should not" do, such as hitting out when he feels anger.

Child. This part of the self contains impulses that come naturally to a person (Natural Child), experiences and parental training that influenced the person (Adapted Child), and the ability to be intuitive, manipulative, and creative (Little Professor). The Child in an adult is often manifested by "leftover" behavior from the childhood. For example, a nurse may experience the following manifestations of the Child within herself during a normal day:

Natural Child—"I'm so tired of these patients—I'd just like to go home and sleep."

Adapted Child—"I can't do that—I'd lose my job."

Little Professor—"I'll use my meal break to rest. That'll make it possible for me to finish the shift."

When a person is feeling and acting much like he did when he was a child, he is in his Child ego state.

Vocabulary of the Child includes: "can't," "gosh," "I'm scared," "look at me now," "help me." Nonverbal behavior includes temper tantrums, raising hand to speak, giggling, pouting, and enjoying puzzles and games. The nurse will encounter the Child in any client who is hurting and freely expressing pain. The Child also is obvious in most high-risk children, particularly in the hyperactive child (Natural Child). Examples of high-risk parents demonstrating the Child readily are the emotionally disturbed parent or an adolescent parent who perhaps has not attained enough maturity to put a child's needs ahead of the Child wants of self.

Adult. This inner "person" is not related to a person's age. The Adult ego state is oriented to current reality and objective gathering of information. It is organized, adaptable, intelligent, and functions by testing reality, estimating probabilities, and figuring mentally. For example, whenever a nurse uses a systematic process for planning care, she manifests the Adult. Dealing on a factual basis, gathering relevant data, and computing objectively are representative characteristics of the Adult ego state.

Verbal expressions of the Adult include: "how," "why," "what alternatives," "what are the facts." Nonverbal behavior includes eye contact that is level, active listening, calm tone of voice, eyes alert, thoughtful facial expression. Most high-risk clients will not demonstrate a strong Adult at the beginning of the nurse-client working relationship. In fact, assisting high-risk children and parents to utilize the Adult in order that they can actively resolve problems and dilemmas is the goal of nursing intervention.

Ego States Picture. Figure 21-1 is a model of the personality structure including the Parent, Adult, and Child ego states. The ego state being expressed is shown in a larger circle which changes as ego states change. The personality model is used to show ego state transactions between people.

Transactions. Transactions refer to how people interact with each other. All interactions involve a stimulus from one of the ego states of the sender and a response from one of the ego states of the receiver. These exchanges occur one after another in conversation, and can be Adult-Adult, Adult-Child, Adult-Parent, Parent-Parent, Parent-Adult, Parent-Child, Child-Parent, Child-Adult, or Child-

Child. Communication from any ego state has its place; however, it is most effective for interactions to be complementary and not crossed or with ulterior (hidden) messages.

A *complementary* transaction occurs when a message sent from one ego state gets the expected response from an ego state in the other person. The same ego state that receives a message sends one out, and when this occurs, the lines of communication are open. Figure 21-2 shows two models of complementary transactions.

A *crossed* transaction is when a response from an unexpected ego state is made to the stimulus, and the lines of transacting between the persons are crossed. At this point, communication is hindered, if not blocked. Figure 21-3 shows two models of crossed transactions.

In an *ulterior* transaction, a hidden or double message is sent along with an overt, verbal message. The covert message is like a "hidden agenda." These transactions are diagramed with a dotted line indicating the ulterior communication in Figure 21-4, which shows two models of this type of transaction.

In delineating and analyzing the transactions

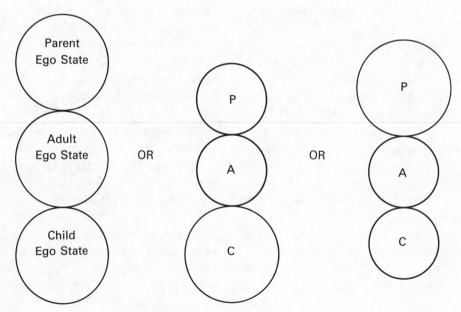

Figure 21-1. Ego State Pictures

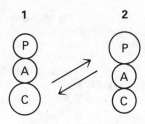

1. Single parent—"It's a heavy load having to be both mother and father."
2. Nurse—"That's understandable. It must be hard for you to find time for yourself."

OR

1. Mother of premature infant (calmly)—"How's the baby doing?"
2. Nurse—"He's doing pretty good. His color is a strong pink and he's handling his feedings fine."

Figure 21-2. Complementary Transactions

of clients, the nurse has a valuable tool for assessment and planning for interventions in high-risk child, parent, and family situations.

Strokes

According to TA, the universal need for touch and recognition can be met by strokes which are acts or feedback that imply recognition of another's presence and value. People need strokes to survive, and as a person grows older, the early hunger for actual physical touch is modified and becomes recognition hunger. Smiles, words, frowns, and gestures begin to substitute for touch strokes. Like touch, these recognitions, positive or negative, stimulate the brain of the receiver and verify for him that he is there and alive.

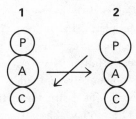

1. Mother of infant with birth defect—"What did the doctor tell you?"
2. Father of infant (scowling)—"You should have been more careful during the pregnancy!"

OR

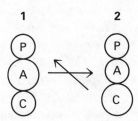

1. Nurse—"Tell me about the baby's intake of food."
2. Mother of failure to thrive child—"I can't remember. Please help me make him stop crying."

Figure 21-3. Crossed Transactions

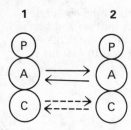

1. Nurse—"Here's the child's medication for his asthma." Ulterior message—wiggles hips, meaning, "See how attractive I am."
2. Single father—"Thank you, Miss Smith." Ulterior message—stares with appreciation, meaning, "I'm interested."

OR

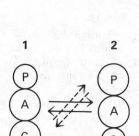

1. Adolescent parent—"I'm sorry I'm late for my appointment." Ulterior message—sighs, meaning, "Punish me. I've done bad."
2. Nurse—"You're too late for us to accomplish anything today." Ulterior message—frowns, meaning, "You are naughty and a bad parent."

Figure 21-4. Ulterior Transactions

While either negative or positive strokes may stimulate body chemistry, it takes positive strokes to develop emotionally healthy persons. Positive strokes leave the person feeling good, alive, alert, and significant; they enhance the individual's sense of well-being, endorse his intelligence, and are most often pleasurable. The feelings beneath positive strokes are of good will and convey a positive position about self and others.

High-risk children, parents, and families especially need positive strokes from each other and helping professionals because their behavior is likely to make giving positive strokes difficult. For example, parents of a hyperactive child may need assistance in balancing their admonitions and "don't's" with praise and encouragement. Also, the nurse may sometimes find it particularly difficult to relate positively to an abusing-battering parent or spouse, or to an emotionally disturbed parent whose behavior is bizarre or repulsive. Even so, positive strokes, specifically in times of stress, should be part of every nursing care plan. At the same time, the nurse should protect his or her own mental health by ensuring an adequate amount of positive strokes for self.

Ways Time Is Structured

According to TA, people function by structuring their time in six possible ways. How this is done depends on the position the person has taken about the self and the kind of stroking the person wants from others. The six ways to structure time are Withdrawal, Ritual, Pastimes, Activity, Intimacy, and Games. All transactions and stroke-seeking can be placed in one of these categories. None of these time structurings is "pathological" unless it severely interferes with a person's functioning and problem-solving. Usually the person is unaware of the way he is structuring time and unaware that there are other alternatives.

Withdrawal. This self-isolation can be physical or psychological, and this behavior can come from any of the three ego states. It is a way of declining to be involved with others, and can be a form of protection from pain or conflict or the result of training. Daydreaming, for example, is one type of withdrawal. A more negative instance of withdrawal would be a terminally ill child or parent pulling away from loved ones, thereby blocking a positive grief process.

Ritual. These are transactions which are simple, stereotyped, and complementary, like everyday hellos and goodbyes. A ritual is a fixed way of behaving toward others that almost everyone uses. If someone says, "Good morning. How are you?," this person is most likely expecting a response of "Fine, how are you?" In this type of encounter, both people get brief, maintenance strokes. Rituals will serve the nurse well in the beginning phase of the working relationship with the high-risk family to convey warmth and caring. Rituals are usually performed quickly and automatically.

Pastimes. These are interactions involving superficial exchanges, often between people who do not know each other well. The transactions are usually pleasant ways of sharing strokes, filling time, and getting to know people. Some pastimes have names, such as "General Motors," in which people talk about and compare cars. "Who Won" is talk about sports, "Wardrobe" about fashions. "Bull sessions" and gossip are examples of common pastimes. Like rituals, pastimes can aid in establishing a nurse-client relationship. However, for effective nursing care and problem-solving, the nurse should minimize pastimes and move beyond them to more in-depth interaction.

Activity. This is a way of structuring time that deals with external reality and is commonly thought of as *work*—getting something done. Activity is usually what people want to do, need to do, or have to do in order to accomplish a task. Since work is often done with others, it is also a way of receiving strokes. The nurse may find it necessary to assist some high-risk clients in building this type of time structuring into their total functioning. Mentally disabled children and emotionally disturbed parents may particularly benefit from learning to include constructive activity in their daily routine.

Intimacy. This meets the greatest need: to be close to someone in a loving relationship. It involves genuine caring and authenticity and occurs in moments free of exploitation or manipulation—those rare moments of human contact that arouse feelings of tenderness, empathy, and affection. Intimacy is sometimes frightening, and involves risk and being vulnerable. Therefore, it may seem easier to a person to avoid intimacy rather than risk feelings of either rejection or affection. The parents of a failure to thrive child for example are often unable to achieve intimacy with each other or the child. Intimacy should be a goal for the nursing care plan for every high-risk child, parent, and family.

Games. Games, the sixth way to structure time, are defined in TA as a series of complementary transactions which seem plausible on the surface, but have an ulterior transaction resulting in a negative payoff that concludes the game and is the real purpose for playing. Another way of stating this is that a set of transactions is a game if it meets four requirements. The players:

1. Have an honest reason for the transaction.
2. Exchange covert messages.
3. Experience a *payoff* or reward for the game.
4. Are usually unaware they are in a game.

Games prevent intimacy and honest, open relationships. Yet people play them because they fill time, provoke attention, provide a way of getting and giving strokes, reinforce opinions about self and others, and even fulfill a sense of identity. People tend to choose a spouse, friends, and even business associates to play the role opposite their own. Games are likely to be repetitious, and are played with different degrees of intensity—from the socially accepted, relaxed level, such as flirting with a gentle brushoff at a cocktail party, to the criminal, homicide-suicide level, such as assault and rape.

Games involve two or three of the roles of Victim, Persecutor, and Rescuer—manipulative roles learned in childhood. Persecutor or Rescuer roles reinforce a negative position about others; the Victim role serves to reinforce a negative position about the self. Each game has its roles, number of players, level of intensity, length, and ulterior message. Each one has its own style and can be played in different settings.

In the game, "Yes, But," one player presents a problem in the guise of soliciting advice. The initiator discounts all suggestions with "Yes, but . . . ," followed by "reasons" that the advice will not work. Eventually the advice giver gives up. This is the payoff, to prove the player's original position. For example, the mother of a failure to thrive infant may ask, "What should I do to care for the baby better?" When the nurse replies to hold the baby close and talk with him, the mother playing the game will respond, "Yes, but I can't because . . . ," rejecting all the advice.

In "Kick Me," a player does something to provoke another player to put him down. The put-down is the payoff and reinforces a negative position about himself. Though he may deny it, a person who uses "Kick Me" tends to attract others who will play the complementary role and are willing to "kick" him. A parent of a birth defect infant may play this game with the nurse to reinforce guilt feelings that something the person did caused the imperfection.

"Harried" is a game acted out to justify a collapse or depression. The player takes on enormous work loads, but eventually his behavior begins to reflect his harried state. He may be disheveled or unable to finish the work, and his physical and mental health deteriorates. He collects and saves up feelings of depression and finally collapses, so depressed he is unable to function. "Harried Nurse" and "Harried Parent" are variations of this game.

"See What You Made Me Do" is played to collect feelings of anger. The initiator, rather than take responsibility for errors or shortcomings, continually blames someone else. If this happens often enough, the purpose of the game is fulfilled— isolation for the initiator. An alcoholic parent may lay the blame for excessive drinking on the spouse; a single parent may accuse the absent parent of causing all the problems.

"Stupid" may be played to collect feelings of inferiority. A player "accidentally" does something incorrectly, and when the mistake is discovered, makes a fuss, complaining, "Oh, how could I have done such a stupid thing!" If the error is genuine, it is not Stupid, but Human, but this player needs to reinforce a negative self-image. An adolescent parent who feels inadequate in caring for a child may play this game; the mother of a fetus at risk might play "Stupid" to explain or excuse her not following a prescription of strict bedrest.

These are only a few common games that are easily recognized. Most games are played unconsciously by the partners. The TA literature describes many more, and the reader is encouraged to explore it for more information.

CLINICAL APPLICATION OF TA STRATEGIES

There are several techniques derived from TA that can be applied to clinical practice with high-risk children, parents, and families. TA strategies focus on both the nurse's and the client's transactions. Figure 21-5 includes a composite list of the strategies.

Use Ego States Appropriately

An important application of the TA framework is to make the nurse aware of all three ego states operating in his or her own personality. Each ego state will be called to action at different times. For example, the Nurturing Parent is appropriate with the premature infant or the failure to thrive child. An emotionally disturbed parent who is careless about taking his medications might elicit the nurse's Critical Parent telling him he "should" take them as prescribed. Even the Child might be utilized if the goal is to teach a high-risk child how to play or express himself. When objective problem-solving is required, the Adult is the best

Figure 21-5. TA Strategies for the High-Risk Family

1. Use Ego States Appropriately
2. Strengthen the Nurse's Adult
3. Reinforce the Adult of Client
4. Determine Client's Personality Structure
5. Analyze Transactions of Client
6. Increase Positive Strokes for Client
7. Explore Time Structuring of Client
8. Discover and Minimize Client's Games

choice. Good nursing judgment is needed to assess the use of ego states and develop interactions based on the most appropriate states.

Strengthen the Nurse's Adult

An individual's Adult ego state is a major asset because it makes effective problem-solving possible. This does not mean that the Parent and Child should be suppressed all the time. They are important also, and should be allowed expression at appropriate times, for example, the Nurturing Parent and the Playful Child. However, dealing with problems in living requires an Adult strong enough to facilitate effective communication, learning, growth and development, decision-making, and adaptive response to stress.

The Adult can be built and made stronger in the following ways.[1] The nurse should:

1. Learn to recognize her Child, its vulnerabilities, its fears, and its principal methods of expressing these feelings.
2. Learn to recognize her Parent, its admonitions, injunctions, fixed positions, and principal ways of expressing these admonitions, injunctions, and positions.
3. Be sensitive to the Child in others, talk to that Child, protect that Child and appreciate its need for creative expression.
4. Count to ten, if necessary, in order to give the Adult time to process the data coming into the computer, to sort out the Parent and the Child from reality.
5. When in doubt, withhold response. One cannot be attacked for something one did not say.
6. Work out a system of values. One cannot make decisions without an ethical framework.

Reinforce the Adult of Client

The ways listed for the nurse to build a strong Adult can also be presented to the client for his use. In addition, the nurse will want to positively reinforce any Adult behavior demonstrated by the client. The client should be praised for effective problem-solving and encouraged to use his strengths in meeting problems and coping with stress. Any person, regardless of how many problems he has, possesses an Adult which, if it is elicited and "nurtured," can be used by the person to meet the demands of living and to gain (or regain) high level wellness.

Determine Client's Personality Structure

The Ego State Portrait is a good assessment technique and will serve to increase the self-awareness of the client.[2] The nurse begins by giving a brief explanation of ego states and what they represent and showing a simple drawing of the personality as pictured:

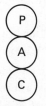

Figure 21-6

Then the nurse instructs the client to draw, by using circles of different sizes, a "portrait" of his own ego states as he sees himself most of the time. The drawing might look something like this:

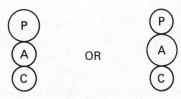

Figure 21-7

After the drawing, the nurse asks the client to consider these questions:

1. Do you see yourself as having a particular way of relating to others?
2. Does your way of relating change with situations? How?
3. Does it change with certain people? How? With whom?

The nurse should encourage expression of other thoughts and feelings as they occur and have each family member do a portrait for himself and one for other members. Then the nurse has the people share the portraits with each other. This will help clarify family relationships and how members relate to each other. The nurse might need to emphasize that *all* three ego states are important and should be acknowledged and given appropriate expression depending on the situation.

This strategy is not appropriate for clients in initial states of a crisis, since this conceptualizing is not a priority at that time. In these instances, the nurse can do an ego state portrait of the client based on her observations and still have an assessment "picture" with which to help plan interventions.

Analyze Transactions of Client

This action requires that the nurse observe for patterns of interaction and identify ego states operating in the patterns, especially for interactions which are nonproductive, destructive, or a hindrance to problem-solving. The nurse observes ego state messages between parents and parents and children, determines if ineffective ego states are blocking communication, and helps the members see the negative effects of their actions on others so they are motivated to change.

This process can be carried out a number of times until the client begins to identify patterns of interaction and ways of relating that are not working in communication and getting strokes for all family members. The nurse might choose to role play transactions with the client to illustrate the interaction and provide a different perspective. For example, the alcoholic parent who blames other family members for his drinking controls the other family members through guilt. Role playing this for the family members may help them see the destructive nature of this game for all family members.

Increase Positive Strokes for Client

The nurse has the person identify and describe how he experiences negative feelings in different situations such as home and work, and instructs him to do the same for positive feelings. Next, the nurse asks the client to identify which he receives more often. Based on the client's responses, the nurse can explore and identify with the client how he can get more positive strokes. The client can then explore others' needs for strokes and how he can give more to partner, child, or other family member.

The nurse can also increase positive strokes for the client by giving as many as possible while working with him. All high-risk children and parents will look to the health professional for approval and reinforcement when they have carried out perhaps difficult, positive health behaviors. The alcoholic parent can well use positive stroking for abstaining; a mentally disabled child will benefit from praise for accomplishing a task such as dressing himself; and the list goes on and on.

Explore Time Structuring of Client

The nurse obtains data on how the client spent his waking time over a recent week and ranks the ways of structuring his time according to how he was most involved: for example, activity, 40 percent; pastimes, 25 percent; and so on. With this information, the nurse can explore with the client whether the way his time is structured is how he really wants it to be. If it is not, the client can identify and explore what he wants to change. The nurse can then assist him to formulate strategies for changing his behavior. A terminally ill child or parent may discover too much time is spent alone (withdrawal); a single parent might realize that too much time is spent working at a job and caring for a child (activity). The result of this strategy should be a more balanced structuring of time and better meeting the needs of self and others.

Discover and Minimize Client's Games

As the nurse observes games, he or she can point them out, explore them, and assist the client in finding new, more rewarding behaviors. The nurse can have the client describe interactions in which there consistently seems to be a negative payoff for him, explore the interactions, and encourage him to devise ways to stop the game playing and meet his needs in more adaptive ways.

Games may be halted by a refusal to play or to give a payoff. For example, not giving advice or suggestions to a "Yes, But" player will stop the game. There are many ways to stop a game. A person might:

1. Give an unexpected response.
2. Stop exaggerating his own weaknesses or strengths.
3. Stop exaggerating the weaknesses and strengths of others.
4. Give positive strokes rather than negative ones.
5. Structure more time with activities, intimacy, and fun.
6. Stop playing Rescuer—helping those who do not need help.
7. Stop playing Persecutor—criticizing those who do not need it.
8. Stop playing Victim—acting helpless or dependent when able to stand on one's own.

The nurse can use these suggestions to help the client stop games and develop new patterns.

Summary of Strategies in a Case Example

Kay, a public health nurse, made a stop at the D family home as a one month follow-up on a premature infant birth. The infant, Gina, seemed to be doing fine, although Mrs. D appeared tired and disheveled. The mother stated that all was going well for the family, which included Mr. D, an auto mechanic, and David, a seven-year-old second grader. After a brief visit, Kay left, but was concerned about Mrs. D's appearance and lack of response to family members' statements. Kay told Mrs. D she would return in a week with some requested information.

Checking with David's school nurse, Kay found that the child was doing fairly well in school. However, he had missed four days in the past

month, and on two occasions had complained to his teacher of being hungry because, "Mommy was too tired to fix breakfast." The teacher had also noted that David appeared more unkempt than usual in the past few weeks. The school nurse had considered the possibility of child neglect; she saw no indication of abuse or battering.

Kay returned to the D home in a week and noted Mrs. D's strained manner. While they were talking, David entered the room. He had not gone to school because, the mother explained, "I think he's coming down with something." David did appear unkempt although he seemed alert and cheerful, and he played quietly with Gina while his mother and the nurse talked. In response to Mrs. D's statement that she had much to do, Kay left, but she felt uncomfortable about how things were going with the D family.

Using TA, Kay attempted to analyze the situation. She recognized that her own feelings were coming from her Parent, both Critical in response to the caring for David and Nurturing in regard to her concern for Mrs. D. For a better appraisal, she moved into her Adult and did a nursing assessment based on her observations and data (Strategies 1 and 2). She concluded that she should visit again, with the goal of sharing her thoughts and feelings about the situation with Mrs. D. This would be a starting point, and further interventions would be based on the results of the visit. By telephone, she arranged a visit a few days later.

On the appointed day, Kay arrived, noting no change in Mrs. D, but added an observation that the middle-income home was neat and clean. David was at school, and Gina was sleeping after a feeding. Kay attempted to relate to Mrs. D's Adult, but twice received responses that seemed to be coming from the mother's Child, "God, I'm tired"; "Am I doing something wrong?" Mrs. D's third response was more Adultlike, "I appreciate your concern. I guess things aren't as fine as I said." Kay stated, "Tell me about what's not going so good," and Mrs. D answered by giving more information and becoming slightly tearful.

Mrs. D explained that she too was concerned

about David and her caring for him. She was feeling much tension concerning Gina, and feared that her attentiveness to her daughter was interfering with her meeting David's needs. She expressed feelings of depression which frightened her because she had experienced a postpartum depression after David's birth. The episode had lasted about two months and cleared almost spontaneously, but was a big part of the D's decision to wait six years before having another child. Mrs. D was determined not to "give in to the blues" after Gina's arrival. Her physician had been, and continued to be, very supportive and helpful, but she offered, "I haven't told him everything I'm feeling."

Mrs. D also expressed some guilt feelings over the couple's decision that she would not return to her job after Gina's birth. They both thought, "I need to be at home with her for at least a year." This meant that Mr. D made every attempt to work overtime, and was considering a second job, to "make up for the lost money." Consequently, Mr. D was usually very tired and away from home a great deal, although "he helps me all he can." The couple had not gone out since a week before Gina was born.

When asked about thoughts and feelings regarding the premature birth, Mrs. D stated, "I don't know why it happened. The doctor couldn't say. She was almost two months early, but Dr. Brown didn't seem too worried. I'm really thankful Gina's done so well. She seems pretty healthy."

Kay reinforced Mrs. D's Adult (Strategy 3) stating that she obviously had done a good job of caring for the infant. Assessing the client's personality structure (Strategy 4), with Mrs. D's cooperation, Kay determined that Mrs. D had little flexibility and continually related in a Parent ego state. Mrs. D felt a need to Parent her husband to an extent, in addition to Gina and David. "He's doing a lot. He deserves to be 'cared for' a little." The result of all this was that Mrs. D's Child was usually suppressed and hurting.

To analyze the transactions of the client (Strategy 5), Kay asked Mrs. D to describe how she related to the other family members. The description supported the idea that Mrs. D related from her

Parent most of the time; however, she had been able to use her organized and intelligent Adult to solve many problems. It remained though that Mrs. D's Child was much in need of expression. "I think I need a little more fun in my life."

In addition to reinforcing Mrs. D's Adult, Kay gave many positive strokes (Strategy 6) as they interacted. This helped to establish rapport, and based on this trust, Kay asked the client to explore how she structured her time (Strategy 7). This activity revealed that Mrs. D spent her waking time in approximately the following ways: activity (work) —80 percent, withdrawal—10 percent; intimacy —5 percent; rituals and pastimes—2 percent; and games—3 percent. With Kay's guidance, Mrs. D was able to identify how she played the game, "Yes, But" (Strategy 8).

The client played "Yes, But" with her mother who called her two or three times a week. Mrs. D would describe a problem and her mother would offer suggestions, all of which Mrs. D would reject. "I think I want her help, but then I keep telling myself I have to solve the problem on my own without depending on Mom." Mrs. D recognized that this game had gone on for several years, but she had become acutely aware of it during her recent pregnancy and after Gina's birth. It bothered her particularly now because she was considering asking her mother to babysit since Gina was doing so well. However, she felt guilty asking a favor because she had not followed her mother's "advice" for so long. With this insight, Mrs. D was able to explore how she could stop the game and perhaps request her mother to babysit.

Kay also had a hunch that Mrs. D played a little of "Harried," but she thought the client had done enough for this visit. She "stroked" Mrs. D for her "work," and asked about the possibility of meeting with the entire family in a few days. Kay's goal for this meeting was to do a more complete assessment of the family and, if it seemed indicated, to make a referral to community mental health resources where they could get long-term assistance. The meeting was arranged, and Kay left feeling that she had used TA to begin assessment of the family's needs and to plan effective interventions that would prevent a severe upheaval in this high-risk family.

SUMMARY

Transactional Analysis is valuable in nursing practice with high-risk children, parents, and families. The nurse can use TA strategies to refine his or her nursing behaviors and to assess, prevent, or reduce family problems for high-risk families.

REFERENCES

1. Harris, T. A. *I'm OK—You're OK.* New York: Avon Books, 1969.
2. Jongeward, D. and M. James. *Winning with People.* Reading, Mass.: Addison-Wesley, 1973.

ADDITIONAL READINGS

1. Babcock, D. E. "Transactional Analysis." *American Journal of Nursing,* 76 #7, July 1976, 1152–1155.
2. Berne, E. *Games People Play.* New York: Grove Press, 1964.
3. Campos, L. and P. McCormick. *Introduce Yourself to Transactional Analysis.* Stockton, Calif.: San Joaquin TA Institute, 1972.
4. James, M. and D. Jongeward. *Born to Win.* Reading, Mass.: Addison-Wesley, 1971.
5. McCormick, P. *Guide for Use of a Life Script Questionnaire in Transactional Analysis.* Berkeley, Calif.: Transactional Pubs, 1971.
6. Wachter-Shikara, N. "Scapegoating Among Professionals: How to Avoid Scapegoating by Using a Transactional Approach." *American Journal of Nursing* 77 #3, March 1977, 408–409.

PERTINENT ORGANIZATIONS

NATIONAL
* *International Transactional Analysis Association*
  3155 College Avenue
  Berkeley, California 94705
  This group can be contacted for more information on the use of TA. Also, it publishes a *Directory of Affiliates and Geographical List of Members* and a *Transactional Analysis Journal.*

* *Transactional Pubs*
  1771 Vallejo Street
  San Francisco, California 94123
  This organization publishes and distributes literature and books on TA. You can write to them for a list and prices.

Teaching Strategies

Priscilla A. Lester, R.N., M.N.

CHAPTER TWENTY-TWO

Health education is not only integral to every nursing intervention, but without it, our practice becomes an unfinished service to individuals and families. Teaching is an important preventive mental and physical health measure. It decreases the anxiety inherent in high-risk situations by making once unfamiliar procedures and concepts understandable to the person involved and, therefore, more comfortable for him to deal with. Teaching provides the family with information which will help them make their own health decisions. Teaching can be very informal and spontaneous, as when a nurse responds to a parent's question, or it can be formal and planned, as with a written program of activities or classroom situations. In either circumstance, there are many alternative teaching methods that are useful for the high-risk family.

Because of the nurse's unique exposure to the patient and nursing's role in assessment of physical and psychosocial aspects of the patient, nurses are best able to evaluate and document behaviors exhibited by individuals which indicate specific family problems. Teaching is one of the most valuable strategies in preventing or reducing the problems for the high-risk family. The nurses in many settings are in excellent positions to provide this teaching.

The stressful, long-term, and family involvement aspects of most high-risk situations make teaching valuable and require well-planned teaching actions. Since most high-risk situations are stressful ones, the nurse plans teaching actions along with crisis intervention and other counseling strategies to help reduce the stress. Because most high-risk situations result in intermittent or long-term family problems, the nurse provides continuity in the teaching plan and coordinates teaching between different professionals. Since most family members are affected by the high-risk situation, the nurse plans her nursing strategies for all the family members.

BASIC TEACHING CONCEPTS FOR THE HIGH-RISK FAMILY

The client's readiness to learn, variables that influence learning, and the types of learning are reviewed briefly in this section. More detailed information on teaching concepts may be found in learning theory references.

Client's Readiness to Learn

Learning occurs when the client is ready to learn. Therefore, before implementing any teaching intervention, it is vital to assess the readiness of the person to learn as evidenced by signs of need, motivation, and ability to learn. Any of these factors may depend on the situation at hand and the emotional reaction to it, as well as past experiences and exposure to various types of learning situations. Other stressors which are related to the situation may also influence learning, such as stress, grief, pain, medications, physical state, and level of alertness.

The teaching plan must be altered to build upon what the client already knows. An example would be a mother who has brought her infant to the emergency room with diarrhea and dehydration. The nurse first assesses what she has tried or been told to do by friends, relatives, or her physician. Perhaps she already knew to withhold solid food and start him on clear liquids a little at a time every hour. Perhaps what she did not understand was the meaning of "clear liquids." The nurse would ask her what kinds of liquids did you try? Or perhaps she did not realize she should give the liquids in graduating amounts so as not to overload the stomach.

The client often identifies his learning needs and communicates them through direct or indirect signals. A direct signal may be a question asking for specific information; on the other hand, indirect signals may be nonverbal communication, such as avoiding a task because the client does not know where to start.

Motivation. Motivation is integral to setting learning goals and is developed before and during the process of instruction. Rewards and outcomes influence motivation. It is important to find a reward or outcome which will motivate that particular individual at a specific time. Often in the high-risk situation the stress itself is enough of a stimulus for the client to want to learn in order to decrease the stress.

For example, a mother of a hyperactive child might be strongly motivated to learn information and behavioral techniques which will enable her to decrease the amount of disruptive behavior exhibited by her child.

Extremely high levels of stress can interfere with the family member's learning. As anxiety increases in severity, an individual's perception and awareness decrease. Since crises of high-risk situations can create extreme stresses and interfere with the individual's perception, crisis intervention may be needed with the teaching strategies.

A lack of motivation reduces learning and may be the result of a difference in value systems and health concepts between the family and health worker. The adolescent parents may be more concerned for their own needs than the baby's needs and less motivated to learn caretaking skills that foster the infant's physical and emotional development.

Variables that Influence Learning

Education should be individualized for each family. To individualize her teaching, the nurse uses an organized system of assessment which includes physical, psychological, developmental, cultural, familial, environmental, and social variables. Each of these variables influences learning and suggests variation in teaching approaches for each family.

Physical variables include physical limitations, level of wellness, including present state of health, adaptation to present situation, and past history of illness. For instance, if a parent is anemic, due to some concurrent illness, his attention span and interest, as well as ability to learn, may be decreased, whereas increasing physical exercise on a consistent basis may increase learning ability.

Psychological variables emcompass past coping mechanisms, cognitive state and level of perception, presence of anxiety, fears, grief, or other unconscious factors. Recent losses, such as divorce, deaths of significant others in last two years, moving, and change of jobs or school, and developmental aspects related to these losses may increase or decrease the ability of the individual to concentrate.

Developmental variables include such things as current level of functioning in relation to age (maturity), the client's caregivers, ability to use language, past interactions with others, and attitude development.

Familial variables include the number of people living within the home and the individual's relationship with them, and problems in the family caused by the individual's illness. They also include stress imposed by these family members.

Social variables incorporates such things as educational level attained, socioeconomic level, neighborhood, occupation, general activities such as hobbies and sports, stress, responsibilities and advantages of roles, and accessibility to medical services (health insurance or transportation).

Cultural aspects may include religion, ethnic background, dietary habits, child-rearing practices, and the many different customs and value systems that are to be expected among members of various cultures and subcultures. Language barriers, of course, can also influence learning. If a foreign language is the client's basic language, it is not unusual for him to find it difficult to communicate in a second language during times of stress. Health professionals often find it neccessary to use interpreters when teaching clients from different ethnic backgrounds. However, even with an interpreter, language barriers can still be a problem because differences in the vernacular of the client and the interpreter may cause confusion and misunderstanding between instructor and learner.

Environmental factors which are important to assess are those relating to the living situation of the individual or family. Teaching must be individualized to the equipment and teaching environment at home or at the agency. Where is the teaching done? Are there other people watching? Is it a quiet room or an ICU? Are there audiovisual aids available. Is role playing used? Is there extra stress imposed by the environment, home, work, or community?

Types of Learning

Learning can be classified in a number of ways. Learning involves acquiring thoughts, attitudes, or behaviors. One classification of types includes cognitive, attitude, psychomotor skills, and operant learning. High-risk families learn in each of these ways.

Cognitive learning is the acquiring and development of concepts. Since concepts order experiences, the nurse bases the concepts on past experiences for the risk family. Some concepts taught high-risk families are hyaline membrane disease, nutrition in pregnancy, effects of alcohol, and other concepts related to risk situations.

Attitude learning is the acquiring of an attitude or emotion. Sometimes in client teaching it may be important to change preexisting attitudes which may have an adverse effect on the health care of the family or individual. In order for the change to take place, it is helpful for the individual to identify for himself how he acquired the attitude. Attitudes may be learned socially, culturally, or experimentally, or they may be derived from generalizations based on what the individual perceives to be true. The nurse carefully assesses if a present attitude is actually harmful to the family members or just different from her attitude. Attitude changes occur slowly through the use of behavior modeling and the families' identification with the attitude of the nurse.

Psychomotor skills are behaviors carried out through the necessary integration of neurological functioning and musculoskeletal coordination. Learning psychomotor skills depends on individual strength, reaction time, speed, balance, precision, and flexibility. An intact, well-developed neuromuscular system is important to learning a skill, as is having a mental image of its performance. Therefore, practice with immediate feedback from the instructor is important to this type of learning. Having an ill infant who needs to be gavage fed is an example of a situation requiring this type of learning.

Operant conditioning, or behavior modification, involves learning a behavior through application of reinforcement theory and is based on the fact that learning can often be motivated by satisfaction. These techniques involve rearrangement of rewards and punishments to weaken or strengthen specific behaviors. The parents of a hyperactive child use rewards and punishments to help the child learn behavior acceptable in the family. More explanation of operant conditioning is in the "Behavior Modification Strategies" chapter.

TEACHING STRATEGIES FOR HIGH-RISK FAMILIES

Teaching strategies depend on the preparation, setting, available resources, and the individual needs of the learner. Many teaching strategies are used for the high-risk family. Figure 22-1 lists the teaching strategies.

Assessing the Client's Needs and Abilities

Just as in the nursing process, it is important in teaching to assess, interpret data, and plan interventions before initiating them through goal setting with the client or family. What are the desired outcomes? How much does the client want to learn? What are the client's resources in time, availability, finances, and lifestyle? What resources are available to the nurse? What is the learning environment? The nurse assesses the needs and abilities of the family members through an assessment guide such as the one in Figure 22-2.

Establishing Objectives. After assessing the families needs the nurse establishes objectives for learning. Objectives are jointly identified, based on the family's present interests and motivation. The objectives describe the desired outcome for the family when the learning has occurred so they will be able to observe their progress. This joint development of objectives is especially important for the family experiencing difficulties from risk situations. For example, with the pregnant adolescent who has low hemoglobin and iron intake, they may jointly agree on an objective of the mother eating at least four ounces of meat twice a day.

Building Teacher's Strengths

It is important for the nurse to recognize strengths and limitations, such as her own level of

Figure 22-1. Teaching Strategies for High-Risk Families

Assessing the Client's Needs and Abilities
   Establishing objectives

Building Teacher's Strengths
   Coordinating other health professional teaching
   Selecting instructional aids
   Developing unique teaching aids

Preparing a Plan of Instruction
   Choosing instructional settings
   Group discussions
   Team teaching
   Choosing teaching methods
   Involving all family members
   Modeling behaviors
   Using rewards
   Communicating with client

Evaluating the Desired Learning

knowledge of the material. If she is not strong in a particular area, it may be necessary to use other nurses' strengths in that area to help her with the planning as well as seeking out learning resources. Enlisting the assistance of others' information or reviewing a teaching plan builds the nurse's knowledge and confidence. Seeking new information is a nurse's strength and not a weakness.

Coordinating Other Health Professional Teaching. Other health professionals are valuable resources for teaching. Occupational therapists, physical therapists, and nutritionists can add to the nurse's teaching. Again, the nurse helps interpret or problem solve after the formal teaching. For example, a nutritionist taught a low carbohydrate diet to a group of patients. The nurse helped the nutritionist to individualize the instruction by sharing medical and cultural aspects of each client with the nutritionist and followed up with individual counseling after the session. Families in risk situations frequently see many health professionals. Coordinated teaching is essential.

Selecting Instructional Aids. A wide variety of instructional aids are available to help the nurse teach the family members. Films, filmstrips, slide-cassettes, charts, diagrams, and pamphlets can be combined with verbal instruction and demonstration techniques for the client, but should *not* be used in lieu of verbal explanation or demonstration

Figure 22-2. Assessment Guide for Learning Abilities and Modes of Teaching

Assessment of
  Needs
  Motivation ——————————→ through the following variables
  Learning ability

1. **Physical**
   Physical limitations—eyesight, hearing, intact CNS, genetic make-up
   Level of wellness —state of health, adaptation to present situation, past history of illness

2. **Psychological**
   Past coping mechanisms
   Cognitive state
   Level of awareness
   Presence of anxiety, fears, grief, etc.
   Recent losses and developmental aspects of the losses.

3. **Developmental**
   Maturity level
   Speaking and language ability
   Interactions with others
   Attitude development—type of home, child-rearing attitudes

4. **Familial**
   People living at home
   Clients' relationship with them
   Problems caused by family, or to them due to stresses of situation at hand

5. **Social**
   Educational level attained
   Socioeconomic level
   Neighborhood, occupation, recreational activities, roles and responsibilities, and stresses imposed by them, accessibility to
     health services, i.e., insurance, transportation

6. **Cultural**
   Religion
   Ethnicity
   Child-rearing techniques
   Value system, mores
   Orientation to time
   Language spoken

7. **Environmental**
   Living situation of client or family
   Location of home within the community
   Milieu of the home, job, and teaching settings
   Stresses imposed by these environments (home, work, community, learning settings)

techniques. Verbal explanation and counseling in-dividualize the material in institutional aids. The specific media chosen depend upon what is being taught and the client's ability to learn. For example, in order to teach a pregnant female about the effects of smoking on the fetus, the nurse may wish to use a diagram and filmstrips which illustrate how the fetus derives its oxygen supply through the maternal blood entering the placenta and how smoking reduces circulation. The nurse can follow the audiovisual teaching session with individual counseling and goal setting to help the mother reduce her smoking.

The library is one of the best resources for locating books, indexes to nursing literature, lay magazines on health issues, and med-line searches on a specific subject area. Some libraries also have facilities for audiovisual searches producing a computer printout of audiovisual materials, films, filmstrips, and so on related to a specific topic. Many professional organizations have catalogs of pamphlets and audiovisual materials available for student, staff, or patient education.

Developing Unique Teaching Aids. Teaching aids can be made through various methods and resources. If the nurse has the equipment available, overhead transparencies can be photocopied from typed materials, diagrams, or hand illustrated materials and mounted on frames to make them easy to handle. The advantage of this method is that the material can be personalized. Charts and diagrams can be put on poster board or photographed for slides by the nurse or the photography department at your institution. If you take pictures and photograph from books or journals to make slides, you must get permission from the book's copyright holder, the publisher, to do so. Pictures from magazines and newspapers, mounted on poster board, can be used for illustrating many things. This is a more economical method.

Presenting videotapes of skills the nurse wants to demonstrate to parents or a group is an alternative way of reinforcing concurrent or past teaching. For instance, if the nurse wants to demonstrate an effective exchange of communication versus an ineffective method as in transactional analysis, she could have staff or expatients act out the scripts and film them with the assistance of an audiovisual department. However, although this results in individually designed material, it may be expensive and requires extra time and training and equipment.

Preparing a Plan of Instruction

After needs and abilities of the client have been assessed and resources explored, the nurse prepares a plan of instruction. The plan includes the desired outcomes of the family members, content to be taught, method of teaching, and time and place of teaching. An individualized teaching plan is very important for the stressed family members.

Choosing Instructional Settings. In a high-risk situation, the choice of settings may be limited by the emergency situation and limited hospital space. If the hospital nurse coordinates her efforts with a public health nurse by planning approaches together, a variety of settings is possible, with the hospital nurse having the institutional setting and the public health nurse able to work in the home and community. It is important to avoid an environment with too many distractors, such as the middle of an intensive care unit, unless the purpose

of the teaching relates directly to the setting (explaining equipment). In hospital settings scheduled classes that meet the needs of a group of clients are often valuable. Groups of families in similar risk situations can benefit from group teaching and discussion if good counseling strategies are combined with the teaching strategies.

Group Discussions. Group teaching can be an effective way of helping family members cope with a risk situation. Group members are chosen for common needs. Members of the group can often help in the teaching. For instance, in a group of women gathered to share a bath demonstration on their new babies, there were several mothers with other children who confirmed ideas expressed by the nurse and helped demonstrate to other mothers.

A group meeting to help family members cope with risk situations focuses on several aspects of the problem: description of the situation and stresses, identification of the family's responses to the stress and resulting difficulties, and discussion of alternate coping actions.

The group should have consistency of leaders and members to allow development of trust among group participants. This is especially important for long-term groups. The group needs to decide in the beginning session whether it is open or closed to new members. New members may be added if no new group is available to them, however, a group must take time and energy to incorporate new members.

When possible, it is helpful to choose group members with similar interests and needs. For example, presenting classes on parenting to a group of single parents with similar interests, needs, and backgrounds can often be more effective in meeting the specific needs of the group than would be possible if the group included married couples or other members whose interest would be different.

The group's time and place for meeting should be open to most group members. A simple survey form can accomplish this goal, giving alternate days, times, and places feasible for teacher and group.

One should also take advantage of "captured" audiences, such as people in waiting rooms of doctor's offices or clinics, or in parents' waiting rooms, where a group is already gathered. These classes must be flexible to allow clients to come and go, since their priority is the appointment they have.

Team Teaching. Nurse-physician, nurse-nurse, and nurse-parent or nurse-public health nurse teams are some types of team approaches. Being in attendance with a physician when explanations are made to patients or families and participating in the overall plan are helpful to everyone involved. The physician may benefit by learning to talk in less technical terms. The nurse will benefit from knowing exactly what aspects the physician has or has not covered. And the individual will benefit by better understanding concepts the health professional is trying to teach. If the nurse is there, she will not have to ask the patient what was explained to him and the patient will not have to reiterate it. An added benefit will be the increased trust between health professionals who gain a better understanding of each other's efforts, attitudes, and skills.

In the nurse-nurse pair, a less experienced nurse who teaches with a more experienced nurse acting as a role model can learn new approaches to patient teaching without expense to the patient.

Nurse-parent teams are sometimes meaningful to other parents. Often, relating to someone who has already been through a similar experience is easier for parents, and it helps increase their confidence in their ability to adapt to a difficult or high-risk situation.

If there is a community professional who will continue to be involved with the family, it is worthwhile to start the nurse-public health nurse team in the teaching prior to discharge from an institution. For example, the Chicago Department of Health employed a community health nurse to work out of Michael Reese Hospital's Special Care Nursery. She has an office on the unit and is able to meet families during the critical hospitalization period. Other community health nurses without this role may be contacted to come to the hospital to meet the family and discuss the continuing nursing care before the discharge.

Choosing Teaching Methods. The choice of one teaching method or a combination varies depending on the situation and the needs of the family. Facts and concepts are basic to cognitive learning and can be taught by written materials such as pamphlets, articles, lecture, discussion, or through audiovisual aids. Attitude learning does not automatically follow from facts or concepts. Attitudes can best be taught through discussion with clients, to help to provide insights and perception of their feelings, as well as through providing a model, to help them imitate those behaviors and attitudes. Psychomotor skills such as percussion, vibration, and nasopharyngeal suctioning of a child with cystic fibrosis are best learned through demonstration and return performance. Combinations of teaching strategies are frequently more effective than one alone.

Explanation and discussion involves introducing a subject, explaining the topic, and discussing the family's reactions. Discussion provides for individualization of the instruction to the family and for evaluation of family reactions.

Pacing is teaching in steps over a period of time determined by the client's abilities. Mastery learning incorporates this concept by not going on to another concept until basic information is achieved. In practical terms pacing means giving the learner several chances to review or practice the material if needed before going on to the next step.

Demonstration provides visual teaching of a skill which can be modeled by the parent. Return demonstrations show how well the parent has learned the skill. If the nurse is teaching a technique to parents such as active and passive exercises for a child with cerebral palsy, she can demonstrate each skill, have the parent repeat the skill, and teach the reasons for it by showing the parents the positive effect of moving and strengthening the target muscle groups.

The clients practice the technique several times until they feel comfortable with their ability to perform it alone. This can occur over a short or long time span. Return demonstration can be immediate, or later, once the client has had a chance to

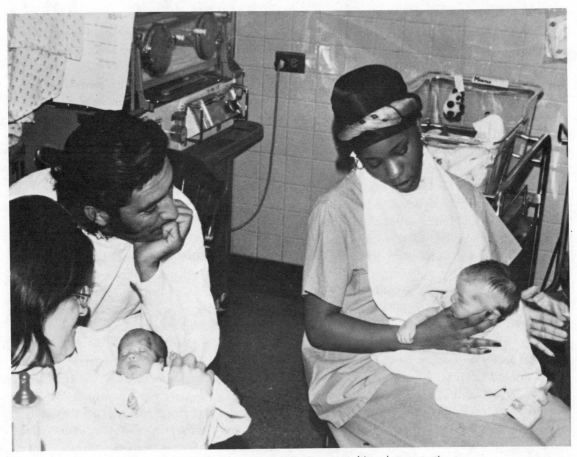

Figure 22-3. High-risk parents returning a teaching demonstration.

review and practice the technique. The parents in Figure 22-3 are returning a feeding demonstration.

Involving All Family Members. The nurse includes all family members in the teaching plan. Involving the parents means encouraging early and continued interaction with their child and allowing them to give whatever aspects of care they feel capable of providing to their child when he is institutionalized. Involving the family means also granting visitation rights to those significant members of the patient's family, such as grandparents who are caretakers, or siblings or children of the affected family member.

Involving parents in a situation, such as a newborn intensive care unit, helps to decrease the normal feelings of alienation that may develop in parents who might feel their child no longer be-

longs to them because his care is totally out of their control. Continued contact also promotes the development of normal attachment behaviors and assists in developing parents who really know their child and are aware of his individuality once he is discharged.

The nurse helps the family control some aspects of their care by encouraging their input in the teaching plan concerning time, space, order of material, methods of presentation, and setting goals and priorities.

Modeling Behaviors. Nurses are role models. Patients watch nurses and look to them for guidance as they are knowledgeable about health care. Other parents can also be role models. One of the most effective ways of teaching parents how to cope with certain situations is to expose them to other parents (in the same room in a hospital, for example) who are effective in their coping.

Using Rewards. Rewards are integral to almost any kind of teaching situation, and are especially important to high-risk parents who frequently have low esteem and confidence.

Verbal cues such as praise can be quite effective, provided they are appropriate to the situation. For example, it would be inappropriate to tell a mother she performed beautifully in a return demonstration of feeding her infant if she did not do it well. Describing the positive result of the behavior, such as a clean child after bathing or a sleeping infant after feeding, provides positive feedback which the parent will be able to recognize by himself in later sessions.

Touch and nonverbal rewards are another means of feedback. A hand on the arm or shoulder, with a smile, can sometimes convey "nice job, well done" as well as the words. Also, there are many ways that people show appreciation without saying words. For instance, a fellow worker may show his approval by performing the same action in another situation, or a parent may not *say* anything, but come in the next day with a box of cookies for the staff.

Timing is another important component in the reward system. Immediate feedback has the greatest effect, and without it, motivation can severely decline.

Parents in a high-risk situation especially need these rewards and feedback. Inherent in many high-risk situations is the feeling of family members that they somehow have failed by not recognizing a problem when it began, not knowing how to cope with it, avoiding seeking help, or doing something they may feel led to the problem in the first place.

Communicating with Clients. The nurse uses concepts and terminology familiar to the family. Not only are there differences in language that affect communication, but also in attitude, perspective, education, and affect which will influence the way they communicate to each other. A nurse should also not feel a failure if she does not always

get along with a client. Some personality differences are unresolvable. She should recognize the limitations of the situation and refer the patient to another willing nurse.

For a parent who is under great emotional stress, as parents in crisis due to risk situations often are, the emotional demands of the situation may block the ability to acquire new knowledge even though he may appear to be attentive. Often the parents of newborns in the intensive care unit need reinforcement as well as reexplanation of terminology that may be foreign to them. Often health workers forget they have a language of their own that is not understood by most of their patients. Also some health workers use technical language to avoid dealing with more difficult issues such as the feelings associated with the situation at hand. Therefore, interpreting explanations which have already been given is often an important nursing function.

The nurse determines if the communication has been effective by setting up a situation where the client will apply the information. When the client states the concept exactly as it was explained, he may have learned the words but not understood the concept. The nurse determines that the communication is successful through application of the concept by the individual family member.

Evaluating the Desired Learning

Evaluating is integral to any teaching plan. Without evaluation, there is no way to assure improvement of teaching content or skills or to assess how much of the information taught was absorbed by the learner. Since high-risk situations are generally stressful, making learning difficult, evaluation becomes even more important.

One method of evaluation is to record the plan for a retrospective look at what information was taught and how. It allows planning and coordination of teaching as well as demonstration. One disadvantage of a record is that professionals frequently assume that if the material was taught once the family knows it and needs no more information in that area. The chart can alert the nurse to assess for the continued retention and application of the taught information and information not yet presented.

Direct feedback from parents on the teaching actions is one of the best means of evaluating the teaching plan. It helps point out where the gaps are, what works, and what does not work. Follow-up phone calls from an index file of families is one way to assure this type of feedback. Another is to check with community service people who have been following the family on a continuous basis after the nurse was involved.

Failure to learn occurs primarily when misinterpretations go unrecognized and unclarified, or under undue stress which may distract the learner. Therefore, reevaluation after each step in teaching is important. Since forgetting occurs soon after learning, providing opportunities for continued use of the skill or information is necessary. Evaluation of learning provides many opportunities to reward the family members for successful learning of new knowledge, skills, or behavior and to reward the nurse for successful strategies.

SUMMARY

Teaching strategies provide creativity for individualized learning experiences for a variety of high-risk families. Teaching strategies are used along with other strategies to prevent or reduce the problems for the family in a risk situation. In order to be effective in teaching high-risk families, the nurse recognizes the individuality of each family member, builds her own strengths, prepares a plan of instruction, and evaluates the desired learning.

ADDITIONAL READINGS

1. Adair, L. M. A. "Patient Education." *Nursing Care*, April 1976, 29–31.
2. Amundson, M. J. "Nurses as Group Leaders of Behavior Management Classes for Parents." *The Nursing Clinics of North America*, 10 #2, June 1975, 319–327.
3. Block, J. H. (ed.). *Mastery Learning.* Chicago: Holt, Rinehart, and Winston, 1970.
4. Ellis, H. C. *The Transfer of Learning.* New York: Macmillan Co., 1965.
5. Hardgrove, C. and A. Rutledge. "Parenting During Hospitalization." *American Journal of Nursing*, 75 #5, May 1975, 836–838.
6. Harrison, L. L. "Nursing Intervention with the Failure to Thrive Family." *Maternal-Child Nursing Journal*, March–April 1976, 111–116.
7. Hogstel, M. O. "A System for Personalized Instruction." *Nursing Outlook*, 24 #2, February 1976, 110–114.
8. Hurd, J. M. "Assessing Maternal Attachment: First Step Toward the Prevention of Child Abuse." *JOGN Nursing*, July–August 1975, 25–30.
9. Jones, M. A. "Reducing Foster Care Through Services to Families." *Children Today*, November–December 1976, 7–10.
10. Jones, P. and W. Oertel. "Developing Patient Teaching Objectives and Techniques." *Nursing Educator*, 2 #5, September–October 1977, 3–13.
11. L. M. "An Ounce of Prevention." Editorial from *Hospitals*, J.A.H.A., 50, May 1976, 51.
12. Murphy, D. A. "A Program for Parents of Children in Foster Family Care." *Children Today*, November–December 1976, 37–40.
13. O'Neil, S. M. "Behavior Modification: Toward a Human Experience." *The Nursing Clinics of North America*, 10 #2, June 1975, 373–379.
14. Redman, B. K. *The Process of Patient Teaching in Nursing*, 3rd ed. St. Louis: C. V. Mosby Co., 1976.
15. Schweer, J. E. and K. M. Gebbie. *Creative Teaching in Clinical Nursing.* St. Louis: C. V. Mosby Co., 1976.
16. Shaw, N. R. "Teaching Young Mothers Their Role." *Nursing Outlook*, 22 #11, November 1974, 695–698.
17. Stone, H. "Introduction to Foster Parenting: A New Curriculum." *Children Today*, November—December 1976, 29—31.
18. Tankson, E. "The Adolescent Parent: One Approach to Teaching Child Care and Giving Support." *JOGN Nursing* 5 #3, May–June 1976, 9–15.
19. Tarver, J. and A. J. Turner. "Teaching Behavior Modification to Patients' Families." *American Journal of Nursing*, 74 #2, February 1974, 282–283.

PERTINENT ORGANIZATIONS

NATIONAL

- *P.E.T.—Parent Effectiveness Training*
  Effectiveness Training, Inc.
  531 Stevens Ave.
  Solana Beach, Calif. 92075
  (714) 481-8121
- *I.C.E.A.—International Childbirth Education Association*
  Various teaching aids
  See local address for your community.
- *ROCOM—Division of Hoffman-LaRoche Inc.*
  (Child care manual)
  P.O. Box 1577
  Newark, New Jersey, 07101

- *Ross Laboratories*
  New Newborn ICU explanation booklet which is excellent for help in explaining special care, has color photos of premies, etc.
- *Health Insurance Institute, Inc.*
  277 Park Avenue
  New York, N.Y. 10017
  For a list of voluntary associations and business firms that have prepared health education materials with addresses provided.
- *Pharmaceutical Manufacturers Assoc.*
  1155 Fifteenth Street N. W.
  Washington, D.C. 20005
  Provide catalog of free publications and 16mm films that may be obtained for patient teaching and the public.

Primary Nursing
Strategies

Kathleen Knudsen DeSantis, R.N., M.N.

CHAPTER TWENTY-THREE

Primary nursing strategies are effective clinical interventions for high-risk families. Primary nursing care individualizes care for a family. *One* nurse is responsible for coordinating all nursing care: the initial family assessment, the planning and implementation of interventions to help the family adapt to the risk situation, the evaluation and assumption of accountability for the outcome of nursing care, and the postcare follow-up. This chapter applies the basic theory and strategies of primary nursing to high-risk families.

Nursing care delivery methodologies have evolved over the years in response to factors present in society and the health care delivery system. *Case modality* involves one nurse caring for one patient for a specified length of time such as an eight-hour shift. Although individual patient care is possible, the modality is expensive with little coordination between shifts. *Functional modality* is the assembly-line approach to patient care with each patient having many nurses responsible for parts of his care. *Team modality* is the care of a group of patients by a different group of nursing personnel each shift. Functional or team nursing has not been effective for providing comprehensive family centered care because when the patient and family are the responsibility of a group of people, they tend to be the responsibility of no one.[5] *Primary nursing* includes 24-hour responsibility and accountability for the nursing care of a small group of patients by one nurse. In this recent clinical mode, since direct patient care is valued, the primary nurse is the bedside nurse. She sets up a trust relationship with the patient and his significant others and coordinates care between shifts or disciplines.

Primary nursing strategies evolved to meet a need recognized by the consumer and the nurse. The consumer is voicing demands for more humanistic, efficient, and high quality care; the nurse is asking to practice professional patient centered nursing. Primary nursing seems to be the answer to both.

BASIC THEORY OF PRIMARY NURSING

Who Is the Primary Nurse?

Every nurse is not suited to function as a primary nurse. The ideal primary nurse is family care oriented. She values holistic care and the nursing process as her methodology of practice. She is competent in assessment, able to make an accurate nursing diagnosis, and willing to prescribe interventions. She can problem solve effectively and has the theoretical background to implement unpredictable or complex nursing interventions. She is willing to accept increased autonomy, authority, and responsibility for her nursing practice.

The primary nurse is empathetic: she is able to feel what the family is experiencing and put herself in their place. She assumes an attitude of advocate for the family. She tries to insure that the family's needs rather than hospital routine and department scheduling are the pivotal point for organization of care.

At present, registered nurses of all preparations and backgrounds as well as some licensed vocational nurses are functioning as primary nurses. Basically, the primary nurse must be capable of designing and managing a plan of total care. Family assignments are made on the basis of family needs and nursing capabilities, the families with the more complex problems being assigned to the nurses with more training and ability.

Where Does the Primary Nurse Function?

Primary nursing strategies have been implemented in all health care settings. The primary nurse who works with high-risk families is frequently found in maternal-child or family practices. In maternal-neonatal settings, the monitrice concept of primary nursing is gaining popularity as more families opt for an awake, aware, participant birth. The monitrice is a specially trained registered nurse (in the United States) who acts as a coach-assistant during labor and delivery.[3] The monitrice

contracts with the parents during the pregnancy to be on call as the delivery date nears. When labor begins, the couple call the monitrice who meets them at the hospital. In collaboration with the physician, she provides total care throughout the labor. The monitrice assesses the progress of labor and suggests appropriate interventions. The father is provided with the same physical and emotional support as mother. The monitrice may continue to function as primary nurse for the family during the puerperium in the hospital and in the home.

Primary nurses are effective in providing comprehensive care to long-term antenatal obstetric patients. The nurse can design a plan of care that promotes family unity despite the lengthy separation. She also serves as a reference person who is most knowledgeable regarding the patient's status, the current medical and nursing care regimens, and future plans for care.

The obstetrical primary nurse is on call for emergencies that occur with her patients. For example, if an antepartum patient with placenta previa begins to bleed and is scheduled for a cesarean section, the primary nurse will be summoned to provide physical and emotional support to the client and the family before, during, and immediately after surgery.

Primary nursing strategies are becoming more popular on pediatric units. Pediatric nurses have long recognized the need to have consistent caretakers for young patients and the importance of involving parents in the child's care. Family centered care and care by parent modalities provide excellent backdrops for primary nursing. Because the primary nurse is present as a bedside nurse and accessible to the family, parents can provide her with information to help her individualize care for the child in a meaningful way. Parents and child are secure in the knowledge that she is *their* nurse and her job is to be there when they need her most. The pediatric primary nurse may work a flexible 40-hour week. She plans to be present and care for the child and family as their needs dictate. When she is not on duty, she delegates care to an associate nurse who makes the routine observations and follows the prescriptions for care. Thus, parents and child are assured of consistent care.

In addition, the primary nurse is becoming more visible in distributive care or primary settings where prevention and treatment of many risk situations occur. The nurse, working under various titles—public health nurse, pediatric nurse practitioner, midwife, family nurse practitioner, alcoholic counselor, school nurse, bariatrics nurse, diabetic nurse specialist, family therapist—is extending the scope of practice to meet the need for community health services. The primary nurse may work out of a clinic, community agency, in a joint practice with a physician, or as an independent nurse practitioner. In these settings, the focus of care is early detection and treatment of medical and or nursing problems or preventive services to maintain a family's present health status.

Differentiation Between Primary Nursing and Primary Health Care

Primary nursing involves a one-to-one relationship at any level of health care, while primary health care is the initial level of service provided to clients including initial assessment and prevention services. Secondary care includes services provided to patients after they have entered a health care delivery system, in which the focus is on restorative and maintenance services.[4] Primary nursing strategies are applicable in any setting because they focus on the patient and family, foster continuity of care, and provide comprehensive care, an opportunity to practice in a professional manner, and a liaison service between the hospital and community. Therefore, the primary nurse can work in any level of health care.

Definition of Primary Nursing

Primary nursing is nursing care that has the following three components:

1. Designation of one nurse who has autonomy, authority, and accountability for all nursing care for her clients;[6]

2. Inclusion of the patient and family in the planning and implementing of care;
3. Coordination of care with other disciplines.

Primary Nurses' Autonomy, Authority, and Accountability. Primary nursing works on the premise that the nurse is a knowledgeable practitioner with something unique to contribute to health care. The primary nurse works autonomously when appropriate to make nursing judgments, has authority for prescribing nursing care, and is accountable for decisions and nursing care.

The *autonomous* primary nurse has control of and is responsible for the nursing care at all times. The care is based on a nursing care plan developed jointly by the primary nurse, patient, and family. When the primary nurse is off duty, associate nurses carry out the care plan, but the primary nurse remains responsible for the prescriptions in the plan. The primary nurse collaborates with other nurses, physicians, and other members of the health team in a colleagial rather than subordinate relationship.

The primary nurse has authority to prescribe for comprehensive nursing care planning and implementation 24 hours a day as long as care is needed. The primary nurse assumes responsibility consistent with authority. She, the patient, and the family make decisions. She is responsible to the patient and the family for the quality of care, meeting care agreements, and continuity of care.

The primary nurse is accountable for all decisions regarding patients in her care. In other modalities the lack of autonomy and dispersion of authority relieve the care givers of accountability for their decisions. In primary nursing, the autonomy and authority result in increased responsibility and increased ability to make changes, guide, and evaluate the nursing care. Since any patient, family, physician, or staff feedback is channeled to the primary nurse, she or he is capable of evaluating and developing sensitive care which would be impossible without this coordination of feedback.

The following case example illustrates the incorporation of autonomy, authority, and accountability into primary nursing practice.

Neal D was hospitalized at eight weeks of age because of a weight loss of one and a half pounds since birth. After a thorough diagnostic work-up was performed with negative results, the primary nurse requested to work with Mrs. D to determine if Neal's problem might be due to maternal deprivation. Utilizing his nursing knowledge and skills, the primary nurse autonomously assessed Mrs. D's handling and feeding techniques, her feelings about and expectations of Neal, and her perception of the problem. Mrs. D felt that she knew how to care for a baby—she had a "healthy, normal" six-year-old daughter—but Neal was difficult to feed: he fussed, squirmed, and regurgitated during feedings. Mrs. D also expressed some jealousy toward the baby, stating that when her husband came home from work he would go to Neal before saying hello to her. The primary nurse discussed his findings with the doctor and together they diagnosed the problem as lack of maternal nurturing due to mother's jealousy of the infant and lack of rewards or reinforcement for mother during feedings. The primary nurse, using his authority, prescribed nursing interventions to be implemented when Mrs. D came to visit or feed Neal. He taught Mrs. D specific feeding techniques aimed at decreasing Neal's fussing, squirming, and regurgitation, and he designed a program in which Mrs. D would be positively reinforced for demonstrating nurturing behaviors. He prescribed that associate nurses would remind Mrs. D of the techniques and consistently reinforce nurturing behaviors when he was off duty. Finally, the primary nurse assumed accountability for the outcome of the care plan. With Mr. and Mrs. D, he evaluated the effectiveness of the feeding techniques and reinforcement program and explored ways of ensuring that Neal's feeding success in the hospital would continue at home. By coordinating feedback from Mr. and Mrs. D, the physician, and the associate nurses, he was able to modify the care plan as Neal progressed and increase the likelihood that he would be accountable for a successful plan of care.

Inclusion of the Family. The primary nurse is aware that the patient is a member of a family and when the patient experiences a crisis, family members with whom his life is closely associated are also affected. So the primary nurse includes the family in her focus and involves family members in the planning and implementation of care. The T family's experience exemplifies how a family may be involved in care.

Mr. T was a 41-year-old Japanese-American who was terminally ill with lung cancer. His family included his wife and four children aged 19, 15, 12, and 9 years. On admission, Mr. T requested that his family be allowed to visit as much as possible, so the primary nurse was summoned to the admitting office to speak with the family. Mrs. T and the children felt that they could be most effective in keeping Mr. T comfortable because they had been caring for him at home and had learned which foods were most easily digested and which bed positions most comfortable. Since the primary nurse believed that Mr. T's need to have his family at his side and the family's need to continue to care for him should be the basis for organization of nursing care, she obtained permission from the hospital administration to waive visiting hour and visitor age restrictions and arranged to have Mr. T admitted to a private room.

At the initial family conference, the primary nurse explained hospital routines, medications, and treatments that would be scheduled for Mr. T. She and the family then discussed the methods by which they could ensure that Mr. T's needs would be met. Mrs. T would come early each morning with a Japanese soup that her husband liked and she would help with morning care. The 19-year-old daughter would come at noon to relieve her mother. She would assist her father with his noon meal and take him to the sun room. Mrs. T and the younger children would come with dinner and Mrs. T and the 15-year-old son would stay and get Mr. T ready for bed. The primary nurse would assist the family as necessary and carry out nursing procedures, such as vital sign monitoring and suctioning that family members were hesitant to perform. When Mrs. T expressed interest in learning these procedures, the primary nurse agreed to teach her. Mr. T was hospitalized for 23 days and his family kept to their schedule with only minor variations. After Mr. T died, Mrs. T and the children asked to see their primary nurse. They thanked her for permitting them to retain some semblance of family life and for allowing them to play the major role in providing care for Mr. T during his final days.

Coordination with Other Disciplines. When a patient and family require services of the interdisciplinary health team to meet their needs, care can become fragmented with each team member caring for "his part" of the family. The primary nurse is in an excellent position to ensure that the patient and whole family are the focus of care. This coordination of care with other disciplines is the third component of primary nursing.

Because of her availability to the patient and family, the primary nurse can coordinate nursing care, medical care (tests and treatments), mental health care, and the special therapies (physical, occupational, respiratory, dietetic) in light of family needs. The interdisciplinary team members usually appreciate the primary nurse coordinating all aspects of care. If a question or problem arises, there is one nurse who is well informed regarding the patient's status, and who will assume responsibility for working out care problems.

The case of 10-year-old Peter, a hyperactive child who was severely injured in a motor bike accident, illustrates the coordinator role of the primary nurse. Because of his many injuries, Peter required the care of the hospital rehabilitation team. The team consisted of a neurologist; physical, occupational, respiratory, and speech therapist; a medical social worker; a home health agency nurse; and the primary nurse. The primary nurse provided team members with the information she had obtained during the family interview so that they were able to schedule their various therapies according to patient and family needs. At subsequent weekly meetings, team members reported on and discussed patient progress in relation to their area of exper-

tise. In addition, the primary nurse kept the team informed of Peter's overall response to the therapies, his adaptation to his changed body image, and the family's questions and concerns. On occasion the primary nurse also served as family advocate suggesting schedule or therapy changes to ensure that the best interests of Peter or his family remained the focus of care.

Difficulties in Implementing Primary Nursing Strategies

The basic difficulty in implementing primary nursing is resocializing nurses to a new role. The initial adjustment to working more flexible hours, going on call, and assuming accountability for all nursing care can be anxiety provoking. Also, primary nurses tend to form close relationships with patients and their families so losses can be more difficult for the nurse to handle. If the nurse allows a normal emotional investment to occur when caring for the patient and family, then inevitably she will experience grief and depression associated with a loss. Primary nurses must consciously design care plans and put them in writing. Many nurses mentally compose care plans but shy away from putting them down in black and white for fear "they are not good enough." Finally, primary nurses may have difficulty accepting themselves and other RNs as authority figures.

An inservice program is necessary to familiarize all appropriate personnel with the primary nursing strategies. The initial inservice should cover primary nursing methodologies, shift changes, nursing process, care plan writing, family theory, family risk difficulties for the frequent clients, and family assessment skills. In addition, the primary nurse requires a greater repertoire of intervention modalities, particularly counseling strategies for developing the nurse-family relationship, and crisis intervention strategies for handling the situational and maturational crises associated with high-risk situations. To provide adequate follow-up care, the primary nurse must be aware of community agencies that provide home nursing care, special therapies and equipment, financial assistance, and health education. Finally, to promote quality control in her practice, the primary nurse should be able to participate in case review conferences and nursing care audits.

Value of Primary Nursing Strategies

Family Acceptance and Satisfaction. In the hospital, families readily accept primary nurses and voice satisfaction with their nursing care. Data was collected on patients' satisfaction with their nursing care according to the method of delivery. Results showed that patients were more satisfied with primary nursing than case method, functional, or team nursing.[6]

In distributive care settings, families express satisfaction in having one care provider and seeing the same person on subsequent visits. Many families felt that the nurse was more interested in them, and they found the nurse more approachable for what they considered trivial information.[1]

Families also show their satisfaction in their behavior. They ring call lights less frequently and make statements like, "We don't have to ask for a thing," "We see our nurse quite frequently and she keeps us informed of what's going on." New parents have commented, "We would have lost control during labor if our nurse hadn't been there." Primary nursing frequently alleviates the situations that precipitate "problem families."

Twelve-year-old Mike was admitted to a team nursing modality pediatric unit for congenital femur defect surgery and was placed in skeletal traction. After two days, he was protesting vehemently that his traction was wrong and no one would fix it, his leg was hurting and the nurses would not give him anything for pain, someone put his tray out of reach so he could not eat lunch, and so on. He phoned his mother five or six times a day to complain and yelled for nurses instead of ringing the call light. The nursing staff investigated his complaints and felt that they were mostly attention-getting devices. His parents, however, went to the director of nurses and the hospital administrator protesting the "atrocious" care their son was re-

ceiving. At this time, the clinical specialist decided to serve as primary nurse for the family. She interviewed Mike and his parents, focusing on their perception of the situation. She explained her role. She would be responsible for Mike's nursing care: ensuring that his traction was correct, helping him get comfortable, making sure his food, water, and call light were within reach. She would investigate and attempt to alleviate any nursing care problems. She left her home phone number with Mike and his parents, instructing them to call if any new problem arose. She agreed to call Mike on her days off that week to be sure that all was going well in her absence. After that, Mike's problem behaviors declined rapidly and he was proud of the fact that *his* nurse had called him and he could call her if someone "gave him a dirty deal." Mike's mother stated that she was pleased that someone was listening to her and doing something about her complaints. Mike's father said, "Now we're getting our money's worth."

Physician Acceptance and Satisfaction. Physicians seem to evaluate nursing care on the skill of individual nurses rather than the mode of nursing delivery.[6] In one hospital study, however, physicians named five advantages to primary nursing care.

1. Stability of nursing staff, with the same nurse caring for the physician's patient day in and day out.
2. The nurse's knowledge of the physician's plans for treatment.
3. Personalized concern and attention to the patient's needs as well as intellectual interest in patients.
4. Good communication from shift to shift and good communication with physicians.
5. Generally good climate to work in because of motivated staff.[6]

In distributive care settings, physicians originally voiced the concern that the primary nurses would "miss something" and the patient would suffer the consequences. However, in a study examining primary care provided by a nurse practitioner, the researcher-physicians concluded that "the nurse practitioner can provide first contact primary clinical care as safely and effectively with as much satisfaction to patients as a family physician."[7]

Nurse Acceptance and Satisfaction. From the nurse's point of view, primary nursing is a satisfying way to practice nursing.[6] Nurses' comments on primary nursing include: "I went into nursing because I wanted to nurse, I didn't want to supervise someone else while they did the nursing." "With primary nursing, I have an opportunity to practice patient-centered nursing." "I find I have more time to work with families." "I have an easier time remembering all the little details about families that help me individualize care; it was almost impossible for me to remember those same details for an entire team of patients."

The primary nurse's high morale and motivation are visible to patients, physicians, and administrators.[6] One young nurse summed up the feelings of many primary nurses: "I feel very good about myself when I know I'm giving good patient care and practicing professional nursing. Several of the patients and families have commented, 'You're always smiling, you must really enjoy your work.' With primary nursing I can honestly answer, 'I certainly do.'"

More Comprehensive Patient and Family Care. Because the primary nurse is responsible for bedside care and focuses on the whole family, the family benefits from increased nurse contact hours. The primary nurse uses a standardized methodology to collect data on family needs, so fewer family needs are likely to be missed. Since the need and goal are diagnosed by the nurse, patient, and family jointly, there is increased likelihood that the goal behaviors will be achieved. Because the primary nurse is aware of the family's capabilities and liabilities for care, her discharge teaching plan is very specific to the family's learning needs, and each family is assured that follow-up care or counseling is available if needed.

Distributive Care Improvements. Families who receive primary care from a nurse practitioner benefit from the nurse's focus on health rather than illness. The primary nurse makes a thorough assessment of biological and psychosocial family needs, looking for actual as well as potential health problems. The family benefits from earlier identification of problems because the primary nurse is familiar with the family and can detect slight behavior changes. As the family comes to trust their constant care giver, they are more willing to provide data to the primary nurse. With a more comprehensive data base, the nurse can assist the family to set realistic goals and can implement a practical plan of care. The primary nurse can follow up and modify the plan of care, again increasing the likelihood that the plan of care will be effective.

Increasing Nursing's Body of Knowledge. When one nurse is responsible for designing a plan of care—diagnosing, writing prescriptions, implementing prescriptions, and evaluating the effectiveness of nursing actions—she learns which nursing interventions are most useful and which are detrimental for particular nursing diagnoses. As the primary nurse has a written rather than a mental plan, there is a record of effective and ineffective processes that can be shared with others and generalized to develop new theories.

APPLICATION OF PRIMARY NURSING STRATEGIES TO HIGH-RISK FAMILY SITUATIONS

Use of the primary nursing roles does not by itself guarantee quality nursing care. The individual nurse's strategies and actions within that role are also important for the success or failure of the primary nursing care. The primary nurse utilizes a process in her practice that begins with client selection and follows through until client needs have been met. The clinical strategies are briefly listed in Figure 23-1.

Organize Primary Nursing Units

The ideal primary nursing unit is staffed entirely by RNs, or RNs and LVNs. Primary nurses usually work during the day or evening shifts, but may work nights depending on patient and family needs. On some units nurses from any shift can

Figure 23-1. Primary Nursing Clinical Strategies

1. Organize primary nursing units
   Determine relationship of primary and associate nurses.

2. Select the appropriate client(s)
   Match client needs with primary nurse's abilities.

3. Pick up the family early

4. Describe the primary nurse role
   Introduce self.
   Set up trust relationship.
   Provide opportunity for family to express fears and ask questions.

5. Assess and diagnose family problems
   Collect objective and subjective family behaviors by observation, physical examination, interview.
   Identify significant variables influencing those behaviors.
   Correlate behaviors with variables and form a conclusion—the nursing diagnosis.

6. Confirm the diagnosis
   Share diagnosis with family via family conference.

7. Develop joint goals
   With family, set goal behaviors.

8. Communicate care plan
   Prescribe nursing action, implementer, and time and frequency of implementation to achieve goal behavior.
   Communicate plan via patient rounds, care conferences and the problem oriented medical record.

9. Individually provide nursing care
   Primary nurse implements nonstandardized or uncommon care prescriptions.
   Primary nurse may delegate common or standardized nursing actions to associate nurses.

10. Evaluate the interventions
    Evaluate effectiveness of nursing actions—was the goal behavior achieved?

11. Follow up on family care
    Collect data to begin discharge plan at initial family interview.
    Provide follow-up care by phone calls, home visits, and/or community agency referral.

choose to be the primary nurse and designate this on the care plan. All units must have specific guidelines for the designation and relationship of the primary and associate nurses. Primary nurses usually carry a caseload of two to four primary patients, and may serve as associate nurses for one to three other patients. Associate nurses care for the patients when the primary nurse is off duty and carry larger caseloads. Shift rotations are arranged at varying times to provide the staff with the time necessary to interview families, write care plans, attend inservice conferences, and provide patient education classes.

Select the Appropriate Clients

A family is selected or assigned with the goal of matching the family's needs with the primary nurse's abilities. The primary nurse functions to meet her client's needs. She carries a caseload of three to six patients and families in the hospital and a much larger caseload in the community. For these clients, she assumes total responsibility in the realm of nursing care. Ideally, in the hospital, high-risk families would be assigned to or requested by the primary nurse who is qualified and enjoys working within the particular risk situation. In the community, the primary nurse would assume care for families who need her particular nursing expertise.

Pick Up the Family Early

The primary nurse picks up the family as early in their health care as possible. In the hospital, the primary nurse may pick up a family before they arrive on her unit. She may meet the family in the physician's office, emergency department, or clinic and serve as a liaison between the initial treatment area and the hospital. In the community, the nurse may pick up a family as soon as a potential risk situation is diagnosed.

Mary, a single 17-year-old, was 30 weeks pregnant with her second child when she first came to the community clinic. She stated that she had gained 40 pounds with this pregnancy and lately had been bothered by headaches, frequent nose bleeds, and shortness of breath. Because of these symptoms and a blood pressure reading of 142/94, she was referred to the high-risk antepartum clinic and picked up by a public health primary nurse. The primary nurse visited Mary in her home several days later. Mary lived in a small duplex with Tom, the baby's father, and her two-and-a-half-year-old son. As Tom was currently unemployed, the nurse was able to interview both parents. Tom expressed concern about Mary's "problems." He had an aunt who had died in childbirth and was worried that Mary might "end up the same way." Mary laughed at this comment and attempted to reassure Tom. She was not particularly worried about her condition. She had had no difficulties with her first pregnancy and felt that if she "took it easy (her) troubles would go away." The primary nurse explained the pathophysiology, symptoms, and importance of early treatment for pre-eclampsia to Mary and Tom. She reinforced the importance of antepartal care and requested that they call her if any new symptoms or problems occurred.

The primary nurse saw Mary at the clinic or visited Mary and Tom in their home until Mary delivered two months later. With close medical supervision and primary nursing care, Mary's pre-eclampsia had been controlled; however, the baby was born with bilateral club feet. Mary experienced guilt feelings regarding her possible role in the defect. By this time the primary nurse was a trusted family acquaintance and was able to reassure Mary that she could not blame herself for the anomoly. As Mary and Tom felt comfortable with their primary nurse, they were able to ventilate their grief feelings with her and utilize the information she provided to help them plan for the baby's future.

Describe the Primary Nurse Role

At the initial nurse-family contact, the primary nurse lays the groundwork for setting up a trust relationship. She sets the climate through words and actions demonstrating her desire to help the family adapt to the situation. She describes her role, making it clear that she is responsible for ensuring that they receive personal, high quality care. She provides the family with an opportunity to express their fears and have their questions answered.

Sharon, an eighteen-month-old, was brought to the emergency department with second and third degree burns of the face, chest and arms. The child had grabbed her mother's teacup from a table, spilling the boiling liquid over herself. The parents were hysterical, blaming themselves for the accident. The staff had focused on the child and were providing intensive care for her injuries. Because of their emotional state, the parents were ushered to another room until the physician was free to speak with them. The pediatric primary nurse was called to intervene with the parents. She introduced herself and stated that she would be caring for Sharon on the pediatric unit. The nurse encouraged them to describe the incident and express their fears and guilt feelings. She described the procedures Sharon was receiving and the purpose for each. By this time the parents seemed much less distraught. The nurse then accompanied them to the treatment room to see Sharon. She remained with them while the child was stabilized and transferred to the pediatric unit.

Assess and Diagnose the Family Problems

After setting the climate for the nurse-family relationship, the next step of the primary nurse process is collecting the data and writing the nursing diagnoses. The family's needs dictate the data that the nurse collects and assessment tools like those in previous chapters are valuable for concise information gathering.

When assessing family behaviors, the primary nurse systematically looks at each family member and then at the family as a group. She gathers data through 1) observation, 2) measurement of internal and external responses, and 3) a family interview.

Observation. The nurse looks at a person's internal and external responses. Specific observation skills include inspection, ascultation, percussion, and palpation. For example, the nurse observes that an infant is pale and limp, his cry weak, and his chest retracting with each respiratory effort. She sees his mother huddled close to his crib, her hands clenched, and her eyes reddened. She sees his father pacing rapidly in the room, frowning, and muttering to himself.

Measurement. The nurse measures a person's internal and external responses, using standardized tools. Some measurements, such as taking a temperature or a blood pressure, are routine nursing procedures. For other responses, such as depression following childbirth or anxiety preceding surgery, measurement tests have not yet been developed. For example, in the family situation described above, the nurse utilizes measurement skills and determines that the infant's heart rate is 180, the mother's weight is 162 pounds, and the father's blood pressure is 140/90 mm Hg.

Family Interview. The family interview reveals important subjective data about the family's reactions to the risk situation. The family interview is potentially the most important assessment tool because responses to illness have a largely subjective element.

The family interview may involve a structured set of questions or may be just purposeful listening throughout the nurse-family interaction. Since the nurse is trying at this point to receive input from the family, she should encourage each member's participation. She does this by directing questions to each person and focusing on their perception of the situation, if they would like to be involved in care and how, and any immediate problems they anticipate because of the situation.

For example, the infant's mother relates during the interview that she has been unable to eat for the last 36 hours. She experiences abdominal pain and nausea when she is forced to watch helplessly as her child struggles to breathe.

Diagnosis. When the nurse completes the initial family assessment, she analyzes the observations, the measured responses, and the family interview data. After analyzing this information, she formulates a conclusion, the nursing diagnosis.

For example, Mr. R is the young father whose child was admitted to the pediatric unit with respiratory distress. The primary nurse observes that Mr. R has been pacing rapidly in the room, frowning, clenching his fists, and muttering, "It's all my fault." In the family interview the nurse notes that Mr. R has had little experience with sick children as his son has never been seriously ill before, he has

no family insurance, and Mrs. R is angry with Mr. R for not letting her call the doctor the day before.

After analyzing the behaviors and variables, the nurse writes Mr. R's nursing diagnoses: anxiety due to lack of previous experience with ill children, financial worries due to no insurance, and guilt feelings due to failure to let his wife call the doctor the day before.

Confirm the Diagnosis

The nursing diagnosis is the nurse's perception of the problem and should be compared with the patient's and family's impression of the problem before the nursing plan of care is prescribed. Frequently the information is best communicated in a family conference. The conference assures that all family members receive the same message. All are made aware of the nursing problems and what can be expected from a plan of care. If inconsistencies in problem perception are encountered, they can be resolved and the nurse avoids a trial and error approach to nursing intervention. The following example illustrates this point.

Mrs. J, a 52-year-old patient in the coronary observation unit, was very conscientious about her appearance. She would don frilly nightgowns, wigs, and use much make-up prior to visiting hours every day. One evening she had a cardiac arrest and her family was quickly summoned. When Mrs. J. became conscious, she saw her family standing about her bed and became quite distraught. The nurses diagnosed her behavior as anxiety over her near brush with death and proceeded to explain that she had use of the latest equipment to detect further problems and the IV medication was very effective in controlling her arrhythmias. The explanations seemed to fall on deaf ears. She refused to talk to or even acknowledge her family. When the family stepped outside for a conference with the physician, Mrs. J related her reason for being distraught. She had never been so embarrassed in her life. The nurses had replaced her nightie with a "tacky" hospital gown. Her make-up was smudged, her wig askew, and her false teeth had been removed! She had kept her false teeth a secret from her children all these years and now the nurses had betrayed her.

Develop Joint Goals

After the primary nurse writes diagnoses, she establishes nursing care goals. Goals generally involve changing a problem behavior to an adaptive behavior and reinforcing or maintaining adaptive behaviors. Goals are written as clear statements of the desired client behavior so that the primary nurse, associate nurses, and others can determine when a goal is achieved. Goal setting is a cooperative effort between primary nurse, patient, and family. This joint goal setting accrues three benefits. If a client and family help identify goals, 1) they will be more likely to accept them as practical and attainable, 2) they are more likely to follow through with prescriptions for implementation of goals, and 3) they achieve an increased sense of control and self-esteem by taking an active part in care.

Communicate Care Plan

When the patient, family, and nurse agree on care goals, the primary nurse prescribes the nursing actions that will lead to goal achievement. Since the primary nurse is responsible for the patient's care on a 24-hour basis, the nursing care plan must be clearly communicated to all health care providers. The nursing prescription includes the nursing action to be implemented, who will carry out the nursing action, and the time and frequency of implementation. The nursing prescriptions are written on the patient's chart, the nursing care Kardex, or even a chart at the patient's bedside. The primary nurse communicates the care prescriptions to the associate nurses at the change of shift report.

It is also important that the physician, primary nurse, therapists, dietitian, and others are kept aware of each other's goals and therapy regimens. Patient rounds, care conferences and the problem oriented medical record system facilitate coordination of care around patient and family problems.

Mr. K, a 34-year-old married father of three, is receiving treatment at a university center outpatient department. An internist, psychiatrist, primary nurse, dietitian, and psychiatric social worker are involved in his care. Mr. K's current problem list includes:

1. Laennec's cirrhosis
2. Malnutrition
3. Unemployment (fired from last four jobs due to "drinking problem")
4. Husband/father role failure
5. Depression
6. Low self-concept
7. Substance abuse (alcohol)

A plan of care is initiated for each problem identified with each care taker contributing his expertise to the solution of the problem. The problem oriented medical record system enhances communication among the health providers because all have a common focus for intervention—the patient and family needs.

Individually Provide the Nursing Care

The primary nurse implements most care prescriptions that she is uniquely trained to do, including those that require modification, have unknown consequences, and are unfamiliar to personnel. Equally important, the primary nurse performs even simple tasks like baths if this contact for observation or support is important for the patient. Ideally, she would perform all nursing care during her shift to foster the one-to-one relationship.

The primary nurse may delegate to associate nurses the implementation of care prescriptions which are common, standardized, and highly predictable in consequences. However, which nursing actions are delegated depends primarily on the ability of the associate nurse to implement them successfully. Before delegating a nursing action, the primary nurse assesses the associate nurse's capabilities that would promote successful implementation and liabilities that would impede successful implementation—lack of sufficient time, other caseload responsibilities, lack of necessary theory base or skill to intervene. Thus, the primary nurse has a rationale for delegating nursing actions and only delegates those which she cannot do because of her workload or off duty time and which could successfully be done by others. Mrs. S's nursing care plan demonstrates appropriate delegation of nursing actions.

Mrs. S is a 26-year-old primapara who delivered a male child with a bilateral cleft lip and palate the previous day. She had voiced much shock, disbelief, and sadness after the delivery but now seemed ready to begin to care for her son. The primary nurse assigned the usual postdelivery procedures such as the postpartum checks and sitz baths to herself so she could work closely with Mrs. S. She also assigned herself to go with the mother to the observation nursery to help her establish contact with her baby and begin to learn the special feeding techniques. On the evening shift the primary nurse delegated the feeding techniques teaching to the associate nurse through the nursing care plan and a short change of shift patient conference.

Evaluate the Interventions

The primary nurse evaluates the effectiveness of nursing interventions. The effectiveness is judged in relation to the patient or family behavior: Was the goal behavior achieved? To answer the question, the nurse uses the same methods she used for gathering data in the initial assessment. If the goal behavior has been achieved and the problem behavior is not likely to recur, that problem can be retired from the active care plan. If a problem behavior continues or the goal behavior is not achieved, the primary nurse reassesses the variables to determine how her nursing approach might be modified to achieve the goal behavior. Evaluation is a continuous process and a crucial tool for updating the nursing care plan and developing new patient care approaches.

The primary nurse and Mr. and Mrs. S, the parents of the baby with a bilateral cleft lip and palate, had established two goals to be achieved the first postpartum day.

1. Mr. and Mrs. S will establish physical contact with their baby in the observation nursery.
2. Mrs. S will feed her son 30–50 cc of formula with a cleft palate nipple at least one time today.

The next day the primary nurse evaluated whether the goal behaviors had been achieved. Did Mr. and Mrs. S touch their baby? Did Mrs. S feed her son successfully? The primary nurse observed the S's stroking their son as he lay in his crib, so she verified that goal 1 had been achieved. The associate nurse reported that Mrs. S began to feed her baby but had become upset and asked the nursery nurses to complete the feeding when the baby gagged and choked on the formula. Goal 2 had not been achieved. After consulting with Mrs. S, the primary nurse decided to modify the teaching approach and remain at Mrs. S's side as she fed her baby. Mrs. S felt she would feel more secure if a skilled baby care provider was with her for the next few feedings. After this modification, Mrs. S was able to achieve the goal behavior and successfully feed her son.

Follow-up of Family Care

The primary nurse has a responsibility to plan for discharge and arrange for follow-up care. Information necessary to begin the discharge plan is collected during the initial family interview, so that while the nursing care plan is being composed, discharge planning begins. During every nurse-family interaction, the nurse identifies learning needs. Having the family participate in care provides a good opportunity to assess particular care capabilities and deficiencies.

When the nursing care plan is formulated, the nurse, patient, and family decide on short-term and long-term goals. For the hospitalized patient, if the long-term goals are not achieved by discharge, the primary nurse arranges to make home visits or refers the family to a community agency. If the family is referred to another agency, continuity of care depends on the ability of the primary nurse and the community agency to work together toward common goals for the family.

The family must be actively involved in planning for discharge. Only they can verify if goals and plans are realistic. Family members are more likely to comply with discharge instructions when they are involved in the planning stage.[2]

Anticipation of discharge and the severing of ties with supportive health team personnel can provoke a variety of feelings in the high-risk family. Some families may demonstrate hostility, stating that they feel rejected now that they no longer need such intensive care. Others attempt to postpone discharge stating that they have forgotten how to provide care or feel they are inadequate to provide special care. The primary nurse can remedy these responses by maintaining channels of communication through phone calls or home visits after discharge. Many families are very relieved to know that *their* nurse is just a phone call away if they need some advice or want to discuss a problem. Other families are pleased to ''report in'' on progress made or just to say hello.

Fifteen-year-old Janet delivered a female infant at 31 weeks of gestation. She had originally planned to place the baby for adoption, but after seeing her tiny daughter decided to keep the baby. Janet lived with her father and stepmother who were home infrequently, two older sisters, and three younger brothers. After talking with Janet during her hospital stay and making a home visit, the primary nurse diagnosed that Janet had a limited knowledge of adequate infant care and no reliable support systems to help her when the baby was eventually discharged. One of Janet's long-term goals was to become a skilled caretaker for her daughter. As the baby's discharge date neared, Janet became progressively more excited about taking the baby home, but remained apprehensive about assuming total care for such a small baby. The pri-

mary nurse arranged for a public health follow-up and, prior to the infant's discharge, discussed the goals and nursing approaches with the public health nurse who would be visiting. The primary nurse decided to make two or three home visits herself the first week after discharge. She also provided Janet with her home and work phone numbers, encouraging her to call if any questions or problems arose. After a difficult first week at home, Janet and her daughter settled into a fairly comfortable routine and the baby developed according to schedule. When they saw the pediatrician for regular check-ups, Janet and her daughter would stop by the hospital to visit their primary nurse and show off any of the baby's new accomplishments.

SUMMARY

Primary nursing strategies are effective clinical interventions for high-risk families. High-risk families need comprehensive individualized care. Primary nursing provides the nurse with the opportunity and the responsibility to meet the needs of the family at risk and practice the patient-centered, professional nursing that is most satisfying for her. Primary nursing places the nurse at the bedside. There she can employ assessment skills and specific nursing strategies that assist the family to return to an optimum state of health. Primary nursing strategies demand more of the nurse, but they allow her to make a socially significant and personally gratifying contribution to the care of high-risk families.

REFERENCES

1. Brown, E. L. *Nursing Reconsidered, Part 2.* Philadelphia: J. B. Lippincott Co., 1971, 360–362.
2. Deakers, L. P. "Continuity of Family-Centered Nursing Care Between the Hospital and the Home." *Nursing Clinics of North America,* 7 #1, March 1972, 85.
3. Hommel, F. "Natural Childbirth—Nurses in

Private Practice in Monitrices." *American Journal of Nursing*, 69 #6, June 1969, 1446.

4. Leininger, M. M., D. E. Little, and D. Carnevali. "Primex." *American Journal of Nursing*, 72 #7, July 1972, 1274–1277.

5. Logsdon, A. "Why Primary Nursing." *Nursing Clinics of North America*, 8 #2, June 1973, 283–291.

6. Marram, G. D., M. W. Schlegel, and E. O. Bevis. *Primary Nursing: A Model for Individualized Care.* St. Louis: C. V. Mosby Co., 1974, 16, 132, 140–141, 153.

7. Spitzer, W. O. et al. "The Burlington Randomized Trial of the Nurse Practitioner." *New England Journal of Medicine*, 290 #5, January 31, 1974, 251–256.

Cultural Strategies

Claudia Anderson, R.N., M.N.

CHAPTER TWENTY-FOUR

Few would argue with the statement that an aim of nursing is to provide optimal care to all. In providing for this care, social, physiological, and psychological factors must be taken into account as the nursing process is instituted. However, the cultural heritage of the client is also very important, and only when cultural aspects are considered can optimal care be a reality.

While culture is an important component of any interaction between the nurse and client or family, it is especially essential in a high-risk situation. The aim of this chapter is to present insights into some situations that may be influenced by culture and to provide strategies that may be utilized to incorporate cultural variations in nursing care for the high-risk family.

BASIC CONCEPTS OF CULTURE

Culture may be thought of as a way of life belonging to a particular group of people. Aspects of culture are learned and handed down from one generation to the next. It is the totality of all learned and transmitted behaviors, attitudes, values, and beliefs of a group of people. Culture influences what foods people eat, the clothes they wear, the religion in which they participate, how they furnish their homes, how they talk, how they wear their hair. As an example, the women in the Mennonite culture cover their hair with bonnets. This group of individuals may elect to forgo such modern conveniences as automobiles and use horses and buggies for transportation. Culture may influence food habits such as fasting for some period or eating a large meal at noon rather than in the evening. Culture may dictate whether one eats such foods as beef or pork.

Of equal importance, culture influences how one views health and illness, health care systems, and health care givers. Members of some cultures may view all health care personnel and medications with great suspicion and distrust, while members of other cultures may view health care personnel as all-knowing. Some members of cultural groups may view illness as punishment from God while others believe it to be caused by witches or another supernatural power. Culture also influences the type of health care sought as well as the decision-making structure within the family.

Culture affects how members view the epidemiology of a disease which is present. It influences beliefs about the nature, course, and probable outcome of that disease. Culture also influences how its members will respond to the disease process. The germ theory is not believed by some cultures. Members of these particular cultures may blame an epidemic on some wrongdoing of the members of the society and will not adhere to isolation precautions.

Culture may affect the way a group of individuals behave in everyday living. For instance, it may be a value in the Anglo culture to practice eye-to-eye contact. People who do not do this may be considered suspicious or mistrusting. On the other hand, this may be seen as a sign of aggression or an invasion of privacy by the American Indian. Norms of behavior such as eye-to-eye contact signifying maternal-child attachment only apply to the culture using that norm.

Further, culture may determine how an individual feels about touch. As with eye contact, touch may be seen as a warm, secure gesture in some cultures, but as a sign of patronizing or aggression by members of another culture. Touch is an important concept in nursing. Generally, nursing students are taught the notion of "laying on of the hands" especially when a client is in crisis. But some cultures view touch as an invasion of privacy or a sign of aggression. If a nurse employs touch frequently as a means of communication, the client may become tense rather than relaxed at times. When this occurs, the nurse can appropriately ask the client if he or she would rather not be touched.

The concept of time may be influenced by one's culture. Many Latin Americans place little value on punctuality. Upon going to a meeting only to find that no one had arrived at the specified time, a friend from Puerto Rico asked whether the meeting was scheduled for nine American or Puerto Rican time. This delay was consistent with her own culture.

Culture dictates interaction between individuals. Members of some cultures may be taught to be submissive to persons viewed as authority figures.

Thus, they may not express their own feelings but attempt to be compliant. For example, the author cared for an elderly Mexican-American gentleman with a potentially terminal illness. This gentleman failed to eat what was considered enough at each meal and frequently sent his tray back to the kitchen barely touched. The nurses caring for the client asked if anything was wrong or if they could bring him anything else to eat. He repeatedly said everything was satisfactory and he was not hungry. Finally, one of the nurses asked his daughter if he had indicated any displeasure with the meal service. The daughter then replied that the man had never eaten anything except Mexican food and was not accustomed to the meats, potatoes, and vegetables that were served him. He was afraid to say anything about this as he felt the nurses might become angry if he complained about the food. Arrangements were made to provide a more culturally routine menu for this individual.

Subcultures. While one belongs to a larger culture, he is also a member of subcultures within that culture. Subcultures have their own sets of values, beliefs, ideology, behaviors, and habits which may or may not mirror those of the larger culture or cultures. At times practices of the subculture may be in opposition to the larger culture. This may lead to a conflict resolution or the subculture may choose to separate itself from the larger culture. The United States has been called the melting pot of the world. This is because of the influx of immigrants on which our nation was founded. Different cultures have lived together, intertwined with one another, and formed subcultures. These subcultures can be either an intermingling of several cultures or units from the larger "pure" culture.

Participation in activities of the main culture may depend upon the degree of acculturation or indoctrination developed by members of the subculture. As an example, a group of individuals who classify themselves as Italian may be citizens of Italy and recent immigrants or descendants of families who migrated from Italy in the early 1900s. They may have descended from families who emigrated to the United States much earlier than the

1900s. The first group may embrace all values and customs which are practiced in Italy while the latter group may celebrate those customs only at holidays.

Individuals who have become acculturated into American ways may have difficulty with parents and grandparents who have not become so acculturated. For example, it may be a cultural practice for a young woman to live at home until she marries. If the young woman desires to work and live in her own apartment following graduation, this could be a source of great conflict within the family. This practice of living at home may be seen as improper by the larger culture but seem acceptable within the subculture.

Culture and Society. Although there is some similarity, one's social standing is different from one's culture. One's cultural heritage may dictate his social status. For example, a new Puerto Rican immigrant without education or employment may be forced into a low social standing. On the other hand, just because one has a Puerto Rican background he is not automatically placed in a lower social status.

Though cultural and social backgrounds are different, they often influence one another. Social standing, for example, may be influenced by one's income, education, and occupation. Opportunities for advancement often are influenced by parents and other family members. For example, if the father in a family has a tenth-grade education, his job opportunities may be somewhat restricted. The mother may or may not have an equivalent education but may not be able to work outside of the home because of a number of small children in the home. Economic opportunities for advanced education may be limited in this family, which prevents the next generation from raising their social standing. This may be influenced by the culture as well. Perhaps the family emigrated from Eastern Europe during the late 1940s. The family may have had no money and the man could have had a trade which was profitable in the old country but, because of industrialization in the United States, is obsolete.

On the other hand, a person may come from a well-educated, prominent, and wealthy British family. Opportunities for this individual to advance and have an upper-middle class social standing are greater than for the individual of the family previously described.

Culture and Religion. Although the focus of this chapter is on culture, one cannot separate religious influences from cultural ones. Whether or not religion influences the culture, nurses consider the religious influences just as they consider cultural ones. Religion has a bearing on both the culture and the health care system—directly or indirectly.

Often religious beliefs dominate or are so thoroughly ingrained in the members of a culture that the religion and the culture must be considered together. In other words, the religion dictates the cultural practice. The Black Muslim religion may be considered to influence its members in this way. Although the organization is a religion, it is also a way of life. One nursing student who belonged to the Black Muslim organization had some conflicts between her religion and her education. The role of women in her religious-cultural group was passive. In her student role, she was expected to be aggressive. Both faculty and the student were frustrated until they began to discuss how her religion influenced her role as a woman.

Though other religions may not dominate the culture, but exist within it, nurses must be aware of their beliefs concerning the health care system. For a Catholic, abortion may be out of the question even though the woman's life may be at risk if the pregnancy is continued. Another example is a Jehovah's Witness, who might risk her own life or that of her child by refusing a blood transfusion. Thus, although the religion does not dominate the culture, it has great bearing on its members' attitudes toward the health care system and those individuals who function within that system.

Culture and the Health Care System. Deciding from whom health care will be sought is often a cultural matter. Whether one seeks a granny midwife, a medicine man, a faith healer, or some other spiritualist, or a physician or nurse may often be influenced by one's culture. When the practitioner is consulted may also be influenced by the culture. People in some groups will seek care only during illness or even into a crisis period. The concept of health maintenance and disease prevention may not be one valued by the particular culture.

Once an individual decides to seek health care, culture will affect how the health care system is viewed. Some cultures may show great distrust of hospitals, doctors, nurses, medicine, and some of the instruments and equipment that are frequently utilized. Some of these notions arise from a mystique about the health care system while others arise out of past negative experiences with the health care system.

Just because a health regimen has been established for a client does not mean that the regimen will be followed. Culture, among other things, may be influential in whether or not the regimen is followed. Distrust of the health care team and system may, for example, prevent a client from taking medication which is deemed essential for him. The way the client views health may also influence his compliance with the regimen. A client may take medication when he feels sick but stop taking it as soon as he feels better. The frequency with which medication is taken may be influenced by sociocultural factors. Medication which is prescribed four times a day may be taken only once a day. This may be because of distrust of the health care system or because of finances. The client may decide to take medication less frequently so that it will last longer.

Some disease processes are more common in some cultures than in others. For example, hypertension and sickle cell anemia are more common among the black population than other cultures. Puerto Ricans have a high incidence of tuberculosis. American Indians have a high incidence of diabetes as well as alcoholism. It is important to assess the community in which the health care facility is located and determine the predominant cultural groups to be served. Health care professionals will then determine diseases common to the various cultures and plan such interventions as detection, screening, and intervention programs.

Perhaps this will gain support from city and county health officials who will expand the programs to include the schools or have mobile vans to take the system to the clients to be served.

It can easily be inferred that culture affects illness behavior. How a client expresses illness, expresses pain, responds to those around him, and follows the prescribed regimen are all influenced by his cultural upbringing. For example, a woman has had both legs amputated for vascular insufficiency. She was a heavy smoker, even though her continuation of smoking jeopardized her future health. Medical and nursing staff constantly attempted to make the woman stop smoking by removing her cigarettes, but she replenished her supply and continued to smoke. Upon investigation it was learned that this woman was from Czechoslovakia. In the woman's culture, supervision and authority were resisted because autonomy is a highly valued virtue. When this was learned, the staff worked with the woman keeping her culture in mind. They no longer demanded that she stop smoking or took her cigarettes away from her. They helped her gather the information necessary to make an informed decision and supported her in choosing for herself whether or not to smoke. Shortly after this approach was taken, the woman gave up cigarettes.[5]

CULTURAL STRATEGIES FOR THE HIGH-RISK FAMILY

In order to practice nursing in a holistic, humanistic fashion, a person's cultural background must be considered when caring for him or his family. Since nurses provide continuing care for families in many settings, they are in a strategic position to utilize their knowledge of a client's cultural heritage to provide optimal care for the client and his family. Figure 24-1 summarizes the nursing strategies.

Nursing care will often be frustrating to the client and the nurse if cultural needs are not attended. This may result in the labeling of a client as uncooperative, a "crock," hostile, stupid, and the like. This may cause the client to withdraw or be-

Figure 24-1. Cultural Strategies
for the High-Risk Family

Acknowledging the Nurse's Cultural Heritage

Avoiding Prejudices and Cultural Bias

Assessing the Client's View of the High-Risk Situation
   Primary health care giver
   Cultural shock related to high-risk situations
   Family role changes

Involving All Family Members

Identifying Significant Others

Avoiding Language Barriers

Using Nutritional Preferences

Evaluating Nursing Actions
   Follow-up

come noncompliant, distrusting, or alienated. When such events occur, the effectiveness of the care giving network is surely weakened.

The following example illustrates the labeling of a culturally based behavior as uncooperative. A patient in his midthirties was admitted to a hospital with an acute myocardial infarction. He was placed on strict bed rest, however was "caught" standing and looking out of his window several times. Upon investigation it was learned that the man was a Muslim and his religion dictated his looking to the east five times a day. When this was learned, the man's bed was turned in the appropriate direction. From that time his "noncompliant" behavior became compliant.[5]

In order to fulfill professional responsibilities to the clients served, nurses must systematically study cultural patterns, especially as they relate to health and illness practices. While it may not be realistic to try to know about all cultures, it is realistic to know about the major cultures served by the employing agency and to have resources for securing information about cultural patterns which are frequently seen. One way this might be accomplished is to identify a family in the community who belongs to one of the dominant cultures and ask them to discuss with the agency their heritage and cultural practices involving health, the health care system, and beliefs about health. This would not only provide resources for the staff but would

also convey to the family that their culture is important and their ideas will be helpful in providing care to members of the given culture. This invitation would serve as good public relations between the agency and the cultural group.

Nurses are further obligated to incorporate the client's values and attitudes regarding health, illness, and activities into the policies and procedures of the health care agency. This requires that nurses be aware of cultural diversity in general and how the culture affects the individual being served. In order to achieve this, it is important to include the client when planning for the care to be given. One way to do this is to ask the client about his preferences and cultural background. The nurse will incorporate this information into the nursing process.

Acknowledging the Nurse's Cultural Heritage

One way to achieve the goal of meeting a client's cultural needs is to acknowledge that we are all products of a culture which influences our habits, beliefs, actions, values, and attitudes. The Protestant ethic is one which values work as good. The nurse who was brought up with this attitude may be in conflict with the client who does not hold this value. The nurse may become angry with the client who receives Aid to Dependent Children. She may believe that this woman is lazy and likes to sit at home doing nothing rather than work. There may be a complex network of factors which the nurse does not understand that influences the lifestyle of the client. Nurses must be cautious in imposing their own values, beliefs, and attitudes on clients. Rather than judging clients by her own cultural standards, health care professionals must view the individual as a member of a culture and a subculture and ascertain how these influence the client's life.

The following example illustrates members of the health team attempting to impose their beliefs on the family. When caring for a client who is a Jehovah's Witness, it must be remembered that these individuals do not accept blood transfusions. They believe the acceptance of blood is against the will of God and that an individual who does accept blood will not be accepted into the Kingdom of Heaven. Although individuals vary in their beliefs, most Jehovah's Witnesses will not accept blood for themselves or their children in any form—whole blood, platelets, plasma, or RhoGam.

The author has worked with a number of these clients and has found them to accept the responsibilities of their decisions. A good number have made elaborate legal documents acknowledging their wishes to refuse blood transfusions. They release medical personnel as well as the hospital from responsibility for their decision. It has been the author's experience that health care personnel do not readily accept the client's decision.

Mary C became pregnant and carefully selected an obstetrician to provide her prenatal care and deliver the infant. She visited this physician only to find that he would not care for her because of her beliefs about transfusions. She subsequently telephoned several other physicians who shared the original physician's attitude. She was referred to a university teaching center for her care.

Prior to the expected delivery date, Mr. and Mrs. C visited a lawyer who helped them draft a document stating that under no circumstances was either she or the infant to receive blood. She and her husband also stated in the document that they exonorated the staff from responsibility should the need arise for blood to be administered. They stated that if blood were administered the body would become impure and the person would never be accepted into Heaven. The document was appropriately signed and copies were delivered to the physician, the hospital, and to Mrs. C's chart.

When Mrs. C entered the hospital in labor, her pelvis was deemed borderline. Although her contractions were strong and close, her cervix did not dilate past four centimeters. The position of the baby remained at a minus three station. After several hours and much consultation, a cesarean was performed. During surgery a uterine artery was severed. Mrs. C lost a good deal of blood and a request was made to Mr. C to administer two units of blood to Mrs. C. The request was denied, so

treatment was continued with Lactated Ringers. Mrs. C did not seem to respond to the therapy. Her hematocrit dropped from a preoperative level of 38 percent down to a level in the twenties. Again a request was made to the family including the woman's husband, parents, and the minister. All said she would die before blood would be administered.

Mrs. C's hematocrit continued to drop and it became imperative to administer blood (or at least packed cells) or she would die. By this time Mrs. C was waking up after surgery. Physicians talked to her and she also said she would die before blood would be administered. By this time Mrs. C's hematocrit was in the low twenties.

During the next few hours, staff became quite frustrated. In their opinion, a life was passing senselessly. Seven hours following surgery the hospital attorney was contacted to see what legal action could be taken to administer blood. It was learned that the document Mrs. C had signed as a legal adult (of 24 years) precluded her receiving blood. Twelve hours after surgery Mrs. C died. Her hematocrit had reached a level of 8 percent.

In talking to her family later, it was learned that they felt it better for her to have died than to accept blood. They felt she would have been condemned had she received blood. They were quite comfortable with their decision even though it created a good bit of anger and hostility on the part of the staff. The staff needed assistance in realizing they could not impose their values on the C's, that the family's decision was based on informed consent and their negative response was preventing them from using their nursing ability to help this family grieve for their loss. It is the responsibility of the nurse to support the family after a decision has been reached—even though this decision is not in accordance with the beliefs of the nurse. Staff also has the responsibility to assist the family in the grief process in a case such as this.

If elective surgery is planned, autotransfusion may sometimes be acceptable. In this situation the client would donate his own blood to be stored until the time of surgery. If conditions warranted, the client could be transfused with this blood. This strategy, while often accepted by members of Jehovah's Witness faith, may be impossible to implement with a pregnant client who may already have a low hemoglobin or hematocrit. It is not always possible to plan ahead for surgery in the pregnant client, such as in cases of women with placenta previa or abruptio placenta.

Avoiding Prejudice and Cultural Bias

In order to individualize care given to the client, the nurse must view him, as mentioned before, as a member of both a larger culture and a subculture or group of subcultures. Nurses must be cautioned against stereotyping an individual as a member of a culture. Although a person may be a member of a certain ethnic group, he may not embrace many of the beliefs held by that culture.

In planning for and instituting the nursing process, nurses assess the client and individualize care based on the assessment and input from the client. The same principle holds for a culture. Just because a person is Oriental does not automatically mean that the person likes to eat with chopsticks. Stereotyping a person may be seen as a form of cultural prejudice. The individual's identity is sacrificed to that of the larger group. This practice must be avoided by members of the health professions.

In caring for clients of various cultural backgrounds, what the nurse brings into the relationship is important to the success of the relationship. Perhaps one of the most important characteristics the nurse has is recognition of her own feelings. A second important characteristic is willingness to allow others a different point of view. The nurse should be open and honest with these feelings. If the nurse is uncomfortable in a situation, the client will sense that discomfort and may withdraw, become aggressive, or attempt to cope in some other manner.

When making a home visit following delivery, a young community health nurse noticed a cockroach crawling from the sugar bowl. The nurse attempted to make light of the situation even though it troubled her greatly. Rather than sharing her discomfort with the client, the nurse tried to act as if this was an everyday occurrence in her life. Later the client relayed her distrust of the nurse. The client stated she did not like roaches any more than did the nurse, and the client would have been more open with the nurse if she had been open with the client.

Identifying what values or ideals a member of a culture has can be done by asking the person. A person from the Mexican-American culture does not necessarily believe in the concept of the evil eye or eat tortillas and beans for every meal. It is much better to ask the client or significant other person directly the meaning of various aspects of his lifestyle than to guess what the client likes or desires. By asking the client to identify certain values or behavior patterns, the nurse shows sensitivity to that client and acknowledges the importance of the client as an individual.

Assessing the Client's View of the High-Risk Situation

It is important to assess what the culture means to the individual, how he, as well as the culture, views the disease process and risk situation, and how he feels about the health care system. Examples of different cultural ways of looking at the risk situations are described here. An assessment guide for determining cultural traits influencing the high-risk situation is in Figure 24-2.

In the following case of a woman from the Gypsy culture who delivered a preterm infant, the

Figure 24-2. Assessment Guide to Incorporate Cultural Traits in the Nursing Care Plan

1. Who makes decisions?
2. Who will care for the family member at risk when he goes home?
3. Who is the primary health care giver? When will different "healers" be sought?
4. What alterations in lifestyle are caused by the hospitalization?
5. How does the family view the high-risk situation?
6. What family role changes may result from the risk situation?
7. Are there other diseases prevalent in the respective cultures which may affect the family?

risk situation meant the "less than perfect" infant could not be incorporated into the community. The Gypsy culture is often thought of as a nomadic one. Frequently a group of Gypsies moves from place to place. When their infants are born, they place a great value on the infant being "perfect"—in size, shape, and form.[1] Anticipating this, it may be wise for the nurse to utilize anticipatory guidance with families and assist families in identifying danger signs and indicate when health care should be sought. It might also be wise to give the family a record of the history and previous intervention, which could be useful if the family leaves the current location and needs health care elsewhere.

The author had the opportunity to care for a Gypsy woman who went into labor prematurely as she and a group of fellow Gypsies were moving across the country. The woman delivered a beautiful baby boy who weighed three pounds, ten ounces. Although he was fine and doing well in every way except for being small, the parents and others within the Gypsy culture viewed him as imperfect. Upon the woman's discharge from the hospital, the Gypsies continued their journey, never to be seen by the hospital personnel again. The infant was placed in a foster home and was later legally adopted after months of investigation to find the natural parents.

A disease may be seen as the work of a spell in some cultures. It may be felt that a witch cast the spell and only a witch can break it. It is unlikely that the family will seek medical attention when they feel the disease is the work of a witch. Similarly, many Mexican-Americans believe in the influence of the mal de ojo, or evil eye, syndrome.[6] This is believed to occur when a person admires an infant without touching it. It can be cured and prevented by having the person touch the infant.

For example, a young Mexican-American couple recently delivered a set of twins. During the immediate neonatal period, both developed vomiting and diarrhea. The couple was becoming acculturated into the urban society and sought assistance from the pediatrician. Both infants were hospitalized. Shortly after the infants were admitted, one of the twins died. As soon as the one infant died, the other was removed from the hospital against medical advice. The infant was taken to a healer (curandera) who placed herbs over the infant and his abdomen was massaged. Within hours the vomiting and diarrhea had stopped. The infant was rehydrated with herbal teas. The couple believes the first twin would be alive if it had been taken to the healer initially. The doctor and hospital are blamed for the infant's death.

Illness may be seen as punishment by God for previous sins. Treatment may be sought by going to a shrine or church and praying for forgiveness. If a baby is born with an anomaly this may be seen as the parent's punishment for an earlier wrongdoing. Because of this, the parent may refuse medical or surgical treatment for the child.

Many members of the American Indian culture do not believe in the germ theory. Elvira F, an Indian woman, developed a case of rubella during the first trimester of her pregnancy. The infant was born with a heart defect and with hearing loss. The family viewed this as being caused by God's will, not by the germ.

The Mexican-American family is quite frequently a believer in folk medicine. Rather than seeking care from a physician or nurse practitioner, the family will often try to treat the ill person with a variety of home remedies which are handed down from generation to generation. Two predominant types of healers exist in the Mexican-American culture. The first type of healer is an espiritista or spirtualist. This person is believed to be capable of putting a person in touch with the dead. The second type of healer is a curandero or curandera. This person is seen when it is necessary to be rid of fright or a frightening experience.[7]

Early ambulation is regarded as instrumental in preventing postpartum complications including phlebitis and urinary and bowel problems. Yet, in some Oriental cultures, a convalescence period of 30 days is deemed necessary to make the baby and mother ready for one another.[3]

Many black people are not likely to seek health care early or to engage in preventive programs.[7] This practice has implications for the importance in health teaching of prevention-intervention and screening programs. Since the client may not see the value in preventive care, she may neglect to obtain prenatal care, return for the six-weeks check up, or take the infant for well-baby examinations. Knowing this, health care professionals may alter their programs to meet the needs of this group. For example, nurses may provide classes which are valued by expectant mothers as a means of getting them in for prenatal visits.

A group of Mexican-Americans do not believe in bathing the infant until it is three days old. It is believed that if the child is bathed sooner than that, a spell will be cast on him. The nurse should include the family in the decision-making process and care-giving plans in order to learn customs such as this.

In some cultures childbearing is regarded as a very normal activity. The American culture may present it as an "illness" during which clients are placed in bed in hospitals away from the home and family. After assessing the client's cultural perspective, it may be possible to assist the client in creating a more comfortable environment within the hospital. Many clients have expressed displeasure in being dependent while in the hospital. Perhaps their independence could be encouraged by assisting them in partial self-care (such as fixing their own sitz baths if desired). Perhaps nurses could also encourage family members or friends to bring in native foods if the client desires. Recent advances in "birthing rooms" with a more informal versatile environment may help, although women with risk pregnancies may need additional medical equipment available.

A common request of the Puerto Rican mother in the early postpartum period is to have a large dosage of castor oil. This may seem like a bizarre request to the care giver; however, a large dosage of castor oil is believed necessary to rid the mother of impurities and to make her ready to accept the neonate. The castor oil is considered to clean the mother's system.

Primary Health Care Giver. It is a mistake to believe that all peoples seek health care through a physician or nurse practitioner. In many cultures the traditional health care services are sought only as a last result. Often families attempt a variety of home remedies and seek the services of a number of faith healers before consulting a physician, nurse, or hospital.

The United States government is realizing the importance of the medicine man in the American-Indian culture. Monies are available from the National Institute of Mental Health to teach present health practices to the medicine men.[7] Professionals should work with these local healers already recognized and trusted by their clients. Consultation between nurses and other healers can be achieved by personal visits and phone calls to discuss clients served by both groups of practitioners.

Some members of various cultures are distrusting and skeptical of physicians, nurses, medications, and hospitals. Before treatment measures can become effective, personnel will have to develop a trusting relationship with the client and family. Treatments can be shared by the nurse, physician, client, family, significant others, and healers that are prevalent within the culture.

Past experience dictates how care is perceived. If a family or friend is reported to have had a bad experience with a hospital or physician or nurse, the current experience will be influenced by that earlier one. This is especially true if a friend or family has had negative experiences from some type of treatment. The entire hospital may be seen in a negative way.

People from some cultures believe in treatments by faith healers. They may see a healer and ingest a concoction made by him. Some healer treatments are effective for some medical difficulties. Many medicines originated from tradition; however, some concoctions may confound the malady or delay the client's seeking medical assistance. This is especially detrimental for rapidly progressing diseases such as infections and cancer. The nurse is often very successful at encouraging cooperative care from both the desired healer and the medical doctor rather than having care only from the physician. Some healers support this concept as well. Nurses can become familiar with the healers and the concoctions they use. It is important to both nurse and client to develop rapport so that all people can work together for the health and well-being of the client.

The medicine man is an important source of support for many American-Indian clients. It is traditional to have a prayer session two months before the infant is due with a prayer and community sing the following night. These two events are thought to ease the delivery and ensure that the infant will be normal.[4] In the Indian culture, medicine and religion may be viewed as interchangeable.

Cultural Shock Related to High-Risk Situations. Brink and Saunders define culture shock as an abrupt change from a familiar to an unfamiliar environment.[2] Being hospitalized in a strange environment surely classifies as a culture shock. Being placed on bed rest, visiting a sick preterm infant in the intensive care unit, or being forced to quit work because of illness all may contribute to culture shock.

Modesty is a highly valued virtue in many cultures including the Mexican-American, Puerto Rican, and Oriental. Modesty may be violated by having a male physician examine a female client. It may be violated when a vaginal examination is performed, a shave is being performed, or the legs are placed in stirrups. Nurses should continue to be sensitive to the clients' need for modesty.

Health care professionals should honor a client's (or family's) need for privacy. It is important to provide space and time for the family to be together, especially in the time of crisis. This may be accomplished by pulling the curtain around the client after a crisis experience, leaving the client and family in the room with the door closed, or sending the family to the chapel. Health professionals should be available but should also provide some time for the client and family to be alone, as desired. The nurse may arrange this by telling the family she realizes that they might like some time alone together but

she is available if they should need her. After some time has been given to the family, the nurse may wish to check in to see how they are and if they need anything. She may also leave the call bell within easy reach of some family member.

Aside from losing their privacy, clients may feel that hospitalization violates their body. They may feel fetal monitoring violates the body of their infant. Certain cultures oppose autopsy because they feel a body which has been mutilated will not be accepted in the next world. If autopsy is acceptable, perhaps all body organs must be placed back into the body for burial. The nurse must assess the individual and cultural practices to determine how hospitalization will affect the family.

Family Role Changes. When a family is involved in a risk situation, generally some role alterations take place. The nurse should assess the type and degree of changes to the family. These changes may be relatively small changes, such as the elderly primigravida who fractured her coccyx during delivery and had to sit on a pillow and change her infant's diapers at a waist level position. On the other hand, they may be drastic adjustments such as finding a babysitter for the older children and both parents spending all free time at the hospital visiting an infant.

One young woman's first pregnancy had terminated in the delivery of an infant at 24 weeks of gestation. The infant expired very soon following delivery. In her second pregnancy, she began to experience contractions at 24 weeks. She was found to have an incompetent cervix, so she spent the next 12 weeks in bed in order to delay labor. A pursestring suture was also placed around the cervix at 24 weeks gestation. Bed rest was difficult for the woman as she was used to a very active life. Because she had so much free time, her mind wandered and she became increasingly concerned about the child.

Martha W delivered an infant with erythroblastosis fetalis. She had two young children at home who had to be cared for. Martha spent a good deal of time at the hospital with the neonate while her mother cared for the children at home. Martha's husband, Charles, was forced to take a second job in order to meet the family's expenses. In addition, he assumed increased responsibilities in the home.

Involving All Family Members

The family is an all too often forgotten source of information to be used in planning care. In many cultures the extended family plays a significant role in one's life. Not consulting this group may mean the difference between a client's adaptation to his condition and a maladaptation.

In addition, the family may be utilized as an interpreter if the client speaks little or no English. The family may translate cultural beliefs and practices which are important in planning for the care of the client. If the family does not readily volunteer this information, the nurse should be assertive enough to ask family members about their cultural preferences.

The family may be involved, with the nurse, in the direct care which is being received by the client. Often parents, spouses, and even siblings feel helpless when the loved one is ill. One way to make the family feel they are being instrumental in assisting the family member to a well state is to involve members of the family in ambulating, bathing, and feeding the client. This does not, however, relieve the nurse from assuming responsibility for the care of the client.

Quite often when a person is admitted to an institution, he feels helpless. The person is stripped of clothes, identity, and familiar surroundings. The food is different, the environment has a sterile appearance, and the bed is high and has a sweaty plastic mattress and strange mechanical features. Visitation by family and friends is restricted. The person is likely to lose his identity and become a mere patient in a bed with a certain disease. It is easy to imagine the fear a client feels under these circumstances.

One way to avoid such feelings of powerlessness is to allow the client to participate in his own care. Hospital routines often seem to be established for the convenience of hospital personnel rather than the client. If a client is used to bathing at night, before retiring, what prevents him from doing so while in the hospital?

On a postpartum unit the staff complained about a new postsection mother who happened to be first-generation Italian. The woman continually pressed her call bell. She requested water, fluffing of her pillows, and rearranging the covers. The client was such a "nuisance" to the staff that they began talking about how to approach the client. Staff members realized they had continually gone into her room saying, for example, "It's time for your bed to be made now" or "It's time for your bath." The medication schedule was somewhat rigid, as well. The next time a nurse entered the client's room, the nurse asked the client, "Would you like to take your pain medication before or after you have the baby in to feed?" The client had a perplexed look on her face and replied, "You mean I have a choice?" When the staff began asking the client how and when she would like things, the client's spirits became elevated and she did not use her call bell as a means of controlling her environment.

Identifying Significant Others

An important factor to keep in mind while working with clients from diverse cultural backgrounds is who makes family decisions in the culture. In the Mexican-American and Oriental culture, the man generally makes the decisions, while in the black culture the woman makes many decisions. In other cultures decision-making may be a joint process between man and woman. From the inception, the nurse should plan to interact with the man (husband, father) as well as the woman in planning or providing care. Certainly the main decision makers should be included when any decisions are being made.

For example, in numerous cultures an unmarried woman's mother is very influential. The relationship between client and care giver will be enhanced if the mother is included in plans from the beginning. Candice L had two children under the age of three years. Candice worked outside of the home and the children were left with the grandmother while Candice worked. One day, Ricky, the youngest of the two, refused to eat his lunch. As punishment for this, the grandmother put the child's hands in boiling water. Family intervention was instituted with a concentration on the maternal grandmother because she was the abuser as well as the primary care giver. Following several intervention sessions, the grandmother was able to alter both her behavior and that of her grandson to the satisfaction of all participants.

Vivian J was born with a myelomeningocele. Her mother was young, 16 years of age. Whenever plans were made for care, surgery, clinic visits, discharge planning, or treatments, the grandmother was included. This was done because Vivian's mother had expressed to the nurse that her own mother would take care of the baby, and including her was much more effective than having Vivian's mother relay messages to her mother.

Over the last few years, visiting privileges during labor have been extended to fathers. In some cultures, such as the Oriental, fathers do not participate in the childbearing process. It is the woman's mother and grandmother who are the support systems. It seems efficacious to allow the grandmother of the infant to be with the mother during labor if this is agreed upon by all participants.

When working with clients whose backgrounds are different from hers, the nurse should use teaching methodology that will fit the lifestyle of the client. One nurse practitioner was concerned with the number of children women in a particular culture had. She held a class on family planning and provided the women with oral contraceptives. Later several of the women were beaten by their husbands. It was learned that the husbands were the family decision makers and they opposed use of contraceptives. The nurse had failed to include the husband as decision maker in her plan.

A common phenomenon among unmarried black women (especially those in their teens) is dependence on their mothers. This includes areas

such as management of the pregnancy and the philosophy of child-rearing. The young woman has probably obtained a good deal of information from her mother and is likely to follow advice given by her mother.

Perhaps an example will illustrate the point. While working as a clinical nurse specialist in a prenatal clinic, the author had the opportunity to work with Elaine T. Elaine was 15 years old and entered the pregnancy somewhat underweight and with a hemoglobin slightly below normal. She failed to gain weight during the first two trimesters and her hemoglobin dropped to a level significantly below normal. After trying a variety of strategies without success, the author asked Elaine to bring her mother in to the next clinic visit. The mother, adolescent, and nurse were able to work together to find a satisfactory approach to Elaine's dietary intake. Elaine's mother had been unaware of the frequency with which Elaine skipped meals. Elaine had fear of gaining too much weight as she believed this would necessitate a cesarean. Decreasing Elaine's fear of eating too much and including the mother in meal planning increased Elaine's consumption of necessary nutrients.

Going along with the idea of including all members in planning care, it is important to identify who the support systems are for the client and family. Different supportive people may be a sister, a faith healer, a distant relative, or a friend. Once this has been identified, plans on how to include these in the risk client or family will be initiated. The nurse must include in this planning any significant others identified by the client.

For example, Virginia W and her sister were very close to one another and Virginia's sister was very supportive to her. Virginia was a single woman having a baby. Hospital policy would only allow either a husband or mother to be with her during labor and delivery. Her sister was prevented from even visiting in the labor room. Since Virginia's mother lived 300 miles away, she was not able to be present with her daughter. Thus, because of inflexible hospital policy, this young woman was faced with laboring and delivering without her major supporter. When Virginia delivered, her infant had a cleft lip and cleft palate. Unfortunately, due to restrictions in hospital policies, this woman had to cope alone with the impact of delivering a defective infant.

In assessing the support systems, it is important to ascertain the family system from which the client comes. In some cultures the nuclear family is of utmost importance. In others, such as the black, the Mexican-American, and the American Indian, the extended family is important. It is necessary to identify the important family members and plan care accordingly. It is necessary to consider the family structure and what it means to the client in our mobile, urban culture. Some couples may rely heavily on their extended families but be separated physically from them. They may feel isolated in times of crisis.

On occasion no one will be present to support the client or family. In this case it is the responsibility of the nurse to develop a trusting relationship. It is also important to provide continuity of care. Nurses giving care to the client who is alone will wish to investigate follow-up by a community health nurse or social service. Perhaps some community based resource will be found for the client as well. This may be through a cultural group to which the client has allegiance. Other counseling and teaching strategies are described in other chapters.

Often prayer rituals are important among the family constellations. Cassandra J became ill with meningitis when she was three months old. Her family was a very religious extended family. This family requested, and was granted, permission to pray for Cassandra at her bedside. The prayer ritual lasted for approximately 30 minutes. By the end of the session, Cassandra's temperature was down to 101°F from 104°. The family attributed her recovery to their prayers.

Avoiding Language Barriers

Communication with members of different cultures is often a problem. The nurse may feel helpless because of the communication barrier. The client may be afraid because he does not understand what is wrong with him or what is happening to him. The failure to communicate may alienate the client and make him seem apathetic or noncompliant to the staff.

Generally there are resources available to the client and the nurse to break this communication barrier. Perhaps the client does not speak any English but the spouse is proficient. The husband is an excellent resource to be utilized as an interpreter. This will also increase the husband's self-esteem (particularly in an obstetrical situation) as he will see himself as directly participating in care given to his wife.

In larger institutions, it is not uncommon to have a variety of bilingual employees. At one university medical center with which the author was associated, many employees served as interpreters to clients. These employees were fluent in languages such as French, Spanish, Portuguese, Persian, and Russian, to name but a few. There were also employees who knew braille and sign language. Personnel kept a list of employees with such talents, and these individuals were frequently called upon.

At times, other clients within the agency will speak the language of the client who does not speak English. Not only can this individual translate the language, he can also assist in translating the cultural beliefs of the individual. The client who acts as an interpreter will have his self-esteem raised by being able to assist the former client as well as the nursing or medical staff.

A fourth alternative is that agencies such as the health department or the welfare department may be of assistance in this matter. These groups may know of individuals or groups who speak the same language as the client who may serve as resource persons. Most likely these individuals would be glad to cooperate with the staff in interpreting needs and desires of the client who is unable to communicate for himself.

If all efforts fail and no interpreter can be found, the nurse will be required to be creative in approaching the client. Perhaps the nurse will point in an attempt to ascertain the needs of the client. Perhaps drawings and diagrams can be made to indicate the nature of the disease process to the client and to explain the planned intervention. However, every attempt should be made to find an interpreter to give the client an explanation of what is happening to him and what is planned for him.

Even if both client and nurse speak English, language may still be a problem because of the colloquialisms used in the hospital setting. Think of the number of IV's we hang, strips we read, preps we do, tubes we use. The language is confusing at times for health care workers. Think about the client who has never heard the terminology before and is acutely ill as well.

A couple from Saudi Arabia were attending a three-month institute relating to the man's job. The woman was pregnant but was to return to her home country ten days before the expected due date. At 38 weeks, however, the woman went into labor. Neither the woman nor her husband spoke a word of English. An individual from the institute attended the delivery with the couple and served as an interpreter.

Using Nutritional Preferences

Culture influences the foods people eat and how they eat them. A good number of cultural groups are vegetarians, including the Seventh Day Adventists, some people from India, and members of subcultures who do not eat meat on moral premises. It is important to learn what vegetarianism means to the client. Some of these individuals will eat milk, eggs, and cheese for their protein while others will eat nothing that comes from an animal. Individuals who do not eat animal products generally eat such things as nuts and soy beans for protein.

Soul food and highly spiced foods generally play an important part in the black culture. When institutionalized, a person who is used to the more spicy foods often finds the food bland. It is hardly fair to expect the client to eat and be satisfied with the typical food served in hospitals. Unless contraindicated medically, it is feasible to include the client in meal planning. Perhaps merely adding tobasco sauce to the food will add enough flavor to satisfy the individual.

One mother recently delivered and was found to be quite anemic during her pregnancy and postpartum period. She was, incidently, a self-prescribed vegetarian who meticulously planned her menu during pregnancy to ensure an adequate, well balanced, diet. She would eat eggs, cheese, and milk. Following her delivery, she ordered a vegetarian diet. Her first tray was delivered on Saturday evening and contained meat. She ate what she could from the tray, but did not send it back. The next morning her tray contained bacon. Again, she ate what she could from the tray. The third tray was delivered and again contained meat. This time she refused the tray and said she would not eat until she received the proper tray. Eventually the dietician came to talk with her and learned that the woman's prehospitalization diet was very adequate. From that point, the dietician worked with the woman to assist her with her dietary preferences. Prior to the nutrition history, the health professionals blamed her diet for her anemia.

It is not always desirable to meet the client's food preferences in meal planning. It may be necessary to provide information to the client. Recently a three-week-old was hospitalized for abdominal distension and irritability. Upon admission, it was learned that the infant's grandfather was feeding the child chocolate doughnuts and barbeque sauce. This practice was stopped when digestion in the infant was explained to the family.

Obesity and malnutrition are common among American Indian women. Starchy foods are a large portion of the diet, due in part to the poverty of many Indians. Another influencing factor is that it is believed that a person will live longer if she is somewhat obese. Diet teaching may be ineffective if the common cultural foods are not included in the diet plan.[4]

Food changes may contribute to culture shock. Consider the individual who did not eat much cheese, eggs, or milk (primarily due to lack of availability of these products). Following delivery she complained of horrible gas and intestinal cramps. It was discovered that these conditions were caused by her dietary changes. These symptoms subsided as her intake of milk, eggs, and cheese was reduced.

Another client was a Korean who had married an American serviceman. She had her first child by cesarean shortly after they came to the United States. She was in a new country, was uncomfortable following her surgery, and had a new diet. Luckily one of the nurses in the institution was also from Korea. When the woman was able to eat, the nurse brought Korean food to the client. This act was warmly received by the client.

Changes in water can also be problematic for clients. It is not uncommon for clients to develop diarrhea from a difference between the water they had in their home and the water they are drinking in the hospital.

In meeting the needs of clients from various cultures, flexibility in the agency is crucial. It may be difficult for dietary departments to accommodate the wishes of all clients but, when consulted as an equal in the health care team, this department probably will see its role in the restorative process and will attempt to accommodate whenever possible. It may not be practical to be served native foods, but the dietary departments generally attempt to individualize their service as much as possible.

Evaluating Nursing Actions

A most important component of the nursing process is that of evaluation. As with other phases, it is important to include the client and family in the evaluative process. Evaluation should include effectiveness of the procedures as well as satisfaction to the client. Evaluations can be assessed in terms of such things as frequency with which clinic visits are kept, subsiding of the symptoms of illness, incorporation of the strategy in the client's lifestyle, and acceptance of the strategy by the client.

It should be remembered that evaluation is an ongoing process and begins with the planning process. Nurses continually evaluate themselves and their strategy to ascertain the degree of their success and acceptance by the client. Strategies and techniques should be evaluated throughout the course of the interaction.

It should be remembered that just because the health team prescribes something for a client or family does not necessarily mean that the idea will be followed by the client. By involving the client and the family in care from the beginning, plans which are in line with the beliefs of the individual and family can be developed. In this way, the health team members can work together with the client for what is seen as a mutual goal.

Renee B's mother had used diethyl stilbesterol during her pregnancy, 26 years previous, to prevent a threatened abortion. As Renee delivered her second child six months prior to her hospitalization, a piece of tissue came out with the infant. This tissue was sent to pathology and was found to be a portion of cervix which was malignant. Following delivery, chemotherapy was instituted.

During this hospitalization it appeared that death was imminent for the young woman. Although she had episodes of depression, her spirits remained high. Staff felt it important to keep Renee sedated. It was noticed that Renee frequently asked that sedation be withheld. When she was sedated, depression followed. In talking with Renee, her husband, and mother, it was learned that she wanted to participate in planning for her children when she died. After this discussion, Renee decided when she would have sedation. She was much more relaxed following this action and her family felt relieved that she was able to participate in the decisions which were being made.

Follow-up. When planning care, provisions should be made for long-term follow-up, since the trust relationship and health behavior changes take time to develop. This should be done by team members who are sensitive to cultural diversity. Strategies used for follow-up include making an appointment ahead because some clients do not have telephones, providing for transportation to clinic visits, if needed, describing the purposes related to helping clients with their identified concerns, maintaining a continued attitude of sensitivity to the client, and allowing the client and family to have a continued say in care.

SUMMARY

In fulfilling professional obligations to clients, nurses must address the cultural backgrounds of clients. This may be accomplished by avoiding transferring their own cultural patterns to others, assessing the client's cultural heritage as it relates to health and health care, refining interventions to adapt to cultural patterns, and evaluating the effectiveness of their actions. In doing this nurses will include the client, the family or significant others, as well as the members of the health team in working toward the goal of optimal health care to all.

REFERENCES

1. Anderson, G. and B. Tighe. "Gypsy Culture and Health Care." In P. Brink (ed.). *Transcultural Nursing: A Book of Readings*. Englewood Cliffs, N.J.: Prentice-Hall, 1976, 256–262.
2. Brink, P. and J. Saunders. "Cultural Shock: Theoretical and Applied." In Brink, P. (ed.). *Transcultural Nursing: A Book of Readings*. Englewood Cliffs, N.J.: Prentice-Hall, 1976, 126–138.
3. Chung, H. J. "Understanding the Oriental Maternity Patient." *Nursing Clinics of North America*, March 1977, 67–75.
4. Farris, L. S. "Approaches to Caring for the American Indian Maternity Patient." *American Journal of Maternal Child Nursing*, March/April 1976, 80–87.
5. Macgregor, F. "Uncooperative Patients: Some Cultural Interpretations." In P. Brink (ed.). *Transcultural Nursing: A Book of Readings*. Englewood Cliffs, N.J.: Prentice-Hall, 1976, 36–43.
6. Prattes, O. "Beliefs of the Mexican-American Family." In D. Hymovich and M. Barnard (ed.). *Family Health Care*. New York: McGraw-Hill, 1973, 128–137.
7. White, E. H. "Giving Health Care to Minority Patients." *Nursing Clinics of North America*, March 1977, 27–40.

ADDITIONAL READINGS

1. Abril, I. F. "Mexican-American Folk Beliefs: How They Affect Health Care." *The American Journal of Maternal-Child Nursing*, May/June 1977, 169–173.
2. ———. "Toward Quality Nursing Care for a Multiracial Society." *Affirmative Action: Toward Quality Nursing Care for a Multiracial Society*. American Nurses Association, 1976.
3. Cadera, M. "The Mexican-American Family and the Mexican-American Nurse." In D. Hymovich and M. Barnard (eds.). *Family Health Care*. New York: McGraw-Hill, 1973, 138–148.
4. Davitz, L., Y. Sameshima, and J. Davitz. "Suffering as Viewed in Six Different Cultures." *American Journal of Nursing*, August 1976, 1296–1297.
5. Hall, E. and W. F. White. "Intercultural Communication: A Guide to Men of Action." In P. Brink (ed.). *Transcultural Nursing: A Book of Readings*. Englewood Cliffs, N.J.: Prentice-Hall, 1976, 44–62.
6. Jackson, R. "Removing Barriers to Quality Care in a Multiracial Society: A Health Care Delivery Organization Perspective." *Affirmative Action Toward Quality Nursing Care for a Multiracial Society*, American Nurses Association, 1976.
7. Johnston, M. "Folk Beliefs and Ethnocultural Behavior in Pediatrics, Medicine or Magic?" *Nursing Clinics of North America*, March 1977, 77–84.
8. Kniep-Hardy, M. and M. Burkhardt. "Nursing the Navajo." *American Journal of Nursing*, January 1977, 95–96.
9. Leininger, M. "Towards Conceptualization of Transcultural Health Care Systems: Concepts and a Model." In M. Leininger (ed.). *Transcultural Issues and Conditions*. Philadelphia: F. A. Davis, 1976, 3–22.
10. ———. "Cultural Diversities of Health and Nursing Care." *Nursing Clinics of North America*, March 1977, 5–18.
11. Parreño, Sr. H. "Unique Needs of Ethnic Minority Clients in a Multiracial Society." *Affirmative Action: Toward Quality Nursing Care for a Multiracial Society*. American Nurses Association, 1976.
12. Primeaux, M. "American Indian Health Care Practices, a Cross-Cultural Perspective." *Nursing Clinics of North America*, March 1977, 55–65.

13. ———. "Caring for the American Indian Patient." *American Journal of Nursing*, January 1977, 91–94.

14. Sparber, J. "Working with Low-Income Families." In D. Hymovich and M. Barnard (ed.). *Family Health Care*. New York: McGraw-Hill, 1973, 149–166.

15. Taylor, C. "The Nurse and Cultural Barriers." In D. Hymovich and M. Barnard (ed.). *Family Health Care*. New York: McGraw-Hill, 1973, 119–127.

16. Tripp-Reimer, T. and Friedl, M. "Appalachians: A Neglected Minority." *Nursing Clinics of North America*, March 1977, 41–54.

17. Willis, W. "Perinatal Loss: Socioeconomic Factors." *Journal of Obstetrical, Gynecological, and Neonatal Nursing*, March/April 1977, 44–47.

PERTINENT ORGANIZATIONS

NATIONAL
- *American Nurses Association*
  24th and Grand
  Kansas City, Missouri 64106
  Has groups of nurses concerned with health care for cultural minorities.

- *National League for Nursing*
  10 Columbus Circle
  New York, New York 10019
  Maintains information regarding health care practices of cultural minorities.

- *Western Interstate Commission in Higher Education (WICHE)*
  P.O. Drawer P
  Boulder, Colorado 80302
  This group has studied cultural diversity in nursing curricula.

LOCAL
On the local level, the nurse is urged to utilize community resources such as clergy, leaders of different ethnic groups, city health departments, county social welfare agencies, and proprietors of ethnic businesses.

Financial Strategies

Marie J. Millington, R.N., M.P.H. and
Leni Wright Ziebell, B.A., B.S.W.

CHAPTER TWENTY-FIVE

Any high-risk situation results in additional expense for families—often great expense. The increased cost intensifies the crisis situation for the high-risk family, which can lead to family disorganization and disruption. At a time when the family's attention is focused on the health situation and they are concerned about what is happening to other members of their family, it may be difficult for them to give sufficient consideration to the financial demands that are developing. Yet the need to deal with them may be quite immediate. It is very important that the effect of this added stress on the family be recognized, so that the nurse can be instrumental in either preventing or assisting the family to deal with it. Nurses are not financial counselors, but there is much that they can do to help the family if they are aware of the financial impact being made. There are many financial strategies that the nurse can employ, which include both prevention and intervention. They will be discussed in this chapter.

National Health Care Costs

There has been a marked increase in the average cost per person for health care in our nation. The $139.3 billion, or $638 per capita, spent on health care in 1976 is a 14 percent increase over that spent the previous year. This includes both physicians' fees and hospital service charges. Hospital care expenditures are the largest item in health care spending. In 1976, $55.4 billion was spent in this category, which was 40 percent of the total.[6] Hospital expenses per patient day have increased 1264 percent since 1946.[5] According to the President's Council on Wage and Price Stability, health care costs are expected to continue to rise sharply in the foreseeable future.[3] Federal expenditures for health are also increasing rapidly and account for a significant part of the federal budget. Last year health expenditures consisted of 11.3 percent of total federal expenditures.[5] It has been determined that causes of increased health care costs are apportioned as follows:

53 percent due to price increases

9 percent as a result of population growth

38 percent from increased use of services and introduction of new medical techniques.[5]

Medical costs have been markedly affected by the exorbitant increase in physicians' malpractice insurance. It is the patient who provides the financial protection for the physician against any legal action against him by paying increased fees for medical care.

The cost of living has increased as well as the cost of medical care, which results in an additional decrease of resources available for a time of crisis. Each family dollar also purchases fewer health support items such as vitamins, bandages, food required for special diets, equipment for rehabilitation, or services such as babysitters for disabled children.

High-Risk Family Costs

A family that is at high risk medically is also at high risk financially because of the need for specialized personnel, complex procedures, and long-term care.

More expensive specialized care is usually required. The care of a mother who has developed a cardiac condition as well as her child who is born with a congenital heart problem is likely to require specialists in a health care center, which is usually some distance from the family's home. Hospital care is given by personnel from a variety of backgrounds—some of whom have received specialized education. This also occurs in the care of a very small premature infant. For example, the cost of room and nursing care for one day for an infant in the intensive care nursery often varies between $49 for observational care to as much as $600 for very intensive care, as compared with $38 for the daily care of an infant in the normal newborn nursery.

Health services are usually required for longer periods of time. Some disabling conditions require continuing care, specialized training or education, or perhaps institutionalization. One premature infant required 42 days of intensive care at $500 per day, 14 days of moderate care at $250 per day, and 21 days of routine baby care at $49, or a total of 77 days costing $25,529. In addition, the disabled child has continued medical, school, and home care costs.

Many risk situations such as congenital anomalies and prematurity are more frequent in low socioeconomic groups. Poverty characteristics such as poor nutrition and housing may precipitate high-risk situations and they in turn precipitate financial difficulties and poverty. For example, a very young couple without income experienced the pregnancy and premature birth of a son two years ago. The child has cerebral palsy and requires special schooling, medical, and social services. Shortly after the child's birth, the father was involved in an armed robbery and imprisoned for one year. Now, on probation, he has found employment which provides a low but steady income with no health insurance benefits. Recently, the mother was referred to a high-risk obstetrical clinic with a complicated pregnancy and many medical, social, and nutritional concerns. The family is once again in financial difficulty with no health insurance and high medical costs.

Financial Difficulties of the Family

The impact of financial stress on the family increases the crisis and possibility of family disruption. The need for the father to take a second job or the mother to work outside the home can put an extra strain on the marital relationship as the couple adjusts to these changes. This increases anxiety and calls for a redefinition of family relationships and can profoundly affect family balance. Possible long-term effects of family imbalance are separation or divorce, "acting-out" of children, or child neglect and abuse. Very often the worries or anxieties of either parent are felt by one or more of the children. Unable to understand the cause of this stress, the child may release his feelings in an unacceptable behavior such as encopresis or abusiveness to siblings. He may also suffer psychosomatic symptoms such as severe headaches, stomach aches, and vomiting. Frequently, the child is hospitalized and undergoes a series of tests only to find that there is no physical basis.

The symptoms of the identified patient in the family may also be symptoms of the entire family's hurt or dysfunction. The nurse's awareness of this possibility can allow early intervention for the family by referral to appropriate resources.

The impact of financial stress also affects the individual parent and his lifestyle. It may necessitate finding a job or an additional job for which he is not specifically qualified or trained. His level of anxiety may be increased by worry over bills, debts, and so on. This may eventually lead to depression or some form of self-destruction such as alcoholism, drug abuse, or mental illness. For example, a couple with a child age one and a half recently found they were expecting twins. Not only was this an unplanned pregnancy, but it is high risk; the previous delivery was premature. The family was in the process of moving and the father was jobless, although highly skilled. The mother, a registered nurse, had to terminate her job because of the pregnancy and need for complete bedrest. The result of these stresses and changes was increased anxiety for each of these parents. The mother was willing to ask for and receive emotional and financial support. But the father became very depressed and temporarily immobilized. His lack of self-confidence increased and he was unable to make decisions, be interviewed for employment, or ask for help. His way of dealing with it initially was increased consumption of alcohol.

FINANCIAL STRATEGIES FOR THE HIGH-RISK FAMILY

The nurse's role in assisting families in which health problems have caused financial problems is outlined in Figure 25-1. Assessment, prevention, intervention, and referral are strategies employed by the nurse. Attention must be given to available resources and services and efforts should be coordinated.

Assessment Strategies

It is important to assess the family's financial situation early to reduce costs when possible. An assessment guide is shown in Figure 25-2.

Establishment of a Trusting Relationship. A

Figure 25-1. Financial Strategies for the High-Risk Family

Assessment Strategies
1. Establishment of a trusting relationship
2. Assessment of family's financial costs
3. Assessment of family's financial resources
4. Estimate of family's ability to cope
5. Evaluation of family's financial status
6. Nursing plan to assist family to find alternative approaches

Prevention Approaches
1. Teaching ways the family can
   a. Reduce health care costs
   b. Decrease insurance costs and evaluate coverage

Referral Approaches
1. Determine when assistance is needed
2. Become knowledgeable about available services
3. Learn each agency's referral procedure
4. Refer families to appropriate sources of care early

Intervention Strategies
1. Reducing health care costs
2. Helping families to cope

Legislative Strategies
1. Plan for comprehensive services with adequate funding for them
2. Actively promote desirable and oppose undesirable health legislation

trusting relationship needs to be developed with the family so that they feel free to discuss the financial impact of the health situation. The nurse works with them by listening, providing information and referral, giving care as needed, and being available to the family. As the relationship becomes more meaningful, a confidence develops in the nurse and in what she has to offer. The family begins to see the nurse as a helping person and they are then likely to bring out other concerns, such as financial matters, which can be explored with them.

When discussing financial problems the family members should be encouraged to verbalize their understanding of what the costs will be. Family members are usually not hesitant to reveal financial information to the nurse if they understand that the information will be used to help them and if they understand how it will be used. The family should be assisted in obtaining more complete information as it is needed, such as length of hospitalization and treatment anticipated, an exploration of what their insurance will cover, and an estimate

Figure 25-2. FINANCIAL ASSESSMENT GUIDE Used in a Clinical Example

Diagnosis of Family Member: Diabetic, pregnant woman, age 28 years, Gravida III, Para I. Severity: Class C Diabetic

I. Estimate of Potential Financial Costs

A. Present Costs

1. Types of medical services needed

a. High risk management of patient during pregnancy (approximately 34 weeks) delivery, and 6 weeks postpartally by obstetrician and internist @

b. Close monitoring of fetal well being during pregnancy and delivery by pediatrician @

c. Initial management of newborn by pediatrician @

2. Types of hospital services needed:

a. **Hospitalization:** of mother and infant for 8 days at time of delivery @

b. **Types of procedures needed:**

1) 5–6 blood sugar tests per month @

2) 1 serum estriol per week for 8 weeks @

3) 6 ultra sound diagnostic procedures @

4) 2 amniocentesis, including procedure and maturity study @

5) 5 oxytocin challenge tests @

6) Cesarean section at 38 weeks gestation @

> **Potential present health care costs—$5,485.**

(Includes prenatal care for 34 weeks, delivery, postpartum care, and infant care in normal newborn nursery)

B. Anticipated Future Costs

1. Types of medical services needed:

a. Management of diabetes by internist at monthly intervals @

b. Continued management of newborn by pediatrician at designated intervals @

c. Possible ophthalmology consultation @

2. Types of procedures needed:

a. Blood sugar tests at monthly intervals @

3. Medication and equipment needed:

a. 100 u. Lente Insulin @

b. Materials for daily urine test @

> **Future potential health care costs for one year—$350**
> **Total potential health care costs—$5,835**

II. Estimate of Family's Financial Resources

A. Insurance: Independent group insurance plan includes hospital/surgical coverage

B. Insurance coverage: $25 deductible for each hospitalization

   1. % of present expenses covered: 80% hospital
                                          100% surgical

   2. % of future expenses covered: no outpatient
                                          80% hospital

C. Community resources: not eligible for financial assistance

D. Approximate costs above—public and private resources: $2,057

E. Savings: $4,000

F. Approximate salary per month after living expenses: $230

G. Large outstanding bills (i.e., previous medical care or other): None

III. Estimate of Family's Ability to Cope

A. Means of coping with previous financial difficulties: paid bills in installments

B. Additional family members employable: none

C. Family's ability to look at alternate financial resources: good

D. Willingness of all family members to help meet financial needs: good

E. Present crisis state: family not in crisis

IV. Approximate costs above salary and savings: NONE

V. Plans

A. Family's plan
1. Family will carefully follow physician's medical diabetic regimen for patient after hospital discharge
2. Patient will keep outpatient appointments regularly, as scheduled

B. Nurse's plan to assist family with alternatives
1. Encourage family to explore the possibility of obtaining additional insurance coverage to meet future needs
2. Refer family to:
   a. State Diabetic Association for literature
   b. Local diabetic group
   c. Community Health Nursing Service following hospital discharge

of what the physicians' and hospitals' charges are expected to be.

Assessment of Family's Financial Costs. The total expected cost of the health care needs to be estimated. What type of medical services are needed at present? Is it general or specialized care? How long will this kind of care be needed? What procedures need to be done? What is anticipated for the future? What will the combined cost of both present and future be?

Assessment of Family's Financial Resources. The family's financial resources also need to be reviewed. What is the total monthly income of all family members? How much has the family been able to place in savings accounts? What types of accounts are these and how available is the money? The insurance coverage should be reviewed by looking carefully at all policies and speaking to the representative of the insurance company, if necessary. What specific hospital and medical expenses are covered? What is the coverage inpatient and outpatient? How long will the insurance provide coverage? Does the family member have Medicare coverage if there is a kidney condition or if the member has been declared disabled? If so, when does the Medicare become effective? Does the family member have coverage by Medical Assistance? Consideration should also be given to public and private community resources that are available to this family. Are the services free of charge or can the rates be adjusted? A multidisciplinary evaluation of a child that is arranged by a local Cerebral Palsy Association is an example.

Estimate of Family's Ability to Cope. The nurse needs to estimate the ability of the family to cope with stressful situations. How have they dealt with financial problems in the past? To what extent have they paid their bills and met their financial obligations regularly? Perhaps they were able to budget and gradually pay the medical bills, or some family members were able to seek additional employment for a period of time without placing undue stress on the family unit. What is the level of education or training of all family members? Are they specifically prepared for certain kinds of employment?

Are they a cohesive, strong family unit in which all members are interdependent and cooperative? If so, one family member may be able to take over responsibilities carried by another member while that member seeks temporary employment, such as babysitting with children so that the mother is able to return to work. How able are they to make other kinds of decisions that do not relate to finances? Are they realistic? Has their judgment been sound? To what extent has their ability to function been impaired by this crisis situation?

Although it is important to assess the family's financial situation early, parents or family members may have difficulty or choose not to deal with financial problems during the initial phase or shock of the health crisis. At that time the total concern is usually a life versus death or normal versus abnormal issue. An example is a young couple who recently experienced the transfer of their three-day-old son from their own hospital to a hospital with an intensive care nursery. The child was acutely ill. The father accompanied the child in the transfer and visited frequently during the first week. He was self-employed as a carpenter and did not have health insurance. During that week he not only wanted to avoid discussion of their financial dilemma but also was unable emotionally to return to work at a time when they needed income the most.

This was not the time to discuss the specifics of finances with this family but to inform them the nurse is and would be available to provide help with assessing their financial problems and resources when they felt the need for assistance with it.

Evaluation of Family's Financial Status. When all of the resources are reviewed and are looked at in relation to anticipated needs, where will the family stand financially? Will the family's regular income make it possible for them to pay for the services not covered by their insurance? Are there public or private services that they qualify for, but have not applied for? What large outstanding bills does the family have?

Nursing Plan to Assist Family to Find Alternatives. After the assessment is complete and findings are evaluated, the nurse makes a plan for intervention (see Figure 25-2). Families whose incomes are just above those who qualify for public assistance will show the greatest deficit when their resources are evaluated in relation to possible costs. Usually they have difficulty paying for private insurance and do not have adequate income to meet the large expenses that they are suddenly faced with. Families in this kind of situation need particular consideration. All available community resources need to be tapped, and special attention needs to be given to the depletion of their resources in relation to their reaching the point where they would qualify for public assistance.

Prevention Approaches

The nurse has an opportunity to teach preventive financial measures to all families with whom she has contact. The best teaching environments for this are clinics, group educational sessions, or community nursing home visits. Teaching and guiding families, both in preventive financial considerations and in money-saving aspects of care is an important function of the nurse, regardless of the setting in which she is employed.

Teaching Ways the Family Can Reduce Health Care Costs. Some community services are available free or with reduced costs for all persons in the community, regardless of their ability to pay, if families are aware of them. Immunization and multiphasic screening clinics are usually offered free of charge by local community health agencies, dental care is available at dental schools at reduced rates, diabetic screening clinics are often offered by general hospitals free of charge, and psychiatric services are provided at local guidance clinics with rates adjusted according to the family's ability to pay. Early and periodic screening, diagnosis and treatment screening of the health status of children who are receiving Medical Assistance is provided throughout the nation by the Early and Periodic Screening, Diagnosis and Treatment Program. The screening is done by community health nurses, with a referral of all children who have questionable findings for diagnosis and treatment by physi-

cians, dentists, ophthalmologists, psychiatrists, and other professional services. One example might be the referral of a child for diagnosis who has been found to have a high level of lead in the blood screening test at the clinic. Both the screening and any resulting diagnosis and treatment are paid for by Medical Assistance. The purpose is to find abnormalities early and obtain their correction early to improve the health status of children in that particular segment of the population. Surveys of the findings in this program reveal that many children screened do have health conditions that need diagnosis and treatment. However, families who are receiving Medical Assistance have most kinds of health care paid for them and therefore usually do not feel the financial impact. It is the families that are just above the eligibility level for Medical Assistance that have the problems.

All of the services just described would aid in reducing overall costs for family health care, although in some instances conditions could be prevented or brought under treatment that would cause or intensify high-risk health situations in families if left untreated. An example of this might be the diabetic screening of children in families in which one or both parents are at risk because of diabetes with complications.

Genetic counseling can prevent certain high-risk conditions. Some of the families that could benefit from this are those in which there has been a previous birth defect which also has implications for future pregnancies. Families may need to consider the outcome of a present pregnancy during which the expectant mother has been exposed to chemicals, has taken medications such as fertility drugs that could affect the fetus, or when there has been a contact with a virus during a certain period of pregnancy, such as that which causes rubella. Some federal funds are available through local Developmental Disability Services. The funds are allocated for counseling at qualified medical centers when there has been an identified need for it. March of Dimes monies are also available for this purpose.

Overuse of medical care can be avoided by learning the normal changes in an infant's developmental behavior pattern, or what to expect from prescribed treatment in relation to health progress. This is particularly true of the mother of a first child. Some of the questions that mothers have can be anticipated by a community health nurse, and she can teach such things as how to follow the physician's recommendations regarding changes in formula or addition of solid foods, normal reactions to be expected from immunizations, and growth and development patterns of children. She can help the mother to determine when a contact with the physician is advisable. Talking with the physician on the telephone can help to determine if a visit to him is necessary, also.

Timely medical treatment will reduce the severity of most conditions such as treatment of the diabetic in order to prevent complications, or early diagnosis and when one of the seven danger signs of cancer occurs. Medical care that can prevent further disability will also prevent greater cost, by reducing the need for services later.

Families need to be taught the importance of certain preventive practices being carried out regularly, they need to learn the technique of those that they can do themselves, and they should be informed of what symptoms should be reported to the physician early. Diseases can be detected early when good preventive care is practiced. Physical examinations that include pap smears, breast examinations, laboratory studies, and other examinations as indicated should be done regularly. Membership in health maintenance organizations provides insurance coverage for preventive care, as well as sick care. It has been demonstrated that persons enrolled in prepaid plans use hospitals less.[5] This might be the person who has a history of gastric ulcers, ulcerative colitis, or hypertension.

Taking advantage of package plans in which a set price is established for a particular kind of care, such as for a pregnancy and delivery, regardless of the number of visits to the physician or the amount of care received, can result in a savings. The increased costs relating to the increased need for care in risk situations are absorbed by the plan and are dispersed among all of the clients of the service.

Presently a need exists for increased insurance coverage for the high-risk pregnant woman who does not have a related medical diagnosis. Some pediatricians offer a one-year service contract for newborn babies, which can be a saving if problems such as a congenitally dislocated hip or a foot deformity are detected within the year. The cost of casts and braces that might be required within the first year would be covered by the service contract for that year.

One of the goals today is to help families assume the responsibility for their own health care. It is important for the family to understand the care that is being provided and the reasons for it, and to retain a file of medical reports and records on all family members. These records can provide valuable information for new members of the health team so that they will be aware of procedures that have been performed and need not be repeated, even though progress reports may not be provided by the previous physician. An example is the child who has been under prolonged treatment for an orthopedic problem or undergone several stages of surgery and rehabilitation for cleft palate whose family moves to another state and has to obtain different specialized medical care and relate to a different state crippled children's service. When the family has a good understanding and record of past health care they can help physicians and nurses to assess their past care and may prevent repeated tests or unsuccessful treatments.

Medications obtained from pharmacies that sell drugs by their generic names and consistently have the lowest prices will provide a substantial savings. If medications are kept safe in the home, it is sometimes less costly to buy the amount of medication that will be needed for one or two months at one time.

Utilization of the kind of care that is appropriate to the need can result in a savings. The family in which the mother has her activity restricted because of a recent heart attack may at a certain time during her recovery be cared for adequately at home. Family members can be assisted with her care by a home health nurse and with grocery shopping, preparation of meals, and light household tasks by a home health aide. When this mother's need for care moves from intensive to regular care in the hospital, and then to home health care, with the amount of service diminishing as her condition improves, the cost will also diminish accordingly. It is necessary that the kind of care needed, in relation to cost, be continually evaluated. Can the health care needs be met adequately at home, is care in an extended care facility or halfway house required, or is hospitalization necessary? Does the condition require the services of a clinical nurse specialist, an outpatient clinic nurse, a community health nurse, or a home health aide?

The purchase of insurance with as comprehensive a coverage as possible will provide the maximum financial protection that the family can afford. The problem that occurs is that the family that can least afford it is the family that needs it most. The family that is just above the level to qualify for Medical Assistance finds private health insurance too costly to purchase. As a result they are not apt to obtain needed health care early and so are more likely to develop serious health problems. They make up the segment of our population that remains uncovered financially until an emergency occurs. There is then a "spend down" of their resources until they reach the level at which they would qualify for public assistance. As the family's level of income rises, they obtain limited hospital and surgical insurance coverage, and the coverage increases as the income rises or as the head of household takes employment where there is good group coverage. The post-World War II development of fringe benefits through collective bargaining and the growth of union-management health and welfare funds have been major forces in a tremendous growth of voluntary health insurance in our country. Almost four-fifths of our national population under 65 years of age has hospital and surgical insurance, but less than half of that same population has coverage for other health services. About 20 percent of the population under 65 years was without any insurance in 1974. It is recognized that a number of people in that category were chil-

dren and were poor, some of whom were covered by Medical Assistance.[5] In a study done in the South Central region of Wisconsin in which 43 parents who had infants in the intensive care unit (ICU) at Madison General Hospital were interviewed, it was learned that the cost of the ICU experience ranged from $1,500 to $13,000. Nineteen had total insurance coverage and five received public financial assistance. Parents paid from 0 to $2,000 for the care provided their infants.[7] By 1975 the government was paying for 40 percent of all health care services, private insurance was paying for 26 percent, and the individual was paying for 33 percent.[5] The cost of dental care has risen at about the same rate as medical care and can quickly deplete a family's budget for health care, particularly if there are a large number of children in the family.[5] Dental care is now being added to insurance coverage, but it is usually in comprehensive policies that have a sizeable deduction. Seventeen percent of the population under 65 years of age who had private health insurance in 1975 had coverage for dental care.[5] Orthodontia is not covered by Medical Assistance, but is sometimes paid for by the state crippled children's service, for example, when dental care is a part of the rehabilitation of children who have cleft lips and palates.

Families need assistance in understanding and following the process required to obtain the reimbursement for health care from their insurance and to declare deductions that are allowed on income taxes. Families need to know the coverage that is available from their insurance. They should review their contracts until they understand it. Classes are offered in some local areas to aid in this. The nurse can help the family to adequately record and report the cost of medicines, transportation to sources of care, telephone calls to physicians, and so on, which are tax deductible expenses for health care.

Teaching Ways to Decrease Insurance Costs and to Evaluate Coverage. Health insurance is a mechanism whereby members pool their periodic payments to meet hospital and medical costs which may be incurred. It is also known as accident health

Figure 25-3. Overview of Private Health Insurance

A. **Major Forms of Health Insurance.** The major forms of health insurance include single or combination coverage of these items:

Hospital—pays hospital bills

Surgical—pays for doctor's operating fees and related care

Regular medical—pays for nonsurgical doctor's fees and nonhospital physician care or care in the home, nursing home, and so on

Major medical—pays for all expenses with co-insurance and deductible designed to cover a major illness

Health maintenance—pays for prevention as well as illness care

Disability—loss of income insurance

B. **Providers of Private Insurance**

Blue Cross and Blue Shield—private nonprofit tax-exempt member corporations functioning under special enabling legislation in most states. Blue Cross is usually a hospitalization plan; Blue Shield usually covers professional services. However, in certain states the distinction does not always apply, since Blue Cross and Blue Shield write policies having both medical services and hospitalization. They furnish mainly service benefits, i.e., direct payment by the plan to the provider for services provided the subscriber, in whole or part. About 35 percent of the U.S. population participates in these plans.

Commercial or profit-oriented insurance companies—offer free choice of the provider with financial indemnification usually of the subscriber for all or part of the expense: for example, agreement to pay the subscriber a specific amount when a service is rendered, i.e., payment to the subscriber of $60 when the hospital charges you $90, leaving you $30 out-of-pocket expense. In 1972 insurance companies had about 60 percent of the gross enrollment.

Independent Companies—community-consumer prepaid group and individual practice plans, employer-employee-union self-insured plans and prepaid group clinic plans are considered independents in the sense that they are not affiliated with or underwritten by the Blue Cross-Blue Shield associations or the commercial insurance companies. They are characterized, usually, without fee for service charges expected by the subscriber of the plan.

HMOs (Health Maintenance Organizations)—first announced in February of 1970 are expected to provide . . . comprehensive quality-assured and economical health services (including preventive care) in return for a predetermined periodic payment.

insurance or disability insurance. Many policies provide little or no benefits in prevention, health education, general medical examinations, and so on. The term sickness insurance would be more appropriately used for most private insurance coverage. An exception is HMOs (Health Maintenance Organizations). See Figure 25-3 for an outline of the major forms and types of health insurance.

Health insurance coverage varies greatly not only in types of policies within a company or corporation but also from company to company. It would be an advantage for the family to compare costs and provisions of plans offered by several companies so that their individual needs can best be met. Rather than being concerned with the least expensive premiums, attention must be given to the provisions. Very often a family will purchase what they think is adequate coverage only to find in a crisis that what they considered to be adequate does

not meet their medical costs. It is extremely difficult at this point to get additional coverage or another health care plan and most families are left with very few options to help them financially.

If a family is purchasing individual family insurance, it is to their advantage to plan for as large a deductible as they can afford in order to get lower rates. A deductible is that portion of hospital or medical charges which an insured person must pay before his policy benefits begin. If possible, the monthly savings from lower rates are saved to cover the deductible if needed.

Premiums paid annually usually cost less to a family than premiums paid monthly. This is usually due to a service charge each month which the insurance company uses to offset the additional bookkeeping expenses on a monthly rate. Again, it is to the family's advantage to save and plan ahead.

Insurance can be purchased from companies

who will pay a fixed rate of insurance per number of days in the hospital rather than actual costs. Premium costs are lower although it does not meet the high cost coverage in a high-risk situation. It is most advantageous as a supplementary insurance. An example would be a plan that would supplement or meet the needs of an individual who has Medicare coverage. Blue Cross and other insurance companies offer this type of insurance.

Group insurance coverage is maximum at minimum cost to the family as high costs for a few members are absorbed by a large number of members. The definition of a "group" which would be eligible for insurance coverage at special rates varies from state to state. Basically, group coverage is provided by employers, schools, and Health Maintenance Organizations. The Kaiser plan in California is a popular HMO health plan. Employees can encourage administrators to arrange group insurance with the best coverage.

An example of an HMO is the Group Health Cooperative of South Central Wisconsin. It is a clinic with salaried physicians and health professionals. In addition to providing complete Hospital-Surgical and Medical coverage, it provides a full realm of benefits in prevention, health education, and well-patient examinations. Some of the services included are psychiatric and family counseling, infertility and family planning, outpatient care and immunizations, eye examinations under age 18, and related medical services such as home health services, services in skilled nursing facility, and health education. The approximate cost in 1978 is:

$28.89/month for an individual

$60.00/month for a family of two

$80.00/month for a family of three or more

Supplementary programs are optional and available in optical, dental, and outpatient drug coverage.

Referral Approaches

Determining When Assistance Is Needed. The nurse should consider the possibility of a need for a referral for financial assistance from the time the patient is admitted to the hospital or the family is admitted to the service of the community health agency.

Some examples of conditions that would warrant this type of a referral are as follows:

1. The family that has no health insurance, has limited savings, and has not applied for Medical Assistance.
2. The family with a member who has a long-term or permanent disability, lacks adequate insurance coverage, and has not applied for aid due to disability.
3. The family in which a member is to have an expensive procedure, such as open heart surgery, and savings plus insurance are not adequate.
4. The family that has used its savings, is continuing to have expenses for health care, and the insurance is limited.
5. The disrupted family in which there is a question of available finances.
6. The family that presents a health need and a related financial need and has not sought help for either.

Becoming Knowledgeable about Available Services. The nurse needs to know what resources are available. They are often compiled in a directory and made available in an agency.

Some of the services that may be beneficial to the high-risk family are described in the pertinent organizations section at the end of the chapter. Some of these services include private insurance companies, Social Security Administration, Visiting Nurse Association, State Crippled Children's Service, and national and state services. In addition there are frequently many local services helpful to the high-risk family with financial difficulties.

Learn Each Agency's Referral Procedure. The referral procedure for each agency is listed in the procedure manual of that agency. The hospital or agency may have a coordinator of patient care or a social worker or a nurse designated to make referrals and channel communications. If that is true, the responsibility of the nurse caring for the patient can vary from just identifying and reporting the need to actually completing the referral and channeling it to the designated person.

Refer Families to Appropriate Sources of Care Early. A referral should be made as soon as specific needs are identified. Telephone referrals speed up obtaining the needed assistance, but should be followed with a written referral.

Intervention Strategies

Nurses can reduce the cost of services that they are providing without sacrificing quality. They can assist the family in coping with financial problems by preventing unnecessary costs and helping the family to respond adaptively to the crisis.

Reducing Health Care Costs. Since the nurse either provides or assists with the provision of most health care treatments, she is in an excellent position to help reduce costs. Using careful techniques so that supplies are not contaminated unnecessarily will limit wastage of materials. Periodic practice with reusable supplies will help to keep skills sharpened so that procedures will not need to be repeated. This could occur with the application of sterile surgical dressings, when catheterizing a patient, or when gavaging an infant. Equipment should be saved for a new nurse to practice with before she performs the procedure. This is just good nursing practice. It assures that the procedure will be performed well in addition to reducing the cost of wasted supplies.

Repeated tests can be reduced if there is knowledge of the results of past tests, such as urinalyses and blood studies. Preparing the patient for tests correctly, such as cleansing the bowel well in preparation for proctoscopy, and carrying out tests accurately, as when doing tuberculin tests, will help to both save materials and reduce costs.

Attempting to prevent or reduce side effects that prolong care by using good techniques not only assures good nursing service to the patient but also helps limit costs. For example, sterility should be maintained to prevent infection, accurate physical assessment should be made as when listening to heart and lung sounds or taking blood pressure, and generally high quality care should be provided.

Periodic evaluation of the kind of care that a patient needs can sometimes result in a reduction of a hospital stay. The nurse in the hospital should assess the family's ability to care for the ill member. It might be a parent who has had surgery and still needs to have the dressings changed periodically due to prolonged drainage, or it might involve the care of a child with congenital anomalies. If it is determined that adequate care can be provided at home, with the assistance of the community health nurse, the patient may be able to be discharged from the hospital early resulting in a reduction in the cost of care.

Sometimes health services need to be developed in areas that are accessible to target populations. This would save both time and transportation costs for families. If the services could then be provided according to the family's ability to pay, there could be further savings available for some families. Examples are satellite maternity, pediatric, and family planning clinics located in areas where they will receive maximum utilization.

Helping Families to Cope with Financial Difficulties. It is important to use interviewing and crisis intervention techniques to help the family identify the financial problem, arrive at appropriate decisions in order to deal with it, and implement appropriate solutions.

Nurses often feel uncomfortable about exploring financial matters with families and therefore avoid doing it. They feel that they are probing in nonhealth matters that are outside of the area with which they should be concerned. However, if financial problems are intensifying the anxieties that are already present in relation to the health situation, the problems need to be explored and then referral made to other services if it is indicated. Motivation to help the family will cause the nurse to move ahead.[2] If a good working relationship has already been developed with the family, as described in Assessment Strategies, the family members already have confidence in the nurse's ability to help them and they are ready to talk openly about their financial concerns. The first goal is to listen to them. What is their perception of the financial situation?

The second goal is to gather needed data to adequately assess the situation. Assessment guidelines were shown in Figure 25-2. The nurse starts where the family is and asks the questions to obtain the necessary information in a friendly way. Insurance policies, community resources, and medical bills can be reviewed together with them to determine the extent of the need. The family may need to obtain further information from the physician, hospital, or insurance company, or perhaps the nurse needs to explore community resources further to provide additional information for the family. The complete data then can be evaluated together with them.

The third goal is to help the family look at the situation objectively.[1] A plan is then developed. They need to be provided with information about resources and they need to arrive at possible courses of action together. What steps can the family take and what functions should the nurse carry out? The family may benefit from a referral to other agencies for service, from materials that could be provided, from nursing measures that will be a savings to them.

The fourth goal in helping the family cope with stress is to provide support.[1] A realistic, but sensitive understanding of the situation is needed. When a sincere desire to help the family is present, it will be communicated to them, and if it is meaningful it will reassure them that someone really is working with them to solve the problems that seem so overwhelming. Support is given by providing quality nursing care that comforts and also by providing information. The nurse should also remain available to the family and maintain contact with them even if she is not visiting them on a regular basis to provide direct service. That will make it possible to continue to assist the family as subsequent issues occur.

After the stress is relieved and the situation has been resolved, the nurse needs to visit them

again and perhaps periodically. It should be determined if the family has returned to a state of equilibrium. What effect has the stress had on the family and what progress is the family making?

Legislative Strategies

Plannings for Comprehensive Services with Adequate Funding for Them. Nurses can have a greater impact on long-term measures that can result in reduction of financial stress on families.

The nurse must participate in the planning and funding of more comprehensive health services. Nurses' involvement in regional health systems agencies that coordinate services is essential. Voluntary work in task groups can lead to more responsible board participation later.

The present patch coverage for specialized programs only meets small segments of the total need. Funds are allocated for prevention and treatment of alcoholism, drug abuse, mental illness, mental retardation, certain specified handicaps of children, and other specific categories. A comprehensive approach is greatly needed in which the different services can coordinate their efforts to provide preventive and therapeutic services for different possibly interrelated problems that the family is having, as well as to approach the effect that one problem has on all family members. The effectiveness with which the family is served is determined by both how funds are allocated and how services are organized and coordinated.

Actively Promoting Desirable and Opposing Undesirable Health Legislation. Nurses need to actively promote desirable and oppose undesirable health legislation. A continuing knowledge of current issues from newspapers and health reports is essential. Sharing of ideas on health issues such as pregnancy being included in disability coverage, national health insurance, and others is important. Each nurse must evaluate all aspects of each issue and have a statement of belief based on facts, experiences, or reason.[4] For example, a nurse's opinion of national health insurance should not be limited to a view that is just for or against it, but should include specific suggestions for the extent of coverage, source of premiums, agency of administration and other issues.

SUMMARY

Health care costs are increasing generally and are expected to continue to increase in the future. Since health problems that place families at risk are particularly costly, their great financial impact increases the already stressful situation for these families. Nurses can help families to prevent and to reduce financial stress by assessing the financial impact on the families, reducing the costs to the family, and providing early assistance with coping. Nurses should be knowledgeable about current health issues and should participate actively in organized health planning and promotion of legislation that will result in better, more accessible health care for all people at a more reasonable cost.

REFERENCES

1. Aguilera, D. C. and J. M. Messide. *Crisis Intervention, Theory and Methodology*, 2nd ed. Saint Louis: C. V. Mosby Co., 1974.
2. Garrett, A. *Interviewing, Its Principles and Methods*, 2nd ed. New York: Family Service Association of America, 1972.
3. Grosswirth, M. "Facing Up to Soaring Medical Costs, Part II." *Parents' Magazine and Better Homemaking*, II #11, November 1976, 62, 114, 115.
4. Johnson, S. H. "Nursing Involvement in National Health Insurance." *Nursing Administration Quarterly*, Fall 1978.
5. *National Health Insurance Resource Book*, rev. ed. Subcommittee on Health of the Committee on Ways and Means, U.S. House of Representatives. Washington, D.C.: U.S. Government Printing Office, August 30, 1976.
6. *Research and Statistics Note*. Washington, D.C.: U.S. Department of Health, Education and Welfare. Social Security Administration. Office of Program and Policy Planning, Office of Research and Statistics. DHEW Publication No. (SSA) 77–1101, Note No. 27, December 22, 1976.
7. "The Impact of Infants' Intensive Care Unit Experience on Families." Unpublished study

done by Mamie Littel, Social Work student. Analyzed by Helen F. Callon, R.N., C.N.M., Madison, Wisconsin, 1975.

ADDITIONAL READINGS

1. Coplan, G. *Principles of Preventive Psychiatry*. New York: Basic Books, 1964.
2. *Disabled? Find Out About Social Security Disability Benefits*. Washington, D.C.: U.S. Department of Health, Education and Welfare. Social Security Administration. DHEW Publication No. (SSA) 76–100068, June 1976.
3. *Helping the Aged, Blind, and Disabled in Wisconsin*. Washington, D.C.: U.S. Department of Health, Education and Welfare. Social Security Administration. DHEW Publication No. (SSA) 76–11144, June 1976.
4. *Hospital Cost Containment*. Prepared by the Staff for the use of the Subcommittee on Health and the Environment of the Committee on Interstate and Foreign Commerce, U.S. House of Representatives. Washington, D.C.: U.S. Government Printing Office, September 1977.
5. *If You Became Disabled*. Washington, D.C.: U.S. Department of Health, Education and Welfare. Social Security Administration. DHEW Publication No. (SSA) 76–10029, June 1976.
6. Interview with representative from Prudential Life Insurance Company, Oshkosh, Wisconsin.
7. Interviews with vice president of Financial Affairs and with personnel from Credit, Business and the Maternal and Infant Intensive Care Center, Theda Clark Memorial Hospital, Neenah, Wisconsin.
8. *Medical Assistance Eligibility Requirements and Benefits*. Division of Family Services. Department of Health and Social Services, State of Wisconsin, January 1976.
9. *Medical Care Expenditures, Prices, and Costs: Background Book*. Washington, D.C.: U.S. Department of Health, Education and Welfare. Social Security Administration. Office of Research Statistics. DHEW Publication No. (SSA) 75–11909, September 1975.
10. *Supplemental Security Income for Retarded People*. Washington, D.C.: U.S. Department of Health, Education and Welfare. Social Security Administration. DHEW Publication No. (SSA) 76–11050, March 1976.
11. *The Size and Shape of the Medical Care Dollar*. Washington, D.C.: U.S. Department of Health, Education and Welfare. Social Security

Administration. DHEW Publication No. (SSA) 76–11910, Chart Book, 1975.

12. *Vocational Rehabilitation for the Blind and Disabled*. Washington, D.C.: U.S. Department of Health, Education and Welfare. Social Security Administration. DHEW Publication No. (SSA) 76–10094, May 1976.

13. Weiner, F. *Help for the Handicapped Child*. Saint Louis: McGraw-Hill, 1973.

14. *Your Medicare Handbook*. Washington, D.C.: U.S. Department of Health, Education and Welfare. Social Security Administration. DHEW Publication No. (SSA) 76–10050, January 1976.

PERTINENT ORGANIZATIONS

NATIONAL

- *American Cancer Society*
219 East 42nd Street
New York, New York 10017
Referrals, literature and films. Local affiliates provide direct services.

- *American Heart Association*
44 East 23rd Street
New York, New York 10010
Research, professional and public education, and community services.

- *American Social Health Association*
1740 Broadway
New York, New York 10019
Resource agency working with and through local organizations. Provides literature. Local associations operate clinics.

- *Association for Children with Learning Disabilities*
2200 Brownsville Road
Pittsburgh, Pennsylvania 15201
Refers inquiries to state affiliates. Provides literature and information about community services.

- *Epilepsy Foundation of America*
1828 L Street, N.W.
Suite 406
Washington, D.C. 20036
Residential care for selected children. Local affiliates provide diagnostic evaluation and vocational rehabilitation literature and films.

- *Muscular Dystrophy Association of America, Inc.*
1790 Broadway
New York, New York 10019
Direct payment for authorized services, referral, public education, literature, films. Local affiliates provide direct service.

- *National Association for Retarded Children*
2709 Avenue E
East Arlington, Texas 76011
Provides information. Local chapters promote but do not provide direct services.

- *National Cystic Fibrosis Research Foundation*
3379 Peach Tree Road, N.E.
Atlanta, Georgia 30326
Coordinates and funds foundation programs for research, education, and care. Direct services provided by local affiliates.

- *National Epilepsy League*
2222 N. Michigan Avenue
Chicago, Illinois 60611
Provides information.

- *National Kidney Foundation*
116 E. 27th Street
New York, New York 10010
Makes referrals to hospitals with facilities for diagnosis and treatment of kidney diseases.

- *National Society for the Prevention of Blindness*
79 Madison Avenue
New York, New York 10016
Public services, education, research.

- *National Tay-Sachs and Allied Diseases Association*
200 Park Avenue South
New York, New York 10003
Referrals to clinics for diagnosis and carrier and prenatal detection. Provides information.

- *National Tuberculosis and Respiratory Disease Association*
1740 Broadway
New York, New York 10019
Referrals, literature, films, professional education, and information research.

- *Social Security Administration*
Financial assistance.

- *The Foundation for Research and Education in Sickle Cell Disease*
421–431 W. 120th Street
New York, New York 10027
Public information, established clinics, referrals.

- *The National Association for Mental Health*
1800 North Kent Street
Arlington, Virginia 22209
Referrals, directs research, public information,

liaison between governmental and private organizations.

- *The National Easter Seal Society for Crippled Children and Adults*
  2023 W. Odgen Avenue
  Chicago, Illinois 60612
  Provides direct services.

- *The National Foundation—March of Dimes*
  P. O. Box 2000
  White Plains, New York 10602
  Supports research, referrals, produces and distributes educational materials, sponsors international, individual, and regional symposia for professionals.

- *The National Hemophilia Foundation*
  25 West 39th Street
  New York, New York 10018
  Public education, stimulates research, referrals to treatment centers. Local affiliates provide literature.

- *United Cerebral Palsy Association Inc.*
  66 E. 34th Street
  New York, New York 10016
  Conducts demonstration projects, provides public and professional educational materials, supports research and professional training.

- *U.S. Department of Health, Education and Welfare*
  Social Security Administration

Washington, D.C.
Research, medical education, provides facilities for research and medical education.

STATE

- *Department of Services for the Blind*
  Counseling of parents and educators of blind children. Financial assistance in some instances.

- *State Department of Vocational Rehabilitation*
  Finances diagnosis, treatment, and education.

- *State Health Departments, State Mental Health Services*
  Consultation, some direct services.

- *State Services for Crippled Children*
  Payment for diagnosis and treatment of selected conditions, operates diagnostic clinics, provides treatment for certain conditions.

LOCAL

- *City and county departments of social services*
  Financial assistance, counseling.

- *City and county health nursing services*
  Direct services, education, equipment.

- *County unified service boards for alcoholism, drug abuse, mental illness, and developmental disabilities*
  Provides professional services in categories named.

- *Visiting Nurses Associations*
  Direct services, education, equipment.

Conclusion: Commonalities and Future Directions

Suzanne Hall Johnson, R.N., M.N.

After describing the family difficulties and nursing interventions for families in the specific risk situations, several questions arise. What are the common family difficulties for the high-risk family? What are the common nursing interventions? What are the priority areas for clinical and research work?

COMMON DIFFICULTIES IN HIGH-RISK PARENTING

Some families are more susceptible to the difficulties related to high-risk parenting than others. There seem to be several common variables that influence the type and degree of problems for the family. These variables are present before the risk situation and include the family's coping abilities in crises, past experiences with health problems, other stress situations and quality of interactions. In determining the family's stresses it is important to identify these family characteristics as well as the characteristics of the high-risk situation itself.

Although the nurse needs to make a specific assessment and problem identification for every high-risk family, there are some common potential problems for any high-risk family. This list of potential high-risk problems is an important guide for the nurse in her assessment of the family. Although the type of stress causing the high-risk situation may vary, it appears that families react in very similar ways to any high-risk situation. For example, parents of a high-risk child, a terminally ill child, or a parent who is alcoholic all experience guilt. Although the underlying stresses are different, the parents' reactions of guilt and possibly anger and blaming of each other are the same.

Any family difficulty can result in either growth or disunity of the family. If the family can work together to identify the problems, generate alternatives, and jointly work to reduce the problem, then the family members experience closeness and satisfaction in dealing with their stressful period. If the family's reaction is to work individually, each person trying to handle his own stress but probably causing more stress for the other family members, disunity of the family is a frequent result. It is the nurse's role to help the family to identify and cope with the family difficulties to assist in growth of the family rather than its disunity.

By looking at the charts of family difficulties in the previous chapters, the common family difficulties become apparent. These include multiple crises, increased separation, inability to express emotional or physical needs, family role changes, and finances.

Multiple Crises

Due to the long-term risk situation and the many stressful times during the risk experience, many families experience multiple crises. For example, for the family with the premature infant the periods immediately following the premature birth when they first see the child, first care for the child, and bring the child home are very stressful. The alcoholic parent who has intermittent periods of inebriation places the family in stressful situations at times over a long period.

The family's ability to cope with stress varies according to their past experiences with crises. Therefore, some families find the multiple crises over time a greater difficulty than other families.

The nurse can help the families by preventing some of the crises through anticipation of the stressful periods during high-risk situations. For example, the nurse can identify the stressful time of an ill child returning home and work with the parents over a period of time as they take more and more responsibility for the care of the child in the hospital. The nurse can also provide positive feedback for the family as they are learning the new caretaking behaviors, so that they become less anxious to be left alone while caring for the child.

Increased Separation of Family Members

Since most of the high-risk situations involve at least one family member with an illness, that family member is frequently separated from the family for medical treatment. This causes increased separation of family members during the stressful time and makes it more difficult for the family to cope with the stress as a unit. The premature infant, the terminally ill child or parent, the child of an abusing parent, the alcoholic parent, and many other symptomatic risk family members are removed from the family during the critical period.

The nurse may be able to prevent some separation of family members by encouraging treatment of an emotionally disturbed parent in an outpatient clinic, for example. In addition, she can decrease the problems of separation by encouraging family members, both parents and children, to visit and care for the symptomatic family member. She can also initiate other means of communication between family members when they cannot visit the ill member.

Inability to Express Their Emotional and Physical Needs

Since the family members usually focus on the symptomatic member in a risk situation, the other family members are frequently unable to identify or express their own emotional needs. For example, the spouse of an alcoholic parent may find it difficult to identify her own feelings of anger and guilt toward the other person. In extreme cases, the parent may actually harm himself or other family members while focusing on the symptomatic member. For example, the mother of a mentally disabled child who is unable to walk may continue to carry the child as he grows older and heavier, until she may injure her own back before identifying her difficulties. The single parent may spend tremendous energy for her child while not having enough time to rest and build up her own energy, thus leading to tremendous tension, tiredness, and even a physical or emotional breakdown.

The nurse can help the family to identify and express their own emotional needs. The nurse must assess the stresses and the coping behavior of each family member during the high-risk situation. Valuable questions are: "How has your life changed since this occurred?" "What things are different at home since this occurred?" "How have other family members changed since the risk situation?" By asking questions about the experiences for each family member and helping to identify their behaviors which show emotional need, the nurse helps the family members to identify their emotional needs and helps them plan ways to meet these.

There are several emotional difficulties common for the high-risk family. These are grief, guilt, low self-esteem, and a lack of energy.

Grief. Parents in high-risk situations frequently experience grief. The grief may be related to an actual loss, such as the death of a child or a parent or it may be related to the loss of an image of the desired family member. Grief due to the loss of the image of a desired family member is shown by the parents' grief following the birth of a deformed child who is different from the desired infant and by the alcoholic parent who is different from the image of the desired spouse. Following the actual loss of a family member or the loss of the image of a desired family member, the parents experience stages of grief including denial, anger, bargaining, depression, and the final stage of acceptance of either the death or the new image of the family member. Each family moves through the stages at an individual rate and in an individual pattern, with some stages possibly very brief and some overlapping.

The nurse helps the family to deal with their grief by helping them to focus the grief on the loss and allowing them to experience the different stages while working with the grief. Toward the end of their grief, the nurse helps the family to look ahead and to focus on the family members' present and future needs.

Guilt. Guilt is a common emotional difficulty resulting from high-risk situations. Due to the complexity of most high-risk situations, there is seldom one clear cause for the high-risk difficulty. Therefore, the family members frequently look at their own behaviors or desires as part of the cause of the problem. This results in their feeling extreme guilt. Family members who have previously had a poor self-image, did things that may have caused the problem, or feel that the high-risk situation is a punishment of God tend to have more guilt than the other family members. The parents of a high-risk infant, such as an at-risk fetus, premature infant, or disabled child, frequently experience guilt and try to think of the things that they did to cause the

child's difficulties. The alcoholic or addicted parent frequently feels guilty for his drinking and addicted behavior, and the abusing parent often feels guilty following the abuse situation.

The nurse helps the family to deal with their guilt following a high-risk situation. The nurse's role is to help the family to understand the probable causes for the situation. This includes describing possible causes not related to the parents' behaviors and identifying parents' behaviors that may have caused the difficulty. For example, the nurse clarifies for the mother of a premature infant that her uneventful airplane ride at three-months pregnancy is very unlikely to have caused the premature birth. The nurse, through genetic counseling, does describe for the family their genetic contribution to the physically disabled child. The nurse helps the family to deal with their guilt feelings by helping them identify what they think were the causes, clarifying whether it is possible that these were the cause, and helping the family members focus on present problems. Regardless of the cause the main focus is now on the care for the at-risk family member and coping with the resulting difficulties. This helps the family to look forward and cope with the present problems rather than dwell on their past difficulties.

Low Self-Esteem. Many parents in high-risk situations experience low self-esteem. The parents are frequently dissatisfied with themselves and their parenting. It appears that the high-risk situation causes stress that prevents the parents from receiving positive feedback from their children and feeling good with themselves and their parenting. The parents of a mentally disabled child may feel dissatisfied. Because of his learning delay they may feel that they are not playing with the child or talking with him adequately. Therefore, they are frequently dissatisfied with their parenting.

Parents in high-risk situations frequently evaluate themselves on criteria that are not related to their parenting. This often leads to their dissatisfaction with parenting. For example, the mother of a mentally disabled child may feel that she is a poor mother because the child is not learning as fast as some of the other children; however, when she focuses on the child's smiling, relaxing, and laughing when the mother plays with her, then her feelings of satisfaction increase. The high-risk parent, such as the emotionally disabled parent or the alcoholic or addicted parent, frequently feels dissatisfied with his parenting because he recognizes how his inconsistent behaviors cause family difficulties.

The nurse can help the parent experiencing low self-esteem by first giving him positive feedback about his parenting and, second and more important, helping the parent to identify reactions of the child or spouse which directly give the parent positive feedback and feelings of satisfaction.

Emotional Weariness. High-risk parents frequently feel emotionally tired and continually worn out, with little energy for themselves and the high-risk member. The tiredness is often due to the amount of stress in high-risk situations when the parents are overwhelmed with difficulties and family needs. Many family members work overtime trying to meet other family members' needs. For example, the mother or father with an ill child frequently continues her or his usual work and housework plus additional visiting and care for the ill child and additional nurturing for the siblings at home. Since many risk situations continue for prolonged periods of time, these parents often experience an emotional tiredness resulting from their worries and the amount of energy they expend to meet all the family members' needs.

The nurse can help the parents to regain energy by first helping them to identify ways to efficiently cope with the most stressful situations without expending unnecessary energy, and then assisting them to gain more energy by discussing their own needs for a quiet time, bath time, or other relaxing time. For example, the single parent frequently spends so much time and energy meeting all the children's household, financial, clothing, and nutrition needs, that he has little energy left. The nurse can help the single parent identify the

value of seeking help from others and setting some time aside to replenish his own energy.

Physical Weariness. Many families experience physical symptoms during a high-risk situation. Most of the difficulties are similar to those experienced at the time of any great stress, crisis, or grief. The parents may experience either sleeplessness and inability to relax from the tension or the opposite—continual sleep and drowsiness as a coping behavior to reduce the stress. Physical ailments related to tension, such as ulcers, muscle sprains, backaches, headaches, nausea, and diarrhea, are possible complaints from parents who are fearful about the health of a family member. These physical ailments not only cause the family members pain and discomfort, but also cause fear about their own health and greater difficulty interacting with family members.

The nurse can help prevent and reduce the family's physical difficulties. Preventing or reducing the impact of the crisis periods already mentioned helps reduce the stress on the family and prevents the physical symptoms. By asking the family if they have had any previous discomfort under stress, the nurse can help identify the presence of early symptoms. To cope with such difficulties, the parents can begin using previously established remedies, such as warm baths for sore back, prescribed diet for the ulcer parent, or medication for a hypertensive parent. For new symptoms or increased or prolonged physical symptoms, the family members should be referred to their own physician and encouraged to describe the stressful situation contributing to their physical difficulties. The nurse can help the family members to recognize that their own health is very important by stressing the importance of keeping all family members healthy in order to care for the symptomatic family member. The nurse should stress that physical difficulties related to stress are very common among parents and not a sign of weakness. Since the physical difficulties should diminish along with the reduction of crisis following the risk situation, the nurse should reevaluate the parents' symptoms after the critical period is over to determine if they need additional medical help.

Family Role Change

High-risk families frequently experience role changes within the family. The death of a child or a parent obviously necessitates role changes for all of the family members coping with the loss of the member. In addition, when one family member becomes ill in a risk situation, that person is often not expected to fulfill his past role, which often leaves family chores to be distributed among other family members. The family role change may be a short-term change during the temporary illness of one family member with the return to the original family roles when the family member recovers. Or the family role change may be permanent, as when a family member dies or suffers a permanent disability. Although some families seem to be very flexible in their roles, interchanging roles almost daily, other families have great difficulty switching roles and helping each other to absorb a role change due to a high-risk situation.

The nurse helps the family identify the role change of the one family member, recognize the need for role changes among the other members, and shift their roles into complementary ones to best meet the family's needs. For families who have previously had difficulty with role change, the nurse uses many of the role theory strategies to help the family become more flexible coping with the changing risk situation and the changing roles within the family.

Discipline. Parents in high-risk situations frequently have difficulties disciplining their children. These difficulties include not enough discipline, too much discipline, inconsistent discipline, and disagreements between parents over discipline. Some parents with an ill child will not set behavior limits on the child, and the whole family will basically run according to the child's needs. Although the parents feel sorry for the ill child and may feel guilty about his illness, the child still needs realistic discipline and limits on his behavior. The child

must still live within the family unit. The nurse can help the parents to recognize the child's needs for limits on his behavior, which will allow other family members to comfortably live within the family.

Too much or too forceful discipline occurs in some families such as the abusive family. Extremely forceful discipline that harms the child becomes a problem in itself for the abusive family. The nurse helps the family to prevent stress situations and to deal with discipline using less forceful means.

The alcoholic or addicted, as well as the emotionally disturbed adult, often provides inconsistent discipline. In this case, the child does not learn to set limits because the limits keep changing depending on the parents' emotional condition. An alcoholic or addicted parent may allow the child to do almost anything while he is in an inebriated state; however, he may use very strict discipline when sober. The nurse works with the family to reduce the alcoholic or emotional problem and to help the parent be more consistent in his parenting.

Sometimes discipline problems in the family produce fighting between the parents. For example, in the situation of a family with a hyperactive child, the high-risk situation would accentuate any differences in the parents' attitudes toward discipline. If one parent was slightly permissive and the other more restrictive in disciplining the child, each could blame the other for the child's disruptive behavior. The nurse helps the family to recognize their differences in discipline attitudes and that the child's behavior is based more on physiological problems than on purely discipline problems. The nurse helps the family to jointly decide on consistent discipline actions.

Sibling Relationships. Sibling difficulties are common in the high-risk family. If one child is the symptomatic family member in a high-risk situation, then most of the family focus is on that child. This frequently results in the other siblings feeling a loss of love and rejection from the parents. It is common for the well brothers and sisters of the high-risk child to display more disruptive behaviors, such as tantrums and intentional misbehaving, to attract the attention of the parent.

The nurse works with the parents to recognize the needs of the well children and to provide explanations to the well children about their parents' love for them. It may not be possible for the parents to spend more time with the well children, however the quality of that time can demonstrate more love and affection to reassure these children of their part in the family and the parents' love.

Finances

Due to the special medical problems of most high-risk situations, the symptomatic person usually requires special medical care and frequently needs long-term medical care. Both the specialized and the long-term care create financial difficulties. The daily charges for hospitalization in an intensive care nursery or an intensive care unit are quite high because of the specialized medical team and equipment. In addition, any special procedures or treatments, including X-rays and lab tests, rapidly increase the bill. The parents receive other bills for phone calls and trips to an often distant medical center. For some families these costs can take a substantial part of their budget. If the child or parent has any remaining difficulties, the family will have continuing medical bills in the future. Although financial difficulties are often not an initial priority problem when the parents' concern is on the ill family member, they can be a major problem later. For families without outside assistance or with insufficient financial assistance, the high-risk situation might end with the family exhausting its savings and energy and going into debt.

Family reactions to the financial difficulties may cause family unity difficulties. A mother may be forced to return to work or the father may be forced to take a second job. Anxiety may increase as parents work harder and cut more corners in their budget.

Fortunately the large bills are often partially or sometimes totally paid by a combination of private insurance, public assistance, and grant monies. Since many of these organizations must initiate coverage during the illness, the nurse must quickly contact the social worker or financial planner to help determine the parents' need for financial help and to initiate outside sources of help.

COMMONALITIES OF INTERVENTIONS FOR THE HIGH-RISK FAMILY

Interventions for the high-risk family have several common factors, including the following:

All interventions are determined through a thorough *assessment*. The nurse does not assume that a potential problem exists merely because a specific high-risk situation has occurred. The nurse determines the characteristics of the high-risk incident, identifies the family's coping methods, and determines the individual family problems. This assessment is the basis for all the interventions.

Interventions are aimed at *all family members*. The nurse identifies the family as the client in the high-risk situation. Although interventions are aimed at reducing the high-risk problems for the symptomatic person, many interventions are also aimed at other family members who are having difficulties related to the high-risk situation.

All interventions are *individualized* to the specific family. Types of nursing strategies such as counseling, behavior modification, and teaching are most useful when the specific nursing actions are individualized for each unique family.

All interventions encourage the family's *own problem solving*. The nurse helps the family to identify their own problems, generate alternatives, select alternatives, perform the actions, and evaluate the strategies. The nurse uses the counseling, teaching, family involving, and other strategies to help the family identify and solve their own difficulties. The family's joint problem solving and success in reducing the difficulties leads to their growth and satisfaction.

Interventions are chosen from a *repertoire* of possible strategies. Rather than excluding many strategies and selecting one to work with high-risk families, the nurse develops a repertoire of many interventions. The nurse chooses the interventions for the individual needs of the family from this repertoire. Many interventions may be used simultaneously or some may be used one at a time and evaluated individually for effectiveness.

All interventions are part of a *team plan*. The nurse's interventions are only part of the health care team plan for the family and therefore must be coordinated with other health care interventions. The nurse must coordinate her interventions not only with the interdisciplinary team but also with other nurses from other shifts or in other settings who are concerned with the high-risk family.

All interventions are *evaluated*. The individual intervention for the specific family is evaluated by determining if the target problem for the family has been reduced. This evaluation helps to refine the interventions and to select the most effective ones for the individual family. In addition, interventions are evaluated among groups of families to determine which interventions work best with that type of difficulty. This type of group evaluation allows generalizations to be formed and identifies types of interventions most useful for specific problems.

All interventions are *refined* based on the evaluation. Nursing interventions undergo continual development and refinement. Refinement of the intervention includes developing guidelines for the use of the interventions, suggesting times or family characteristics where the interventions are most or least useful, and suggesting very specific plans for use of the interventions. In the evaluation the nurse focuses on very specific behaviors and symptoms of the problem so that she can determine when the behaviors have changed and the problem has been reduced.

FUTURE DIRECTIONS

Suggesting future directions for clinical, education, and research practice helps to place the money, time, and energy into the areas of priority that are most likely to help the high-risk family. The future directions must be based on the present information and practice and must identify the next steps in the development of clinical practice, teaching of clinical practice, and the questions to be studied in research. Directions also help to coordinate the work so that there is no duplication of work, no gaps in important areas of clinical practice, education, or research. One of the nursing practice priorities identified by the American Nurses Association Commission on Nursing Research is "to improve the outlook for high risk parents and high risk infants."[1]

According to the present practice and suggestions for the future in the previous chapters, the following areas are priority. These priorities incorporate all three nursing roles—clinical practice, education, and research.

Determine the Causative Factors for the High-Risk Situations. Although some causative factors have been identified for some of the high-risk situations, many of the contributing factors have not been identified. Determining the causative factors is essential in later preventing the occurrence of the risk situation. For example, determining various family situations leading to alcoholism and abuse could help to reduce the incidence of the risk situation.

Prevent Risk Situations. For risk situations with known causes, the nurse needs to reduce the causative agents and prevent the problems from occurring. For example, stressful crises at home frequently precipitate the battering of a child. Establishing day care centers where families can leave a child for care on a particularly stressful day helps to reduce child abuse.

Prevent Family Difficulties. Since the high-risk situations cannot all be prevented at this time, the nurse needs to develop additional ways to prevent the family difficulties from occurring after the risk incident. For example, if the death of a terminally ill child cannot be prevented, the nurse can develop additional interventions for helping the family to grieve and adapt to the death of the child.

Identify Early Signs of the Family Difficulties. The nurse needs to develop very sensitive assessment guidelines to determine early symptoms of family difficulties. With early diagnosis of the family difficulties, interventions may be instituted to reduce the problem in its initial state, before other complications and family difficulties have resulted. For example, if poor maternal attachment is an early sign for potential child abuse, then early interventions to foster maternal attachment will reduce the later problems of child abuse.

Develop Specific Nursing Actions. The nurse needs to refine present interventions, try present interventions in new situations, and develop new effective actions to reduce the family difficulties. Developing specific actions includes suggesting criteria in a protocol to determine when a nursing action is needed, describing specific guidelines for exactly how, when, where, and by whom an intervention is to be carried out. For example, for the adolescent mother, general nursing actions describe the need for teaching the mother about nutrition, while very specific nursing actions include exactly how the teaching will be carried out (in a one-to-one setting), who the most useful nurse would be, what types of teaching tools would be useful, what the most effective timing of teaching would be, and other specific factors in the interventions.

Determine Effective Administration of Nursing Care. Determining more effective means of providing nursing care for the high-risk family is important. Determining the effectiveness of community health centers, primary nursing, the multidisciplinary team, and the home visit is important in providing care for the high-risk family. For example, for the family with a premature infant transported to a regional center, administration of nursing care can be a problem. Evaluation of the effectiveness of counseling from the regional center, and coordination between the specialty nurse in the regional center and the community health nurse in the community center need to be further developed.

Evaluate Nursing Actions. The nurse needs to determine which actions are most effective in reducing the family difficulties and must determine how her role is significant in helping the family. Evaluation of nursing care by determining what changes have occurred in the family as a result of the nursing care is an important priority. For example, evaluating strategies to help the family grieve over the loss of a parent would include comparing the outcomes of the grieving for the parents provided with the nursing counseling with those not provided with the nursing counseling.

SUMMARY

There are many potential difficulties for the family in a high-risk situation. Although the difficulties are unique for each family, there are many common characteristics and problems for families in any high-risk situation. The nursing interventions that are individualized for the family based on an assessment of all family members and evaluated for their effectiveness are the most effective for the high-risk family. Although there are many effective interventions presently available for the nurse to help the high-risk family, the nurse can further develop her interventions to prevent, identify, reduce, and evaluate the problems of the high-risk family. The nurse has a significant role in the present care of the high-risk family and in developing new health practices for these families.

REFERENCE

1. "ANA Commission on Nursing Research States Priorities," *Nursing Research*, September/October 1976, 357.

Appendix:
Self-Study
Course Guidelines

High-Risk Parenting is a text that can be used as the content for classroom or self-study learning. The following guidelines should be used when using the book for approved continuing education credit.

Continuing Education Approval and Contact Hours

The home study course, *High-Risk Parenting*, has been approved for nine contact hours of continuing education for nurses. The American Nurses Association approved the course itself. The Florida and California Boards of Registered Nursing and the Colorado Nurses Association, which is ANA accredited, approved the author's organization, Health Update, as an approved provider of continuing education for nurses. These approvals are recognized in most states. The course will be submitted for approval each year.

Prerequisite Knowledge

This course focuses on the effects of the risk conditions on the family rather than the pathophysiology and physical care related to the disease itself. This information is important but is learned in other courses or through clinical experience.

Some clinical experience with families with a family member at risk is helpful for this course since it helps the learner apply the information to actual families. For learners with no previous clinical experiences with families at risk, these experiences can be set up during this course. However, the risk situations described in this text are so common in any type of nursing specialty that most nurses with clinical experience in school or as graduate nurses will be able to recall past clinical experiences.

Objectives

By the end of this course the nurse will be able to:

1. Define the term "high-risk parenting."
2. Describe at least five common potential difficulties for any high-risk family.
3. Describe at least five strategies for high-risk families, including why the strategies are useful and how they are most effective for this type of family.
4. Apply the concepts to clinical practice by developing the nursing care plan for an actual high-risk family by:
   —assessing and identifying problem behaviors of the mother, father, or child.
   —analyzing the family interactions to describe at least three family problems using descriptive observations such as behaviors or statements.
   —selecting three interventions for each family difficulty in the objective above.
   —evaluating the interventions by describing desired changes in the behavior or statements from the initial assessment.

Directions

1. Complete the following required readings:
   —"High-Risk Parenting," introductory chapter.
   —any one chapter in the High-Risk Child or the High-Risk Parent section.
   —any one chapter in the Nursing Strategies section.
   —"Commonalities and Future Direction," last chapter. Each reading takes approximately 2 hours for a total of 8 hours.
2. You may complete additional readings from any section or from the bibliographies or suggested organizations presented in each chapter. This additional reading is optional.
3. Complete the post-test including all blanks and questions. The post-test takes approximately one hour (making 9 total hours).
4. Mail the post-test and $15 in check or money order for evaluation and continuing education credit to **Suzanne Hall Johnson, RN, MN, c/o Nursing Division, J. B. Lippincott, East Washington Square, Philadelphia, PA 19105.** Each test will be individually reviewed and commented on by Suzanne Johnson, the author, using criteria based on the content of this book.

POST-TEST

Clearly Print the Following Information.

Name_____   Soc. Sec. #_____

Address_____   Nurse License #_____

City/State_____   License State_____

Zip Code_____   License Expiration Date_____

Phone #_____   Employer_____

Signature_____   Position_____

Class: High-Risk Parenting: Home Study
Contact Hours: 9 Home Study Contact Hours

Date of the Post-Test:_____

Complete all of the questions. You must meet all the objectives as measured in these post-test questions.

1. What does the term "high-risk parenting" mean and what is the value of this concept?

2. Describe at least five common potential difficulties for any high-risk family.
    1.

    2.

    3.

    4.

    5.

    Other:

3. List five strategies for high-risk families, then describe why the strategies are useful and how they can be used most effectively for these families.

Strategy 1:
  Why:

  How:

Strategy 2:
  Why:

  How:

Strategy 3:
  Why:

  How:

Strategy 4:
  Why:

  How:

Strategy 5:
  Why:

  How:

For questions 4-7, select a high-risk family from your own clinical practice for the remaining questions. Plan the nursing care for the family using the following care plan format to answer the questions. What is the risk condition for this family:

_____ .

    4. In assessing the family members for problem behaviors, identify in the assessment section below any mother, father, or child behaviors showing potential problems.

    5. Analyze the family interactions, then describe at least three family problems using actual descriptive behaviors or statements, in the section below.

    6. Describe at least three interventions for each of the family problems in question 5.

    7. Evaluate the interventions by describing desired changes in the behavior or statements from the initial problem identification in questions 4 and 5.

4. Assessment	5. Problem Identification	6. Interventions	7. Evaluation
	1.	a. b. c.	
	2.	a. b. c.	
	3.	a. b. c.	

You may use extra paper if needed.
Mail the post-test and $15 to Suzanne Hall Johnson, RN, MN, c/o Nursing Division J. B. Lippincott, East Washington Square, Philadelphia, PA 19105.

Index